Foundations of Abnormal Psychology

CONTRIBUTORS

W. Ross Ashby	*University of Illinois*
Albert Bandura	*Stanford University*
L. Douglas DeNike	*University of Southern California*
Roy C. Hostetter	*University of Illinois*
Jerry Hirsch	*University of Illinois*
Philip W. Jackson	*University of Chicago*
Jerome Kagan	*Harvard University*
Perry London	*University of Southern California*
Brendan Maher	*Brandeis University*
Willard A. Mainord	*University of Louisville*
Samuel Messick	*Educational Testing Service*
Leslie Phillips	*Boston College*
David Rosenhan	*Center for Psychological Studies, Educational Testing Service*
Norman Tiber	*University of Southern California*
Michel Treisman	*Oxford University*
Crayton C. Walker	*University of California at Los Angeles*
Edward Zigler	*Yale University*

edited by

PERRY LONDON
University of Southern California

DAVID ROSENHAN
Center for Psychological Studies
Educational Testing Service

Foundations of Abnormal Psychology

HOLT, RINEHART AND WINSTON, INC.
NEW YORK CHICAGO SAN FRANCISCO ATLANTA DALLAS
MONTREAL TORONTO LONDON

Library of Congress Catalog Card Number: 68-11410
2561603
Printed in the United States of America
1 2 3 4 5 6 7 8 9

Preface

It is sometimes alleged that psychology has two voices. One speaks of its experimental aspects, its research with animals or humans in areas of learning, physiological, perceptual, social, and personality psychology. The other voice is reserved for abnormal psychology, and for abnormal psychology alone. Although they ultimately share the same concern—the understanding of man in the full measure of his experience and behavior—these voices seem hardly to be coming from the same organism. The experimental one speaks of man in the language of science in terms of research and research design, of experimental method and outcome, of carefully stipulated theory and precise measurement. The other speaks of *Man* in rich and strong prose, in language that both shapes and is shaped by the culture, in dramatic themes that are compelling if not yet convincing. The sense of large understandings is what the latter voice offers. The experimental psychologies, on the other hand, are concerned with progress—slow, often painfully tedious—but progress nonetheless.

These psychologies—let us call them the general and the abnormal for brevity's sake—have not much cared for each other. Although the psychopathologist would occasionally claim that psychopathological phenomena were exaggerated outcomes of quite normal processes, he would then go on to invoke theories and language that could be applied only with great difficulty to the normal human being that all of us are familiar with. And if he was primarily concerned with psychotherapy, he did not commonly turn to the general psychology of attitude and behavior change for his hypotheses and operational tools. For a long time, the psychologist concerned with psychopathology marched his own lonely road, often with a few brothers, but far away from the extended family.

Much the same has been true for the general psychologist. When his concerns ran to sensory psychology, he rarely saw hysterical anesthesia as an interesting boundary condition. If he was interested in perception, psychotic hallucination was rarely a phenomenon of *his* concern. And much as psychotherapists were rarely interested in the social psychology of attitude change, so research in attitude change rarely reflected the experience of successful psychotherapists.

Our intent in preparing this volume was to bring together materials from various domains of psychology that might have fruitful bearing on the study of abnormality, to create a dialogue between general and abnormal psychology. The endeavor was exciting for all the participants. Whether it was successful, however, is another matter. In some regards it could not fail to be useful. The recent advances in social and developmental psychology, in behavior theory and genetics, in learning, perception and neurophysiology cannot but have critical bearing on abnormality. Man is, after all, of a piece. But if the reader is convinced that a marriage between general and abnormal psychology is necessary, let him not imagine that it was easy, or that the immediate road ahead is blissful. Often enough, the *immediate* relevance of the general domain to abnormality is not distinctly apparent. A direction is suggested, a vague hint, as it were, and nothing more. For some readers, the absence of an apparent close relationship between the first section ("General Foundations") and the last ("Negative Abnormalities") will be disconcerting. For others, however, the same state of affairs will prove exciting. Not all of the seams and rough edges have been concealed; not all of them should or could be concealed. Many questions remain unanswered; some are not even raised. Such is the current state of the discipline, and students will have been well served if they become aware of these problems.

Though it may not seem so to the beginning student, the borders of psychology are expanding swiftly. There is, we think, little question that the theories of psychology that seemed sufficient to account for abnormal behavior a few years ago are much in need of modification today. And those that seem sufficient today are likely to be replaced by more comprehensive views tomorrow. The situation is at least as troublesome for those who require firm truths about abnormality as it is delightful to those who enjoy the pursuit and expansion of knowledge. This book is clearly addressed to the latter. It does not pretend to clear, loud answers regarding all issues in abnormality, and the truths it offers are admittedly tentative, willingly subject to modification. It does, we hope, describe the status of the field at the present time.

It may be useful to stipulate at the outset the major ways in which *Foundations of Abnormal Psychology* departs from most books that have preceded it. In the first place, *Foundations* is multi-authored. The decision to bring together a number of authorities in the preparation of this book was at least as much a matter of finding the degree to which various views could be integrated as of presenting those views authoritatively. In the matter of integration we were more successful than we dreamed possible. Although the contributors to the book work in different traditions, there is considerable consensus among them regarding the nature of abnormal phenomena and the dynamics that create and propel them. There are, however, the differences of opinion and view that are to be expected in any field whose final horizons are yet quite distant.

In addition to attempting to relate the mainstreams of scientific psychology to those of abnormal psychology, we have taken some liberties in defining the domain of abnormal psychology. We enter into this problem in some detail in the first chapter, but the reader may want to be forewarned that we do not equate abnormal with psychopathological. Rather we believe that *abnormal*, in its useful meaning, is most like the word *unusual*, and if psychopathology is unusual, so is creativity, genius, and positive social character. Thus, a section of the book is devoted to positive abnormalities, much as one is devoted to negative abnormalities, or psychopathologies. This somewhat broader conception of abnormality proves to have some usefulness, not the least of which is that it allows for a consideration of *normality*. In Chapter 5 we take up this problem and offer what we think is a compelling and novel view of this much-thought-about, but not often examined, problem.

In a rapidly moving field, the state of knowledge always moves faster than anyone's attempt to summarize it. Any author who has endeavored to write a textbook knows that by the time he has finished, his work is dated. If this is the case with a single-authored textbook, it is most certainly true for one that is authored by a dozen people and integrated by two. Many of the contributors completed three or four drafts of their chapters, often engaging in revisions in order to integrate their work better with the total project. The work of the editors was considerably expanded to better knit together the entire endeavor. These matters took time, more time than might ordinarily be required to produce such a volume, with the result that the views of some of the authors have been modified between the time of writing and that of publication. This is especially true of the views expressed in Chapter 9 by Bandura, and in Chapters 8 and 15 by Rosenhan and London. The student, however, should be neither distressed nor alarmed by this fact; he has never read a scientific treatise that was completely "up to date," but he has nevertheless profited from his reading. Our intent in mentioning this fact is less to reassure the student than to notify the scientist who may peruse this volume that the views of some of the authors may have undergone modification.

A book such as this owes much to many minds and hands. Our largest debt is to the anonymous colleagues, students, and secretaries of the individual authors, without whose efforts the pleasure and utility of this endeavor might have been greatly reduced. Among those whose efforts are known, the editors are especially indebted to Professors James H. Bryan, Louis Costa, Joseph T. Hart, William Meredith, and Silvan S. Tomkins for their comments on various parts of the manuscript. Michael B. Davenport was enormously helpful both in Los Angeles and in Princeton in organizing and checking the manuscripts, and in generally facilitating the editorial process. Our thanks goes also to Ruth Boyatt, Anne Burrowes, Janet Cuca, Irene Kostin, Jessica Lipnack, Vivian London, Ruth Mannes, Carol McPherson, and Edward C. Nystrom for specific assistance with various parts of the manuscript, and to Joyce Crossland and Annette Hamarman, who typed various drafts. The efforts of all participants are gratefully acknowledged.

January, 1968

PERRY LONDON
DAVID ROSENHAN

Contents

Foundations of Abnormal Psychology

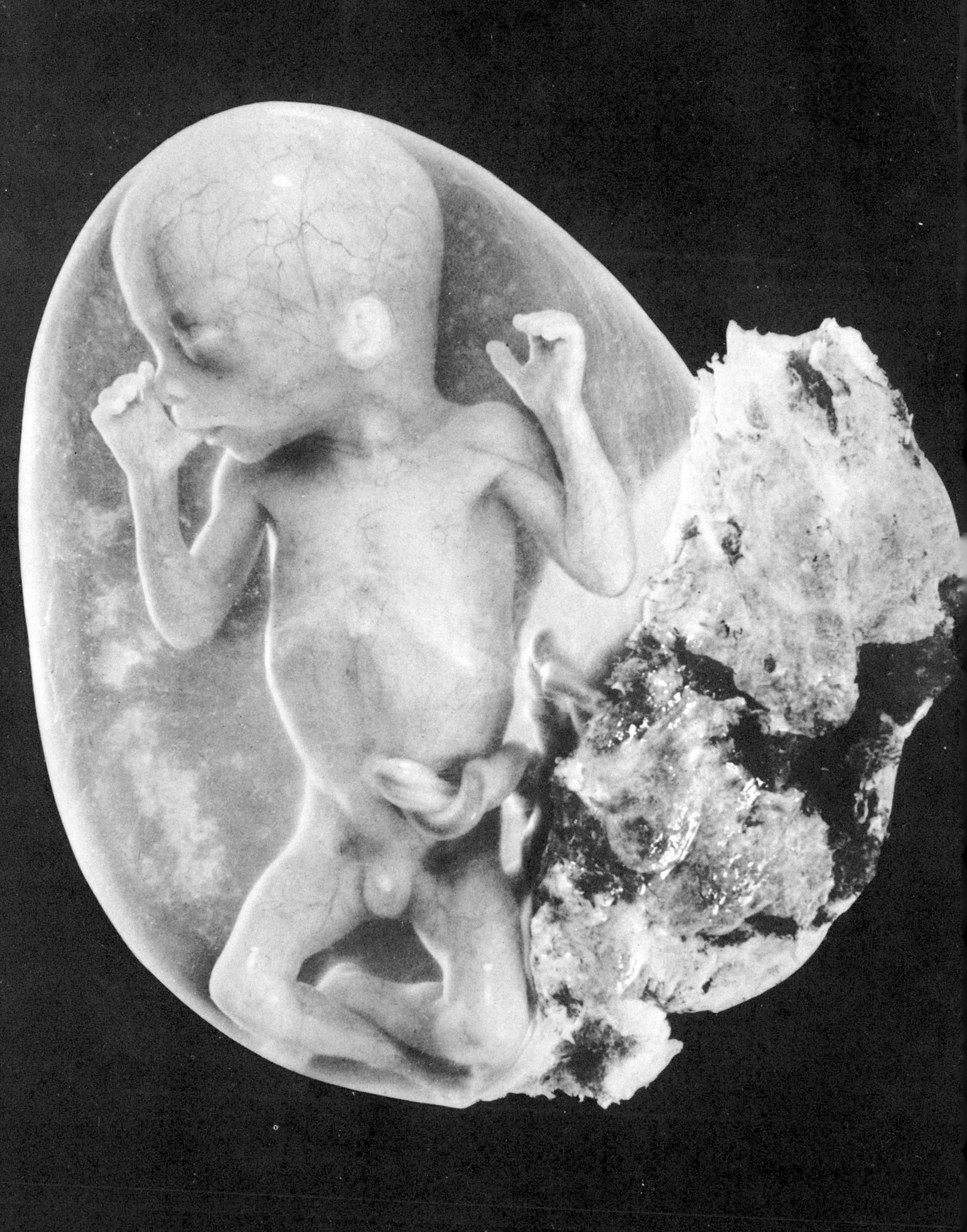

SECTION I

General Foundations

A fetus seen in the womb. Photo © Lennart Nilsson, courtesy *Life* magazine.

I

The Meaning of Abnormality

PERRY LONDON

DAVID ROSENHAN

It must be sometime around the high school years that young people begin to use the word *normal* both to reassure themselves and to question their own and other people's sanity. In almost any situation where they discover feelings in themselves with which they have previously been unfamiliar, observe their own swings of mood, or notice seemingly inexplicable inconsistencies in their own or other people's conduct, they wrestle with the question, "Is this normal?" From then on, the word seems to become a fixed part of their vocabularies and, like much of many people's vocabularies, is sometimes used as a convenient substitute for thought, a kind of intellectual reflex that can be used to label behavior whenever understanding it is too much trouble.

STATISTICAL CONCEPT OF NORMALITY

Normality as Conformity, Consistency, or Morality

Used unreflectively, *normal* has a number of meanings which, though they differ somewhat from each other, all refer to whether or not a particular manner of thinking, feeling, or acting is acceptable. What people mean by *acceptable* is not always clear to observers, nor is it necessarily any clearer in the minds of those who worry about their normality in the first place, but there are a few general things that can be said about it.

In the first place, people often think that their behavior is acceptable if it is common or usual, that is, if it conforms to the behavior of others. Used this way, when people ask themselves if they are normal, they are really wondering if they are sufficiently conventional, if their behavior is acceptable to others, if it conforms to the manners or morals that define proper conduct in their society. In a peculiar but accurate way, they are asking if their behavior is invisible, undistinguishable from that of their peers. The assumption on which this notion of normality is implicitly based is that conventional behavior is itself acceptable, that is, that the common practices of most people in a society are a reasonable basis for setting one's own standards of behavior.

People are often concerned with normality of a somewhat different kind, however, though it is still related to acceptability and to what is usual; they ask whether they are normal in their own eyes. In this case, the standards of acceptability are not the conventions of behavior of other people, but the standards of what is acceptable to one's own self. Most people consider their own behavior normal in this sense if it meets three criteria: (1) *intelligibility*—we feel we understand the nature and motives of our behavior; (2) *consistency*—we feel that our behavior is predictable on the basis of what we know about ourselves; and (3) *control*—we feel that our behavior is subject to our wishes so that we may either produce or prevent a particular behavior at will. This use of *normality* derives from such questions as, "I wonder why I did that?" (intelligibility), "How is it that I felt one way yesterday but quite differently today?" (consistency), and "Why can't I cut that out?" (control).

Finally, in addition to socially oriented and self-oriented definitions of *normality*, people commonly use a moralistic or idealized one. Here the standards of acceptability are neither common practices nor one's common expectations of himself, but rather the moral or idealized norms which are believed to characterize all right-thinking, -feeling, and -acting. This point of view starts with the idea, for example, that people *ought* to behave in a certain way, whether they really do or not, and concludes that it is normal to behave in the way one ought to. It is normal, this view would argue, to love and to work, to believe in a supernatural God, to be neither overly constrained and shy nor overly impulsive and socially aggressive.

Each of these concepts of *normality*—the socially oriented, the self-oriented, and the idealized moral—has some merit as a standard against which one's behavior can be described. On the other hand, common use of the term "normality" is not so much descriptive as evaluative. In other words, the meanings attributed to it are not intended merely to compare, but are ways of passing judgment, especially negative judgment, on behavior. This becomes most clear if one thinks about the implied meanings, in each context, of the companion term "abnormal."

In the first case, where *normality* means "conformity," it is abnormal to be unconventional. In the second, it is abnormal to behave inconsistently, in an uncontrolled way, or in a manner which we do not ourselves understand. Finally, it is abnormal to behave immorally or to fall too short of the ideal. In each instance, given the pertinent definition of *normality*, the statement defining *abnormality* is quite literally correct. But the implication of any of these statements as they might be made in ordinary conversation is surely that it is undesirable to be abnormal. Indeed, in the common parlance of much of our society, *normality* has become synonymous with *goodness*. By the same token, "abnormality" has become a polite term for all manner of erratic, bizarre, or otherwise undesirable behavior which, if not downright wicked, is still better done without.

Regardless of the precise meaning intended at any time, *normal* always has the general connotation of that which is expected, routine, or ordinary, and *abnormal* conversely always connotes the unexpected, extraordinary, or unusual. These are essentially correct, if imprecise, uses of the words. There are, however, two connotations in this ordinary usage that are quite incorrect. First is the idea that these concepts can be used loosely to describe a person; in fact they are only applicable to traits that a person may have in greater or less degree. Second is the idea that there is anything inherently good or bad about being normal or abnormal in any particular way; the actual desirability of being more or less normal in a given respect depends entirely on the particular conditions the observer is interested in satisfying.

Acceptance of a new understanding of the concept of normality in psychology will probably require a good deal of rethinking on the part of many people, whose use of the term has become habituated to the common errors of meaning associated with it. Abnormal psychology, for example, is usually thought of as the psychology of insanity and emotional disorders (psychopathology), and insofar as these conditions are relatively unusual, they are properly considered abnormal. But other, equally unusual psychological states are also properly within the province of abnormal psychology, such as extraordinary intelligence, creative ability, strength of character, and the like—aspects of human behavior that must also be explored if an understanding of this science is to be achieved. To explore them properly, moreover, it is necessary to understand the concept of normality somewhat more precisely than in oversimplified terms of the ordinary and the extraordinary. Such an understanding in turn requires an immediate digression on *probability* and *continuity* or, more colloquially, the problems of gambling and of measuring.

Probability

Suppose you were a gambler engaged in the simplest of all gambling contests, the kind in which you win or lose according to how well you guess whether a flipped coin will land with "heads" or "tails" up. If the coin is tossed fairly, it has an even chance of showing either heads or tails on each toss, and it is safe to say that, if it is tossed enough times, about half the throws will show heads and half tails. What is of special interest to a gambler, however, is the fact that it is possible, within reason, to estimate the likelihood that two tosses in a row will show heads, or that three in a row will, or four, or any number, and he can use such estimates or probabilities to adjust the size of his bets. A mathematical expression that most American children learn by their freshman year in high school was invented for the specific purpose of aiding gamblers in this task. It is called the *binomial distribution* or *binomial expansion*, and it works in the following manner.

Each time the coin is tossed, it will show either heads (H) or tails (T), and only one of the two possibilities will actually occur. Because these possibilities are mutually exclusive, we say there is a "one in two" chance (1/2) that heads will show and the same "one in two" chance (1/2) that tails will appear, or that the odds are "fifty-fifty" for either heads or tails, meaning that each has a 50 percent chance of appearing on a single toss of the coin (Table 1.1).

Table 1.1
Single Toss of Coin

Possibilities	Chances
H	1/2
T	1/2

The second time the coin is tossed, however, the question is: how likely is it to come out the way it did the first? Adding the possibilities of the first and second toss together, there are now four possible outcomes, only one of which will actually occur. As Table 1.2 shows, there will either be heads both tosses (H^2), tails both tosses (T^2), heads the first toss and tails the second

Table 1.2

Second Toss of Coin

Possibilities		Chances
Toss 1	Toss 2	
H	H = H^2	1/4
	T = HT	1/4
T	H = TH	1/4
	T = T^2	1/4

toss (HT), or tails the first toss and heads the second toss (TH). Since there are now four possibilities, the likelihood of obtaining any one of them is "one in four" or 1/4. But note that HT and TH are identical in the sense that they are both mixtures of heads and tails. So if we are not concerned with the order in which they occur but only with the total number of heads and tails in the two tosses, we can combine HT and TH and say: the probability of obtaining a head *and* a tail on two flips is 1/4 + 1/4 = 2/4 or 1/2. The probability of obtaining two heads in a row or two tails in a row is 1/4 in each case.

The probabilities for the third toss are shown in Table 1.3. There are now eight possibilities. The chances of getting three heads in a row is, then, 1/8. The chance of getting two heads and one tail are, however, 3/8 since there are three different ways in which that combination can arise. Likewise, the chances of getting two tails and one head are 3/8, while the probability of obtaining three tails is 1/8. Here is another way of saying the same thing:

$$(1)H^3 + 3H^2T + 3T^2H + (1)T^3$$

For the two-toss situation (Table 1.2) we would write the probabilities like this:

$$(1)H^2 + 2HT + (1)T^2$$

The general equation that describes the probability events we have been discussing is called the binomial expansion, and it is written:

$$(a + b)^n$$

where a and b are the two events (heads and tails) and n is the number of tosses.

Table 1.4 shows the results of the binomial expansion for several tosses of the coin. Note that as the number of tosses increases, the probability of getting relatively large numbers of either heads or tails decreases markedly. For six tosses, the chances are 1/64 that you will get six heads, and only 6/64 that you will get five heads and one tail. The chances are 1/128 that you will get seven heads (or

Table 1.3

Third Toss of Coin

Possibilities				Chances
Toss 1	Toss 2	Toss 3	Total	
H	H	H	HHH = H^3	1/8 or 0.125
		T	HHT = H^2T	1/8 or 0.125
	T	H	HTH = H^2T	1/8 or 0.125
		T	HTT = T^2H	1/8 or 0.125
T	H	H	THH = H^2T	1/8 or 0.125
		T	THT = T^2H	1/8 or 0.125
	T	H	TTH = T^2H	1/8 or 0.125
		T	TTT = T^3	1/8 or 0.125

Table 1.4
Binomial Expansions

No. of tosses (n)	Expansions	Total possibilities
1	$a + b$	2
2	$a^2 + 2ab + b^2$	4
3	$a^3 + 3a^2b + 3ab^2 + b^3$	8
4	$a^4 + 4a^3b + 6a^2b^2 + 4ab^3 + b^4$	16
5	$a^5 + 5a^4b + 10a^3b^2 + 10a^2b^3 + 5ab^4 + b^5$	32
6	$a^6 + 6a^5b + 15a^4b^2 + 20a^3b^3 + 15a^2b^4 + 6ab^5 + b^6$	64
7	$a^7 + 7a^6b + 21a^5b^2 + 35a^4b^3 + 35a^3b^4 + 21a^2b^5 + 7ab^6 + b^7$	128

seven tails) in seven tosses. Expansion of the binomial term makes an endless network of combinations of a and b, until there is eventually no place except the end points that does not have some of both letters, and until the probability of having a great deal of one and very little of the other becomes increasingly small.

When the binomial is endlessly expanded, the total pattern which results is called the *normal distribution*. If one is to be literal about it, normality is a purely mathematical event and is, like all mathematical phenomena, a mere figment of the imagination. For the normal distribution is a continuous one, and *true* continuity does not exist in connection with the things that students of normality are generally interested in. But this hardly matters for practical purposes. Even where true continuity does exist, it is not very useful, for it makes no use of discretion, and discretion is the soul of understanding. Time is truly continuous, for example, but we make use of it only by acting as if it were discrete, that is, as if it could be marked off into separate pieces. Otherwise, we could never tell anyone the correct time, for as we announce it, it has already changed. And while the philosopher Heraclitus observed that it was impossible to step into the same stream twice, for practical purposes we all do.

The Normative View of Normality

There are many events which, though truly discrete, like Mendel's peas or the heads and tails on a coin, occur in such an enormous variety of combinations that, taken all together, they form a pattern which looks like the normal distribution. This *apparent continuity* depends on the number of tosses to be made. Biological species, because of their reproductive nature, make plenty. Some such natural coin tossing, highly romanticized, is as familiar to most students as the binomial expansion itself—illustrated by Mendel's laws (see "Mendelism" in Chapter 2). A large number of biological events have this characteristic, like height or eye color, and so do a lot of derivative psychological ones, like intelligence (see Chapter 2) or manual dexterity. For our purposes, talking about normality is, in the broadest sense, talking about biology.

Take intelligence, for example. In a book that was wonderfully reasoned for its day, *Hereditary Genius*, Galton (1880) described his studies in the nature of intelligence, particularly that of eminent genius. Without the use of IQ tests (they were invented by Binet some twenty-five years later) he established that although there are all grades of genius, truly eminent genius is quite rare:

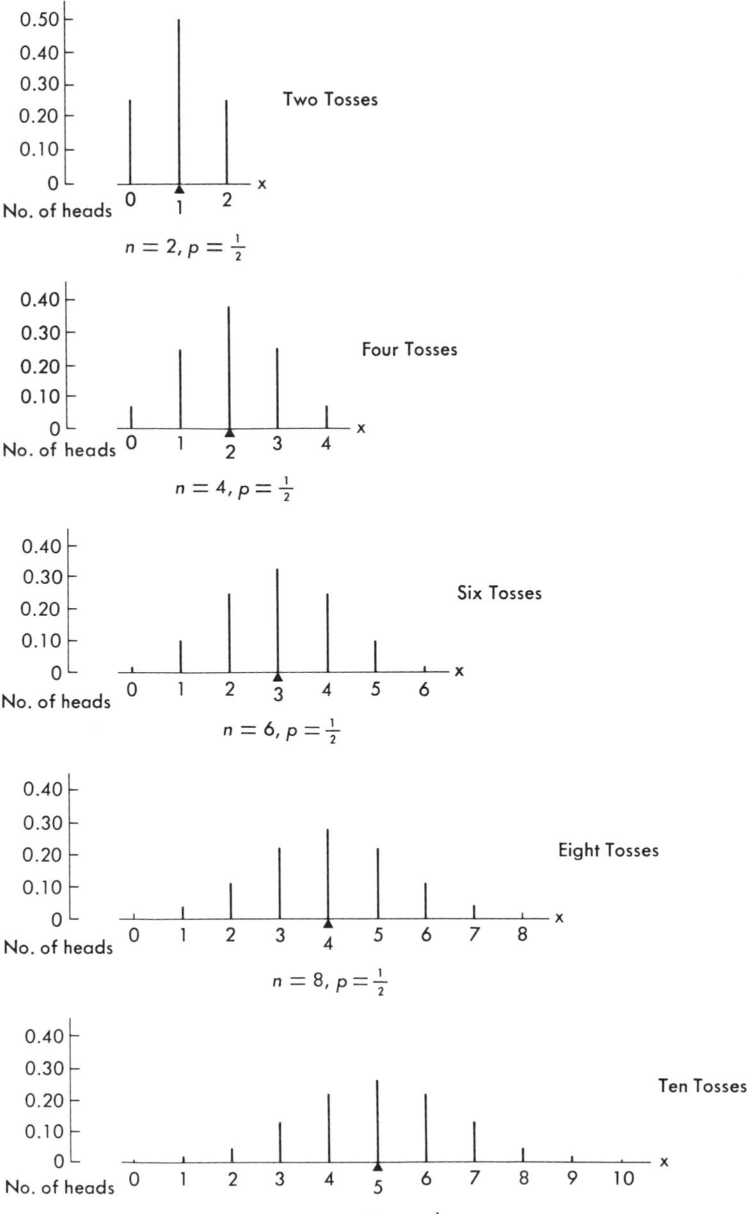

Figure 1.1 As the number of incidents ("tosses") increases, the normal distribution becomes wider and flatter. From Mosteller, Rourke, and Thomas, *Probability: A First Course*, 1961, Addison-Wesley Publishing Company, Reading, Mass.

> When I speak of an eminent man [Galton wrote], I mean one who has achieved a position that is attained by only 250 persons in each million of men, or by one person in each 4000. Four thousand is a very large number. . . . On the most brilliant of starlight nights there are never so many as 4000 stars visible to the naked eye at the same time. . . . This is my narrowest area of selection. I propose to introduce no name whatever into my lists . . . that is less distinguished.
>
> The mass of those with whom I deal are far more rigidly selected—many are as one in a million, and not a few as one in many millions. I use the term "illustrious" when speaking of these. They are men whom the whole intelligent part of the nation mourns when they die. (Galton, 1880, pp. 10–11.)

Notice that Galton had already introduced distinctions among several kinds of genius—one in four thousand, one in a million, one in many millions. He subsequently distinguished lesser geniuses, men who may have made enormous contributions but who did not merit the honorific of eminence. There are more of these latter men, he held, as there must be, because intelligence, like height, is normally distributed and the further one departs from the very end of the curve, the more permutations of chance (genetic materials, favorable environment, and the like, in the instance of intelligence) one will find. Put differently, most people will be found near the average, be it in height or weight or intelligence. The more one moves away from the average, the fewer people one will find. This notion is as applicable to genius, Galton found, as it is to idiocy: idiots are as rare as eminent men, but Galton was not much concerned with idiots. (The inheritance of intelligence is discussed in detail in Chapter 2, and current thinking on mental retardation in Chapter 14. The term *genius* is used here in a statistical sense, but it is treated quite differently in Chapter 6.)

Figure 1.1 describes for two, four, six, eight, and ten tosses of a coin the likelihood that ten, nine, eight . . . through zero heads or tails will be observed. A similar figure can be drawn to describe human fortunes in longevity and illness, height and girth, intelligence and personality traits. It hardly matters for the present what causes the regular curve that begins to emerge after ten tosses—whether it be heredity, environment, or simple luck (whatever that is). What is critical for the present discussion is the curve itself.

Notice the shape of the curve that normal distribution yields (Figure 1.2). It is commonly called "bell shaped" and it indicates that after ten tosses the greatest probabilities are that there will be equal or nearly equal mixtures of heads and tails. It is a rare series of tosses that will yield ten or nine heads in ten tosses, or one or zero heads, much as it is a rare man who is entirely white or black, possessed of sterling character or none at all, uniquely intelligent or dumb, entirely organized or disorganized in thought, completely introverted or extroverted. *It is this rareness that is of special interest and is called abnormal.* Rareness defines what is abnormal in the statistical sense. And rareness occurs at both ends of the normal distribution. If it is rare to obtain only heads in a series of ten tosses, it is equally rare to obtain only tails. If it is rare to find many geniuses among a large group of people, there will not be many idiots either. The same is true for great beauty or great ugliness and for being very tall or very short, alert or phlegmatic, and so on. The essence of the notion of normality includes the existence of positive as well as negative abnormalities. Rareness in this scheme is a two-sided thing. (The social implications of *normality*, used in this sense, are the main subject matter of Chapter 5.)

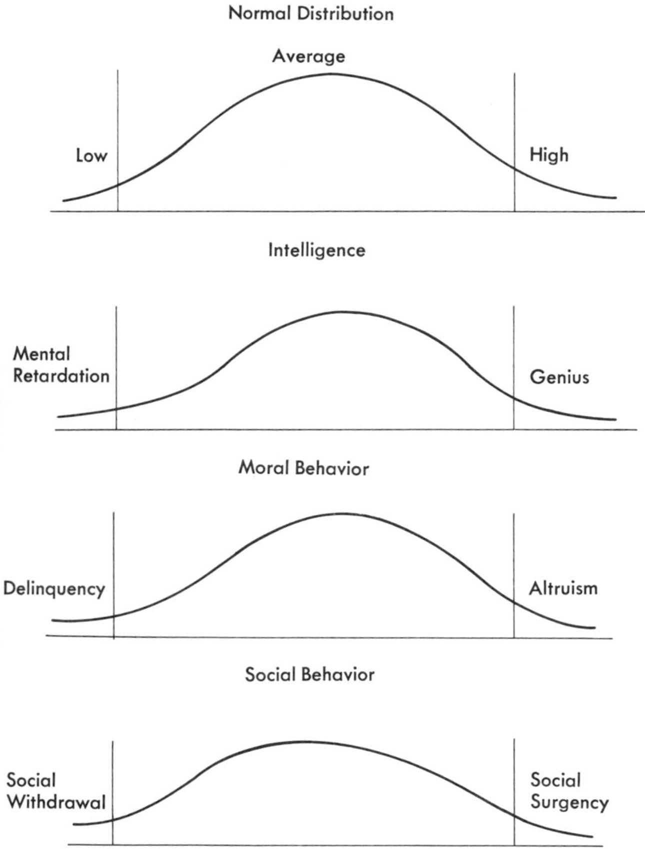

Figure 1.2 The normal distribution curve and normally distributed traits and behaviors.

Obviously when we talk about normality in people, we cannot speak of a person as being normal in general, for normality refers to events and traits, not to people.

It is a *statistical characteristic* of a *kind* of event which is, to begin with, capable of occurring in either one of only two ways and in a great variety of combinations of those two ways. There are all kinds of *traits* to which this concept properly applies, as Allport (1937) has argued, but it is *the trait* which is normally distributed among people, not people who are truly normal or not. In the statistical sense, *normal* really refers to the distribution of some kinds of traits. In loose use, when we say a person is normal, we really mean he is about average with respect to a trait which is normally distributed among people. For any trait to qualify, it must be present to some degree in everybody.

Looking back again to the normal distributions shown in Figure 1.1, and imagining that they refer to personality traits rather than to tosses of a coin, when we say that a person is normal with regard to a trait, we mean that if it is possible to have as much as ten and as little as no degrees of that trait, the person in question has four or five or six. He is about average. He is undistinguished with regard to the trait in question.

It is also important to realize that this conception of normality and abnormality suggests that abnormal traits are cut from the same cloth as normal ones, so that the same laws of learning, of development, and of genetics apply to both. This may seem simple and straightforward in the present context, where it is clear that the binomial distribution dictates what is normal and abnormal, but it was not always so obvious among students of behavior and it is not so in everyday popular opinion even now. "Abnormal people" were once, and probably still are, considered a group quite apart from the rest of us. They were either infested with demons, or infected with disease, or (where neither of these views were known or applicable) so clearly different from the rest of us as to be operating in terms and under principles that were entirely their own. The madness of the schizophrenic was rarely seen as an extreme case of our own madness, while mental retardation was called mental defectiveness, implying that mental retardates lacked what the rest of us had. Such a view of abnormality, we believe, facilitated (if it did not promote in the first place) a treatment for such people that was inhuman and very much different from treatment accorded to so-called full-fledged members of the human race.

The Sequential Dependency of Psychological Traits

Until now, we have applied our statistical concept of abnormality to the question of how rare a trait is among different people. But it is important to recognize that rareness also refers to the presence or absence of a trait *over time* in the same person, that is, to the persistence or constancy of a person's behavior. One might argue that *one* rare act on someone's part, whether it is desirable or not, is not by itself abnormal. Abnormality implies that the act or trait is of a more or less constant, hence predictable, sort.

Return for a moment to our gambler's dilemma. He might ask two questions. First, what is the probability that *time after time* seven heads (HHHHHHH) will arise from seven flips of a fair coin? And second, what is the probability that another pattern, such as HTTHTHH, will arise? The chances for *any* pattern of events to arise are identical: 1/128 for seven tosses, and much smaller for a larger number of tosses. Now the gambler may consider that only a string of heads is "significant" or "lucky" and that other patterns are simply random, but we understand that the same laws of sequential probabilities underlie all such patterns of events.

Now consider the same problem as it might be posed by a psychologist. What is the probability, he might ask, that a person will always offer one of two equally probable responses to a series of seven similar situations? And what is the probability that he might offer one response on the first occasion, its opposite on the second and third, the original response again on the fourth, and so on? The probabilities are identical, as we have seen above. But if he gave the same response on all seven occasions, and if it was one that is not ordinarily elicited with such frequency, the psychologist would take note (as would any perceptive observer) of its *persistence*.

The relevance of *trait persistence* to abnormality is illustrated in Figure 1.3. Imagine six situations that are roughly similar in social characteristics, say situations where the central actor is a person in authority. And suppose, for the sake of this example, that there are only two equally probable responses to this actor: a frown and a smile. We might expect that whether one or the other of these responses appears would depend on some additional characteristics of the situation, such as whether the person in authority is himself smiling or frowning. By and large, the hypothetical people in Figure 1.2 meet our expectations: sometimes they are angry and sometimes they are smiling. In the first situation, all are smiling except Person 5. Person 5 is thus deviant with regard to this situation, but not yet so deviant that we would want to label his behavior abnormal in general. In the second situation, Person 5 is still angry, but so are many others—all of them, in fact, except Person 1. Looking across the six situations we find that Person 5 is constantly angry, that his anger persists even when others are smiling. We now have some basis for suspecting that his response may be abnormal. So too for Person 1, whose constant smile alerts us not only to his deviance in any particular situation, but also to the inflexibility of that response. If there were even more situations in which the responses of anger and joy were equally probable, and in which Persons 1 and 5 maintained their characteristic responses, we would have strong evidence for trait abnormality.

Persistence means much more to the psychologist than it does to the coin gambler, for when psychological traits persist they acquire interesting characteristics. In the first place, they "harden"—

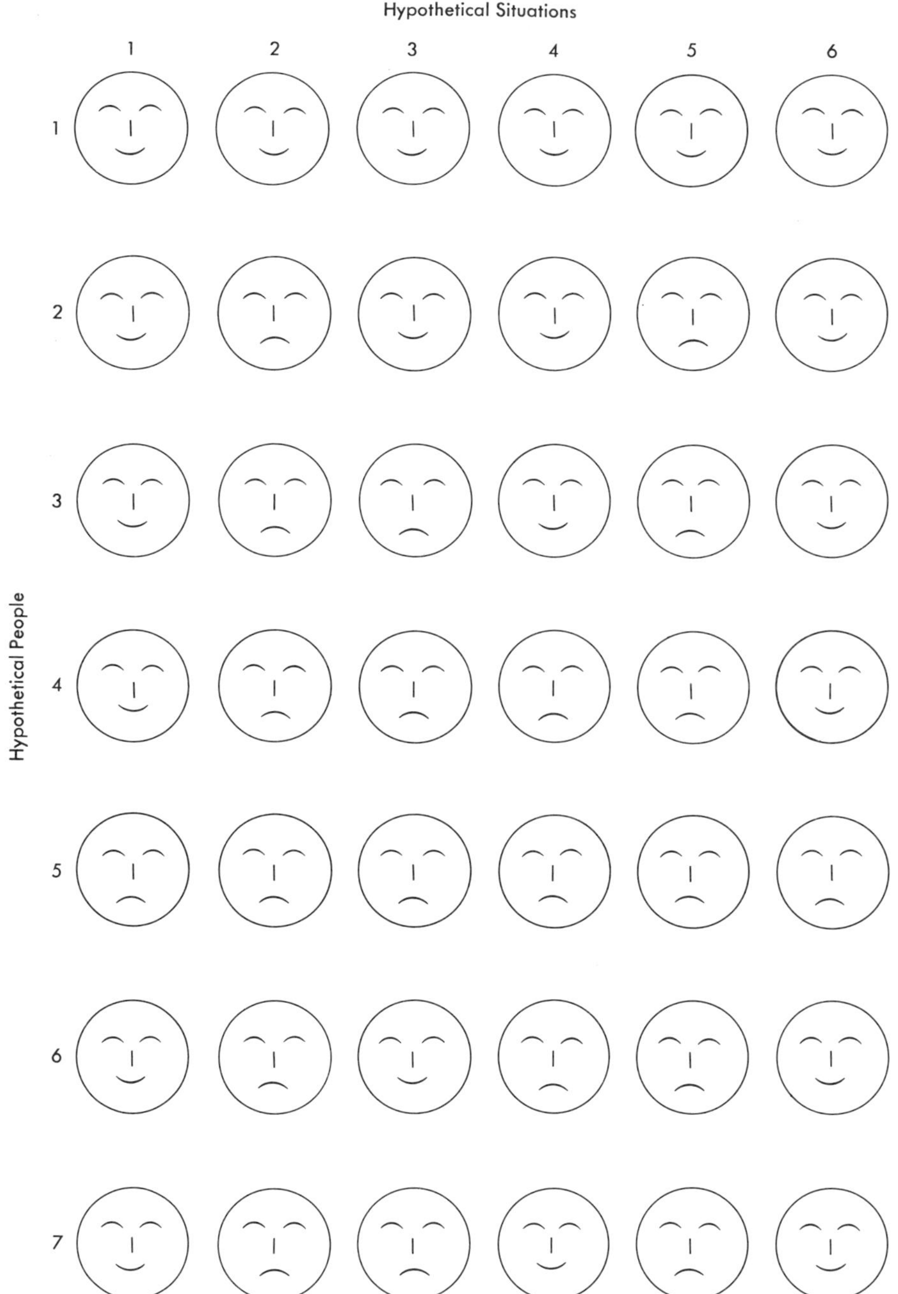

Figure 1.3 A hypothetical illustration of abnormality.

that is, become habitual—and thus become more likely to occur in subsequent situations. This permits greater predictability than is the case with coin tossing. Moreover, this persistence is likely to make the trait socially more salient, and thereby contribute to others' view of the trait as abnormal in either the positive or the negative sense. This may best be made clear in two examples.

1. A person who is abnormally shy tends to withdraw in social situations. One social consequence of his behavior might be that, sooner or later, people will begin to ignore him, perhaps forget to invite him, or having invited him, not have much to say to him. The psychological consequence for the shy person might be that he would feel disliked, and this might depress him. He might further begin to wonder what people are *really* thinking about him. Both depression and self-doubt might have bad effects on his work or study habits and might, in fact, serve to make him more shy than he was at the outset. In short, the persistent shyness is now seen to have effects on thinking, on affect, on social and work behaviors, and on the intensity of the shyness itself.

2. To consider a positive abnormality, a person who responded to a series of situations with honesty and courage when the prevailing pressures encouraged more deceptive behavior might become socially salient on that count alone. He might also find that, rather than subjecting him to more intense social pressures, or punishing him for his gentle deviance, many people were now coming to see things his way, seeking his counsel rather than seeking to shape his opinions and behaviors. He might thereby feel reinforced not only in his honesty and courage, but also, say, in his capacity to make sensible decisions and in his self-esteem, as well as in other traits. All of this might make him more likely to respond confidently with similar behaviors in subsequent situations. (Such means of self-enhancement are discussed at length in Chapter 5.)

The upshot of all this is that, quite apart from the statistical properties that make particular traits abnormal, there are psychological and social factors that perpetuate these traits, increase their predictability, and give them ramifications that extend to other traits, to ideations and affects, and to others' responses to the person in question. These interdependencies of persistent responses and consequences, which we observe as loose constellations of associated behaviors, are called *syndromes*. Studying them allows us to go beyond the matter of individual traits and to understand people in terms of personality styles and dispositions.

Two Complementary Methods of Assessing Normality and Abnormality

Treating normality as a statistical concept, as we are doing here, and recognizing that it applies only to traits which everyone has to some degree, there are at least two different ways of using this statistic to study traits. We can look at many different people to see how much of a given trait occurs in each one, or we can look at a single person to see how often and how much it occurs in him. The first way is called the *normative* approach, and the second is known as the *ipsative* method. Both approaches are described in detail by Allport (1937). Each of them is valuable in some situations and probably obscures understanding if it is used in others; in still other situations, neither approach is very meaningful unless it is used in conjunction with the other.

Normative methods are most commonly used for studying characteristics which can be more or less clearly identified in people and, therefore, readily compared from one person to another. Many anatomical features—such as height, weight, color of eyes, hair, or skin—can be easily and satisfactorily studied in this way. Even though features like height and weight change as a result of growth, illness, or other things, they are still easily compared from one person to another because, at any given time, they are apparently quite stable. It is relative stability that permits the use of the normative method, for unless there is some reasonably fixed position or base point applicable to everybody, it is hopeless to try to make comparisons.

Ipsative methods, on the other hand, are applicable to precisely those events or characteristics which are slippery and unstable, in the sense either that they change rapidly in a fairly brief time span or that they occur in a single individual in so idiosyncratic or peculiar a form that there is no meaningful point of comparison between him and others with respect to that trait.

The appropriateness of one or the other method depends on the use to be made of the information. The ipsative method might be more useful to a doctor who is concerned about the blood pressure of a patient, but the normative method is more valuable for predicting the course of an infection.

Two general statements can be made about the methods. (1) The more complicated the characteristic under study, the more necessary the ipsative approach becomes to a full understanding of it. If one wishes to understand the work of creative artists, for example, he must examine them individually over a period of time rather than compare them in some across-the-board fashion with most other people. Most other people do not, on the whole, compose symphonies, paint pictures, or write novels, so there is not likely to be any meaningful basis of comparison. (2) In practice, the normative approach generally antecedes the ipsative one. In other words, the peculiar characteristics of one person are inevitably variants of characteristics which, in less specialized form, occur in everyone—and it is reasonable to attempt to identify the broader characteristic, and the norms of its occurrence, before concentrating on the narrower one. In some situations, moreover, it may be indispensable to do so. If, for example, one wishes to study the characteristics of Mozart's musical genius, it is reasonable to begin by studying the elements which antecede musical composition, like ability to repeat tones, to remember tunes, and the like. These simpler elements exist to some degree in everyone and can be examined by normative methods. Indeed, if one wished to select children for training as composers of music, it would be quite necessary to begin with this approach, because it is unlikely that a child could ever learn to compose music if he could not learn to recognize the harmonic differences between one sound and another.

The uniqueness of every human being is an offshoot of the common condition of man.

PERSPECTIVES ON ABNORMALITY

The concept of abnormality applies to events which are studied by both normative and ipsative methods. For the former, *abnormality* means that which is unusual relative to others and for the latter, that which is unusual relative to one's self.

The definitions of *abnormality* here sound like the common uses of the term described at the beginning of the chapter, and in fact, there is only one vital respect in which they are different. As used here, *abnormality* has no bearing at all on acceptability, and it no more implies anything inherently undesirable than do other descriptive adjectives like *tall*, *short*, or *purple*. As we use it, *abnormal* is always a functional rather than an evaluative label, describing the factual character or nature of an event or characteristic but implying nothing one way or the other about its desirability.

Functional and Evaluative Criteria and Their Ambiguity

Desirability, or goodness, is a meaningful idea only in relation to some criterion by which achievement can be measured.

Legal, ethical, and religious codes of behavior all have different criteria of goodness or desirability, which usually revolve respectively around how well a person obeys the law, follows the ethical tenets in question, or observes the adjurations and prohibitions of the religious doctrine at hand. In each case, moreover, the criteria of good behavior are justified or rationalized by appeal to some superordinate goal, usually the preservation of order within a society for lawyers, consistency with some defined good for philosophers of ethics, and compliance with the will of a supreme being for clerics.

For scientists, the most generally accepted criterion of desirability is efficient function, or utility. In other words, the scientific standard of value generally wants to know how efficiently an event serves some specific purpose. In the case of human behavior, the scientific criterion of goodness has nothing to do with how normal or abnormal a trait is, but only with how well it aids a person to accomplish some goal or achieve some purpose. Characteristics that help a person to achieve what most of us consider evil or repulsive purposes nevertheless satisfy the functional criterion of desirability. This criterion is therefore not an altogether sufficient guide in deciding whether a particular characteristic is desirable or not. Functional criteria can never be used to give *final* answers to such questions, for the notion that something is good for a certain purpose is of no use in deciding whether the purpose is itself any good. And if one then attempts to find a functional criterion for judging the purpose, he comes up with another purpose, and on and on in infinite regress.

The only alternative to functional criteria, however, are dogmas of the kind espoused by legal, ethical, and religious systems. It is probably necessary to invoke such dogmas at one or another time if people are to have decent and humane relations with each other, but only functional criteria have meaning in science. The moral is that science alone does not make a human being, but that is not our immediate problem.

Even strictly functional criteria of desirability are ambiguous, however, because the same trait which functions as an asset to a person in one situation may be a grave liability in another situation. Boundless good cheer is a wonderfully endearing quality at a party, but it does not wear well at funerals. And the dull sobriety which makes some boy unbearable to a coed cheerleader may inspire confidence, good will, and nudgings toward the altar from her mother. Similarly, a single trait may serve the purposes of one person very well and those of another very ill. Happy undertakers and lugubrious obstetricians may both have business troubles resulting from mismatching of mood with trade.

Functional criteria for evaluating behavior have the positive value of permitting one to see what the consequences of particular behavior characteristics are likely to be. Whether those consequences should be sought or avoided is a decision which scientists are no better qualified to make than anybody else. But unless the consequences of behavior patterns can be known, nobody else can make very intelligent decisions about them either. Behavioral scientists have the responsibility of discovering and communicating what the implications and consequences of behavior are; everybody has the obligation to understand those consequences and to decide how some behaviors ought to be dealt with.

Positive Abnormalities

From almost any point of view—scientific or moral—some behavior characteristics are more desirable than others because, by permitting an individual to function more effectively, they increase his possibilities of contributing to the welfare of society. Even from an individual point of view, some traits are more valuable than others because, rather than being assets in one situation and liabilities in another, they have positive value in almost any situation. To the extent that such attributes are normally distributed, their possession in unusual degree is abnormal. For our purposes, traits of this kind concerning which functional and evaluative criteria tend to conjoin favorably are called *positive abnormalities.*

Well-known traits that fall in the category of positive abnormalities are very high intelligence or uniquely well developed talent in some specialized area of human invention or performance. These traits are sometimes labeled "genius" or "creativity," and they are most commonly attributed to people of high achievement in scientific or intellectual pursuits, to writers, artists, and musical composers and performers. Another set of positive abnormalities which usually goes under different popular labels includes characteristics like leadership ability, persistence in the pursuit of goals, great endurance in the face of stress, and adherence to principles in spite of temptation or danger; these behaviors are generally identified as "character." Genius, creativity, and character are all discussed in great detail in later chapters of this book.

Historical Notes

In any discussion of positive abnormalities, it is important to bear in mind that the positiveness which attaches to them cannot be divorced completely from the cultural setting in which they occur. Skill in physical performance, particularly in athletics, was highly idealized in classical Graeco-Roman civilization. Intellectual accomplishments were valued also, but less universally, as witness the divergent fates of Socrates and Aristotle. Artistic achievements were even more variably regarded, and artists, who were among the most lionized figures of Periclean Athens, did not, for the most part, attain equal status in the Roman Republic. The classical ideal type, moreover, both in democratic Greece and republican Rome, was always held to be the "good citizen," who, whatever he may have had or lacked as athlete, artist, or intellectual, possessed traits of character which made him a reliable and loyal member of the body politic, ready to devote himself to its interests above all merely personal concerns—including those of his family—and unhesitatingly prepared to die for its welfare should the need arise.

In contrast, consider the idealized criteria of personal accomplishment among the ancient Jews, whose civilization, in terms of modern ideals of political and social equality, was even more advanced than that of the Greeks or Romans. Performance skills in athletics were demeaned as having relatively little value (except in war), artistic accomplishments were, for the most part, beneath mention in any context but a religious one, and intellectual achievements that did not pertain directly to the ethical imperatives of the traditional religion were, with almost no exceptions, buried in the course of Jewish history. Even citizenship had no value in this thoroughly theocentric culture unless its expression suited the prophetic religious temper which claimed sole right to evaluate it. The prophet Jeremiah, who, in a Hellenistic society, would have been excoriated as a traitor to his state, was revered by the Jews for his steadfast adherence to his inspired message that God willed the destruction of his state.

Quite probably, many of the same personal characteristics made possible the behaviors of Jeremiah in Judea and of Horatius at the bridge in Rome, but the precise valuation placed on the behaviors differed according to the dominant values of the cultures in which they occurred.

With the advent of Christianity as the dominant source of value judgments in Western society, the classical ideal of the broadly developed individual, multiply skilled in the facets of human potential, gave way for a thousand years to the doctrine that since this world was only a preparation for the next, it mattered little what humans tried to accomplish. The Italian Renaissance, however, beginning around the end of the thirteenth century, restored the classical ideal and, itself producing a large number of geniuses in many branches of the arts and sciences, laid the groundwork for the modern veneration of men of outstanding ability.

Although the recognition and appreciation of meritorious individual accomplishment was more or less legitimized by the Renaissance, it was not made the subject of scientific inquiry until the end of the nineteenth century, at which time Sir Francis Galton, generally regarded today as an intellectual genius in his own right, began a more or less systematic study of the genesis of genius in an attempt to identify the hereditary components which contributed to the development of this positive abnormality. His results, to which we referred earlier, were published partly in 1869 as *Hereditary Genius* and in 1883 as *Inquiries into Human Faculty*. These were probably the first major works of their kind since Plutarch's *Lives*, some 1800 years earlier.

Even more systematic inquiry became possible with the invention of the modern intelligence test by Alfred Binet and Théophile Simon in France in 1905. In 1916, Lewis Terman, an American psychologist at Stanford University, published a translated and revised version of the Binet-Simon scale called "The Stanford-Binet Test of Intelligence," on which very high scores were considered to indicate "genius." With this term, used only as a convenience for discussing the implications of IQ (intelligence quotient) test scores, Terman put the concept of genius for the first time into a more or less formal quantitative statement. He also pioneered the study of other desirable traits of character, and was, in a very real sense, the father of the scientific study of positive abnormal psychology.

It is interesting to note that, especially in very recent times, interest in the study of positive abnormalities, particularly in methods of developing them in young children, is again rationalized in terms of social necessity and competitive national goals. Not only do politicians, educators, and social scientists justify their interest in these phenomena by citing the potential value of positively abnormal people to the struggle of democracy against its detractors, but agencies of both federal and local government invest large sums of money in scientific investigations of genius and creativity, as well as of character traits like leadership ability.

Despite current interest, however, positive abnormalities have received less scientific attention than negative ones; yet their great potential value to mankind in general, let alone to the individual, makes them worthy of more attention. The entire second section of this book (Chapters 5 through 8) is concerned with positive deviations from the normal.

Negative Abnormalities

Just as traits like creative ability or intelligence function in a generally positive way to benefit the individual and, potentially, society, others have characteristically negative effects on both. These traits, when possessed in marked degree, constitute the *negative abnormalities*. Discussion of them takes up the third section of this book (Chapters 9 through 16), but they are the entire subject matter of most abnormal psychology texts.

The conventional subject matter of abnormal psychology deals with negative abnormalities that, taken together, are often called "psychopathological states" or *mental illness*. Four kinds of disorders are usually included under this heading: (1) organic damage, (2) psychoses, (3) neuroses, and (4) character disorders. At least two other major categories of negative abnormality are commonly recognized, however; these are mental retardation—that is, abnormally low intellectual functioning—and antisocial patterns of behavior, such as delinquency and criminal occupations. Because antisocial behavior is often associated with a particular character disorder, especially so-called psychopathic or sociopathic personality, it is usually dealt with under that heading.

Organic damage refers to bodily conditions from which behavior disorders result. Several kinds of disorder result from physical damage to the brain caused by accident or illness. Still others come from imbalances in body chemistry or destruction of critical tissue, especially nerve tissue, in other parts of the body. Organic disorders are true mental illnesses, involving both disturbances of functioning and physical disease or damage. In this book, they are discussed chiefly in Chapter 13 ("Body, Mind, and Behavior") along with so-called psychosomatic conditions, though there are some references to organic disorders with a strong genetic component in Chapter 2 and to others in Chapters 11 and 14.

The other three common categories of psychopathology are much more ambiguous and harder to define. Roughly, *psychosis* corresponds to what is commonly called insanity; it refers to behavior patterns which suggest that a person has lost touch, either intellectually or perceptually, with reality. *Neurosis* is applied to less pronounced disorders in which an individual who is otherwise apparently sane persistently behaves in ways inappropriate to his situation or suffers a great deal of anxiety. *Character disorder* is applied to behavior that is clearly disturbed in a person who is neither organically damaged nor surfeited with anxiety and who, in many cases, seems to have been as he is for a very long time.

Psychotics are often identified by dramatic symptoms like delusions and hallucinations, or by less dramatic but equally ominous tendencies to be completely withdrawn emotionally from other people. Common neurotic symptoms include distressing obsessive thought patterns about irrelevant or unnecessarily disturbing things, compulsive behaviors, or unexplained attacks of anxiety. Character disorders, like organic damage, may be revealed by any of these patterns or yet others.

What makes these many disorders difficult to define with any precision is the fact that they are not really mutually exclusive categories. The symptoms of almost any of them may, at one or another time, be seen in people who are thought to belong essentially in another category. This makes it difficult to classify disorders even for purposes of description. Chapter 10 restricts itself to a discussion of conditions which are commonly associated with neurosis, but Chapter 11 discusses both psychoses and character disorders, and Chapter 9, in an effort to describe the learning conditions which help give rise to various disorders, discusses all three.

To confuse matters still more, the nature of a particular disorder is misleading with respect to its origin, and the origins of many such disorders are little understood. *All* psychopathological conditions, by definition, are disorders of functioning, but some of them have an organic basis and some are learned as unfortunate habits; in many instances, it is very difficult to know which are which, and experts commonly dispute whether pathological states can be understood best in terms of the model ordinary physical diseases offer or of that which can be constructed from the study of the learning process. Some of this conflict is reflected in the different approaches to negative abnormalities taken in subsequent chapters.

Historical Notes

The ancients studied positive abnormalities under names like "virtue," "citizenship," and "artistic inspiration," but their concerns with the negative abnormalities now called mental illness were not awfully different from our own. In early Greek civilization, it was generally believed that madness and insanity were supernaturally caused afflictions, as it is probably still more widely believed than confessed even in modern America. Characters in Greek mythology who offended the gods, for example, might be punished with insanity, which could be cured only with the help of a priest who could influence Aesculapius, the god of healing. At temples of Aesculapius, sick people made offerings, fasted, prayed, and awaited the arrival of a divine vision (sometimes aided by a priest disguised as a god, who would appear at night).

Hippocrates (460–377 B.C.E.[1]), who lived during the golden age of Pericles, made the first modern approach to mental illness by insisting that such disorders were caused by natural rather than supernatural events. To those who considered epilepsy a sacred disease, he responded:

> It is not, in my opinion, any more divine or more sacred than other diseases, but has a natural cause, and its supposed divine origin is due to men's inexperience, and to their wonder at its peculiar character. (Veith, 1965, p. 14.)

Hippocrates believed that the origins of mental illness were to be found in abnormal conditions of the brain, a very modern view, but his ideas about what these abnormalities are like were wildly wrong. Aretaeus (30–90 C.E.) and Galen (130–200 C.E.), however, were even more wildly wrong, though they too had organic rather than supernatural theories of mental illness.

Hippocrates also recorded some of the earliest formal descriptions of mental disorders, including psychotic depression, and began the practice of compiling psychiatric case histories, noting symptoms, course of illness, and final outcome. His treatments were no better than the priests', but neither were anybody else's except those of Soranus, 400 years later.

Soranus has been called the forerunner of Pinel, who originated modern methods of psychologically treating mental illness. Soranus was the first to propose humane treatment of severe disorders, such as providing some amount of comfort for the ill. He also made a critical point which receives much attention today, namely that it is important to keep a patient's vocational interests alive during treatment. He recommended, for example, that "a laborer should be engaged in conversation about the cultivation of the fields, and a sailor in discussion of navigation" (Zilboorg and Henry, 1941, p. 83). These humane and commonsensical views of treatment were rare after Soranus almost until today.

Galen (130–200) was the last important physician of classical civilization to write about mental illness. He contributed little new in the way of descriptions or suggested new treatments, but he was particularly knowledgeable about what we would today call psychosomatic disturbances, and he accomplished the feat of collecting and summarizing the bulk of medical knowledge existing in his time. After him the world entered a twilight which is commonly called the Dark Ages.

During the first two or three hundred years of the Christian era, the writings

[1] The abbreviations C.E. and B.C.E. represent *Common Era* and *Before the Common Era.*

of early Greek and Roman scholars fell into disrepute. The Christian church, growing in power and strength at that time, encouraged this process. When Christianity was established as the state religion of Rome in 313, for example, the study of Plato and Aristotle was banned. Christian scholars such as St. Basil and St. Jerome asserted that classical writings were pagan and heretical. One consequence of these events was that the works of earlier Greek and Roman physicians, such as Hippocrates and Soranus, were no longer read, and the belief that insanity should be the concern of the medical profession rather than of religion was discredited. The responsibility for interpreting and treating mental illness was almost completely transferred from physicians to theologians and monks. When Michael Psellus wrote his encyclopedia in the eleventh century, the section on mental illness was entirely devoted to a "detailed account of the hierarchy of demons who are troubling and vitiating the functioning of the human soul" (Zilboorg and Henry, 1941, p. 116). Nowhere in Psellus' work was there an account of early Greek and Roman writings on this subject.

As it became widely accepted that mental illness was caused by evil spirits, Christian monks gradually took over the care of disturbed people. Several monasteries functioned as early mental hospitals. At first, the monks relied mainly on exorcisms to heal mental disorders. They recited prayers and incantations over the patient with the aim of scaring away the demons. Later, however, exorcisms were supplanted by much harsher methods, namely, torture and burning at the stake. Ostensibly directed at fighting witchcraft, these methods were applied to large numbers of the mentally ill and to others who showed any kind of behavior deviations from the majority of people. The manual in widest use for identifying witches was the work of two Dominican monks, Johann Sprenger and Heinrich Kraemer, who were both members of the Inquisition; it was called *Malleus maleficarum*, the "witches' hammer" (1494).

From the intellectual vantage point of either the twentieth century or classical times, the attitudes and teachings of the Middle Ages with regard to mental illness are simply incomprehensible. They appear to reflect a complete abandonment of concern with the nature of reality, the kind of concern that was so apparent in the work of Aristotle, Hippocrates, and Galen. In the Middle Ages, nothing is unknown; the answers to all questions—physical, theological, and psychological—are derived from what is already believed to be true.

Hysteria, like other dramatic forms of neurosis, is seen as the workings of devils and demons, *incubi* and *succubi*, witches and their curses. The origins of these ideas reach into the Old and New Testaments: "A man, also a woman, that hath a familiar spirit, or that is a wizard, shall surely be put to death. They shall stone them with stones. Their blood shall be upon them" (Lev. 20:27). They were amplified and exemplified by Christian scholars. Augustine's belief in the existence of demons, his tales of miraculous cure, his damnation of lust and sensual pleasure, and his belief in magic and magicians were major authority for later writers, who expanded and expounded upon his work, amplifying his concerns and suggesting new remedies based on his.

Although almost everybody believed in the power of witches during this period, a few softly dissented. One of these, Johann Weyer (1515–1588), had little influence during his life but became influential more than a century after he died. Weyer attempted to make mental illness once more the concern of the physician. His major work, *De Praestigiis*

Daemonum, was written when witch burning was at its peak. In it, he insisted that the great majority of "witches" were sick, innocent people who needed medical treatment. Their confessions should be considered symptoms of mental disturbance, he maintained, and not be taken literally.

Although with the advent of the eighteenth century, the mentally ill were no longer tortured or burned at the stake, neither were they given adequate care or treatment. Frequently they were simply thrown out by their families and left to wander through the countryside. This way of life, however, was often more beneficial than the treatment they received in institutions designed to house them, such as Bethlehem hospital in London (from which the word *bedlam* comes) and Bicêtre in Paris. The major function of these institutions was to remove the mentally ill from the rest of society, not to help or cure them. Only a few humane institutions for the mentally ill existed anywhere, and only the very wealthy could afford them.

The reformation of mental institutions in France was begun by Philippe Pinel (1745–1826). Although many in France had spoken out against the miserable conditions in these institutions, only Pinel actually did something about them. After becoming chief physician, first of Bicêtre, then of Salpêtrière, he removed the chains from the inmates, noting the reactions of the patients as he went along. Some were soon well enough to be discharged. Some who had been quite violent became calm and relaxed after they were freed, suggesting that their violence was not so much a part of their illness as a reaction to cruel treatment.

In addition to Pinel, two other individuals were prominent in the fight to improve conditions in mental hospitals. These were William Tuke (1732–1822), a Quaker merchant in England, and Dorothea Dix (1802–1887), an American schoolteacher.

Hippocrates' custom of taking the patient's history was reintroduced by Pinel, and the observation involved gave rise once again to description and classification of mental illnesses. Eventually, descriptions and classifications which have stood the test of time were devised. During the nineteenth century, general paresis, a neurological disorder resulting from syphilis, was described and differentiated from other mental disorders by Fournier (1857–1914) and Krafft-Ebing (1840–1902). The mental and neurological psychosis that can result from chronic alcoholism was outlined by Korsakov (1854–1900) by the end of the nineteenth century. At about the same time, German psychiatrists described the symptoms of what we know today as "paranoia," "catatonia," and "hebephrenia," all psychoses.

Rather than describe new disease entities, Kraepelin (1856–1926) grouped previously identified syndromes into two major categories: (1) dementia praecox, "characterized by symptoms found in catatonia and hebephrenia and also . . . auditory hallucinations and perhaps persecutory trends" (Zilboorg and Henry, 1941, p. 456); and (2) manic-depressive psychosis. These categories were based on the evidence of an impressive amount of data from thousands of case histories covering not only the course of the illness, but also the patient's background and a follow-up report on his activities after leaving the hospital. Kraepelin's categories remain the major basis for classification of mental disorders.

Scientists of the eighteenth and nineteenth centuries continued the search for organic causes of mental illness. Morel (1807–1873), a French psychiatrist, proposed the following possible organic causes: heredity; toxins (such as alcohol, narcotics, metal poisoning); and primary brain disease, which resulted in disorders called "sympathies." Maudsley (1835–1918), a British psychiatrist, added several factors to Morel's list: anemia, circulatory defects, and infections. The German psychiatrist, Greisinger (1817–1868), stressed only one variable as a major cause of mental disorders, namely, brain pathology. Occasionally, psychological factors like disappointment in love, financial worries, and overwork were suggested as causative variables. The search for organic causes bore fruit with the discovery of general paresis, Korsakov's psychosis, and certain abnormalities of the brain clearly associated with senile psychosis.

The importance of psychological factors in mental illness was emphasized, toward the end of the last century, by the work of Charcot (1825–1893), who was able to remove many symptoms of hysteria by hypnotic suggestion. Furthermore, through hypnosis, he could induce the patient to adopt new symptoms. Thus, the specific symptoms of hysteria were found to be maneuverable by suggestion, indicating that they were not caused by local bodily injury. Nevertheless, Charcot thought that hysteria resulted from some organic disorder which he was unable to identify.

Pierre Janet (1859–1947), a student of Charcot, developed a new and original way of understanding hysteria as a disorder resulting from the dissociation (separation) of an idea system from the rest of the personality. Without the restraining influence of other elements in the personality, a dissociated idea system could receive direct, physical expression in the form of an hysterical symptom. Janet believed that dissociation could be traced to hereditary weakness in the capacity to organize experience.

An alternative theory explaining why some ideas become dissociated and buried from the rest of the personality was offered soon afterwards by Sigmund Freud (1856–1939). According to Freud, ideas and memories are not separated off because of some neurological weakness, but are actively buried from awareness (repressed) by certain powerful forces within the personality because they are associated with painful conflicts. In addition to a theory about the formation of hysterical symptoms, Freud, with his early associate Breuer (1842–1925), also proposed new methods of treating hysteria. These methods eventuated in the development of free-association techniques and psychoanalysis (see Chapter 15).

At around the same time, Ivan Pavlov (1849–1936), who had just won the Nobel prize in physiology and medicine (1904) for his work on the digestive system, was completing the first of a series of brilliant experiments in Russia from which an important technology of mental treatment was gradually to arise in competition with psychoanalysis (see Chapter 15).

It is obvious that the negative abnormalities, especially mental illness and related disorders, have received a great deal of attention during much of history. But it is only in very modern times that significant strides have been taken toward scientifically understanding these problems or doing effective work to resolve them. And to this day, relatively little, by comparison with almost any physical disorder, is known of them, even relatively little about how they ought to be studied and researched. Thus, even though negative abnormalities have been studied much more than positive ones, they require much more study in their own right, for there is a great deal to do before they will be truly understood and controlled.

Mental Health, Mental Illness, and Magical Thinking

The study of negative abnormalities at this time in history must inevitably involve the student in a thoroughly confusing disputation which has increasingly preoccupied psychologists, psychiatrists, and other users of behavior science since midcentury. It is the problem of whether mental illness is really illness of a kind that needs medical treatment or whether it is a reflection of peculiarities in a person's learning experiences that requires something more like education for its relief. In some respects, this is a foolish argument: as we have intimated in the previous section, some disorders arise from organic problems and others seem to have their basis in learning disabilities, and as we shall see repeatedly from Chapter 2 on, some problems can be treated best by medical or surgical means and others by psychological and educational methods; there are still others for which no effective treatment is yet known. The statistical concept of normality used in this book comprehends all these conditions.

On the other hand, there has long been a tradition, particularly in psychiatric medicine, that mental illness is simply a special case of infectious disease, and this point of view is explicitly or implicitly rejected by all the contributors to this book. Though some infectious diseases produce profound behavior aberrations, it is not a corollary that most behavior aberrations result from infections. Conditions like neuroses, character disorders, and probably psychoses are particularly unlikely to arise from infectious processes. Is it, then, reasonable to regard functional behavior deviations as illnesses? If so, perhaps we should also consider criminals mentally ill, since their behavior deviates quite sharply from most peoples'. If not, and we cannot consider behavioral deviates mentally ill, then what do terms like "mental health" and "mental illness" really mean? Perhaps they are altogether meaningless as we commonly use them, and perhaps their use even distorts our perceptions of the true conditions we mistakenly call by these names.

This notion has been brought to professional attention most forcibly by a psychoanalyst, Thomas Szasz (1961). Critiques, based largely on his work, of the so-called medical model of mental illness are presented in some detail in Chapters 5 and 9. Chapter 16 concerns itself at length with the problems of defining what can be usefully incorporated within the concepts that we clumsily and in part erroneously label "mental health" and "mental illness." Meanwhile, it is important to realize that the concepts have some meaning even if the current terminology is poor. *Mental illness* is not like smallpox or polio, and perhaps a term like "behavior disorders" or "deviations" would be more precise. But such terms have their own inaccuracies. In any case, it is more important to recognize and understand the aggregate of human miseries that are subsumed by any of these terms than to ruminate endlessly on the inadequacies of the labels.

By the same token, "mental health" is also an ambiguous label, just as the entire concept, *health*, is ambiguous, implying both "the absence of illness" and "the presence of a state of well-being." Unfortunately, we have no adequate terminology for describing the conditions which concern us in this book. But this is not a crippling disability; an understanding of the subject matter should not be hindered by the sometimes obsolete medical language which has been handed down to psychiatry from Hippocrates to Freud.

DETERMINANTS OF INDIVIDUAL BEHAVIOR

Whether a particular behavior trait is evaluated positively or negatively with respect to individual or social functioning, and regardless of where it falls on the scale of statistical normality, the same classes of events can be said to underlie or determine its development. Some of these determinants of behavior are biological; others are the results of educational processes, formal or informal, which the individual absorbs directly through interactions with other people or indirectly through communications media. Still other determinants of behavior belong to the immediate situation in which the individual finds himself.

Biological Determinants

Biological determinants of behavior fall into two general classes: (1) genetic and physiological variables, and (2) parental influences. A considerable number of negative abnormalities result more or less directly from genetic and physiological events; an example is phenylketonuria, a type of mental retardation. Also included in this category are congenital physical disorders which may have pronounced influence on the development of behavior, such as neonatal blindness or deafness and other debilities that occur in embryos because of maternal illness or drug-induced conditions. By the same token, severe illness in infancy or childhood may be taken as a physiological determinant of behavior patterns, subject to the rule of thumb that the earlier such events occur, the more serious their potential consequences.

Discussions of genetic determinants of behavior often focus upon unfortunate genetic events. But the pendulum swings in both directions. Very high intelligence may be as genetically determined as mental deficiency. The ordinary events of development are no freer of genetic and physiological influences than the extraordinary ones. Physical appearance, energy level, and even some aspects of mood and disposition, called temperament, are relatively direct expressions of such influences. Many details of the implications of genetics for behavior are discussed in Chapter 2, and physiological bases for behavior disorders constitute the main subject matter of Chapter 13.

Parental influence is not usually considered a biological determinant of behavior, but from an evolutionary viewpoint, the extensive period of helplessness which human infants undergo by comparison with other animals throws on the parents the biological goal of sustaining life and fostering the best (or worst) conditions of development. There is some reason to believe, moreover, that nursing patterns have a critical effect on the development of such unlikely things as intelligence (Ribble, 1943), alertness (Spitz, 1945), and later tendencies to become anxious or maintain equanimity in trying situations (Sullivan, 1953). Influences of child-rearing patterns are discussed chiefly in Chapters 4, 8, 9, and 10.

Psychodynamics

Learned determinants of behavior are often called "psychodynamic" because they refer not to stable events, such as genetic and some physiological ones, but to the constantly shifting patterns of interaction between an individual and others which result in his learning to react to such patterns of stimulation with particular patterns of response. For most purposes, the most critical sources of learning are other individuals—in early life, parents and siblings, and in later childhood and after, peers, mentors, and other members of society. Chapters 3 and 4 discuss the dynamic bases of behavior.

Situational Determinants

The combination of physiological and psychodynamic determinants, each with its own tremendous potentiality for variability, helps explain why there are such vast individual differences in the behavior of different people. But a very large part of behavior is determined by the interaction of the individual's established patterns and characteristics with the unusual or unique circumstances which immediate situations confront him with. The variety of situational determinants that influence behavior is so great that, taken with the variety of established behavior patterns, it is often impossible to assess personality and make very dependable statements about different types of people or their characteristic behaviors, even when reliable typologies can be found. These difficulties become most apparent in connection with negative abnormalities, as indicated in Chapters 9, 11, and 16.

The upshot of all this is not that it is impossible to understand human behavior, but rather that there may be severe limits to how well the behavior of any single individual or even type of person can be predicted. Even so, it will help understanding greatly to try to approach those limits, and this cannot be done unless the main determinants of behavior patterns can be understood. The remainder of this section discusses some of the critical determinants of individual behavior that underlie both the positive and the negative abnormalities which occupy the rest of this book.

SUMMARY

Normality is used casually by most of us to describe how acceptable our behavior is to ourselves and others, either in terms of its *conformity* to expectations, its *consistency*, or its *morality*. In this book, the word is used more precisely to mean the correspondence of an individual's behavior to that of others or its consistency over time, without implying that either conformity or deviation is inherently desirable. The concept of normality, as used here, refers to the *statistical* notion of the *normal distribution*, which is based mathematically on the expansion of the binomial distribution and takes the graphic form of a bell-shaped curve. From the point of view of this formulation, *abnormality* means relative rareness, which, in psychology, refers to the deviation of an individual's behavior from that of others or from his own accustomed patterns. It is the behavioral characteristic, or trait, which is abnormal, not the person. Also, from the perspective of social desirability, some abnormalities are positive, like high intelligence, good character, and creative genius, while others are negative, like neuroses, psychoses, and mental retardation. There is no technical term for the positive abnormalities, but many of the negative ones are referred to as *psychopathology* or *mental illness*.

There are two fundamental methods of assessing behavior traits. The first, the *normative* method, involves studying many different people to see how much a given trait pertains to each one; it is concerned with the individual differences among people. The second, the *ipsative* method, involves studying a single individual over a long period of time to examine the patterns and variations in his behavior. Ipsative methods tend to be most useful for studying very complicated behavior, and normative ones for studying simpler and more stable kinds of behavior.

There are also two kinds of standards commonly used to evaluate behavior, the *functional* and the *evaluative*. The former are generally used for judging scientific work; in connection with human behavior, they can only examine how well a person's behavior serves his goals, not whether his behavior is good or evil, which is the province of evaluative criteria.

Positive abnormalities characteristically help a person to function more effectively and, in so doing, permit him to contribute beneficially to the welfare of society. The traits considered positive abnormalities vary with cultural setting. In classical antiquity, good citizenship was an ideal of behavior, whereas in the Judeo-Christian tradition, intellectual and ethical accomplishments were exalted above good citizenship. Modern studies of positive abnormality may be said to begin in 1880 with Sir Francis Galton's investigation of genius and the work of Lewis Terman on intelligence. In general, the positive abnormalities have received less attention than the negative ones.

Negative abnormalities characteristically involve both social and personal disabilities and often much personal anguish as well. The major categories of disorder under this heading are (1) organic damage, (2) psychoses, (3) neuroses, (4) character disorders, including antisocial behavior, and (5) mental retardation. These categories are somewhat ambiguous and overlapping, so that symptoms of one disorder often occur along with symptoms of another. Formal study of negative abnormalities began as early as Hippocrates, but modern treatment of mental illness really began with Pinel in the late eighteenth century, and modern psychiatry with Kraepelin in the middle of the nineteenth.

Two different directions have developed in modern psychiatry: one seeks the roots of behavior disorders in organic processes, and the other in psychological ones. Partly as a result of these differences, modern students of behavior disorders are not sure to what extent it is reasonable to describe them in terms of a medical model of illness or a psychological model of peculiarities of learning experience. There is no clear resolution of this problem. Some conditions reflect roots primarily in organic disturbances and others more clearly in the social learning history of the individual.

GLOSSARY

Abnormal—generally, unexpected, extraordinary, or unusual; technically, deviating from the average; colloquially, unconventional, inconsistent or uncontrolled, immoral or falling short of the ideal, erratic, bizarre, or otherwise undesirable (especially behavior).

Binomial expansion—an algebraic expression of the sum of two terms raised to any power; the algebraic approximation of the normal curve.

Catatonia—a behavior disorder characterized by either general inhibition of overt response or excessive motor activity and excitement.

Congenital physical disorder—disability present in an individual at birth, possibly but not necessarily innate.

Continuity; continuous distribution—uninterrupted succession, connection, or relation of events: time is continuous.

Dementia praecox—obsolescent term for schizophrenia.

General paresis—a neurological disorder resulting from syphilis.

Ipsative method—a method of measuring traits which uses the individual's own behavior as the standard of comparison (see *normative method* for comparison).

Negative abnormalities—traits which have characteristically negative effects on personal and social functioning.

Neurosis—an ill-defined personality disorder that is less disabling than psychosis (see Chapter 10).

Normal—generally, expected, routine, or ordinary; in statistics, following a frequency distribution characterized by the large central portion of a bell-shaped curve; moralistically, acceptable; psychosocially, "invisible" (see Chapter 5).

Normative method—a method of measuring traits which uses the behavior of known groups of people as the standard of comparison (see *ipsative method* for comparison).

Organic damage—impairment of function due to impairment of physiological structure; physiological conditions from which behavior disorders result.

Phenylketonuria—a type of hereditary mental retardation.

Positive abnormalities—behavior characteristics which enable an individual to function much more effectively and to contribute more to the welfare of society than the "average" man.

PROBABILITY—the likelihood that an event will occur.

PSYCHOSOMATIC DISTURBANCE—persistent physiological symptoms or impairments that originate in psychological distress.

SENILE PSYCHOSIS—a chronic severe disorder of the aged manifested by bizarre behavior and thinking with accompanying impairment of brain tissue.

SYNDROME—a pattern of symptoms.

REFERENCES

Allport, G. W. *Personality: A psychological interpretation*. New York: Holt, Rinehart & Winston, 1937.

Binet, A., and T. Simon. Methodes nouvelles pour le diagnostic du niveau intellectual des anormaux. *Année psychologique*, 1905, **11,** 191–224.

Galton, F. *Hereditary genius*. New York: D. Appleton & Company, 1880. (Originally published 1869.)

———. *Inquiries into human faculty and its development*. London: Macmillan & Co., Ltd., 1883.

Ribble, Margaretha A. *The rights of infants*. New York: Columbia University Press, 1943.

Spitz, R. A. Hospitalism: An inquiry into the genesis of psychiatric conditions in early childhood. *Psychoanalytic Study of the Child*, 1945, **1,** 53–74.

Sullivan, H. S. *The interpersonal theory of psychiatry*. New York: W. W. Norton & Company, Inc., 1953.

Szasz, T. *The myth of mental illness*. New York: Harper & Row Publishers, 1961.

Terman, L. M. *The measurement of intelligence*. Boston: Houghton Mifflin Company, 1916.

Veith, Ilza. *Hysteria: The history of a disease*. Chicago: University of Chicago Press, 1965.

Zilboorg, G., and G. W. Henry. *A history of medical psychology*. New York: W. W. Norton & Company, Inc., 1941.

SUGGESTED READINGS

The question of what constitutes normality and what abnormality is still a matter of intense debate among psychologists and psychiatrists. Many definitions have been offered, but none seems yet to have captured the consensus of professionals working on these matters. Many of these theories fuse normality with mental health and, consequently, abnormality with mental illness. The result is an idealized notion of normality that we have tried to avoid, but that the student may want to familiarize himself with. Some of the issues are taken up in the following books:

1. Jahoda, M. *Current concepts of positive mental health*. New York: Basic Books, Inc., 1959. One of the important volumes that emerged from the considerations of the Joint Commission on Mental Health and Illness.
2. London, P. *The modes and morals of psychotherapy*. New York: Holt, Rinehart & Winston, 1964. An analysis of both statistical and "dynamic" theories of normality.
3. Offer, D., and M. Sabshin. *Normality: Theoretical and clinical concepts*. New York: Basic Books, Inc., 1966. An integrated survey of opinion on mental health.
4. Szasz, T. *The myth of mental illness*. New York: Harper & Row, Publishers, 1961. A vigorous attack on the entire notion of mental illness and, implicitly, on our conceptions of normality.

Studies of positive abnormalities are, as we have noted, less frequent than those of negative abnormality. Interesting volumes that consider the former are:

1. Galton, F. *Inquiries into human faculty and its development*. London: Macmillan & Co., Ltd., 1883.
2. Terman, L., *et al. Mental and physical traits of a thousand gifted children*. Stanford, Calif.: Stanford University Press, 1925.
3. Terman, L. M., and Melita H. Oden. *The gifted child grows up*. Stanford, Calif.: Stanford University Press, 1947.

Several works are concerned with one or another aspect of the history of negative abnormality. Among these are:

1. Dain, N. *Concepts of insanity in the United States: 1789–1865*. New Brunswick, N.J.: Rutgers University Press, 1964.
2. Veith, Ilza. *Hysteria: The history of a disease*. Chicago: University of Chicago Press, 1965.
3. Zilboorg, G., and G. W. Henry. A *history of medical psychology*. New York: W. W. Norton & Company, Inc., 1941.

2

Behavior Genetics

JERRY HIRSCH

ROY C. HOSTETTER

Behavior genetics is by no means a new area of interest in the study of human behavior or of abnormal psychology, although recently interest in it is greater than at any previous time. The importance of animal genetics and the practical uses to which knowledge of it can be put have been apparent almost since the beginning of civilization, long before any formal knowledge of the subject existed. For as long as man has been domesticating animals, he has been using one of the methods of behavior genetics—selective breeding. He needed no knowledge of biology to learn to protect animals he could live with safely, and their offspring, and to kill wild and dangerous animals. The maintenance and breeding throughout many generations of animals suitable to man's needs led to the development of domesticated breeds of dogs, cats, and other pets and, more importantly, to the breeds of animals that supply our meat today. These animal species are still selectively bred. Dog and cattle breeders maintain elaborate pedigrees which contain a wealth of information not only about the physical characteristics of each animal and its family, but also about their performance.

THE SCIENCE OF GENETICS AND THE STUDY OF BEHAVIOR

Behavior genetics can be defined as the study of the genetic aspects of behavior variations. Individuals of every species differ in behavior from each other as well as from members of other species. Some of these differences are the result of experience in the environment, which always differs somewhat from one individual to another, even in the same family. But many individual differences are the result of differences in genetic structure, and behavior genetics is concerned with discovering which are which. More precisely, behavior genetics seeks to identify the genetic correlates of behavior and how they operate, leaving the effect of experience on behavior to the student of behavior dynamics and development (Chapters 3 and 4).

Behavior genetics uses methods developed in genetic investigations of lower organisms—some a lot lower, like fruit flies, and some as advanced as cattle. Major differences between human behavior genetics and the behavior genetics of lower organisms are (1) the difficulty of controlling human breeding and (2) the difficulty of classifying human behavioral traits into mutually exclusive categories. The basic principles of genetics must therefore be drawn largely from animal genetics, but the same principles apply to human behavior genetics.

The Darwinian Revolution

Much of the history of man's reflections about himself in relation to the other animals has been dominated by the idea that there are unlimited qualitative differences between his mental functions and those of animals. It is no surprise that this was believed in Western classical antiquity; Plato and Aristotle were not altogether convinced that *women* had souls, let alone dogs, cattle, and swine. As recently as the seventeenth century, Descartes (1596–1650) wrote that animals were automata, devoid of a soul, and this belief was supported by the Church. In 1859, however, Darwin's theory of evolution raised doubts in the scientific community that all the previously assumed differences between man and the lower animals were real. The implication of Darwin's theory was that man and the lower animals differed only by virtue of having taken different evolutionary paths, more or less by accident, from similar ancestries. This idea was carried further in *The Expression of Emotion in Man and Animals* (1872), where Darwin tried to show that many human facial expressions of emotion were homologous to those shown by animals in times of stress. The idea that man and other animals possess a common ancestor in the ancient past is at odds with church dogma that each living thing was the object of a special creation. For this reason, the theory of evolution is still opposed by some churches.

The theory holds essentially that (1) more individuals are born than can reach reproductive age; (2) in each generation there is heritable variation among members of a species; (3) individuals whose heritable variations allow them to adapt better to their environment produce more offspring that grow to maturity; and thus (4) a species that is well adapted to the environment is propagated. As this process continues over many generations, different organisms become adapted to different aspects of the environment. Then, as the environmental conditions themselves change, the organisms best adapted to them become accordingly different (see Figure 2.1). When enough differences have accumulated between two groups of organisms to prevent breeding between them, a new *species* has been formed. In the case of man and the great apes, for example, the theory would suggest that sometime in the ancient past some organism existed which was capable of evolving into two *genera* (groups of species), the apes and man. The idea that man and the animals are part of the same biological system makes it seem plausible that the relations found among biological structures and behaviors across many different animal species might have some application to the study of similar relations among men.

One of the first areas in which the theory of evolution had a pronounced effect was the study of the inheritance of human abilities. Galton's study of the familial relationships of eminent men (see Chapter 1) may be considered the first modern research in human behavior genetics. One of the outstanding biologists

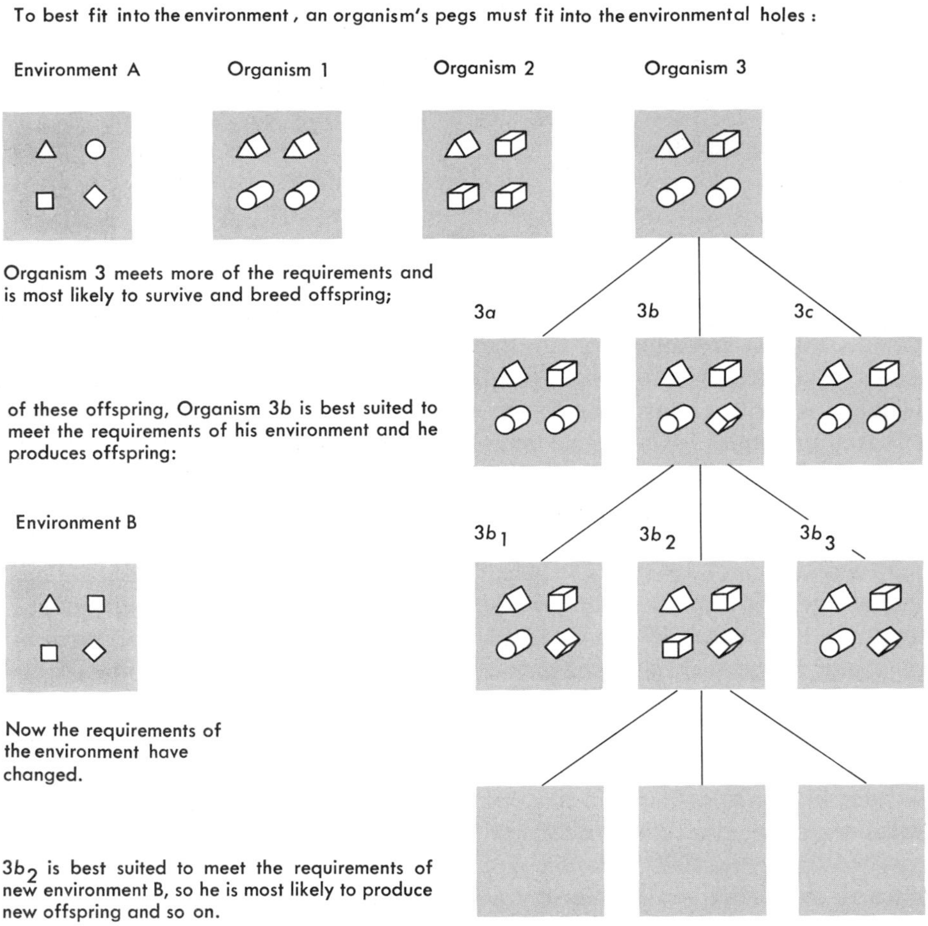

Figure 2.1 Evolution.

of the nineteenth century, Galton (1822–1911) was a firm believer in the dominance of nature over nurture. In 1869 he wrote:

> The instincts and faculties of different men and races differ in a variety of ways almost as profoundly as those of animals in different cages of the Zoological Gardens.

His investigations of genius showed that intellectual superiority tended to run in families. Of course, this classic study suffers from the same chief shortcoming that still besets genetic studies—the inability to separate the influences of a common heredity from those of a common environment—but its conclusions nevertheless seem to hold to this day.

Galton was criticized because he could not rule out the possibility that men were eminent because they came from superior social and cultural environments rather than because they were the heirs of a favorable biology. He had several answers to this criticism: (1) In America, where education was available to all (he thought), there were not a large number of superior individuals, as one would expect to find if environmental conditions alone could produce superior intelligence. (2) Some of the eminent men he studied came from impoverished homes, but inherited abilities allowed them to rise above environment. (3) The relatives of the Pope, who were accorded all the social advantages, were not uniformly superior individuals. How to separate the effects of environment from those of heredity has been one of the biggest problems in investigating genetic correlates of human abilities. Some research techniques for handling this problem are discussed below under "Research in Human Genetics."

The profound impression Darwin's theory made on the scientific world was presently accentuated by the recognition that very little was known about actual biological processes and mechanisms of inheritance. Two principal questions are to be answered in this connection: *What* gets transmitted from one generation to the next, and *how* does the transmission occur? The most popular answers in the nineteenth century, one attributed to Lamarck (1809) and the other to Darwin himself, were both wrong.

Lamarck is generally considered the proponent of the theory of the inheritance of acquired characteristics, although many pre-Mendelian biologists held some version of it. In essence, it states that, as an organism strives to overcome obstacles in its environment, physical changes occur in its structure, and the changes thus acquired are passed on to its offspring. To Lamarck's credit is the fact that this was the first self-consistent theory of evolution which derived man from animal ancestors; it was only his mechanisms for explaining evolution that turned out to be wrong. He believed that the environment directly altered heredity, so that bodily changes that were responses to environmental contingencies passed directly to the next generation even though it did not undergo the same life experience.

Darwin believed that Lamarck was generally correct and tried to understand how the transmission occurred, since he believed the only direct communication from one generation to the next to be through the sex cells. Only 150 years earlier it had been thought that a homunculus (little man) containing all the cells of an offspring was preformed in the sex cells of the parent, but this theory had long been discredited. The substitute theory Darwin proposed was called "pangenesis." It alleged that each cell in the body contained a small copy of itself called a "gemmule." In adulthood, the cells discharged these gemmules, which passed through the body into the gonads, where they were transformed into sex cells. Later they were retransformed into new body cells, which changed as the new offspring developed, and as gemmules were in turn passed on to the gonads.

Before the end of the nineteenth century, Weismann was able to demonstrate more or less conclusively that Lamarck was wrong and to provide a reasonable explanation, also wrong, of why acquired characters were not inherited. Lamarck's theory is so plausible on the face of it, however, that it is still popularly believed in many places. In fact, Lysenko, recapitulating Darwin without acknowledging him, made the theory the "official truth" of Soviet biology in 1950.

The actual facts were already available, while Darwin was still working on pangenesis, in the then unknown writings of an Austrian monk named Gregor Mendel, whose hobby was breeding pea plants. Mendel published two papers on the morphological (structural) character of pea plants in 1866 and 1869, but their importance did not become apparent until his work was rediscovered at the beginning of this century. His interpretations of the results of his experiments in crossbreeding set the stage for the full development of the field of genetics as it is now known, and indeed they are valid to this day.

The two "laws" attributed to Mendel, "segregation" and "independent assortment," are still the basic laws of genetics; they are described in detail later in this chapter. Mendel proposed that each genetic factor is represented twice in an individual's hereditary complement. One representation comes from each parent. The important difference between the Mendelian idea and those current when his work was rediscovered was his demonstration that each genetic factor was a distinct particle which always maintained its integrity, remaining whole within the organism, and which could be recovered in unaltered form in the next generation. The theory that preceded Mendel's "particulate theory" was the "blending theory" of heredity which proposed a chemical fusion of hereditary materials in the progeny instead of a transitional mixture of the genetic elements contributed by each parent. The idea of blending probably arose because the traits studied were of a continuous nature; that is, like height or intelligence they existed in degrees or amounts which were distributed continuously in the population (see the discussion of probability in Chapter 1). When individuals with different degrees of expression of such traits mated, the offspring often appeared to be intermediate with respect to these traits between the parental values. It thus appeared as if the hereditary elements had blended to produce some intermediate expression of the trait. Mendel, on the other hand, restricted his work to traits that had discrete distributions, that is, traits that could be assigned to only one of two possible phenotypic (observable) categories, like the color of pea plant blossoms.

After the rediscovery of Mendel's papers, the biologists who accepted the particulate theory disagreed with those who continued to support the blending theory. The particulate theory was strongly supported when advances in cytology (the study of cells) made it possible to observe bodies (chromosomes) in the cell nucleus that obeyed Mendelian principles. As we will see later, genetics today is concerned with both discrete and continuous characters, because it is possible now to understand how heritable characters that are continuously distributed can result from several genetic factors that, individually, obey the basic Mendelian laws.

These two important developments—Darwin's theory of evolution and Mendel's pea plant experiments—have been the basis of many important developments of modern biology. Our understanding of the biological processes underlying genetics is still not complete, but it is growing with enormous speed. We are on the threshold of dramatic breakthroughs. In very recent years, Watson, Crick, and Wilkins won a Nobel prize for their work on the structure of genetic elements, and more recently, Jacob, Monod, and Lwoff were awarded a Nobel prize for their work on the functional properties of genetic material. Much has been learned about the chemical nature of hereditary material since 1944, when O. T. Avery and his colleagues studied the properties of DNA (deoxyribonucleic acid), and now man is coming very close to unlocking the secrets of life as a result of research in genetics.

Early Issues

The study of psychology and of many more critical and immediate aspects of the conduct of human affairs, like race relations and politics, has been clouded for a long time by a misunderstanding of heredity. Before considering the details of the genetic process or its relevance to either positive or negative abnormality, therefore, it is important to clarify the issues in the principal debate on which genetics bears, namely the conflict between *heredity* and *environment* as the controlling factor in human personality, or what Galton called *nature* versus *nurture*.

Since the seventeenth century our ideas about individual development have been largely dominated by the *tabula rasa* (empty slate) theory of John Locke (1632–1704), which asserts that infants come into the world free of instincts and inclinations of any kind, so that their eventual development into one or another kind of adult depends only on their life experiences or interactions with the environment. From Locke's point of view—and that of the Associationist (or Fourierist) philosophers, who heavily influenced the thinking of America's founding fathers—all men are created equal in a biological as well as a political sense, so that there is no possible justification for one group of men to dominate another by virtue of an inherent superiority. This "environmentalist thesis" has been a keystone of modern political democracy, and the alternative notion that some men are inherently superior has been embraced chiefly by those who wished to enslave and subdue others. In modern times, the latter position was formulated most cogently by the French historian Comte de Gobineau in his *Essay on the Inequality of Human Races* (1855). Gobineau argued that all mankind's achievements have come from various branches of the Nordic races of Northern Europe, to which he by chance belonged; these races dominated the classical civilizations of Greece, Egypt, and China until miscegenation between themselves and their subjects (perhaps the only flaw in the Nordic character) led to the decline of their domains. This thesis reached its insane culmination in the murder of millions of innocent "inferior" people in Germany under Hitler. More politely expressed, it has also been an important basis for the oppression of colonial peoples throughout the world and for the subjugation of America's Negro population.

It is easy to see why conscientious students of human behavior, especially if they are decent people, must be wary of accepting hereditarian theses lightly when history demonstrates so clearly how easily they can be used to subvert human rights. The truth should not be overlooked either, however, and the truth is that *both* organic structures (inherited) and the contingencies of life experiences (environment) together determine the course of individual behavior.

Genotype and Phenotype

The biological inheritance of every person consists of genes, and the totality of the genes is the *genotype*. To designate the sum total of the observable characteristics of an individual, Johannsen (1903) proposed the term *phenotype*. The phenotype changes with time as a result of experience, whereas the genotype does not change. An organism's appearance and behavior are both aspects of its phenotype. *The phenotype is not inherited*; it can only develop as life goes on. The genotype interacts with the environment, and the outcome is the process of development, through which the phenotype of an individual is manifested. The phenotype is determined by the genotype and its interaction with the environment. There is no organism without a genotype, and no genotype can exist without an environment (Dobzhansky, 1962).

In the relationship between heredity and environment, heredity (the genotype) sets the limits of possible development, and environment determines the extent of actual development (the phenotype) within those limits. It is misleading, therefore, to generalize about the effects either of environment or of heredity, for neither one really has an independent existence. It is largely because of our political experience that we are tempted, when individual differences are observed, to explain them only by differences in developmental environment. Differences between environments, however, can only be evaluated for one genotype at a time. Therefore, we now think about the heredity-environment relationship in terms of the *norm of reaction*. Each unique genotype has its own distinctive norm of reaction, that is, a range of phenotypes it can produce in different environments. Because different genotypes often produce different phenotypes in the *same* environment, we cannot generalize easily about the effects of any particular environment. The differences we observe about people are phenotypic differences. They may result more from genetic or more from environmental influences or from the equal interaction of both, but they are never the exclusive product of either one.

Environmentalists and hereditarians still hotly debate the nature-nurture issue, and extreme positions are still maintained by both sides, but the dichotomy between environmental and genetic traits is as invalid as the division of men into inferior and superior races: the debate is meaningless. What we want to know are the relative magnitudes of the genetic and environmental components in the observed variations of a given trait. The problem is one of measurement (Dobzhansky, 1962).

It first became evident when people analyzed Galton's research that the problem is not an easy one to solve, especially when we are concerned with human abilities rather than those of other animals. Early in this century, influential studies on the hereditary nature of feeble-mindedness were made by H. H. Goddard and A. H. Estabrook. These were the case histories of the "Jukes" and the "Kallikak" families, whose abilities were at the lower and less desirable end of the scale from those Galton studied. The Jukes family was traceable back to five sisters, whose descendants after 130 years numbered 1258 living people, all of whom Estabrook (1916) reported to be social misfits of one kind or another. He did not assign primary causation to either heredity or environment, however, but, quite modern in viewpoint, indicated that both environment and heredity had some part in determining these personality types.

Goddard (1912) made a stronger case for hereditary determination of social undesirability in his report on the two Kallikak families. He traced both back to one man, whom he called Martin Kallikak (Greek for "good-bad"). As an Army officer during the Revolutionary War, Kallikak had an affair with a feebleminded barmaid who consequently gave birth to a son, after whom came a family of social misfits which included 480 descendants very much like the Jukes family. When Kallikak returned home from the war, he married a "normal," upper-class girl and sired a family of average and superior individuals. Both families were begun by the same wealthy man, and the social misfits occurred only among the descendants of the impoverished feebleminded girl, but Goddard concluded that inheritance of feeblemindedness, not of social deprivation, was responsible for the degenerate family.

These studies of families suffer from the handicap common to all work in human genetics: the effects of heredity and environment cannot be completely separated. Members of the same family share not only a common ancestry but also a common environment. In trying to overcome this difficulty, investigators long ago began to use twins as their subjects. Here it seemed was a clearcut way to separate heredity from environment. The twin method is discussed in more detail under "Research in Human Genetics."

Now we move to a discussion of current ideas about the workings of the basic unit of biology, the cell. Cell reproduction is the crucial biological event in inheritance, and an understanding of biological inheritance is indispensable to the student who wishes to evaluate the results of studies of human behavior genetics and their theoretical interpretations.

BASIC CONCEPTS OF MODERN GENETICS

Genetics can be, and often has been, studied without attention to events within the cell. Mendel's experiments, which first revealed two of the fundamental laws of heredity, were performed before the mechanics of cell reproduction were understood. Today, Mendelian experiments have become standard laboratory exercises in high school and college; they can be performed and understood without first-hand knowledge of cellular processes. But some knowledge of the architecture of the cell and the functioning of its component parts enhances understanding of the genetic basis of individual differences and also helps to eliminate biologically unsound research from the behavioral sciences (Hirsch, 1963).

Cell Structure

Observation with a standard microscope shows the cell interior to be divided into sections, some appearing amorphous and others evincing a definite and relatively stable structure (see Figure 2.2). The area containing little obvious structure is called the *cytoplasm*. Examination with an electron microscope, however, reveals a world of structural detail in this seemingly formless mass. There is a network of interwoven membranes which are usually lined with dense particles, the *ribosomes*. These small particles are related to the function of the gene.

The areas of well-defined, visible structure within the cell are the *Golgi apparatus*, the *mitochondria*, the *centrosphere*, and the *nucleus*. The *Golgi apparatus*, it is currently thought, serves as a collection area for the synthetic products of the cell just before their release into the intercellular environment. The *mitochondria*, rod-shaped bodies enclosed by a double membrane, are being actively studied. They are found most abundantly in cells that utilize large amounts of energy. Cells of the flight muscles of insects and cells that actively transport molecules and ions across their membranes (nerve and kidney cells, for example) have a generous supply of mitochondria. Most of the chemical reactions that convert the energy of nutrients—fats, carbohydrates, and proteins—into forms which can be utilized by the cell occur within the membrane of the mitochondria.

The *nucleus* is the largest constituent of the cell; it contains the genetic material, which controls the major share of the cell's activities. The microscopic appearance of the genetic material varies with the different stages of the life of the cell. When the cell is not actively dividing, the nucleus looks like a network of fine tangled thread. It can be seen when the cell is stained with chemicals which indicate deoxyribonucleic acid (DNA) and certain types of protein. For this reason, the genetic material is thought to be a complex of DNA and a specific protein. When the cell is dividing, the genetic material untangles and individual *chromosomes* (rodlike bodies in the cell nucleus that are considered to be the seat of the genes) appear as separate, threadlike units (Figure 2.3). These changes are described more fully in the discussion of meiosis.

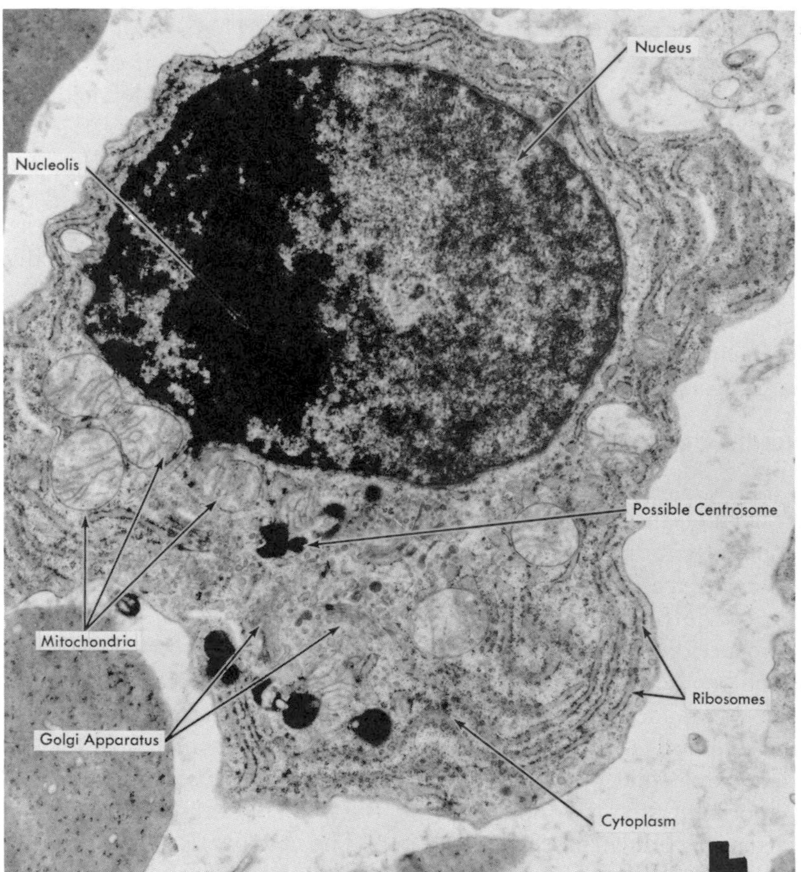

Figure 2.2 Electron microscopic photograph of cell. Magnification, 25,000. Photo © WESKEMP "Ferguson."

Adjacent to the nucleus is usually found a clear area, the *centrosphere*, which contains the *centrioles*. These are two bodies that can be stained very darkly and that look like short cylinders closed at one end. They characteristically have eleven rings—nine of outer and two of inner fibers. Although the part these small bodies play in the functioning of the cell is not entirely understood, several bits of observational evidence indicate that the centrioles are very important: (1) In animal cells, they form the poles towards which the chromosomes move during cell division. (2) Like the chromosomes, they appear to undergo self-replication. (3) One centriole is carried in the head of the sperm and is transmitted into the egg. This centriole divides and forms the poles for the first division of the new individual. (4) They form the basal body out of which grow the cilia (hairlike processes) in ciliated cells, and they form the base of the sensory cells of the eye. While much is still to be learned about the centrioles, we know that they are one of the important cellular *organelles*, or anatomically distinct structures.

Reproduction

Cells have several ways of reproducing themselves. One of these is *mitosis*—a division of the nucleus into two daughter nuclei with identical chromosome complements. Another type of cell reproduction occurs only in bisexual species. Two cells of complementary specialization, the egg and the sperm, are produced, one by each sex. These fuse to form a single cell (*zygote*) which develops into a new individual. The cellular divisions which lead to the production of these specialized sex cells are called *meiosis.*

Mitosis. Because a detailed knowledge of mitosis is not necessary for understanding genetics, we attempt here only to clarify the differences between it and meiosis. Figure 2.4 shows the chromosome events involved in mitotic division. Each chromosome duplicates just before the cell divides mitotically. When the cell divides, one half of every doubled

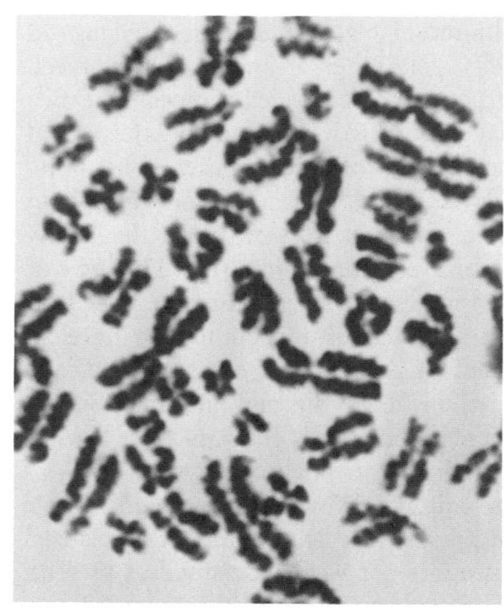

Figure 2.3 Human chromosomes. Photo © WESKEMP.

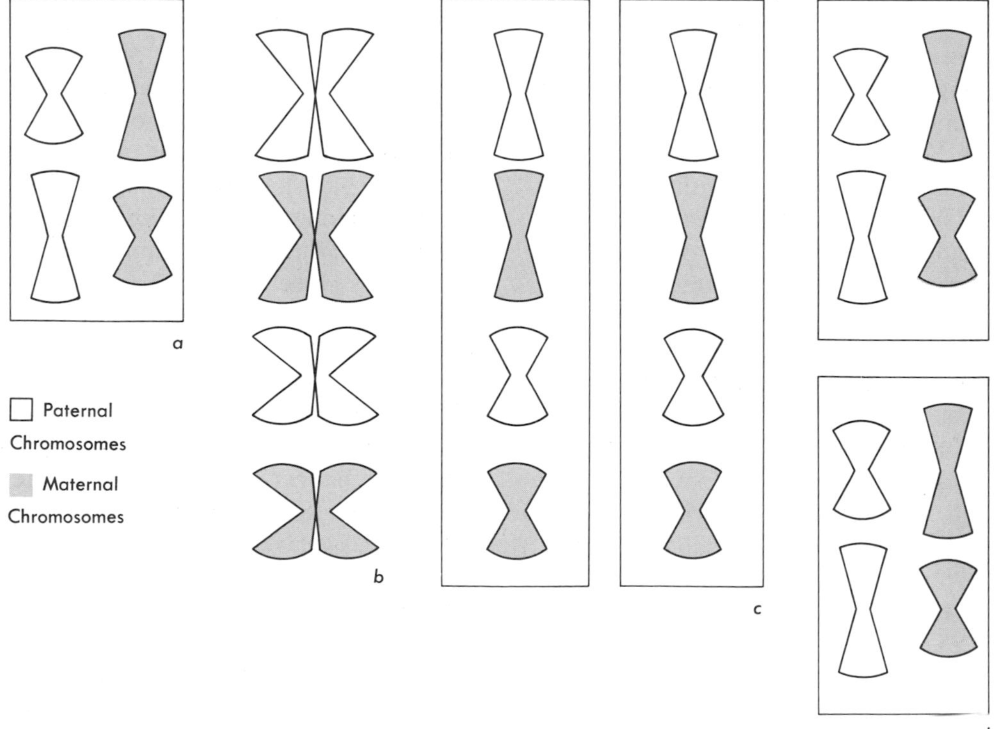

Figure 2.4 Chromosome events of mitosis: *a*, the cell before mitosis; *b*, the chromosomes replicate; c, each doubled chromosome divides; *d*, the two daughter cells have the same genetic content as the original cell.

chromosome goes to each of the *daughter* cells. The other organelles (distinct cell structures) are divided between the two daughter cells in an approximately equal but less systematic manner. The mitochondria, Golgi apparatus, and cytoplasm then increase in size until the newly formed cells reach maturity. This type of division is characteristic of single-cell organisms and of the embryonic development of multicellular organisms. Mitotic division keeps the chromosome complement of body cells constant. The process by which the single-cell zygote develops by mitotic division into a multicellular organism with many kinds of specialized tissues is not well understood at present. The problem of differentiation and specialization of cells is the center of much current research (Flickinger, 1963).

Meiosis. Cell divisions which lead to the production of *gametes* (specialized sex cells: *egg* and *sperm*) do not maintain the genetic status quo, as mitosis does. On the contrary, they appear to be a most efficient machinery for generating variations. Since egg and sperm arise from cell divisions that are alike with respect to what happens to the chromosomes, these divisions are discussed here as a phenomenon that is common to both sexes. Differences between egg and sperm production appear when the functional gamete is formed. In the egg cell, most of the cytoplasm is confined to one of the four possible gametes, but in the sperm cell, most of the cytoplasm is eliminated. The sperm is thus mostly nuclear material surrounded by the cell membrane. Figure 2.5 shows a schematic diagram of the nuclear divisions during meiosis.

The important events in meiosis are as follows: (1) Each chromosome pairs with the corresponding chromosome from the other parent. (2) The chromosome complement is reduced from diploid (a double occurrence of each chromosome) to haploid (a single occurrence of each chromosome) because each gamete receives only one member of each pair of chromosomes. (3) Because the orientation (positioning) of the members of each pair is random, at the first division each new cell gets a random sample of maternal and paternal chromosomes. (4) Since there are only two divisions in meiosis these divisions yield four cells. In the male, all four cells become mature sperm. But in the female, only one cell becomes an egg; the other three become polar bodies which later disintegrate.

When the sperm fertilizes an egg, a *zygote* is formed with the full complement of chromosomes common to the species. One member of each pair is contributed by each parent. The independent meiotic assortment of the chromosomes is one of the mechanisms that maintains genetic variability. The number of unique chromosomal combinations possible in a gamete (sex cell) depends on the number of chromosome pairs typical of the species. This number may be represented by 2^N, where N is the number of chromosome pairs of the species. In man, since $N = 23$, 2^{23}, or 8,388,608, different chromosomal combinations are possible in a gamete. A mating pair of human beings is able to produce $8{,}388{,}608^2$, or over 70 trillion, unique zygotes. These calculations are based on the assumption that individual chromosomes maintain their integrity over generations, but in the case of many species, many factors, including mutation (changes in the gene), generate endless genetic variety upon which natural selection can act.

Genotype-Phenotype Relations

As we have indicated, the phenotype consists of those aspects of an individual that can be observed. Body size, eye and hair color, reactions to various pharmacological agents, and behavioral adjustments to the environment are phenotypic characteristics. The genotype is the ge-

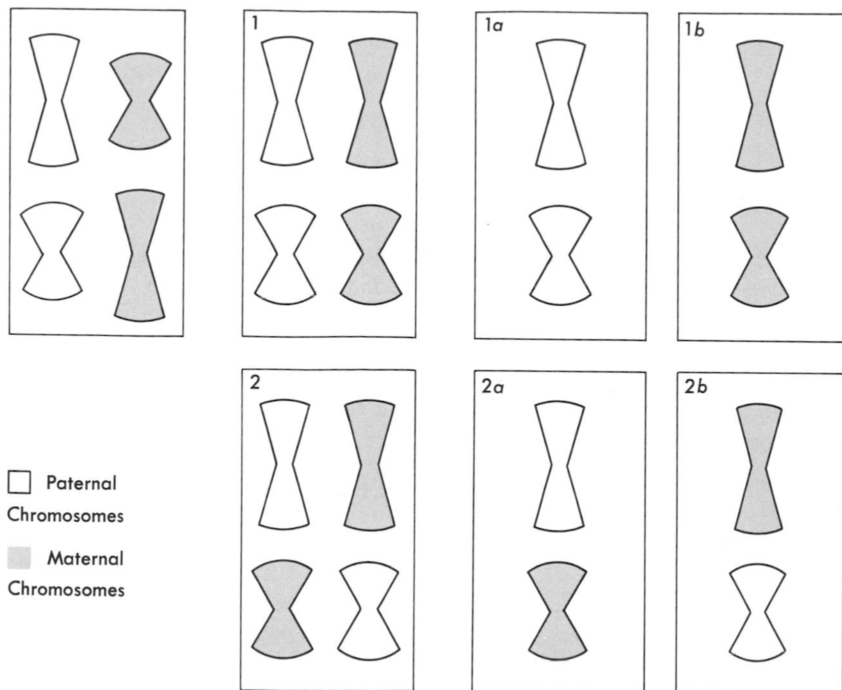

Figure 2.5 Chromosome events of meiosis: *a*, the cell before meiosis; *b*, possible arrangements at division; *c*, four unique chromosomal arrangements can be produced.

netic constitution of the individual. Because it cannot yet be observed directly, the genotype of a particular individual can only be inferred from observations of the phenotypes of his relatives. The first requirement for analyzing genotype-phenotype relations is to find a reliable system for classifying the phenotype, for inferences made about the genotype are no more dependable than the scoring of the phenotypes. This problem assumes particular importance in the study of heredity and behavior in man because we cannot control breeding as we can in plant and animal studies.

The second requirement is to know the true mating and breeding system and the relationships among the individuals studied. The investigator of human behavior genetics must use family histories and must perform his genetic analyses after the breeding has actually occurred.

Because most genes are represented twice in the genotype—one *allele* (gene form) on each member of a chromosome pair—there may not be a one-to-one correspondence between genotype and phenotype. For a given gene, an individual may have the same allele on both members of a chromosome pair, or he may have different alleles. In the first case, he is said to be homozygous for that gene and in the second, heterozygous. Thus, where two alleles exist, there are three genotypic possibilities: two ways of being homozygous and one way of being heterozygous. If we have two alleles, A and O, and if a person with the genetic composition *AA* or *AO* exhibits the phenotypic characteristic A, then we say A is *dominant* and O has no effect, or is *recessive*. In order for the phenotypic characteristic O to be exhibited, the genetic composition must be *OO*. If the genetic composition *AA* exhibits the phenotypic characteristic A more strongly than the composition *AO*, then we say that A is an *intermediate* gene.

We have been concerned with phenotypic characteristics which can be related to a single gene. Mather (1949) and others have labeled genes with a clearly distinguishable effect on the phenotype *major* genes. The traits controlled by such genes are usually classifiable into two or three exhaustive and mutually exclusive categories. The major gene probably has one locus, or position on the chromosome, and a limited number of alleles, each of which produces a distinguishably different expression of the phenotype. This model is consistent with Mendel's laws of genetics.

Mather used the *polygene* concept in order to include quantitative characters in the framework of Mendelian principles. In the polygenic model, many different genes are involved in the expression of a character. Each one makes a small positive or negative contribution to the phenotypic score. The phenotypic score for an individual is the algebraic sum of the effects of all the genes associated with the trait. Each one of the polygenes obeys the Mendelian laws and, in this way, is no different in its basic biological properties from a major gene. The main difference between the two kinds lies in their effects on the phenotype. Because polygenes adhere to Mendelian laws, it is possible to predict the distribution of phenotypic scores for the offspring of specific matings. Shields and Slater (1961) give an example based on the assumption that height is determined by three pairs of genes, *A* and *a*, *B* and *b*, and *C* and *c*:

> We will suppose that the capital letters tend to cause tallness, the lowercase letters shortness, that there is neither dominance nor recessivity, that all genes are equally common, and that mating is taking place at random. Then the tallest individual we can find, with the constitution *AABBCC*, will be relatively uncommon; for every one of him there will be six individuals one degree less tall: *aABBCC*, *AaBBCC*, *AAbBCC*, *AABbCC*, *AABBcC*, *AABBCc*. . . . It is readily seen that the commonest group will be the middle group, with average height, . . . and, in fact the population, graded by height, will be distributed according to the terms of the expansion of $(\frac{1}{2} + \frac{1}{2})^6$. (P. 309.)

And as the number of genes involved in the determination of the trait gets larger and larger, we get an approximation of the normal curve.

Therefore, if we find phenotypic characters with a distribution which approaches a normal curve, we will say that they are a result of multifactorial or *polygenic* inheritance. Because a number of environmental conditions may cause the same distribution, we cannot say that a characteristic is the result of polygenic inheritance simply because it exhibits a distribution approaching a normal curve, but, rather, we must also observe

> a regression equation linking the deviation from average values shown by a series of subjects with the deviation shown by their relatives. As an example, we may take the case of intelligence. As is well known, the Binet IQ is normally distributed. . . . If we measure the intelligence of a series of school children, and also those of their sibs, it will be found that the correlated data are fairly well described by a linear equation: the IQ of the sib will tend to deviate from the mean in the same direction as that of the original subject. (Shields and Slater, 1961, p. 310.)

Therefore the concept of polygenic inheritance can be used to describe the genetic basis of intelligence; this material is discussed more fully in Chapter 14.

Phenocopy. The fact that two genotypes can yield one phenotype and that many phenotypes are the result of polygenic inheritance makes the genetic anal-

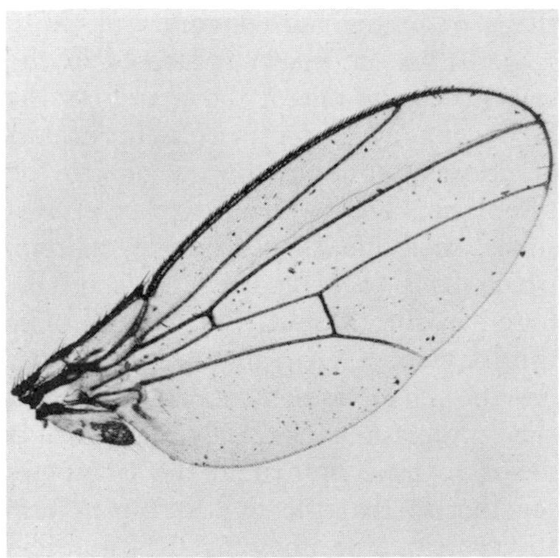

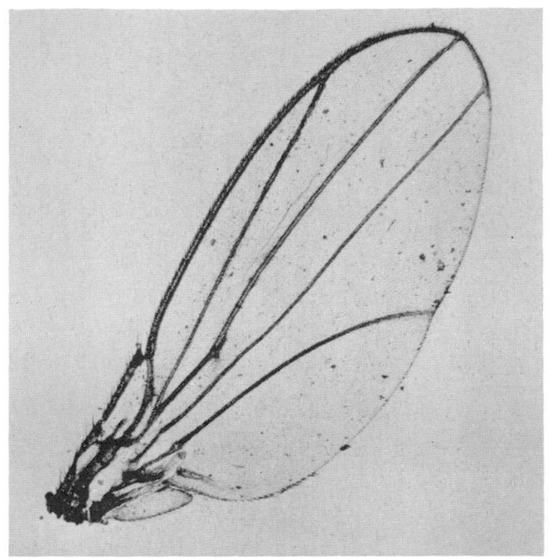

Figure 2.6 Drosophila exhibiting phenocopy: *a*, normal phenotype; *b*, crossveinlessness. Photo © Walter Dawn.

ysis of phenotypes difficult. When the environment is not the same for all genotypes, the problems of genetic analysis may be further complicated by interaction between genotype and environment, as in the case of *phenocopy*, a special kind of phenotype. Sometimes a genotype that ordinarily produces one kind of phenotype is exposed to special environmental conditions that cause it to produce a phenotype characteristic of another genotype under what, for it, would be standard conditions. The phenomenon has been well documented in experiments with Drosophila (fruit flies). For example, animals who are heterozygous for a recessive mutation (crossveinlessness) which produces flies without certain wing veins will not show the trait under normal laboratory temperatures. But if these heterozygotes are subjected to heat shock during the larval stage, they will develop like the homozygous recessive; that is, they will show the crossveinless phenotype (see Figure 2.6).

In the case of man, an analogous situation occurs with the successful treatment of *phenylketonuria*, a form of mental deficiency accompanied by high concentrations of phenylpyruvic acid in the urine. The phenylketonuric individual carries two recessive alleles and can be identified by biochemical and behavioral tests. If this genotype, however, is allowed to develop in an environment that presents a low concentration of the amino acid, phenylalanine, in the diet, the homozygous recessive individual may develop normally.

The realization that genotype-environment interactions exist becomes especially important in the study of human behavior genetics, where it is impossible to control experimentally either genotype or environment.

Gene Expression and Structure of Genetic Material

The actual transmission of genetic information from parent to offspring takes place by means of the material within the chromosomes. The chromosome contains a complex of *protein* and *deoxyribonucleic acid* (DNA). Since both of these chemicals undergo the replication and division of meiosis, either might be

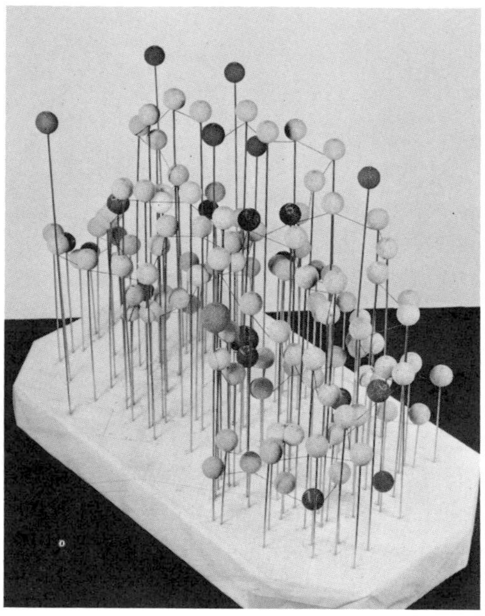

Figure 2.7 Model of the molecular structure of the enzyme, ribonuclease. Photo © Roswell Park Memorial Institute.

considered the carrier of genetic information. The experiments of Avery *et al.* (1944), however, showed that purified DNA alone could accomplish the transfer of genetic information. The chemical structure of DNA is only gradually coming to light, but its most important characteristic is the ability of its molecules to replicate accurately. Thus DNA performs the primary function of hereditary material, which is self-replication.

The determination of the structure of the DNA molecule and the demonstration that DNA is the mode of transfer of genetic information led to the discovery of how the genes work. The primary effect of genes, it seems, is to specify the sequence of amino acids in protein molecules: the DNA specifies the chemical composition of ribonucleic acid (RNA), which, in turn, specifies the sequence of the amino acids which constitute the protein. Three types of RNA serve three different functions in the synthesis of protein (see Figure 2.7). *Messenger-RNA* (m-RNA) is formed in the cell nucleus on one of the strands of the DNA. It provides for an efficient transfer of information from the nucleus to the cytoplasm. *Transfer-RNA* (t-RNA) is a single molecule shaped like a hairpin, which coils back on itself; it is usually found in the cytoplasm of the cell. The third type of RNA is found in ribosomes on the endoplasmic reticulum, within the cytoplasm. The only function it seems to have is to hold the ribosomes together so that the m-RNA's can form the protein. The ribosomal RNA-protein complex appears to function only as a workbench where the proteins are assembled.

In some fashion which is still not completely understood, the sequence of chemical bases in DNA provides the "code" which determines the sequence of amino acids in protein. Recently, theoretical models have been developed which attempt to explain this relationship. Eck (1963) has developed one which accounts for most of the already demonstrated relations between the chemical bases and the amino acids and which also predicts the relationships between specific amino acids and bases for which experimental evidence is still lacking.

It is in this way that genes are now known to function. Any behavioral variations which are inherited must reflect variations in protein structure. *Behaviors themselves, of course, are not inherited: what an individual receives from his parents are molecules of DNA and protein.* From these develop the form of the body and the structural basis of all behaviors.

Mendelism

Segregation. Somatic cells contain a diploid (paired) set of chromosomes. One member of each pair comes from the male parent and the other from a female. Since the genes are carried on the chro-

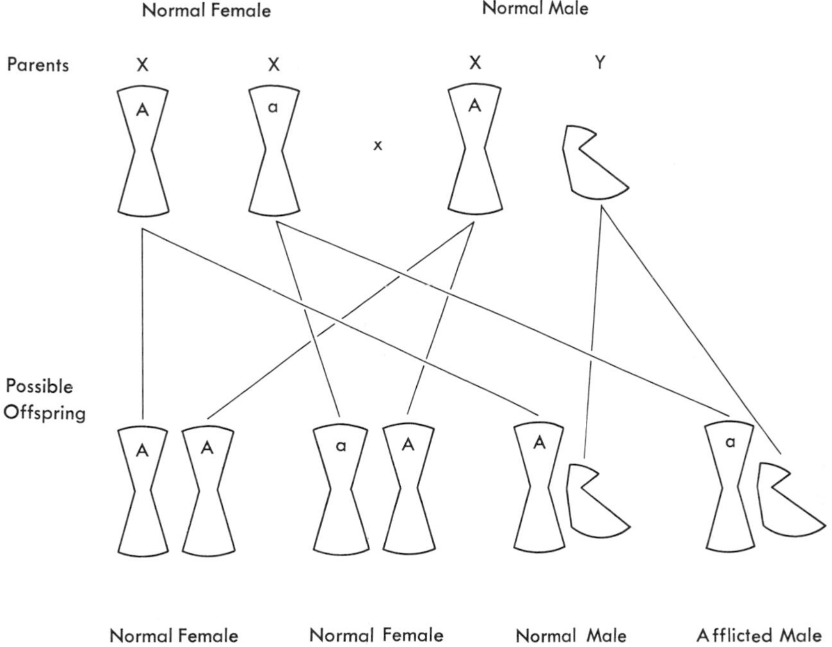

Figure 2.8 Inheritance of a recessive allele on the *X* chromosome. *A* is dominant over *a*.

mosomes, each parent normally contributes one allele of every autosomal gene in the species. The pattern of inheritance for genes carried on the sex chromosomes is somewhat different from that of genes on the chromosomes which are not involved in sex determination (the autosomes).

In man, the segregation of alleles (gene forms) is most easily demonstrated with sex-linked characters. One pair of chromosomes differs from the others in that the two members of the pair are not the same in males and females. In the female, both members of this pair are alike; they are called X chromosomes. In the male, they are not alike; the larger one is the same X chromosome that appears in the female and the smaller one is the Y chromosome that ordinarily appears exclusively in the male. Where there is a single chromosome and therefore only one allele for each of its genes, there is a one-to-one correspondence between genotype and phenotype. Hence, in the male phenotype, the X chromosome genotype lies exposed for observation.

Figure 2.8 shows the mode of inheritance of a recessive allele that is located on the X chromosome. If red or green colorblindness is contributed by a colorblind male marrying a female with two normal alleles, all male offspring will be colornormal and all female offspring will be phenotypically normal but genotypically carriers. If colorblindness is contributed by the female, two possibilities exist. If she is heterozygous, half her sons will be colorblind and half will be normal. Her phenotypically normal daughters will be half heterozygous carriers and half normal homozygotes. If the female is homozygous for the colorblindness allele, both she and all of her sons will be colorblind while all her daughters will be heterozygous carriers.

This demonstration of how alleles segregate may now seem superfluous in the light of modern cytological evidence from the direct observation of chromosomes; but it was considered important enough, at the time of the rediscovery of Mendel's work, to be proclaimed a law: the law of segregation of alleles. It was important because it disproved the widely held blending theory of inheritance accepted by Darwin. It showed that genes are particulate and that they maintain their integrity as they pass from one generation to the next, whatever may have been their associations in a particular genotype and the development of its phenotype.

Independent assortment. Mendel's second contribution to formal genetics was the law of independent assortment. He studied two characters simultaneously and observed that segregation of the alleles for one character occurred independently of segregation of those for the other character. Consideration of two characters at once yields certain characteristic genotypic ratios. If individuals homozygous for contrasting alleles at the two loci, or positions on the chromosome, are crossed (*AABB* x *aabb*), their offspring must be heterozygous for both loci (*AaBb*). When heterozygotes intermate (*AaBb* x *AaBb*), they produce four types of sex cells or gametes (*AB*, *Ab*, *aB*, *ab*), which can combine at fertilization to produce nine genotypic classes of individuals in the ratio: 1 *AABB*: 2 *AABb*: 1 *AAbb*: 2 *AaBB*: 4 *AaBb*: 2 *Aabb*: 1 *aaBB*: 2 *aaBb*: 1 *aabb*. Grouping these genotypes into phenotypic classes depends upon the presence or absence of dominance between alleles. Of course, completely independent assortment can only occur for genes located on different chromosome pairs. For several reasons, traits may sometimes be correlated rather than independent, but we will see that correlation does not invalidate Mendel's second law.

The work of Galton and others, on characters which appeared to be inherited but did not segregate into the Mendelian ratios, posed problems for the particulate theory of inheritance. The problems arose because variations in the characters investigated, like height and weight, could not be classified into a few discrete categories but were distributed along a more or less continuous scale. Many behavioral traits, such as intelligence or energy level, also show continuous variation. This gradation of expression led many students to think that such characters demonstrated a blending type of inheritance.

Mendel's laws of segregation and independent assortment still provide the basis for defining a gene. For a gene to be detected by the methods of genetics, it must take at least two allelic forms; that is, it must show segregation when the appropriate matings occur. And for two genes to be distinguished, they must be separable; that is, their segregating alleles must assort with some degree of independence.

Correlated characters. There are two events that may interfere with the usual independent assortment of hereditary traits and give rise to *correlations* between characters. One is *linkage* and the other is *pleiotropy*. The genes on a chromosome are *linked* together and form a kind of chain. When two chromosomes lie next to each other in a pair, parts of either one may break off and join on to the other, exchanging positions with comparable parts of the other. The part may be a single gene, but it is more commonly a group of genes, a segment of the entire chain. The presence of one gene in the new chain is correlated with the presence of several others because all of them *crossed over* to the chromosome at the same time.

The phenomenon of *crossing-over* is quite common. Because genes cross over

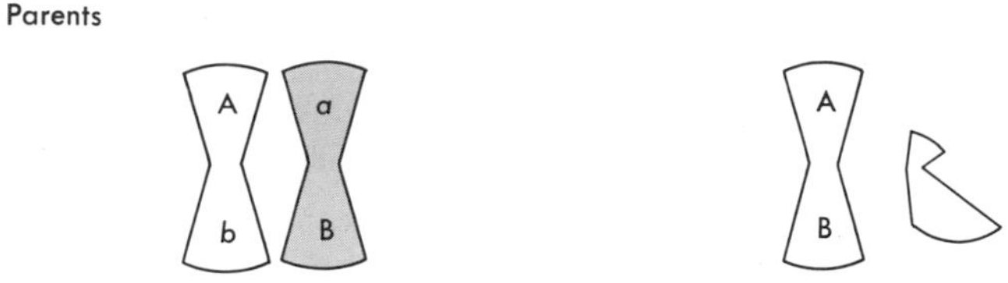

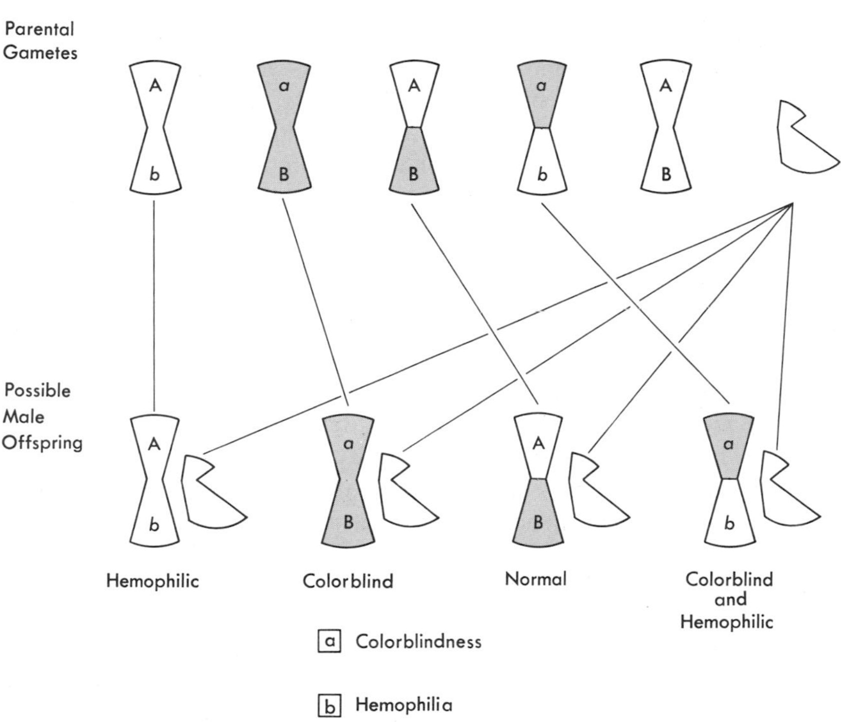

Figure 2.9 Crossing over in the *X* chromosome of a female with two heterozygous loci.

with those lying near them in the chain, by looking at a great number of chromosome pairs it is possible to estimate the location of genes in a linkage group and to determine the distances between them. In mapping the exact location of genes on a chromosome, estimates of distances between genes are based on the relative frequency with which the linkage breaks. In humans, the first chromosome to be successfully mapped will undoubtedly be the X chromosome because of the ease of identifying the X chromosome genotype in the male. Figure 2.9 shows the gametes and the progeny phenotypes which can arise as the result of crossing over between two heterozygous loci on the X chromosome genes of a female. The various combinations of alleles of the X chromosome genes would be detectable in the male offspring because of the lack of comparable loci on the Y chromosome. Given a number of such heterozygous women with enough sons, it would be possible to estimate the distance between the two genes. If a whole series of loci could be used, it would be possible to map the entire X chromosome.

Crossing-over also increases genetic variability. Stern (1960) calculated that if he assumes 10,000 different loci, 2 percent heterozygosity, and one crossover event per chromosome, the number of chromosomal combinations from one human jumps from 2^{23} to $2^{22} \times 10^{23}$. The number of eggs produced by a female (about 400) and the number of sperm produced by a male (maybe one trillion) are very small indications of the possible genetic combinations.

When a correlation among traits is due to multiple effects of a single gene, that gene is said to be *pleiotropic* in its effects. Gruneberg (see Sinnott *et al.*, 1958, p. 352) has shown how one gene may influence an entire series of traits. In his well-analyzed study of the phenotypic effects of a single mutant allele, he has shown that a cartilage anomaly appears early in development. Rats carrying the allele for this defect develop various feeding and breathing difficulties, which together eventually lead to death. In man, we can expect analogous conditions to exist, many of which may lead to maladaptive behavior patterns.

GENETICS AND HUMAN BEHAVIOR

The discussion of cellular genetics and of research methods thus far has concerned the entire field of genetics. Human behavior genetics, however, is a somewhat specialized field because it is limited to a very few specialized research methods. These methods must be generally understood before we can discuss the actual human behavioral aberrations which result from genetic events.

Research in Human Genetics

We can select and inbreed animals which differ in their expression of some phenotype, and then examine the progeny to see if their characteristics conform to the predictions of our genetic models. Human beings are less docile, however, and fussier about choosing their own mates. In the absence of inbreeding and controlled matings, investigators of human traits have turned to correlational studies and complex statistical variance analyses, to twin studies, and to pedigree analysis in their efforts to understand the genetic basis of human behavior.

Correlational analysis. The method of inferring genetic bases of human traits that is perhaps most common—correlational analysis—has been carried out on a number of traits involving familial relationships. The genetic correlation between related individuals can be determined by considering the meiotic events (the degree of blood relationship) that separate them. The genetic correlation between parent and offspring, for example, is exactly 0.50 because the offspring receive one half of their genes from each parent. The genetic correlation between siblings, on the other hand, varies from 0.00 to 1.00. Only its average is 0.50.

Since the degree of meiotic relationship gives us the general genetic correspondence among individuals in a family, we can infer the genetic status of a behavior trait from the relationship of its distribution among the members of a family to the general distribution of known genetic traits in the same family. Figure 2.10 illustrates how this has been done in studying the relationship between heredity and tested intelligence. It presents the distributions of correlational measures collected in studies over the past half century.

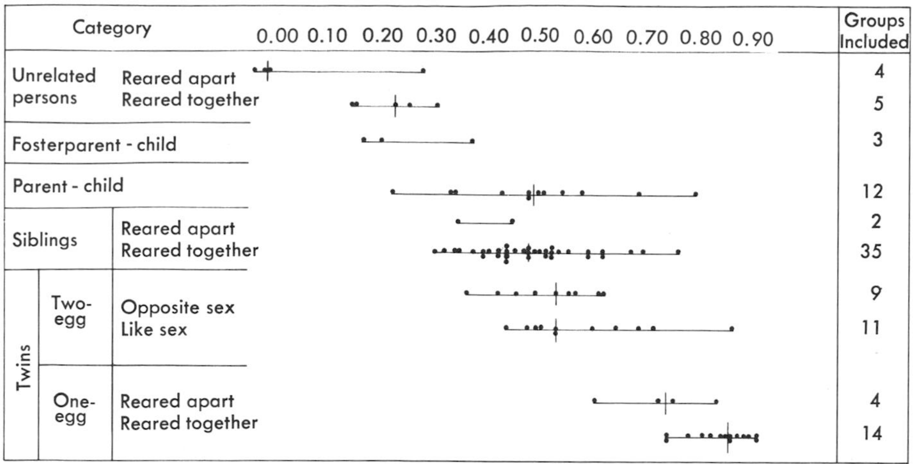

Figure 2.10 Correlation coefficients for "intelligence" test scores from fifty-two studies. Coefficients are indicated by solid circles, and medians by vertical lines intersecting the horizontal lines, which represent the ranges. From L. Erlenmeyer-Kimling and L. F. Jarvik, "Genetics and intelligence: A review," *Science*, Vol. 142, pp. 1477–1479, 13 December 1963, © 1963 by the American Association for the Advancement of Science.

> The 52 studies . . . yield over 30,000 correlational pairings. . . . The investigators had different backgrounds and contrasting views regarding the importance of heredity. Not all of them used the same measures of intelligence, and they derived their data from samples which were unequal in size, age structure, ethnic composition, and socio-economic stratification; the data were collected in eight countries on four continents during a time span covering more than two generations of individuals. Against this pronounced heterogeneity, which should have clouded the picture, and is reflected by the wide range of correlations, a clearly definitive consistency emerges from the data. (Erlenmeyer-Kimling and Jarvik, 1963, pp. 1477–1478.)

Twin studies. In man, the study of monozygotic (MZ) siblings (identical twins) represents the only known possibility of a controlled genotype. In the rare cases where twins have been reared apart, comparison of like-sex dizygotic twins (DZ, fraternal twins) with MZ twins reared apart and with MZ twins reared together permits us in a limited way to control and measure the effects of both environment and heredity. In the early work, determination of zygosity was mainly impressionistic and uncertain, but today, twins can be compared on a large series of characters that are known to be controlled by single genes. Because the genetic correlation between siblings can vary over a wide range of values, it is impossible to ascertain monozygosity with absolute certainty. The probability of correctly detecting the zygosity, however, has increased greatly with the increase in the number of traits compared.

The rationale of twin studies assumes that (1) with environment held constant, if discordance in the trait studied is greater among DZ (fraternal) than among MZ (identical) twins, the difference is attributable to heredity; (2) with genotype held constant, if discordancc among MZ twins reared apart is greater than among MZ twins reared together, the difference is attributable to environment; and (3) if discordance is greater among MZ's reared apart than among DZ's reared together, environment is more important than heredity, whereas if concordance is greater, heredity is more important than environment.

With the objective of partitioning the observed variance of a trait into its genetic and environmental components, Cattell (1953) has developed an analytical method which can process measurements on pairs of individuals ranging through all degrees of genetic relationships from MZ twins to unrelated individuals randomly selected. Should this approach apply to enough conditions and problems, some day it may become standard procedure for investigating human genetic backgrounds.

Pedigree analysis. Since controlled breeding of men is not possible in a free society, pedigrees are often used for the analysis of particular characteristics. A pedigree is a "family tree." Analysis of one usually begins with an individual manifesting the trait we are interested in and proceeds to all the relatives that can be examined or about whom there is information concerning expression of the trait. After data on trait expression and individual relationship in a family have been gathered for two or more generations, an attempt is made to fit a genetic model to the observations.

The pedigree in Figure 2.11 is from a rather extensive study of Huntington's chorea, a deadly disease of the nervous system producing uncontrolled movement: impairment of memory, attention, and judgment; irritability; and depression. There is no effective treatment, and the afflicted individual may progressively deteriorate for ten to twenty years until death. The pedigree in Figure 2.10 shows that this disease is probably due to a dominant allele, although occasionally, when the genetic model predicts an affliction the individual does not show the disease. Absence of the disease might, however, be explained by the late age of onset; some people carrying the dominant allele might have died of other causes before the syndrome developed. If Huntington's chorea is associated with a dominant allele, then in principle, anyone carrying that allele will develop the disease.

When a recessive allele is involved, the genetic model is more difficult to discover because fewer individuals show the critical phenotype. Traits associated with recessive alleles only come to light when an individual receives the same allele from both parents. This event is relatively rare because only one fourth of the offspring of two heterozygous normal parents will have the genotype (see Table 2.1, Case 4). Such rare traits cannot be traced in many families. Since members of the same family usually have more like alleles than the general population has, recessive alleles come to light more often when there is some inbreeding (matings between closely related individuals). Clearly, when recessive alleles are rare, absence of inbreeding will greatly reduce the chance of discovering the trait and analyzing its genetic basis.

Although in many instances there may be no alternative to pedigree analysis, it has several disadvantages. First, it is often necessary to depend upon people other than the investigator for some of the observations. Man's long life-span and deferred reproductive age make it almost impossible for one investigator to observe personally more than three generations. Often information must be obtained from ill-informed family members. The use of data from such observers is particularly undependable in the study of mental disorders (Neel and Schull, 1954). A second difficulty of pedigree analysis is that the environment—both physical and psychological—changes from generation to generation. The phenocopy phenomenon is a reminder that changing environmental conditions can change phenotypes. Even

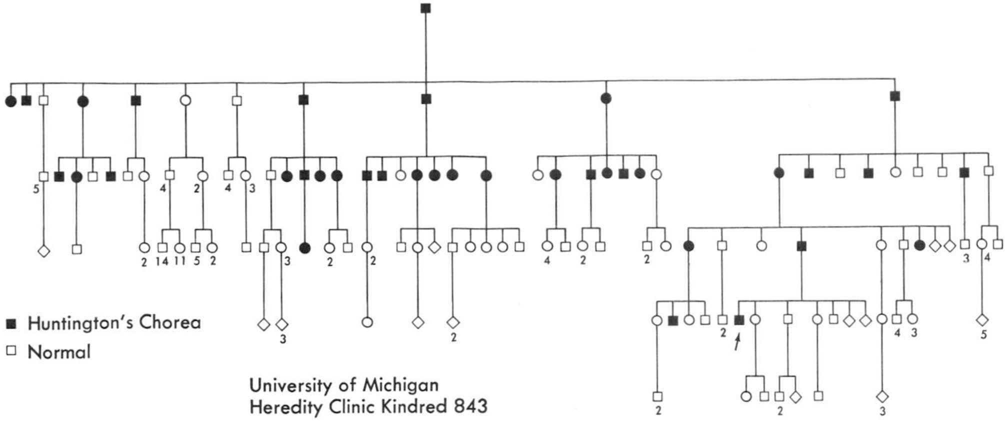

Figure 2.11 A pedigree of Huntington's chorea. A single dominant autosomal gene is responsible for the onset, at about thirty to forty years, of the degeneration of various areas in the brain. Many pedigrees appear deficient in affected persons because of the death of carriers of the gene before the age of onset. From J. V. Neel and W. J. Schull, *Human Heredity*, University of Chicago Press, 1954.

Table 2.1

Dominant Inheritance

Phenotypes *Aa* and AA are indistinguishable and normal; *aa* is abnormal.

	Types of Matings			Gametes		Types and Frequencies of Offspring Genotypes
	♂		♀	♂	♀	
Case 1	AA	x	AA	A	A	All AA
Case 2	*Aa*	x	AA	½ A ½ *a*	A	½ AA ½ A*a*
	AA	x	A*a*	A	½ A ½ *a*	½ AA ½ A*a*
Case 3	A*a*	x	A*a*	½ A ½ *a*	½ A ½ *a*	¼ AA ½ A*a* ¼ *aa*
Case 4	AA	x	*aa*	A	*a*	All A*a*
Case 5	A*a*	x	*aa*	½ A ½ *a*	*a*	½ A*a* ½ *aa*
	aa	x	A*a*	*a*	½ A ½ *a*	½ A*a* ½ *aa*
Case 6	*aa*	x	*aa*	*a*	*a*	All *aa*

where traits are phenotypically related in a single pedigree, a common genetic mechanism cannot be assumed without analyses based on population studies.

For all these reasons, pedigree studies are probably most valuable only in the early stages of analysis. They may suggest genetic models to be tested on larger populations. They also provide a basis for beginning investigations into the biological nature of the observed variation. Ultimately, however, any variations in functioning that are inherited must probably be traceable to variations in the DNA which one generation gives to the next, and that is a problem for biochemists, not behavior scientists.

Whenever the question of the relative importance of heredity and environment arises, it must always be remembered that heritability is a property of populations as well as of behaviors. More precisely, heritability is relevant to the particular population in which phenotypic measurements are obtained and to the variety of environmental circumstances in which the individuals of that population developed. An increase in environmental heterogeneity will decrease heritability just as will a decrease in genetic heterogeneity. A more uniform environment will increase heritability just as will greater genetic heterogeneity. Because it is population-, situation-, and generation-specific (that is, peculiar to a particular population, situation, and generation), we must never expect to find only a single value for the heritability of a character in any species.

Genetic Determinants of Human Behavior

The methods of investigation of human behavior genetics have generally been applied to negative abnormalities more than to positive ones, although Galton's pioneering work in the field was concerned with genetic disposition towards high intelligence. There are many certain, and many more probable, genetic bases to such positive attributes as high intelligence, artistic ability, good health—that is, high resistance to infection, high energy level, stamina and endurance, and many aspects of what is generally labeled temperament, not to mention physical beauty, some components of which are obviously genetically determined. Behavior geneticists ordinarily pay no very great mind to the problem of identifying the particulars of any of these because nothing urgent needs to be done about them. Nobody wants to do away with beauty, intelligence, or artistry, and nobody wants to be forced into breeding for them, however desirable they may be. The problems of negative abnormality are more urgent, and behavior geneticists study them in more detail, with a view toward eliminating or controlling their unhappy effects on human behavior.

The research methods already described have given us some idea of genetic influences on human aberrations, but the preponderance of environmental influences on phenotyping makes the results of many studies inconclusive. Still, they serve the purpose of indicating possibilities. Disorders that are thought to have a genetic basis can be classed in five groups, according to cause: (1) *chromosomal aberrations*, nonlethal changes in the structure and number of chromosomes; (2) inheritance of *dominant* genes; (3) inheritance of *intermediate* genes; (4) inheritance of *recessive* genes; and (5) *polygenic* inheritance.

Chromosomal aberrations. It has been known for some time, from work on experimental animals and plants, that some nonlethal changes occur in the structure and number of chromosomes. Individuals with unusual chromosome sets are not always fertile. Because of meiotic accidents, sperm or ova are sometimes produced with either more or less than a haploid chromosome set. When these exceptional gametes are involved in fertilization, they produce zygotes (fertilized eggs) with either a deficiency or an excess of chromosomal material. If the resulting genetic imbalance is not too great, the zygote may develop into a mature organism, but any such imbalance is usually sufficient to produce a phenotype easily classified as "abnormal."

Recent advances in the study of cells have enabled us to identify three human syndromes correlated with chromosomal aberrations. One involves excess autosomal materials and the other two involve aberrations of the sex chromosomes.

Down's syndrome, (Figure 2.12) formerly called mongolism, was long thought to be genetically determined. It showed a higher concordance between identical twins than between fraternal twins, and certain aspects of the syndrome occurred more frequently in the families of afflicted individuals than in the general population. With improvements in human cytological techniques (that is, techniques for studying cells), evidence began to accumulate that afflicted individuals usually have more chromosomal material than normal individuals: They usually have three chromosomes instead of the normal two in one of the sets.

Other diseases associated with chromosomal aberrations involve abnormal distribution of the sex chromosomes. People with *Turner's syndrome* (Figure 2.13) are completely lacking one sex chromosome; they appear to be female but have no ovaries, or only rudimentary traces of them. These people are usually small and show infantile development of the mammary glands (Sohval, 1963). An excessive number of sex chromosomes, on the other hand, results in *Klinefelter's syndrome* (Figure 2.14). These people appear to be males, but they have a defective hormonal balance and underdeveloped testes, which usually lack mature sperm.

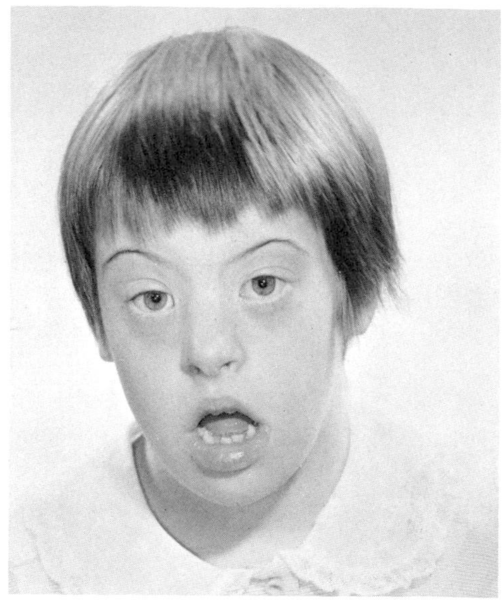

Figure 2.12 Down's syndrome. Courtesy Dr. Herman Yannet, Southbury Training School.

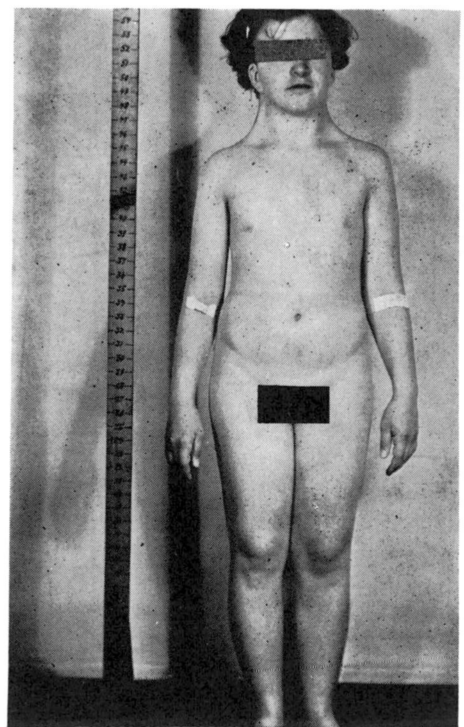

Figure 2.13 Turner's syndrome. From *Clinical Endocrinology,* Ed. 3, by Paschkis, Rakoff, Cantarow, and Rupp, Hoeber Medical Division, Harper & Row, 1967.

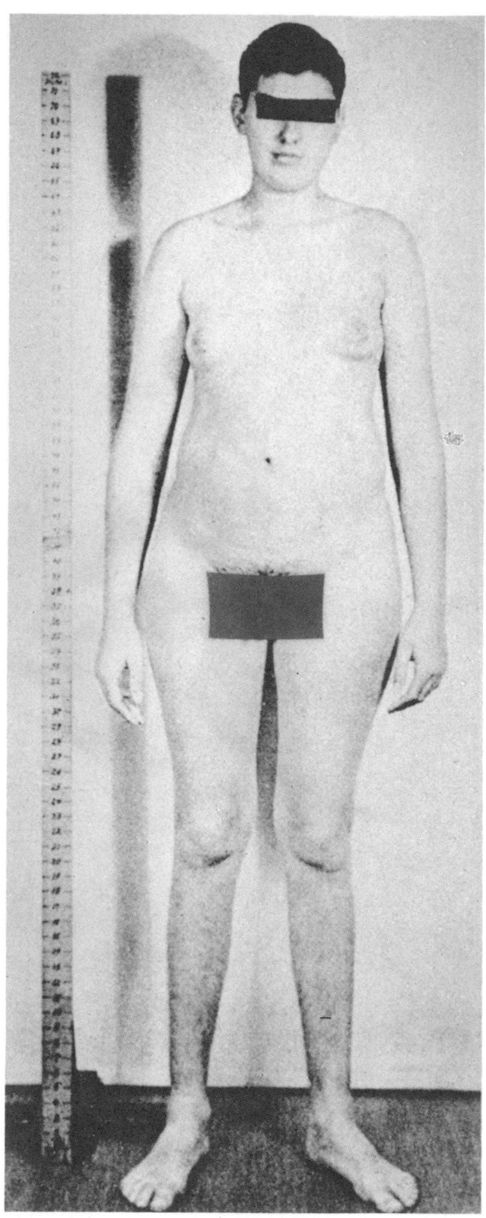

Figure 2.14 Klinefelter's syndrome. From *Clinical Endocrinology*, Ed. 3, by Paschkis, Rakoff, Cantarow, and Rupp, Hoeber Medical Division, Harper & Row, 1967.

It may be useful here to point out the distinction between genetically based behavior disorders in which the disturbance of behavior is immediate and direct and those in which the behavioral aspect is mostly a product of the social consequences of the genetic misfortune. Down's syndrome, phenylketonuria, and Huntington's chorea all illustrate the former; the problematic behavior follows inevitably from the genetic problem. Aberrations of sex structures, as in Turner's and Klinefelter's syndromes, however, do not inevitably prevent their victims from functioning effectively in society any more than baldness or skin color do. It is true that inability to reproduce sexually is likely to result in social difficulties and thus in psychological problems, the importance of which must not be minimized. But so does baldness in a woman or dark skin color in Alabama. The genetic event has a problematic quality more because of its social consequences than because of any inherent dysfunction it forces on the individual.

Dominant inheritance. Referring back to our discussion on the inheritance of dominant genes and to Figure 2.7 let us assume that *D*, a dominant allele, causes an abnormality or defect, and that its complementary recessive allele, *d*, is normal, which here means "predominant in the population." Most people, by definition, will have a *dd* genotype and will be normal, and some will have the *Dd* genotype and will be disordered. The *DD* genotype will be rare, perhaps even incapable of surviving, and therefore may be ignored for all practical purposes (Shields and Slater, 1961). If we have a mating between a normal and an abnormal person, we can expect that half the offspring will be normal and half will be abnormal. The normal ones will be homozygous (*dd*), and the abnormal ones will be heterozygous (*Dd*) and capable of transmitting the abnormality to the next generation. Theoretically then, if we find a person with a dominantly inherited abnormality, we can expect to find that one of his parents (50 percent) and 50 percent of his siblings will also be abnormal (correlational analysis).

Pick's disease, a form of presenile dementia, is a dominantly inherited disorder that usually develops late in middle life. Sjögren *et al.* (1948), by investigating the relatives of affected persons, found that the disease affects only 19 percent of the parents and 7 percent of the siblings, instead of the expected 50 percent. They concluded that most carriers do not develop the abnormality because they are protected by genes that modify the effect of the abnormal gene.

Epiloia (*tuberose sclerosis*), another presenile dementia, causes brain tumors, general mental deficiency, and epilepsy. It appears in early childhood, and the affected person is usually institutionalized before he has children. Gunther and Penrose (1935) estimate that about one case in four is the result of a new mutation (see Shields and Slater, 1961).

Congenital word blindness and *congenital tone deafness* are perceptual abnormalities that may have a dominant genetic basis. Despite normal intelligence, people with congenital word blindness have difficulty learning to read and write. Hallgren (1950) concluded that this abnormality is the result of a single dominant gene because he found that 50 percent of siblings with one affected parent developed the abnormality. Kalmus, using a series of tests devised to measure ability to sing in tune and to recognize commonly known melodies, concluded that tone deafness was probably caused by a single dominant gene (Shields and Slater, 1961).

Uncertainties in the methods of human behavior genetics extend to the area of psychiatric disorders, as we shall see in more detail in the third section of this book. As a result, we do not know the causes of many behavior disorders, including the two most common patterns of psychosis, *manic-depressive psychosis* and the many variants of *schizophrenia*. Most students of these disorders are convinced that they are functional, that is, learned through experience and not caused either by genetic or other organic causes. But the methods of behavior genetics, especially correlational analyses and twin studies, have been applied to them, with the result that some scholars believe a dominant gene is somehow involved. Slater in 1938 (see Shields and Slater, 1961), Kallman (1950), and Stenstedt (1952) found a high incidence of similar psychoses in the parents, siblings, and children of manic depressives (Shields and Slater, 1961). Leonhard in 1934 (see Shields and Slater, 1961) observed that "atypical" psychosis (which even psychiatrists have not been able to relate to other conditions) also appears often enough in parents and siblings of affected persons to be dominantly inherited.

Schizophrenia may include a much more complicated set of conditions than manic-depressive psychosis does. In any case, the evidence is fairly substantial that at least some kinds of schizophrenia have some kind of genetic basis. Böök (1953) studied families in a small northern Swedish community and concluded that schizophrenia results from a dominant gene that is weak and variable in its manifestations (see Shields and Slater, 1961). Six major twin studies of schizophrenia made between 1930 and 1961 and neatly summarized by Rosen and Gregory (1965, pp. 324–326) strongly suggest a genetic component. Its precise characteristics and the mode of transmission remain unclear, but a single dominant gene is probably not responsible.

Recessive inheritance. Recessive genes are protected against elimination by natural selection because the carrier himself suffers no ill effects. From the example above, under "Genotype-Phenotype Relations," we found that a carrier (AO) of a recessive gene (O) exhibits the characteristics of the dominant gene (A). If two carriers have offspring, one child may receive a recessive gene from each parent. He will then have the genetic composition OO and will exhibit the recessive characteristic. But because each child of an affected individual (OO) inherits the recessive gene, the genes spread widely through the population. Muller (1950) estimated that everyone carries eight pathogenic (disease-causing) recessive genes. Penrose in 1938 (see Shields and Slater, 1961), after classifying 1280 mentally deficient patients with diseases of the nervous system, suggested that recessive genes make a significant contribution to the lower grades of mental deficiency. Recessive abnormalities seem to be of earlier onset and more stable in their effects than dominant abnormalities (Shields and Slater, 1961).

Familial amaurotic idiocy, a severe mental defect which usually leads to early death; *microcephaly*, mental retardation resulting from arrested development of the brain and failure of the cranium to reach normal size; and some cases of *spastic paraplegia* have been thought to evince the characteristics of recessive inheritance (Penrose, 1954).

That *blindness* may be recessively determined has been shown by studies of the offspring of cousins, which revealed a high proportion of blind or partially blind people (Shields and Slater, 1956). Many cases of *deaf-muteness* may also be recessively determined (Shields and Slater, 1961).

Intermediate inheritance. There is no certain case of intermediate inheritance in psychological pathology. Possibly, though, one or more of the genes which are conceivably involved in the causation of schizophrenia is of this kind. For example, if a recessive gene causes schizophrenia in the homozygote (AA), it may cause only a slight (schizoid) deviation in the heterozygote (AO).

Polygenic inheritance. Although intelligence has already been used as an example of polygenic inheritance, it would be wise to expand and explain more. Roberts (1950, 1952) studied the siblings of children with low IQ scores (mean, 77.4) on the Stanford-Binet and found that the mean score of the siblings was 88.1, a significant digression towards the standard mean IQ, 100. Terman and Oden (1947) found that children whose parents had IQ's above 140 had mean scores of 128, a digression towards the standard mean. Roberts also found that siblings of idiots and imbeciles (IQ of 45 or less) showed no comparable regression. These studies seem to indicate that intelligence is polygenically inherited at both ends of the scale, except in cases where injury, disease, or abnormalities caused by dominant or recessive genes become the determining factors of intelligence.

Many feel, though, that predispositions to neuroses and some psychoses may be polygenically determined. Rosen and Gregory (1965) suggest, on the basis of correlational evidence, that polygenic inheritance is much more likely in schizophrenia than the more popular notions of dominant or recessive inheritance.

> The observed frequencies are lower than would be expected for simple recessive inheritance and much lower than expected for inheritance via a single dominant gene. The observed frequencies are more nearly consistent with a hypothesis of polygenic transmission. One of the implications of a polygenic mode of transmission is that schizophrenia could not be rapidly reduced by eugenic control as it theoretically could be if the mode of transmission were by a single dominant gene. (P. 325.)

The Limits of Prediction: A Genetic View

The search for the genetic principles which underlie much of behavior is part of the general search for laws of behavior.

Our increasing success in finding these genetic principles suggests that we will be more and more successful in uncovering the behavioral laws they help to determine. But this does not imply in any way that we will be able to predict every aspect of behavior with great ease or to exert unlimited control over behavior. If there is any single thing to be learned from a careful analysis of genetic principles and of the genetic basis of behavior, it is that every individual is unique in some important ways and that the very laws which underlie his behavior guarantee his uniqueness. As a result, there are probably built-in limits on the extent to which we shall ever be able to predict and control individual behavior.

SUMMARY

Human beings exist as members of populations that are intrinsically heterogeneous. The nature of this heterogeneity has yet to be fully described. Confining our discussion to the genotype, the following picture emerges: Human beings are a sexually dimorphic (bisexual) species. Because of the diploid nature of our chromosome sets, populations are polymorphic (have many forms) with respect to every gene that segregates and assorts by Mendel's laws. For such genes there are at least three genotypically recognizable classes: when there are two alleles to a gene, any union of gametes can produce either of two possible homozygotes or a heterozygote. Genes on different chromosomes generally assort independently of one another (Mendel's second law). The number of human genes can be conservatively estimated at no less than 10,000; even without considering linkage and crossing-over, then, man's twenty-three chromosome pairs can generate over seventy trillion different genotypes. In view of the fact that gene recombinations actually occur, however, if we assume that there is an average of only four alleles at each locus, the number of potential human genotypes reaches the astronomical figure of $10^{10,000}$!

One of the most important implications of this vast genetic potential for diversity, let alone the enormous variety of environmental conditions an individual may experience, is that laws of behavior, at best, will be more general than specific and more probabilistic than mechanical. If that is the case, much of the pleading of eugenicists for controlled breeding of human beings is scientifically as well as politically misplaced. The genetic determinants of most characteristics are so complex that we would probably either do no better with selected mates or we would purchase the genetic benefits of controlled mating in one trait with equivalent detriments in another.

In any case, the more we know about the structural basis of behavior, the more certain we become that enormous heterogeneity is built into the species. Williams (1956) has catalogued human and animal variety with respect to physiological, anatomical, biochemical, and behavioral phenotypes. He points out that in all fields of study—medicine, the social sciences, the humanities, and others—there is an unfortunate tendency to divide people into two classes, the normal and the abnormal. Implicit in our common use of *normal* is a reference to some region of a statistical distribution which is arbitrarily designated as not extreme—for example, the middle 50 percent, 95 percent, or 99 percent. We choose such a region for every trait. Anyone whose measurement puts him outside that region is therefore arbitrarily regarded as a deviate. But, as Williams says:

> If we consider . . . that among the numerous measurable attributes that human beings possess there may be many which are not mathematically correlated, we are confronted with an idea which is opposed to the basic dichotomy of normal and abnormal mentioned above. If 95 percent of the population is normal with respect to one measurable item, only 90.2 percent (0.95^2) would be normal with respect to two measurable items, and 60 percent (0.95^{10}) and 59/100 of 1 percent (0.95^{100}), respectively, would be normal with regard to 10 and 100 uncorrelated items.
>
> The existence in every human being of a vast array of attributes which are potentially measurable, . . . and often uncorrelated mathematically, makes quite tenable the hypothesis that *practically every human being is a deviate in some respects.* (1956, pp. 2–3.)

All the evidence derived from the infinite variety of genotypes (Stern, 1960) and of phenotypes indicates that each member of our species is unique, a true *individual.* In spite of this evidence, most laws of behavior—whether they are laws of learning, perception, mental disorder, or therapy—falsely assume a typical man. The fact that everyone is an individual must not be ignored when we attempt to understand causes and find cures of abnormal behavior patterns.

GLOSSARY

ACQUIRED CHARACTERISTICS, LAMARCK'S THEORY OF—the theory that physical changes made in response to the environment are passed on to succeeding generations.

ALLELE—gene form.

AUTOSOME—a chromosome other than a sex chromosome.

BEHAVIOR GENETICS—the study of the genetic aspects of behavior variations.

BLENDING THEORY—the theory of heredity that proposes a chemical fusion of hereditary materials in the offspring.

CELL MEMBRANE—cell boundary.

CENTRIOLE—one of two cylindrical bodies in the centrosphere; although their functioning is not completely understood, it is apparent that they are important cellular organelles.

CENTROSPHERE—a clear area in the cell adjacent to the nucleus and containing the centrioles.

CHARACTER—the observable effect of a gene or genes.

CHROMOSOMAL ABERRATION—nonlethal change in the structure and number of chromosomes.

CHROMOSOMES—rodlike bodies in the cell nucleus that are considered to be the seat of the genes.

CONGENITAL WORD BLINDNESS—a perceptual abnormality that causes difficulty in learning to read and write.

CONTINUOUS DISTRIBUTION—uninterrupted succession, connection, or relationship; height and weight are continuously distributed.

CORRELATE—either of two things that are related.

CORRELATED CHARACTERS—characters related in such a way that one does not occur without the other.

CORRELATIONAL ANALYSIS—method for inferring genetic bases of human traits.

CROSSOVER—the exchange between two chromosomes, of comparable parts.

CYTOLOGY—the study of cells.

CYTOPLASM—the amorphous substance of a cell, excluding the nucleus.

DAUGHTER CELLS—the two cells resulting from the mitotic division of a cell.

DNA (DEOXYRIBONUCLEIC ACID)—a chemical found in the chromosome that performs the primary function of hereditary material, which is self-replication.

DEVIATE—a person differing considerably from the average or the standard in some respect.

DIMORPHIC—characterized by two forms.

DIPLOID—having each chromosome represented twice in the nucleus.

DISCRETE DISTRIBUTION—a frequency distribution which consists of distinct, separate steps; eye color is discretely distributed.

DIZYGOTIC TWINS—fraternal twins.

DOMINANT GENE—the member of a pair of alleles that predominates and is responsible for the phenotype of a heterozygous individual; if we have two alleles, A and

O, the individual's genetic composition is AO, and if the individual exhibits the phenotype A, A is called the dominant gene.

DOWN'S SYNDROME—mongolism.

DYNAMICS—the complex forces which make behaviors moving, constantly changing phenomena.

EMPIRICAL—related to facts; based on experience; nontheoretical.

EPILOIA—a form of presenile dementia which causes brain tumors, general mental deficiency, and epilepsy.

EVOLUTION, DARWIN'S THEORY OF—the theory that living forms evolve chiefly as the result of natural selection, according to their relative abilities to survive the hardships of their environment.

FAMILIAL AMAUROTIC IDIOCY—a severe mental defect which usually leads to early death.

FEEBLEMINDEDNESS—mental deficiency or retardation.

FUNCTIONAL PSYCHOSES—psychoses believed to be caused primarily by learning and experience and not to have a large genetic, intrauterine, or physiological basis.

GAMETE—specialized sex cells: egg and sperm.

GEMMULE—in Darwinian theory, a small copy of a cell contained within each cell.

GENETICS—the laws of inheritance of traits.

GENOTYPE—the sum total of the inherited characteristics of an individual.

GOLGI APPARATUS—bodies which serve as a collection area for the synthetic products of the cell.

GONADS—sex glands: ovaries and testes.

HAPLOID—having each chromosome represented only once in the nucleus: the normal condition of gametes.

HERITABLE VARIATION—the within-species variation that is transmitted by the genes.

HETEROGENEITY—marked dissimilarity.

HETEROZYGOUS—having different alleles on the members of a chromosome pair.

HOMOZYGOUS—having the same allele on both members of a chromosome pair.

HOMUNCULUS—according to folklore, a little man endowed with magical powers.

HUNTINGTON'S CHOREA—fatal disease of the nervous system.

INSTINCT—the native or hereditary factor in behavior.

INTERMEDIATE GENE—one that exhibits the phenotypic characteristic more strongly in a homozygous individual than in a heterozygous individual; if the genetic composition AA exhibited the phenotypic characteristic A more strongly than the composition AO, A would be called an intermediate gene.

KLINEFELTER'S SYNDROME—a disorder in which individuals who appear to be males have a defective hormonal balance and underdeveloped testes.

LINKAGE—a chainlike connection between two or more genes which increases the probability that they will be inherited together.

MAJOR GENE—a gene that has a clearly distinguishable effect on the phenotype.

MEIOSIS—cell divisions which lead to the production of the specialized sex cells, the eggs and the sperm.

MENDELIAN LAW OF INDEPENDENT ASSORTMENT—Mendel's observation that the segregation of the alleles for one character occurs independently of their segregation for other characters.

MENDELIAN LAW OF SEGREGATION—Mendel's observation that genes are particulate, meaning that each genetic factor is a distinct entity that maintains its integrity from one generation to the next; the law was important because it disproved the widely held blending theory of inheritance.

MENDELISM—laws of heredity based on Mendel's principles.

MESSENGER RNA—a type of ribonucleic acid which provides for transfer of information from the cell nucleus to the cytoplasm.

MICROCEPHALY—mental retardation resulting from arrested development of the brain.

MITOCHONDRIA—rod-shaped bodies within the cell that are responsible for the conversion of the energy in nutrients into forms which can be utilized by the cell.

MITOSIS—a division of the cell nucleus into two daughter nuclei with identical chromosome complements.

MONOZYGOTIC TWINS—identical twins.

MORPHOLOGY—the study of bodily forms and structures.

MUTATION—change in the gene.

NATURE-NURTURE ISSUE—the issue of the relative influences of heredity and environment in the development of individuals.

NEGATIVE ABNORMALITIES—marked traits which have characteristically harmful effects on an individual's personal and social functioning.

NORMALITY—generally, expected, routine, or ordinary; in statistics, following a frequency distribution characterized by a bell-shaped curve; moralistically, acceptable, according to particular beliefs.

NORM-OF-REACTION CONCEPT—the idea that each genotype has its own distinctive range of phenotypes that can be developed in different environments.

ORGANELLE—an anatomically distinct cell structure.

PANGENESIS—Darwin's theory of the transmission of characteristics through sex cells.

PARTICULATE THEORY—the theory that each genetic factor is a distinct particle that can be recovered in unaltered form in the next generation.

PATHOGENIC—causing disease.

PEDIGREE—family tree, genealogy.

PEDIGREE ANALYSIS—method used for the analysis of particular genetic characteristics.

PHENOCOPY—a distinctive phenotype that develops under special environmental conditions and is characteristic of a genotype other than its own.

PHENOTYPE—the sum total of the observable characteristics of an individual.

PHENYLKETONURIA—a type of mental retardation, usually considered hereditary, that becomes evident only under certain environmental conditions.

PICK'S DISEASE—a form of presenile insanity.

PLEIOTROPY—the expression by a single gene of multiple phenotypic effects.

POLAR BODY—one of the minute bodies of an ovum that separate from it during maturation.

POLYGENE CONCEPT—a concept introduced by Mather to include quantitative characters in the framework of Mendelian principles; in the polygenic model, many different genes are involved in the expression of one phenotype.

POLYMORPHIC—having many forms.

POSITIVE ABNORMALITIES—behavior characteristics that enable an individual to function much more effectively and to contribute more to the welfare of society than the "average" person.

RECESSIVE GENE—the member of a pair of alleles that is subordinate and is not expressed in the phenotype of a heterozygous individual; where the individual's genetic composition is, say, AO, and the phenotype A is exhibited, O is the recessive gene.

REGRESSION EQUATION—a formula for computing the most probable deviation from average of one variable from the known value of another variable.

RNA (RIBONUCLEIC ACID)—a chemical that works in conjunction with DNA in the transfer of genetic information.

RIBOSOMAL RNA—a type of RNA that serves as a workbench where the proteins are assembled.

RIBOSOMES—small particles in the cytoplasm that are related to the function of the gene.

STATISTICAL VARIANCE ANALYSES—methods for determining whether the score differences of individuals within a group could have occurred by chance.

SYNDROME—a pattern of symptoms.

TABULA RASA, DOCTRINE OF—the view that the mind is a "blank tablet" at birth to be written on by experience.

TRANSFER RNA—a type of ribonucleic acid found in the cytoplasm of a cell; it has not been associated with an anatomically distinct cell structure.

TURNER'S SYNDROME—a disorder of individuals who appear to be female but have no ovaries.

X CHROMOSOME—the female sex chromosome.

Y CHROMOSOME—the male sex chromosome.

ZYGOTE—the cell formed when the sperm fertilizes the egg; the zygote is diploid.

REFERENCES

Avery, O. T., C. M. MacLeod, and M. McCarty. Studies of the chemical nature of the substance inducing transformation of pneumococcal types: Induction of transformation by a desoxyribonucleic acid fraction isolated from pneumococcus Type III. *Journal of Experimental Medicine,* 1944, 79, 137–157.

Böök, J. A. A genetic and neuropsychiatric investigation of a North Swedish population: I. Psychoses. *Acta Genetica et Statistica Medica,* 1953, 4, 1–100.

Cattell, R. B. Research designs in psychological genetics with special reference to the multiple variance method. *American Journal of Human Genetics,* 1953, **5,** 76–93.

Dobzhansky, T. *Mankind evolving.* New Haven, Conn.: Yale University Press, 1962.

Darwin, C. *The expression of the emotions in man and animals.* London: John Murray, 1872.

Eck, R. V. Genetic code: Emergence of a symmetrical pattern. *Science,* 1963, **140,** 477–481.

Erlenmeyer-Kimling, L., and L. F. Jarvik. Genetics and intelligence: A review. *Science,* 1963, **142,** 1477–1478.

Estabrook, A. H. *The Jukes in 1915.* Washington, D.C.: Carnegie Institution, 1916.

Flickinger, R. A. Cell differentiation: Some aspects of the problem. *Science,* 1963, **141,** 608–614.

Galton, F. *Hereditary genius.* London: Macmillan & Co., Ltd., 1869.

Gobineau, J. A., Comte de. *Essai sur l'inegalité des races humaines,* 1853–1855.

Goddard, H. H. *The Kallikak family.* New York: Crowell-Collier and Macmillan, Inc., 1912.

Gunther, M., and L. S. Penrose. The genetics of epiloia. *Journal of Genetics,* 1935, **31,** 413–430.

Hallgren, B. Specific dyslexia ("congenital wordblindness"): A clinical and genetic study. *Acta Psychiatrica et Neurologica Scandinavica,* Suppl. 65, 1950.

Hirsch, J. Behavior genetics and individuality understood. *Science,* 1963, **142,** 1436–1442.

Johannsen, W. Heredity in populations and pure lines: A contribution to the solution of the outstanding questions in selection. Gena: Gustav Fischer, 1903. Translated and reprinted in J. A. Peters (ed.), *Classic papers in genetics.* Englewood Cliffs, N.J.: Prentice-Hall, Inc., 1959.

Kallman, F. J. The genetics of psychoses: An analysis of 1,232 twin index families. In *Congrès International de Psychiatrie, Rapport VI.* Paris: Hermann, 1950, pp. 1–27.

Lamarck, Jean Baptiste Pierre Antoine de Monet, Chevalier de. *Philosophie zoologique,* 1809.

Mather, K. *Biometrical genetics.* London: Methuen & Co., Ltd., 1949.

Mendel, G. Versuche uber Pflanzen-Hybriden. Zwei Abhandlungen. First published in *Abhandlungen des Naturforschenden Vereines in Brunn.* Vol. IV, 1865; Vol. VIII, 1869. (Vol. IV translated as "Experiments in plant-hybridization," in *Journal of the Royal Horticultural Society,* 1909, **26,** 1.)

Morgan, T. H. Sex limited inheritance in Drosophila. *Science,* 1910, **32,** 120–122.

Muller, H. J. Our load of mutations. *American Journal of Human Genetics,* 1950, **2,** 111–176.

Neel, J. V., and W. J. Schull. *Human heredity.* Chicago: University of Chicago Press, 1954.

Penrose, L. S. *The biology of mental defect.* London: Sidgwick & Jackson, Ltd., 1954.

Roberts, J. A. F. The genetics of oligophrenia. In *Congrès International de Psychiatrie: Rapport VI.* Paris: Hermann, 1950, pp. 55–117.

Roberts, J. A. F. The genetics of mental deficiency. *Eugenics Review,* 1952, **44,** 71–83.

Rosen, E., and I. Gregory. *Abnormal psychology.* Philadelphia: W. B. Saunders Company, 1965.

Shields, J., and E. Slater. An investigation into the children of cousins. *Acta Genetica et Statistica Medica,* 1956, **6,** 60–79.

Shields, J., and E. Slater. Heredity and psychological abnormality. In H. J. Eysenck (ed.), *Handbook of abnormal psychology.* New York: Basic Books, Inc., 1961.

Sinnott, E. W., L. C. Dunn, and T. Dobzhansky. *Principles of genetics,* 5th ed. New York: McGraw-Hill, Inc., 1958.

Sjögren, T., H. Sjörgen, and A. G. H. Lindgren. Morbus Alzheimer and Morbus Pick: A genetic, clinical and patho-anatomical study. *Acta Psychiatrica et Neurological Scandinavica,* Suppl. 52, 1948.

Sohval, A. R. Chromosomes and sex chromatin in normal and anomalous sexual development. *Physiological Review,* 1963, **43,** 306–356.

Stenstedt, A. A study in manic-depressive psychosis. *Acta Psychiatrica et Neurologica Scandinavica,* Suppl. 79, 1952.

Stern, C. Principles of human genetics, 2nd ed. San Francisco: W. H. Freeman and Company, 1960.

Terman, L. M., and M. H. Oden. *Genetic studies of genius,* Vol. 4: *The gifted child grows up.* Stanford, Calif.: Stanford University Press, 1947.

Williams, R. J. *Biochemical individuality.* New York: John Wiley & Sons, Inc., 1956.

SUGGESTED READINGS

An overview of the field of genetics, particularly one that stresses the interplay of biological and cultural events is presented by:

Dobzhansky, T. *Mankind evolving: The evolution of the human species.* New Haven, Conn.: Yale University Press, 1962.

Three excellent summaries of the effects of genetics for both normal and abnormal behavior are found in:

1. Fuller, J. L., and W. R. Thompson. *Behavior genetics.* New York: John Wiley & Sons, Inc., 1960.
2. McClearn, G. E., and W. Meredith. Behavioral genetics. *Annual Review of Psychology,* 1966, **16,** 515–550.
3. Shields, J., and E. Slater. Heredity and psychological abnormality. In H. J. Eysenck, (ed.), *Handbook of abnormal psychology.* New York: Basic Books, Inc., 1961, pp. 298–343.

3

Behavior Dynamics

BRENDAN MAHER

Human behavior is the product of many complex and variable influences that are constantly combining and changing. It is this complex of influences that we must study if we wish to predict a single person's behavior in a particular situation. Four classes of information are most useful in this regard: (1) the attributes of the external situation; (2) certain stable facts about the person's biological makeup; (3) the person's past history of rewards and punishments in similar situations; and (4) his present state of motivation, that is, of "needs" or "drives."

The elements in these four groups cannot be well understood independently of each other. The biological characteristics of a person, for example, influence his susceptibility to different kinds of motivation. By the same token, the external environment may arouse particular kinds of motivation, or his state of motivation, on the other hand, may very well determine which parts of the environment he perceives. Despite this interdependence, it is reasonable to single out one factor at a time, to analyze and study it, and to consider the others in relation to it. This chapter focuses on the realm of motivational variables and their effects upon behavior.

THE MEANINGS OF MOTIVATION

The term *dynamics* in the title of the chapter is meant to convey the idea that behavior is a moving, constantly changing phenomenon. The forces that set it in motion and sustain, or "energize" it, are variously called motives, drives, or needs. Behavior itself is observable, but motives can only be inferred. We *see* a man raid the refrigerator; we only *infer* that he is hungry.

To take a more complicated example, suppose a student in a library goes to the bookshelves and starts thumbing through one book after another, examining the titles and replacing the books. He moves from book to book with increasing speed,

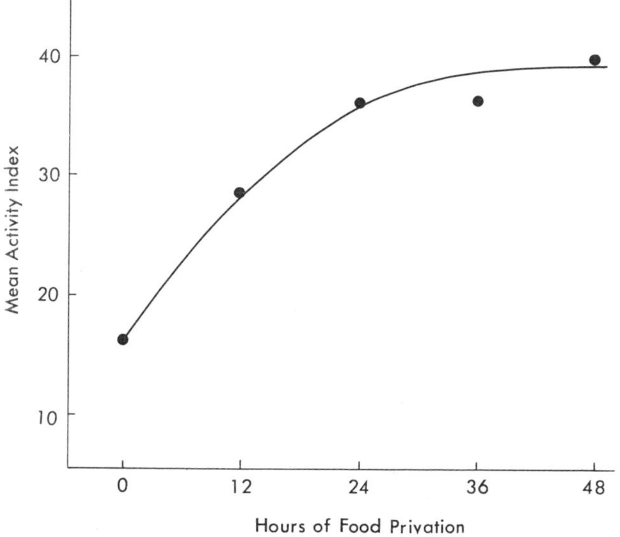

Figure 3.1 Relationship between gross bodily activity and the number of hours of food privation. From Siegel and Steinberg (1949).

then stops, scratches his head, and goes to the card index. He pulls out a card, writes a number on a slip of paper, returns to another shelf, removes a book, and then sits quietly with it in a chair.

From this sequence of acts, most observers would infer a motive: that the student "wanted" or "needed" a particular book. Failing to find it easily, he undertook a second kind of search, which succeeded. Once he had the desired object in hand, the initial sequence of behavior (searching) ended and a new sequence (reading) began.

This example indicates certain properties every motive shares: it *arouses* activity, it determines the *direction* the activity takes, and it *terminates* the activity when its object or goal is achieved. Most current definitions of motivation incorporate all these properties. For example, "Motivation is the process of arousing action, sustaining the activity in progress, and regulating the pattern of activity" (Young, 1961). Or "[Motivation is] the combination of forces which initiate, direct and sustain behavior toward a goal" (Lindsley, 1957). Both of these definitions mention the *energizing* or *arousing* function of a motive and the *directive* or *regulative* function. The distinction between the two is not merely plausible; it has actually been demonstrated in some formal experiments.

Energizing function. The simplest illustration of how motives energize behavior is the common experience of an increase in bodily activity when one is motivated. An experiment (Siegel and Steinberg, 1949) demonstrated this fact in measurable terms by showing that, when rats were deprived of food, and thus motivated by hunger, their bodily activity increased in direct proportion to the number of hours of food deprivation. Figure 3.1 shows the general form of these results without indicating the precise details of the relationship between motivation and activity, which are quite complex.

Directive function. A good illustration of how motives direct behavior, as well as energize it, is seen in "selective attention," where, for example, a hungry man is more attentive to the sights and smells of food than to other things around him. This phenomenon was studied formally by Lazarus *et al.* (1953), who found that very hungry people were quicker to identify pictures of food than pictures of other things. Here, too, although the general relationship between motivation (estimated by hours of food deprivation) and perception (speed of recognizing pictures flashed rapidly on a tachistoscope) was clear, it was complex, rather than simple and additive. Clearly, however, our motives serve to direct our attention towards some particular things in the environment and away from other things. Selective attention has the effect of limiting and guiding our responses in the direction of a goal.

The goal. We have described "motive" as that which initiates (energizes) and guides (directs) a sequence of behavior. Whatever serves to bring that behavior sequence to an end is called the goal or object of that motive. Food is the goal of the hunger motive, drink of the thirst motive, and orgasm of the sex motive. But it is important to recognize that most human motives are not so elementary as these and therefore do not have such simple physical goals. Prestige, affection, knowledge, and many other complex states may also be goals.

The particular act that achieves the goal is called the *consummative response* (eating food, attacking an enemy, copulating with a sex partner), whereas the various acts that precede consummation and make it possible are called *instrumental responses.*[1]

At this point, we may define a motive as a *state of an organism that can be inferred from behavior sequences directed towards a particular class of goals whose attainment leads to the termination of the sequence.*

Motivation as inference. Our definition suggests that since observation of behavioral sequences is the only way to study motives, the value of any measure of motivation depends on how well it *assesses* or *predicts* those sequences. One measure of hunger is only *better* than another, for example, if it predicts precisely the eating or food-seeking behavior that we observe. Motives, in fact, are ideas or *constructs* which represent our conceptions of the relationship between certain measurable events. These events fall in two classes; one may be called *antecedent* or *input* events, and the other may be called *consequent* or *output* events. In hunger, things like the number of hours of food deprivation, amount of weight loss, and changes in the blood sugar level and the rate of stomach contraction can be classed as input events. Speed and strength of seeking food, the persistence of the search, and the gusto with which it is eaten once it is found, on the other hand, are instances of output events.

All these events are susceptible to measurement by one means or another. The "input" events, often manipulable and measurable in the laboratory, might be considered loosely *to cause* the sensation of hunger. "Output" events, on the other hand, change or vary only as a result of input changes, and might therefore be said *to be caused* by hunger. We can measure the events that occur "before" and "after" hunger, and by way of these measures arrive at a network of relationships to which we assign the shorthand name: *the hunger motive.* When we call the motive a "force" that "drives" the individual, we are only speaking figuratively; it is misleading to use this sort of language literally, as some motivational psychologists tend to do. The study of behavior dynamics is largely concerned with unraveling the relationships between input and output events and with understanding the processes which mediate or govern them.

To understand human behavior, we must distinguish between two broad classes of motives: (1) motives which seem to originate in the biological nature of the human species, and (2) motives which appear to derive from the individual's own experience, especially within a particular culture. The first group is called *biological* or *primary* motives, and the second has been variously labeled *learned, acquired, social,* or *secondary* motives. You will recall from the previous chapter, however, that a person's appear-

[1] Notice that *response* here is synonymous with *behavior*. This usage is common in technical writing about psychology; it emphasizes the general belief of psychologists that behavior does not occur spontaneously and inexplicably, but is always stimulated by something.

ance and behavior—his phenotype—is determined by the interaction of his biological inheritance, or genotype, with the environment. This says, in effect, that there is a biological component even in the learned motives. To be more accurate, therefore, we shall label as *biological* those motives in which biological factors are the major determinants of behavior, and as *biosocial* those motives in which biological variables play only a relatively minor part.

THE BIOLOGICAL MOTIVES

The biological motives include the avoidance of hunger, the avoidance of pain, and the need for sexual release. Most scientific knowledge about these motives, like our knowledge of genetics, comes from experiments with animals (see Chapter 2), but we shall try to present human data wherever possible. As with breeding, we cannot exert the same degree of control over the motives of human beings as over those of animals, especially with respect to such elemental needs as hunger, freedom from pain, and sexual gratification. And since the validity of our measures of motivation depends on their agreement with observed behavior, we must be very cautious about inferring the motivations of human beings from the observations we make of lower organisms.

Hunger

When a living organism is deprived of food for very long, certain bodily changes take place. These are (1) contractions of the digestive tract, (2) reduction in the level of blood sugar, and (3) increased activity in part of the central nervous system. Each of these variables is an input event for the hunger motive, but their correlation with food-seeking behavior is complex.

Gastric contractions and behavior. It is popularly believed that hunger is caused by, or depends upon, stomach contractions, but this is not true. Wangensteen and Carlson (1931) describe a patient who underwent a total gastrectomy (stomach removal), but reported afterwards that he felt hunger sensations just as usual. Rats whose stomachs were removed, moreover, responded to food deprivation with the same "hungry behavior" as normal controls (Tsang, 1938). This general finding has been separately confirmed by Bash (1939) and by Morgan and Morgan (1940), who even after severing the nerves from the stomach to the brain found that their subjects acted as if they were hungry.

Stomach contractions do have something to do with hunger, however; Quigley (1955) has shown that increases in food deprivation are accompanied by increasing stomach contractions. The fact of the matter seems to be that stomach contractions are not a *necessary* input event for the hunger motive, but rather one of several variables that usually combine to produce hunger.

Blood sugar level. Many experimenters have found that increases in the level of blood sugar are followed by decreases both in stomach contractions and in subjective feelings of hunger (Carlson, 1916; Stunkard and Wolff, 1954, 1956; Mayer and Bates, 1952). Evidently, a decrease in the blood sugar level is another event in the complex network of input variables for hunger.

Central nervous system. The brain, through the hypothalamus, seems also to take part in the control of eating. Hypothalamic surgery on laboratory animals produces overeating (hyperphagia) or undereating (aphagia), depending on the location of the surgical incision or lesion. Brobeck (1955) suggests that one part of the hypothalamus (the lateral) activates hunger while another (the medial) inhibits it. Thus, when food is eaten, the body instructs the brain to depress appetite by both actively inhibiting the medial hypothalamus and failing to stimulate the lateral hypothalamus. As the food is metabolized and its nourishment dispelled, these bodily signals disappear and hunger is no longer inhibited. Food is sought and eaten, and the cycle is repeated.

Again, the process is more complex than that. Animals with brain lesions causing aphagia can relearn normal eating habits if they are kept alive by artificial feeding until the habits are formed. Like gastric contractions and blood sugar, the nervous system is not the exclusive regulator of hunger, but only one part of the network of input variables.

Food deprivation and weight loss. The two input events most frequently used to study hunger are duration of deprivation and amount of weight loss. Both are easy to manipulate and both correlate highly with the output events that characterize hunger. By controlling them, it is possible to make very accurate predictions of an animal's eating behavior, its general activity level, and the amount of pain (electric shock) it will withstand to reach food. There is, as one might expect, a strong relationship between weight loss and eating (Ehrenfreund, 1959) and between weight loss and general motor activity (Moskowitz, 1959; Treichler, 1960).

Hunger and learned modifications. So far we have talked about hunger as if it were a simple biological fact, but anybody who tends to be overweight knows that hunger is anything but simple. The evidence shows that its effects upon behavior are greatly changed with experience. Thus, when rats are placed on a regular deprivation schedule with feeding at the end of each period of deprivation, after only a few sessions they will eat a stable amount of food each time instead of gorging as much as possible. One investigation (Lawrence and Mason, 1955) adds the observation that if the experimental feeding period coincides with an accustomed mealtime, the animals will eat more than if the feeding is dissociated from regular mealtimes.

Most people tend to have regular mealtimes, and many of us often eat out of habit without feeling particularly hungry. It seems reasonable to say that eating behavior can be evoked by external stimuli, like a noon whistle, as well as by internal ones, like a playful hypothalamus. A regular schedule of eating can serve as a training regimen, as illustrated by the finding of Cofer and Appley (1964) that eating increased after deprivation if an animal *anticipated* feeding.

Hundreds of animal studies, beginning with Pavlov's famous dog, indicate that many aspects of behavior that seem to depend on biological hunger can be induced by outside, goal-related stimuli. Hunger has often been cited as the prototype of a biological motive, but even so fundamental a motive as this is related to behavior by many complicating mediating links, some biological and some learned. At least as many complications will show up with the other motives we consider.

Pain Avoidance

When a living organism experiences or anticipates pain, certain behavior takes place. A response that removes the sufferer from the pain is called *escape behavior*, while a response that prevents contact with anticipated pain is called *avoidance behavior*. Avoidance is usually learned very quickly in response to events that have previously been associated with pain. Our purpose here is to study the motivation for avoidance behavior and to see how it works.

Virtually all studies of pain have been done with laboratory animals, the most popular components being a caged rat, a light or buzzer, and an electric shock. In a typical situation, a buzzer sounds for a few seconds before the electric shock is turned on. During this buzzing period, a door opens, permitting the rat to get out of the cage before he gets shocked. After a few shocks, the animal learns to head for the exit as soon as the conditioned stimulus (the buzzer) starts to sound. The initial escape response had an obvious biological basis in the internal effects of pain; but somehow the rat learns to continue the response when there is no painful input, but only a buzzer. One explanation of how this learning occurs might be that the buzzer has developed the power to elicit some of the painful bodily changes produced by the electric shock—enough to bring about an avoidance response. Such changes occur mainly in the *adrenergic* or *sympathetic* division of the autonomic nervous system, and include, for example, an increase in heart rate and a reduction in skin resistance.

The trouble with this explanation is that autonomic changes occur much more slowly than avoidance responses. Solomon and Wynne (1953) found that dogs react to conditioned avoidance stimuli at a high rate with no sign of autonomic changes. But autonomic changes are not the only effects of pain. Simple sensory input to the brain probably occurs instantly, or at least more rapidly than the motor avoidant responses, and the buzzer may produce the reaction by means of this process. But because it is almost impossible to measure these events, there is no empirical support for either hypothesis, and the behavior remains unexplained.

Regardless of how it gets learned in the first place, once avoidance behavior is learned, it is very difficult to "extinguish," or remove. Extinction is normally achieved by removing the reinforcements or rewards that have followed a particular response. For the hunger motive, for example, a food-seeking behavior would be extinguished by seeing to it that the response in question does not lead to food. But it is more difficult to extinguish habits of pain avoidance, for the individual never waits to find out that the pain is no longer there: the animal in our example is safely out of the cage as soon as the buzzer sounds and will never know that the shock would not follow after all. There are three ways of attempting to extinguish conditioned avoidance behavior. One is restraint—for example, closing the exit. A second is to provide a strong approach stimulus to compete with the avoidance one—for example, giving a reward such as food when the buzzer sounds. A third is to punish the avoidance response—for example, shocking the animal if he *leaves* the cage. The latter two methods create a conflict of motives that fosters its own problems, as we shall see later in discussing conflict. In the case of everyday human behavior, all three methods are very difficult to arrange practically. Restraint, especially, is not readily available. Under the circumstances, it is not surprising to find that fearful avoidance behavior may be continued when it is no longer appropriate.

We shall examine the implications of inappropriate avoidance behavior in discussing anxiety later in this chapter. For now, we should note mainly that much motivation for avoidance behavior is acquired or learned, even though the basis of this behavior rests with our biological disposition to avoid painful experience.

Sex

Some psychological theorists, especially psychoanalytic ones, regard sexual motivation as fundamental to most others, especially to social or acquired motives. In Western society, sexual behavior is subject to many restrictions and is strongly punished under all but a few specific, socially accepted circumstances. Thus, it is no surprise that children develop conflicts about sexuality and that some later maladjustments can be traced to these conflicts.

The biological sources of the sexual motive, especially the internal stimuli that elicit sexual behavior, are even more complicated than those involved in hunger and pain avoidance. Understandably, therefore, the interactions of the sexual organs, the brain, and the sex hormones with human sexual behavior are more complicated too, and the modifications that learning exerts are even greater on sex behavior than on hunger or avoidance.

Sexual biology and behavior. The general relationship of sexual biology to behavior seems to be that sex organs and hormones play their major role in the development and initiation of sexual activity rather than in maintaining it. This is less clearly the case with the brain.

The bulk of evidence on the role of the genital organs indicates that sexual behavior survives their loss provided that the individual was sexually experienced beforehand. Money (1961) reviewed cases of patients who had lost external sex organs and found that both arousal and orgasm continued to occur even in paraplegic patients who had no neural connections between their genitals and brains.

Investigations of the behavioral effects of sex hormones point up even more clearly how important learning is to the sex motive. If pituitary and gonadal hormones are given to animals, increased sex activity results or, where none existed before, sex activity begins. But castration, the reverse of hormone dosage, only reduces sexual activity in animals who have not had sexual experience. The hormones are necessary, in other words, to start sexual responses, but once the responses have been learned, they may be maintained even without hormonal activity. In the higher species, in fact, and most of all in human beings, changes in sex hormones are not likely to change established sexual behaviors very much. Ford and Beach (1951) found that impotent men were not helped by doses of androgen (a male sex hormone), while male homosexuals who were given androgen showed increased sexual arousal—but only toward their homosexual partners!

In lower species, at least, the brain does little to hinder sexuality—especially in females! Beach (1940, 1943) found that rats, cats, and guinea pigs can copulate as usual with large parts of the cortex destroyed. This is less and less true, however, as we climb the phylogenetic scale. In humans, contrary to the opinions of the parents of American college students, the higher brain centers are very much needed for sex.

Learning factors. From the detailed studies of Kinsey *et al.* (1948, 1953), we know that specific patterns of sexual behavior differ significantly among different social classes and from one human culture to another. Beach has pointed out the role of external stimulation in producing sexual arousal in people, emphasizing the fact that sexual responsiveness may become conditioned to specific partners, particular locations, or other special stimuli. In general, adult human sexual behavior is greatly modified by learning, in which endocrine factors are much less important and brain centers much more important than in animals. These conclusions appear to apply more to males than to females, however, perhaps partly because men lack the cyclic sexual biology which menstruation universally imposes on women.

Sexual activity and guilt. Studying the sex motive, we must take into account how guilt complicates sexual behavior. In our culture, severe punishment for early signs of sexual interest may make people fearful and conflicted about sex later in life. In some cases, not only are overt responses (such as masturbating or reading "dirty books") punished, but so are evidences of sexy thinking and fantasy (having a "dirty mind"). The punishment of sexual fantasy is typically quite a different thing in our society from the punishment of a drive like aggression. *Overt* aggressive acts are often punished, as are overt sex acts, but a child is rarely punished for having an "angry mind." Consequently, one is less likely to avoid thinking about hostile topics than about sexual topics. The effects of such punishments upon future conflicts are explored later in this chapter.

We have seen in our discussion of the biological motives that hunger, pain, and sex all have learned components. Let us turn now to a consideration of motives that are *primarily* learned and do not stem directly from known biological sources.

THE BIOSOCIAL MOTIVES

In sexual motivation, learning plays an important part in determining the choice of goal, the kind of response, and the likelihood of any response at all. But the form of the consummative response itself—that is, copulation with a partner—is comparatively stable across many cultures and, indeed, across many species. This is true of hunger and pain avoidance as well, so that we can make some gross predictions about behaviors motivated by hunger, pain avoidance, and sex regardless of the specific effects of learning in any given case. Psychologists are also interested, however, in the dynamics of many kinds of behavior for which biological determinants seem to be minimal or lacking. Such motives as power, achievement, affiliation, dependency, prestige, and security have all been studied in many ways.

These motives are called *learned, acquired,* or *social* to emphasize the importance of socially determined rewards and punishments in shaping the behavior patterns that stem from them. The problem for psychologists has been to identify consistent patterns of response that would define each acquired motive. The motive of dependency, for example, might be inferred from a great many items of behavior, like actively seeking help, suffering distress when left on one's own, or readiness to obey a leader. For all these responses to reflect a single motive, however, they must be elicited by the same stimulus with great consistency in the same person. In other words, the likelihood that one response will occur should be highly correlated with the likelihood that others in the group will occur. Otherwise, each response would represent a different motive, and it would be meaningless to assign the entire group to a single motive.

The high intercorrelation of response patterns within individuals is only one of the typical characteristics of biosocial motives. Typically also, when one of the responses in a pattern is blocked, it is more likely to be replaced by another response from the same pattern than by one from outside the pattern. By the same token, if one goal is unattainable, another goal of the same general type is likely to be substituted. People differ, for example, in their power motives, that is, in the strength of their need for power. A person who wants political power very much would probably first seek it by open election. But if that fails, and the motive is strong, he may turn to another power-seeking response, such as violence. On the other hand, if the goal of political power is unavailable, he may turn to other power-related goals, such as economic or administrative power. In any case, all of these alternative responses and goals can clearly be assigned to a single motive—power.

Learned motives and satiation. Hunger is typical of biological motives in that food *satiates* it; after eating, in other words, the motivation is reduced. Learned motives do not always parallel biological ones in this way. On the contrary, attainment of the goal often elicits new stimuli that serve to increase the original motive. Winning a minor position of power brings the person into closer contact with people holding positions of even higher power, and thus greater power seems desirable. The changes in consumption habits that come with increased wealth expose the newly successful person to more expensive styles of living than he may ever have desired, but he then strives to achieve them.

This paradoxical situation, where attainment of a goal serves to intensify rather than satisfy the drive, applies more to positive or "approach" motives than to negative or avoidance motives. We want more of things we desire in the first place (our motivation is increased), but when we can successfully avoid a fearful or unpleasant situation, our concern about it diminishes (the avoidance motive is reduced).

The strength of learned motives. The study of personality is very much concerned with assessing the strength of learned motives in individual cases. The strength of biological motives can be measured, as we have seen, by manipulating input variables, such as duration of deprivation, and measuring output, such as activity levels. But for learned motives the input variable is generally less clear because it does not reside in the immediate tissue needs of the individual but in the history of rewards and punishments that have led to the acquisition of the motive. This cannot be measured easily. To assess it, the investigator must try to concoct an input situation which will arouse the motive and to select some appropriate response which will permit him to measure its strength. Generally, he must attempt to evoke a moderate "amount" of the response, because if he uses too much or too little stimulation, he will obtain no measurable differences between subjects: either all or none of them will respond. In measuring anxiety, for example, we do not want to scare everybody, nor do we want to amuse everybody. We want to present a threat of intermediate strength and see who gets scared—and how much—and who does not. The strength of anxiety in any individual is then measured by the amount of threat needed to evoke a response, or by the amount of response elicited by a certain threat.

The origin of learned motives. By definition, a newborn infant has no learned motives. The learning that occurs during infancy must be guided or mediated by rewards and punishments relating to the biological motives. The only tools of control a parent has are to give or withhold food, to change or fail to change wet diapers for dry, to alleviate or inflict pain, and to provide or fail to provide the comforts of physical contact and personal presence. By manipulating these tools, a parent may establish long sequences of learned behavior in the child. These processes will be dealt with later.

In practice, we may study learned motives without knowing about the biological situation in which they emerged. We say that a learned motive has been established whenever a goal evokes consistent responses that are not connected to any biological drive. For example, if parental approval initially was required for satiation of a hunger drive ("You can't have your dinner unless you behave"), then the development of a learned need for approval is demonstrated when the person responds to a new situation where the only goal is approval. The fact that it originated in connection with food is of minor importance at this point.

Early investigators of acquired motives sometimes had very limited notions of the possible range of unlearned motives; they often assumed that things like needs for physical affection or parental closeness arose because of their connection with feeding during infancy. Today this view is questioned because of evidence showing that needs for physical contact and affection are themselves biological and do not depend on learning for their origin. Rewards and punishments are just as effective in developing learned motives when connected with these needs as with hunger or pain.

Before we take a detailed look at some learned motives, we will examine the general subject of how motives, which energize behavior, are themselves aroused.

MOTIVATION AS AROUSAL

The State of Arousal

When an individual is responding to a stimulus, we say that he is in a state of *arousal,* or *activation.* The source of stimulation may be external, as pain often is, or it may be internal, as hunger always is. The responses that define arousal fall into three general categories: autonomic, cerebral, and behavioral. In a sense, we may say that the individual is always in some state of arousal as long as he is alive, because responses are always going on in his brain, autonomic system, or behavior. Sleep and deep coma represent the lowest extremes of a continuum of arousal states.

The state of arousal depends on a very complex series of events in the nervous system. Our understanding of these events has been made easier in recent years by the discovery that a single brain structure appears to control them; it is called the *reticular formation.*

The reticular activating system. Some years ago two neurophysiologists, Maruzzi and Magoun, discovered that when very mild electric stimulation was given to the reticular formation in the brain stem of a sleeping cat, the animal woke up. Electrical recordings taken from the brain showed that it was going through the same changes that occur when an animal wakes up normally. This discovery led to the speculation that the reticular formation was responsible for activating the animal's cerebral cortex, and so it was named the *reticular activating system* (RAS). It was already known that all incoming sensory nerve tracts had connections with the reticular formation in addition to their connections with the brain cortex, but Maruzzi and Magoun were the first to shed light on what was happening there.

It now appeared that the RAS was the "switchboard" responsible for alerting the cortex to the fact that a sensory message was coming. That is, an incoming sensory impulse—visual, tactile, and so forth—would not only go directly to the appropriate area of the cortex, but would also pass through the RAS, which would arouse wide areas of the cortex to receive the impulse. The general form of this sequence is shown in Figure 3.2.

In addition to its arousing function, the RAS also includes an inhibiting mechanism which sees to it that some stimuli are selectively screened out and do not arouse a response. This makes it possible for a mother living in the middle of a large city to sleep peacefully through continual traffic uproar but to awaken instantly if a child cries. The arousing and inhibiting functions of the RAS work together to bring about many familiar features of behavior.

The first behavior we are likely to notice in someone receiving a stimulus is that he will stop, look, and listen; that is, he will pay *attention.* Doing so involves the inhibition of one line of activity and the activation of another. Another term for this same sequence is the *orienting response* (or orienting reflex). The orienting response is the basis of curiosity and to some extent of all learning, which makes the discovery of its physiological key in the reticular activating system of great importance.

If a stimulus is repeated often enough, it gradually loses its power to arouse the

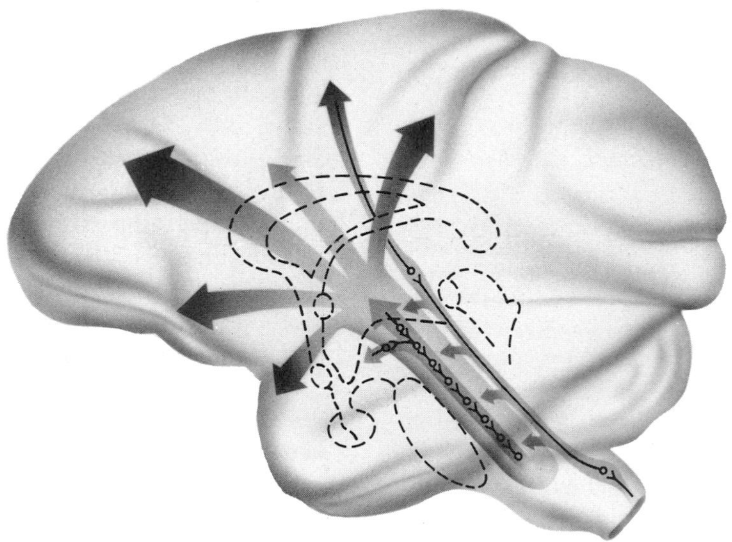

Figure 3.2 Lateral view of the monkey's brain, showing the ascending reticular activiating system in the brain stem receiving collaterals from direct afferent paths and projecting primarily to the associational areas of the hemisphere. From H. W. Magoun, "The ascending reticular system and wakefulness," in J. F. Delafresnaye (ed.), *Brain Mechanisms and Consciousness*, 1954, F. A. Davis, Philadelphia.

organism, and we say that *adaptation* has taken place. The adapting mechanism makes it possible for us to ignore irrelevant aspects of our environment and to get on with important things. Adaptation is at least as important as attention in enabling us to behave in an integrated way. The mechanism that controls adaptation is the inhibiting function of the RAS. It is important to realize that adaptation is not simply a matter of the arousal system "running down"; rather, it involves the active prevention of a response. Jasper (1958) explains it this way:

> The function of the reticular system in normal adaptive or integrative behavior may be more in the nature of a prevention of a general arousing reaction to all stimuli, with a control of selective responsiveness to significant stimuli. . . . This implies that inhibitory rather than excitatory functions may be most important, either during sleep or wakefulness (P. 322.)

Our discussion of arousal began with a statement that the stimulation may be either external or internal. The adaptation process must work differently for these two classes of stimuli, however. After all, we do not respond to continued hunger by getting used to it. Obviously, inhibition of such biological stimuli would not be good for the survival of the individual or the species, and so the adaptive mechanism must somehow be capable of differentiating the kinds of stimulation it repeatedly experiences.

Measures of Arousal

Several methods of producing and measuring arousal are in use in the laboratory. One is electrical stimulation and another is administration of certain drugs, notably amphetamine and atropine. The processes for measuring arousal differ for each response category: autonomic, cerebral, and behavioral.

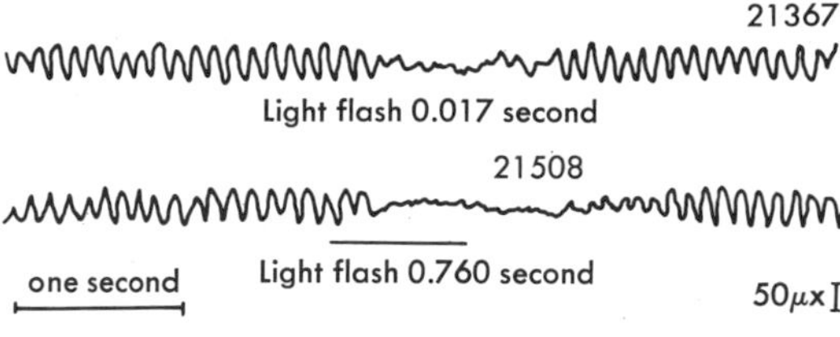

Figure 3.3 Alpha rhythm "blocking" by light. From Donald B. Lindsley, "Electroencephalography," in *Personality and the Behavior Disorders,* edited by J. McV. Hunt, copyright 1944 The Ronald Press Company, New York.

Autonomic bodily changes related to arousal are studied chiefly by two devices. The most familiar of these is the *polygraph,* colloquially (and wrongly) known as the lie detector. A more recent device is the miniature radio transmitter, which permits a process called *telemetry,* that is, measuring from a distance without hooking the subject up to wires. These devices are sensitive to perspiration, electrical conductance of the skin, changes in heart rate and blood pressure, muscle tension, and respiration rate—all common correlates of arousal.

Cerebral measures of arousal depend chiefly on the *electroencephalograph* (EEG), an instrument for measuring electrical activity on the surface of the brain. As a person passes from deep sleep to high alertness, there are consistent changes in the forms of his brain waves, and these changes are recorded upon a graph such as the one pictured in Figure 3.3.

Behavioral measures of arousal are taken by observing a person's general activity level and by noting the presence of the orienting response. Irwin (1932) observed that infants are increasingly active as time passes between feedings. The same has been observed of hungry animals (Hall and Hanford, 1954); here, even more activity takes place if the hunger is accompanied by external sensory stimu-

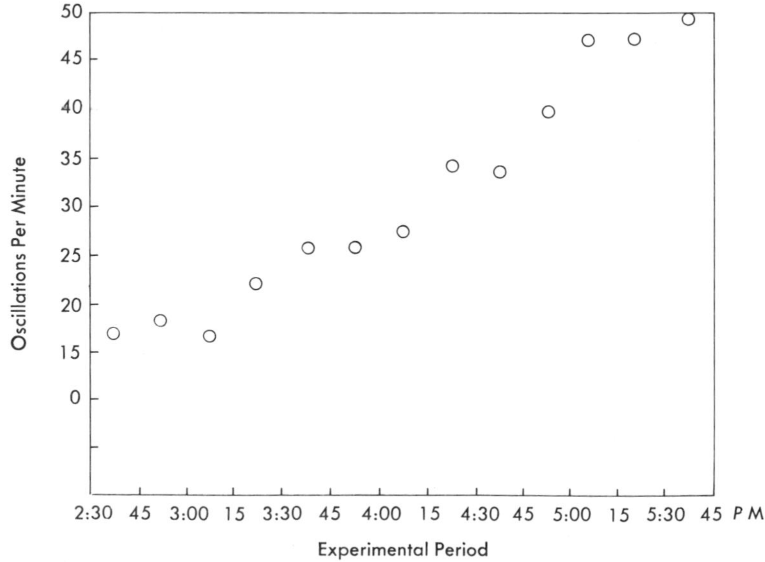

Figure 3.4 Motility of seventy-three infants between two consecutive feedings. From Orvis C. Irwin, "Changes in activity between two feeding periods," in *Readings in Child Psychology,* Ed. 2, Wayne Dennis, Editor, © 1963. Reproduced by permission of Prentice-Hall, Inc., Englewood Cliffs, New Jersey.

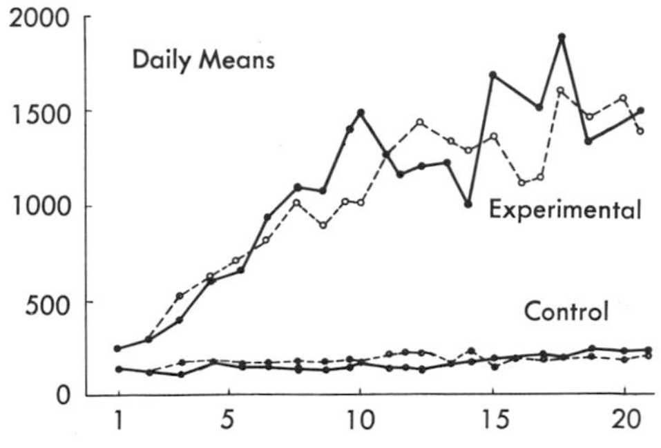

Figure 3.5 Mean daily running activity, in percentage of base rate. Data from two experiments. From Hall and Hanford (1954).

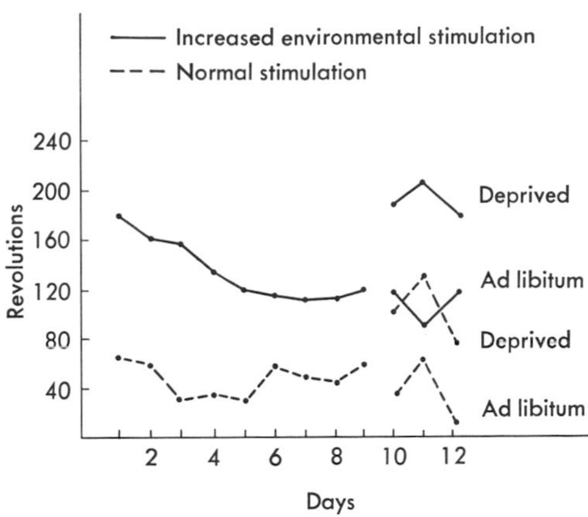

Figure 3.6 Effect of increased environmental stimulation and food deprivation on activity. Reprinted by permission from *Psychology of Motivation* by John F. Hall, published by J. B. Lippincott Company. Copyright © 1961 by J. B. Lippincott Company, Philadelphia.

lation (Hall, 1956) (Figures 3.4, 3.5, 3.6). Pavlov in 1910 observed the orienting response when his dog typically pricked up his ears and turned toward the source of sound.

Individual Differences in Arousal

The measurement of arousal brings us to the question of whether there are stable individual differences in arousability. This question takes several forms. We may ask whether the details of a person's autonomic response pattern are stable, and we may be concerned with differences in *arousal threshold,* that is, the amount of stimulation required to produce an arousal response, regardless of its exact pattern.

Investigations of individual differences in autonomic arousal have used the concept of *autonomic response specificity,* or tendency of the same autonomic components to respond uniquely to various stress situations. Lacey and his colleagues (Lacey, 1950; Lacey *et al.,* 1953) found that individuals tend to respond with maximal autonomic activation in the same physiological system, whatever the arousal stimulus. In addition, there is a strong tendency for the entire pattern of autonomic activation to be reproduced from one stressing stimulus to another. They describe this phenomenon as follows:

> The autonomic nervous system does indeed respond to experimentally imposed stress "as a whole" in the sense that all autonomically innervated structures seem to be activated, usually in the direction of apparent sympathetic dominance. But it does not respond "as a whole" in the sense that all autonomically innervated structures exhibit equal increments or decrements of function. Striking intraindividual differences in the degree of activation of different physiological functions are found when the different reactions are expressed in equivalent units (Lacey *et al.,* 1953, p. 8.)

Similar findings of specificity have been reported by Wenger (1948) and Malmo (1959), and profiles of response patterns to different stresses by Bindra (1959) and by Schnore (1957).

But negative evidence comes from Kaelbling *et al.* (1960), who, after an exhaustive analysis of a variety of autonomic responses in twelve tested and retested subjects, were unable to find stable specific patterns. Their experiment is important because it raises the question of individual differences in the threshold for arousal. An experimental stress that is intense for one subject may not be so for another. Under extreme stress, in fact, response specificity tends to disappear altogether. It is quite possible that reliable differences among response patterns can generally be found only under moderate stresses. Under very high or very low conditions of arousal, all responses may be uniformly high or low.

Experimental investigation of this kind of proposition has been difficult because of the obstacles to producing intense stresses in a laboratory. However, with the advent of telemetric methods for monitoring autonomic responses at a distance, the possibilities of gaining data on this issue have improved immeasurably. In general, there are two ways in which we might evaluate a person's response to stress. First we may use the peak level reached by a response; for example, we note that heart rate reached a peak of 120. Secondly, we may ask to what extent this figure differs from the average response in the general population. Both of these measures may be used intelligently by comparing them to the initial resting value of the measure (the value before exposure to stress)—thus, a gain of ten heart beats per minute may have a different meaning when the resting rate is seventy than when the resting rate is forty-five. Complex scoring devices have been developed for both kinds of measure. According to Lacey's terminology, the absolute gain is recorded as an *autonomic tension* score, while the relative changes are termed *autonomic lability* scores.

Arousal and Fantasy

We have been discussing arousal as a biological state, but it is important in psychological phenomena as well. Aroused motivational states are commonly accompanied by fantasy or daydreaming. Experimental investigation of fantasy has relied largely on the use of thematic tests: the subject tells a story about pictures that are shown to him, and the story is examined for content relating it to the motive under scrutiny. Such experiments usually involve manipulation of the subject's motivational state by deprivation or other means. His thematic responses are then compared with those of nonmotivated control subjects.

Fantasy productions are frequently used as a measure of motive strength. The major work on this topic has been done by David McClelland and John Atkinson and their associates and has been primarily concerned with measuring learned motives such as achievement and power. But in the first such study of importance hunger was the motivational variable. Atkinson and McClelland (1948) deprived subjects of food for one, four, and sixteen hours and then asked them to write stories about six pictures involving food—eating, deprivation, and so forth. The stories were scored for various kinds of imagery, and the general conclusion was that an increase in food imagery accompanied increased deprivation.

Power as a motive, and its effects upon fantasy, has been studied by Veroff (1957), who tested the fantasy productions of candidates for university student government positions while they were awaiting results of the balloting—when their power motivation presumably was maximally aroused. He compared the results with those of controls tested in a classroom situation and found, as expected, that the election candidates told more stories with power motive content.

Achievement motivation has been investigated in the same way as power. One early study of achievement involved presenting subjects with a task and varying the explanations of its purpose. One group was told it was helping to provide normative data for some graduate students, another that scores reflected leadership ability, intelligence, and so forth. After completing the task, the subjects wrote stories about a series of pictures, and

Table 3.1

Effect of Relaxing versus Achievement-arousing Instructions on Production of Achievement Fantasies[1]

	Relaxed ("You are helping to provide data for graduate students.")	Achievement-arousing ("Your scores reflect leadership and other related abilities.")
Achievement-related themes	63.5 percent	84 percent
Unrelated themes	36.5 percent	16 percent

[1] From Atkinson's *Motives in Fantasy, Action and Society*, © 1958, D. Van Nostrand Company, Inc. Princeton, New Jersey.

the stories were scored for content related to achievement, deprivation, obstacles, and the like. The percentages of these themes produced under the two different conditions of achievement arousal are shown in Table 3.1, which indicates a relationship between fantasy themes and the different instructions the experimenters gave.

The foregoing examples indicate a fairly simple relationship between fantasy and the aroused motive state. When the behavior normally evoked by a motive has previously been punished, however, a more complex relationship develops between the strength of the motive and the content of the fantasy. Examples of this relationship are found in studies of the fantasies people give when they are sexually aroused or in aggressive states.

Direct and overt expression of *sexual* fantasy is generally susceptible to social disapproval, if not legal punishment. We should consequently expect, when sexual motives are aroused, that overt sexual themes will be avoided unless the environment is one that has permitted or reinforced overt sexual discussion in the past. An important demonstration of this relationship has been reported by Clark (1952, 1955), who recorded the stories of male college students. One group was shown life-size slides of nude females in a classroom, while another group was shown the same slides at a fraternity beer party. Both groups were evidently aroused sexually, but the group in the classroom was presumed to be in an environment where overt sexual fantasy might be punished. As expected, stories told under classroom conditions were low in manifest sexual content while those told in the fraternity situation had considerable overt sexual content.

Many more examples could be cited here, but the point should be quite clear: motivational arousal serves to shape the intensity and the content of fantasies, unless punishment is associated with overt expression of the motive.

SOME CENTRAL HUMAN MOTIVES

Thus far, we have discussed motivation in general, identifying the broad categories of biological and biosocial motives and describing how all motivation may be viewed as arousal. While observation and measurement of arousal contribute to our understanding of how all motives operate, we have yet to examine some specific motives that make up the rich network of human behavior. We turn now to some of the major learned motives in human behavior, particularly guilt and aggression. These motives are important in the development of several negative behavior deviations and are therefore of special interest to students of abnormal psychology. We then discuss dependency and the need for achievement and competence, the first because it is generally important in human development, and the second because it exemplifies the kind of motivation which underlies the positive abnormalities.

Anxiety

It is easy enough, when we see someone trembling and fearful, or listen to him talking about his fears, to understand that his behavior is motivated by anxiety. But for the most part, people experience anxiety in subtler and more refined ways, making it necessary to infer anxious motivation from a number of different kinds of response. There appear to be four classes of response that indicate anxiety. These are (1) overt behavior that takes the person away from some stimulus; (2) bodily changes, chiefly in the autonomic nervous system; (3) involuntary movements, such as trembling; and (4) subjective feelings of fear or worry, which may be reported verbally to an observer.

If a psychologist wishes to discover how anxiety motivates behavior, he must have at his command a good measure of anxiety. All four kinds of anxious response can be tapped for useful information, but none of them is entirely adequate to the subject. Consequently, the investigator usually uses a variety of observations drawn from several of the response classes. By pooling or combining several measures, he hopes to approximate an understanding of anxiety more closely than any single one would allow.

The problem of measurement is perhaps more critical with anxiety than with any other central human motive, not because anxiety is more difficult to study than others, but because it may be more important. As will become apparent to some extent in the next chapter and next section, but even more in the chapters on functional negative abnormalities (neuroses, psychoses, and the like), it is widely believed in the mental health professions that anxiety is the key motivation of much psychological disorder. Many explanations of the origins of these disorders attribute them to unsuccessful attempts to deal with anxieties, and many important therapeutic methods are essentially techniques for uncovering anxiety or otherwise dispelling it. With all of this attention (by now almost three generations of it), it is still not very clear exactly how anxiety works. That problem, as you can see, is largely one of measurement. Most of our discussion will be concerned with the effort to track anxiety down.

Anxiety Measures

Investigators have developed three kinds of instruments to get at the four kinds of anxious responses described. These are: (1) *verbal measures,* including formal questionnaires and projective tests; (2) *biological measures,* which include both drugs and polygraph recordings, and (3) *behavioral measures,* which measure nonverbal responses.

Verbal measures. By far the best known verbal measure of anxiety is the Taylor (1956) Manifest Anxiety Scale (MAS), a questionnaire on which the subject answers *true* or *false* to several statements of self-description. The statements, selected from the Minnesota Multiphasic Personality Inventory (MMPI), include items which experienced clinicians believe to indicate anxiety, such as physical tension, feelings of apprehension, and many common worries. Some typical items are

I worry over money and business. (True)
I hardly ever notice my heart pounding and I am seldom short of breath. (False)
I shrink from facing a crisis or difficulty. (True)

Each item answered in the anxiety direction (indicated here in parentheses) receives one point, and the total is the subject's anxiety score.

The Manifest Anxiety Scale has been used principally in two ways. One has been to compare it with other measures of anxiety. When such comparisons yield high correlations, we say an instrument has high *concurrent validity*, which means simply that it tends to get at the same thing some other instrument does. The MAS has been compared both with physiological measures (Runquist and Ross, 1959) and with other verbal measures of anxiety (Korchin and Heath, 1961) and the correlations have tended to be statistically significant, but not terribly high.

Another use of the MAS, and that for which psychologists have found it most valuable, is the prediction of certain kinds of behavior that we could logically expect to be related to anxiety. Successful predictions of this kind establish for a test what is called *construct validity*. Taylor (1956) has pointed out that the MAS may be used as a measure of anxious motivation and that predictions about learning may be made from it. In fact, most studies of the effect of anxiety on behavior have concerned the relationship of high MAS scores to learning and performance, and some interesting general findings have been reported. Of particular interest are the ideas that people high in anxiety acquire conditioned defensive responses faster than those low in anxiety and that there is a generally positive, though complex, relationship between high anxiety level and high efficiency in learning and performance. The experiments on conditioned defensive responses have used very simple measures, like the speed with which eye blinking can be conditioned, and have not always shown precisely the same effect (Bindra *et al.*, 1955). The relationship between anxiety and efficiency, moreover, varies with things like the complexity of the task to be done. Overall, efficiency increases as motivation increases up to a point, but decreases beyond that point as the task becomes more complex or difficult, perhaps because, as Sarason (1960) observed, complex tasks may be somewhat threatening even when no special noxious stimulus is involved. The disorganization of behavior that occurs in complex tasks thus may be due, at least in part, to their inherently stressful character.

Experiments with the MAS illustrate that, apart from its relationship to fear and avoidance behavior, anxiety may also be seen as an instance of high arousal that shares some of the general properties of arousal.

True-false statements are not the only verbal measures used to study anxiety. Renner *et al.* (1962) have devised a sentence completion test for this purpose. In it, the subject completes some sentence stems in any of several ways and is scored according to how much anxiety his sentences reflect. For example:

I feel:	tense, from too much worrying.	2 points
	uneasy when I first enter a crowd.	1 point
	fine.	0 points
I can't:	concentrate very well.	2 points
	seem to find myself.	1 point
	play the piano (other specific skill).	0 points

High scores indicate high anxiety. The validity of this kind of test has been assessed by correlating it with other measures like self-descriptions, descriptions by friends, and the MAS. Such correlations, while statistically significant, have indicated some relationship but not a great deal (Maher and Repucci, 1964).

Projective tests like the Rorschach inkblot test have also been used as measures of anxiety. *Shading* responses on the Rorschach test, in which the subject likens the inkblot stimulus to "clouds" or "smoke," require a minimum of imagination and are thought by many users of the Rorschach to reflect anxiety. Empirical evidence to support this conclusion is still lacking, however, and the general value of projective tests for studying anxiety is still uncertain.

Biological measures. Anxiety is biologically measured in two ways. In one, threatening stimuli, or "stressors" are applied to individuals and the bodily changes that result are measured. Another approach looks for bodily responses that are correlated with verbal expressions of anxiety or with overt avoidance behavior. Most investigators use combinations of these measures for different purposes. In general, biological aspects of anxiety are more complicated to measure than verbal aspects because the biological systems involved are many and complex.

When a person faces a threatening situation or the stresses of fatigue, extreme temperatures, or bodily injury, certain physical changes occur. One of the major biological systems involved in generating these changes is the *pituitary-adrenal axis.* The pituitary gland secretes several hormones whose chief function is to produce reactions in different bodily organs and systems. One of these, adrenocorticotropic hormone (ACTH), is released by threat or by stress and stimulates the *cortex* of the adrenal gland (next to the kidney). The same threat or danger simultaneously activates the sympathetic division of the autonomic nervous system (ANS), which arouses the adrenal *medulla.* In both instances, hormones are released into the blood stream that produce a variety of local effects all over the body. Bodily response to danger or to anxiety can thus be measured either by the amount of these substances in the blood, by the amounts of their metabolites, or byproducts, excreted in urine and other body fluids, or more directly by local effects at many sites on the body surface.

When stimulated by ACTH, the adrenal cortex produces substances called *corticoids,* whose major function seems to be regulation of inflammatory reactions to infection or wounds. Their presence is indicated by the secretion of certain metabolites in the urine, chiefly two types of compounds called 17-ketosteroids and 17-hydroxycorticosteroids. Stress, among other things, brings about an increase in both of them.

A second physiological consequence of stress is the reduction in number of a type of blood cell known as *eosinophils,* so that lowered eosinophil count is an additional measure of stress. Yet a third measurement involves the storage of adrenal ascorbic acid, which is depleted as a result of stress. This measurement can be made only with animals, however, since present techniques for obtaining it require the destruction of the adrenals, which is always fatal.

When the adrenal medulla is activated, it secretes three substances called *catecholamines.* Two of them, epinephrine and norepinephrine (adrenaline and noradrenaline), are important to us. Increased epinephrine production causes heart rate to speed up, the peripheral blood vessels to constrict, the bronchia of the lungs to dilate, the contractions of the stomach to stop, the mucosa of the nose to dry, and the pupil of the eye to enlarge. Some of these changes can be measured by the polygraph, an instrument for recording autonomic changes related to arousal.

Many polygraphic measures reflect general arousal, however, and it is difficult to define specific response patterns for anxiety that distinguish it from other emotions, such as anger. Some observations of such distinct patterns have been reported by several investigators, though, especially in studies using the drug Mecholyl.

Mecholyl causes a rapid drop in blood pressure that is soon followed by a return to normal levels. Several types of reaction to this drug are known (Funkenstein, 1955), but our main interest concerns two reaction patterns that occur when the injection of Mecholyl is preceded by an injection of epinephrine or of norepinephrine. When epinephrine precedes the Mecholyl, the fall in pressure is slighter and the recovery is more rapid than when norepinephrine is given. Funkenstein found that when normal subjects, not under drug influence, were verbally ridiculed, some became angry with the insulter while others reacted with self-blame and anxiety. He called the former pattern "anger-out" and the latter "anger-in" or anxiety. Angry subjects showed the typical noradrenaline pattern when they were given Mecholyl, while anxious ones produced the adrenaline response. Ax (1953) found essentially similar results when he exposed subjects to the threat of an electric shock from an allegedly defective circuit. But in Ax's experiments, the same subjects showed different biological reactions to fear and to anger. When frightened, the epinephrine response was prominent; when the same person was angry, the norepinephrine response was prominent. Thus, even though one or the other catecholamine may dominate in a person's system and may dictate his response in situations where either anger or fear is possible, his experience of the second emotion is mediated by the dominance of the second chemical.

We have attempted to offer a brief outline of the major trends of work in this area, in part because such work constitutes an important part of present research in behavior dynamics and in psychopathology, in part also because we all know that there are physiological concomitants to anxiety. But the issues are by no means clear. In the first place, despite the intense search, few differentiators between one emotional experience (say, fear) and another (say, anger) have been uncovered. And in the second, where one experimenter has found differentiators, others have not been able to replicate or reproduce them.

The current state of research in this area has led some writers to consider that anxiety is a joint function of *both* physiological arousal *and* cognition. Schachter and Singer (1962) demonstrate, for example, that mere elevation of epinephrine in the circulatory system does not at all guarantee the experience of anxiety, *unless the person is in anxiety-provoking circumstances.* The same elevation of epinephrine, if it occurs while one is watching a funny movie, yields joy and hilarity; on a lovely moonlit evening, with an attractive date, it might yield attraction, even love. Epinephrine, by itself and in neutral circumstances, provokes no affect at all.

The significance of this approach is that it questions the utility of searching for specific differentiators of emotion and tries, rather, to find the joint physiological and cognitive determinants. Where there is no cognition, as in the neutral circumstance mentioned above, there will be no affect. And where there is no physiological arousal, there can be no affect either, regardless of how powerful the cognitive aspects are. Thus, it is possible that psychopathic criminals experience little anxiety, not because they are blind to the realities of their circumstances, but rather because they have a very high threshold for physiological arousal (Schachter and Latané, 1964).

Behavioral measures. The main nonverbal behavioral indications of anxiety are avoidance responses. Because it is difficult to measure direct physical movement away from a situation, research on this issue has concentrated upon avoidance in the sense of misperception or denial. Maher and his students (Otto, 1963; Menaker, 1964) have studied such avoidance responses with a device which shows pictures of stimuli that vary in their degree of repugnance. The subject can turn off the pictures by means of a simple switch connected to a timer. Tension-producing pictures tended to be turned off very quickly. Examples of high- and low-tension pictures are given in Plate 1, together with the average viewing times they elicited.

It is much more complicated to cope with threatening stimuli which cannot be "turned off" directly. Lazarus *et al.* (1951) played recordings of sentences having either sexual, aggressive, or neutral content, at the same time hindering audibility by means of static. Accuracy of recognition was measured, as well as the appearance of hostile and sexual themes on a sentence completion test. Two general patterns of response emerged: one group was much less accurate in its perception of sexual or hostile sentences than in its perception of neutral ones, while subjects in the other group were *more* accurate in their perception of these presumably threatening items. The investigators termed these two groups *repressors* and *intellectualizers* respectively. Clearly, we cannot infer anxiety in any simple fashion from two such opposed patterns of response, even if one of them is frankly avoidant!

The problem that faces the psychologist here is that the individual is likely to have adopted as habit any one of many different responses that have in the past rid him of anxiety or reduced it to bearable proportions. On the face of it, sensitivity to anxiety-arousing stimuli instead of denial of them seems to be self-defeating; it seems to indicate an approach to threat rather than an adaptive escape from it. Byrne (1966) has suggested that such sensitivity is just as indicative of maladjustment as denial is and therefore just as indicative of anxiety. No clear rationale has yet been developed to account for this, however, and it is still difficult to see how the approach response of the intellectualizer could be a measure of anxiety.

Throughout the foregoing discussion, we notice that there are two implications about the concept of anxiety as a human motive. It is assumed to be arousable by certain kinds of stimulus, and it is also assumed to differ from one person to another, so that some will respond anxiously to stimuli that others will consider relatively harmless. Some measures, such as the MAS and the sentence completion test, depend on the subject's ability to report a kind of *chronic* anxiety pattern. Others, especially biological measures, tend to generalize from the subject's responsiveness to *specific* threats presented by the investigator. For most purposes, and especially for understanding psychopathology, the development of chronic anxiety is of major theoretical importance, and we shall now consider some of the major hypotheses on this point.

Origins of Anxiety

Most ideas about the origins of anxiety are derived from some theory of conditioning or learning. Perhaps the most widely accepted hypothesis is that anxiety originates in the fear that accompanies pain or the threat of pain. If so, all the anxiety of the adult human being would be a special instance of conditioned reactions to pain, and the laws governing its development or extinction could be studied in the laboratory with the use of painful unconditioned stimuli like electric shock as the major tool.

Anxiety and pain. There is no doubt that pairing a neutral stimulus with a painful stimulus produces autonomic bodily changes in the subject, rapid learning of any response that ends the pain, and avoidance of the hitherto neutral (now conditioned) stimulus on future occasions.

This laboratory model of avoidance learning parallels clinical aspects of anxiety in many respects, but it is still only an experimental analogue. Anxiety responses also occur when there is no evidence of previous painful stimulation. Wild animals, for example, show avoidance and escape behavior and other signs of distress when faced with predators even though they have had no previous painful experience with the predator. Similarly, distress responses occur in newborn humans startled by a loud noise, or when physical support is suddenly removed.

The strongest evidence against the pain-anxiety hypothesis, however, is provided by cases of congenital analgesia, a disorder causing complete insensitivity to pain from birth. This condition (apparently of genetic origin) may lead to burns and injuries because its victim has not learned to avoid stimuli that are painful to the normal person. But since Kessen and Mandler (1961) point out that children with the disorder develop anxieties nevertheless, it is difficult to defend the idea that all anxiety develops from some original *painful trauma.*

Anxiety and the inhibition of distress. Kessen and Mandler (1961) have suggested the term *fundamental distress* in connection with their theory of the origin of anxiety. Their position is described as follows:

> It is our contention that a non-traumatic theory of the sources of anxiety can be defended and, further, that anxiety may be reduced or terminated by devices other than escape from or avoidance of threat. These alternative formulations are proposed as a supplement to, rather than substitutes for, the archetypical theories of anxiety.
>
> The schematic model suggested here for the occurrence of anxiety in distinction from the classical model of the organism fleeing the association of pain is the cyclical distress of the human newborn. There may be antecedent events which could account for the crying and increased activity we recognize as distressful in the young infant—for example, food privation, shifts in temperature and such—but *it is not necessary to specify or even to assume such a specific antecedent event.* (P. 399.)

Viewing the distress of the human newborn as a fundamental phenomenon which does not require explanation in terms of some prior event, Kessen and Mandler suggest that some specific fears which do not get conditioned to *pain* are actually conditioned forms of *fundamental distress.* Distress is a condition which accompanies many other conditions of the organism besides pain. When a child is cold, he is also distressed; similarly, when hungry, he is distressed, and when pained, he is distressed; in fact, *any state of need or drive may be accompanied by distress.*

This model assumes, clearly, that physical states such as hunger, cold, or pain, are separable from distress, so that, in any such painful situation, the individual's response pattern will include some responses which are made to the condition itself and some which evidence the distress accompanying it. They also propose, however, that certain special events have the power of inhibiting distress and that these inhibitors reduce distress regardless of the situation that generated it. Examples of such specific inhibitors are non-nutritive sucking in the newborn (for example, sucking on a rubber nipple stuffed with cloth—a "pacifier"), being rocked, seeing an adult face, and various kinds of rhythmical stimulation. In the presence of these inhibitors, distress responses tend to be reduced, but when the inhibitor is removed, distress returns unless it is prevented by some new calming state, like sleep.

By the usual processes of conditioning, any stimulus which has been associated with the action of a specific inhibitor might acquire *secondary* inhibitory properties; that is, it might gain some inhibiting power of its own. The sight of the rocking chair, for example, might become a conditioned distress inhibitor, tending to soothe the person much as rocking itself originally did. Likewise, neutral stimuli associated with the termination of a specific inhibitor might acquire the power of eliciting distress. These proposals do not replace or contradict the pain-anxiety theory, but they offer a broader range of situations that may be operating to produce human anxieties than the traditional pain-anxiety model does.

Anxiety as overarousal. Still another hypothesis comes from Malmo (1957), who has suggested that clinical anxiety is a "disease of overarousal." Prolonged exposure to arousing stimulation, he argues, may lead to critical change in a person's capacity to inhibit arousal. As indicated in the discussion of arousal earlier in this chapter, *inhibition* refers to an active process, not simply to the "absence of arousal."

Brief elevations in the level of arousal ordinarily are followed by inhibition and the return of the arousal level to the resting state. Malmo hypothesized that continuous and protracted arousal leads to an overuse of the inhibitory mechanisms that ultimately weakens them. He suggests that inhibition is mediated by a chemical "transmitter" substance which loses effectiveness in prolonged anxiety. From his model, we should expect that arousal measures would not distinguish between anxious and nonanxious subjects when both groups are in a resting state. The occurrence of arousal stimuli, however, should produce differences between them.

Malmo also observed that pathologically anxious subjects should respond anxiously to any arousing stimulus, whether or not it resembles those which generated anxiety in the first place. Cameron (1944) illustrates the same point:

> It will be noted that nearly all such patients [with anxiety states] complain that they cannot go into crowded places or into any situation where sustained efforts will be required of them. Their symptoms are made more severe by anything which elicits emotional reactions, such as altercations or participating in a discussion of illness. Nearly all find, at least at first, that their symptoms are increased by visiting their former places of employment or meeting fellow workers. In other words, their symptoms are exacerbated by anything which serves to increase tension. *Emphasis should be placed on the fact that their symptoms are* ***elicited*** *or* ***intensified****, not primarily by the reactivation of any conflict situation which may exist, but literally by everything in the course of the day which serves to increase tension.* (Pp. 56–57; italics added.)

A related observation of interest here is that a critical change in the inhibitory process after prolonged arousal may permit arousal to occur at levels of stimulation too low to arouse a normal subject. Clinical or pathological anxiety then would be characterized by a low threshold for arousal and an extremely slow return to a resting state.

While these three hypotheses do not by any means exhaust current thinking about the origins of anxiety, they are typical of the models used, and the kinds of problems posed by the phenomena of anxious behavior.

Guilt

The concept of guilt has been used for a long time to explain some kinds of negative abnormalities, particularly disorders involving states of depression, but it has not received very careful scientific attention until quite recently. Most discussions of guilt relate it to the concept of *conscience* or, in psychoanalytic terms, *superego*. Conscience is aroused when a person commits some act he knows is forbidden or fails to perform some act to which he is obligated; the activity of conscience then produces feelings of guilt.

This description parallels the private experience of most people, but it does not tell us very much about the nature of guilt or of conscience. The important problems in this connection are: How does conscience develop and operate, and what are the effects of guilt feelings on human behavior? The details of the developmental process are attended to in Chapter 4, and the consequences of conscience and of guilt for positive and negative behavior patterns, respectively, are described in discussions of character (Chapter 8) and of the functional neuroses and psychoses (Chapters 10 and 11). We shall only introduce the subject here by indicating some definitions and problems connected with analyzing and understanding these central but complex motivations.

The Criteria of Conscience

Sears *et al.* (1957) have suggested three criteria that indicate conscience in a child. These are (1) *resistance to temptation*; (2) *self-instruction to obey* the rules of behavior; and (3) *overt evidence of guilt* when the child has broken the rules. These behaviors, they say, indicate that a child has "internalized" control which was previously exercised by external punishments and rewards.

The idea of "internalizing control" is essentially picturesque but not really explanatory. Behavior is controlled by stimuli which may occur in the environment of the child, may be provided by his own actions, or may occur as internal bodily responses such as emotions. Hill (1960) has given a particularly penetrating analysis of the three criteria of Sears *et al.* from the viewpoint of current knowledge of learning. Let us examine these.

Resistance to temptation. We say that a person demonstrates resistance to temptation when he fails to approach a stimulus that entices him but that is regarded as wrong or immoral by his culture. For the failure to approach to qualify as "resistance to temptation" rather than simple avoidance, not only must the stimulus be enticing, but the behavior should occur even when there is little chance that actual punishment would follow yielding. In other words, the person must decline to perform the act even though he believes he could "get away with it." From a learning viewpoint, the most probable interpretation of this kind of behavior would be that the approach response is inhibited by some aspects of the stimulus situation that really have been connected with punishment in the past, even if these aspects are not obvious to an observer or to the individual himself. Resistance to temptation would thus be a special case of avoidance learning in which the cues for avoidance are concealed. The child who has been punished for stealing may have a chance to steal something under circumstances where detection is almost impossible. He may become anxious and inhibit the response as soon as he recognizes that the thing is desirable, or when he is planning how to steal it, or when he actually makes some preliminary moves toward doing so. The point at which he becomes anxious in such a sequence depends largely upon the typical point at which he has been punished in the past. If punishment has been infrequent and long delayed, resistance to temptation may not develop at all.

Self-instruction. Hill (1960) suggests that self-instructed obedience to moral principles is learned from the verbal principles which parents enunciate. The major principle to account for such learning is *imitation*, or *vicarious learning*. A child may fail to learn this kind of self-instruc tion either because the principles are never verbalized to him by parents or because conditions necessary for imitating his parents did not exist. For this reason, children raised in foster homes or institutions which provide no stable parental figure to imitate may have more difficulty than others in learning moral principles.

Overt evidence of guilt. The term *guilt* really refers to several different behaviors, including emotional (visceral) responses, verbalizations of guilt feelings, and perhaps most important, a tendency to seek punishment. One would think that people always try to avoid punishment, and seeking punishment sounds paradoxical. If we consider, however, that in many situations, especially in the lives of children, punishment is followed by the restoration of affection or some other token of forgiveness, then we can understand how seeking it is analogous to the behavior of an experimental animal who crosses an electrified floor in order to reach a goal beyond it. A child's misdemeanor is often followed by scolding and the withholding of love until some punishment has been inflicted and endured. If this sequence has occurred often enough, the child may learn that, upon performing some forbidden act, the easiest way to retain his parents' love is to confess, take whatever punishment is given, and "get it over with" without delay. The expectation of rejection and seeking of punishment following the breach of a moral rule is what the individual himself would describe as the feeling of guilt.

When a child grows up and leaves home, he may still feel guilt for violating parental rules even though he no longer risks punishment. To relieve this guilt, it is sometimes necessary to confess or to seek punishment, or both, even to the extent of punishing oneself if no substitute parent (such as society) obliges. If it becomes clear, however, that no punishment is forthcoming for certain kinds of adult immorality, the anticipation of punishment gradually weakens until it is extinguished; a necessary ingredient of the feeling of guilt thus disappears. For most adults, guilt is likely to be maintained at an adaptive level, increasing or diminishing in proportion to the real likelihood of punishment.

Pathological guilt. The foregoing analysis has used the principles of avoidance learning, but it does not differ very much from the conception of guilt offered by psychoanalysts. Psychoanalytic writings have been concerned mostly with "pathological guilt," that is, the behavior of persons who seem repeatedly to seek punishment but gain only momentary relief from it. Hendrick (1934) summarizes the psychoanalytic position thus:

> Analysis . . . discloses that a painful experience may be unconsciously self-induced, for many individuals find it easier to endure a pain inflicted from without than to withstand the pressure of unconscious phantasies, which, if they do break into consciousness, are perceived as torments of conscience or feelings of worthlessness. For example, a man who suffers the abuse of an "impossible" spouse may be praised by his comrades for his goodness in enduring all and sacrificing everything for her, while analysis reveals that she is endured because the suffering she causes satisfies such an unconscious "need of punishment." Sometimes it will be observed that the death or divorce of such a spouse results in a marked exacerbation of a psychoneurosis, which previously had been absent or mild, because the unconscious guilt was satisfied by the marital suffering. (Pp. 70–71.)

The continual endurance of punishment in social or interpersonal situations does not prove that the victim is suffering from guilt, but we can see that a person who repeatedly breaks some social prohibitions might well have a history of punishment-seeking.

Empirical research on the problems of guilt is far less advanced than work on the comparable problems of anxiety. The nature of the analysis presented here, however, suggests that such research should focus on the cognitive components of guilt, much as research on anxiety is focused on the autonomic components of anxiety. The visceral components of guilt are probably the usual elements of autonomic arousal, but verbal descriptions of anxious and of guilty feelings may differ in important respects.

Hostility and Aggression

Psychologists have given considerable attention to hostile and aggressive behavior. By aggression we mean behavior *intended* to injure or distress another person, not behavior in which injury is incidental to the attainment of some other goal. Symbolic or substitute forms of aggression, like telling aggressive stories or drawing aggressive looking pictures, are often studied in research on this subject. The main questions addressed by such research and by theories of aggression is how stimuli acquire the power to arouse aggression, and how aggression, once aroused, is expressed.

Aggression as a response to frustration. One of the classic hypotheses about the instigation of aggressive behavior was advanced by Dollard *et al.* (1939) in a monograph entitled *Frustration and Aggression.* Based on some earlier ideas of Freud, it argued that aggression is a consequence of frustration. Frustration in turn is defined as anything that interferes with "an instigated goal response at its proper time in the behavior sequence" (see Figure 3.7). There are many possible sources of interference with attainment of a goal. Obstacles may be external—something may physically prevent one from reaching his goal; they may be internal—the goal object may be forbidden and the approach thus hindered by fear of punishment; or the individual may lack the skill or talent to reach his goal and thus meet continual frustration in his effort.

These kinds of frustration do not necessarily lead *only* to aggression. Berkowitz (1962) classifies six different responses to frustration:

1. Reversion to some other goal once preferred at an earlier stage of development (*goal regression*).
2. Shifting to earlier immature techniques to secure the frustrated goal (*instrumental-act regression*).
3. Constructively seeking alternate routes to the goal.
4. Repetition of the ineffective technique (*fixation*).
5. General behavioral disorganization resulting from anxiety aroused by the frustration.
6. Attack upon the frustrating obstacle (*aggression*).

The frustration-aggression hypothesis proposes that frustration tends to instigate aggression by stimulating the motivational state we call "hostility." Whether or not aggressive behavior actually occurs, however, and the form in which it occurs depend upon a number of other factors, like fear of retaliation or punishment.

These observations make necessary some modification of the original frustration-aggression hypothesis (Dollard *et al.*, 1939), which assumes that "aggression is always a consequence of frustration" (p. 1) and that "the occurrence of aggressive behavior always presupposes the existence of frustration" (p. 1). But questioning both these assumptions provides some focal criticisms of the hypothesis.

The first problem is whether or not all aggression can be attributed to frustration. For one thing, it is difficult logically to prove that something cannot happen (in this case, that aggression cannot occur unless produced by frustration). Sec-

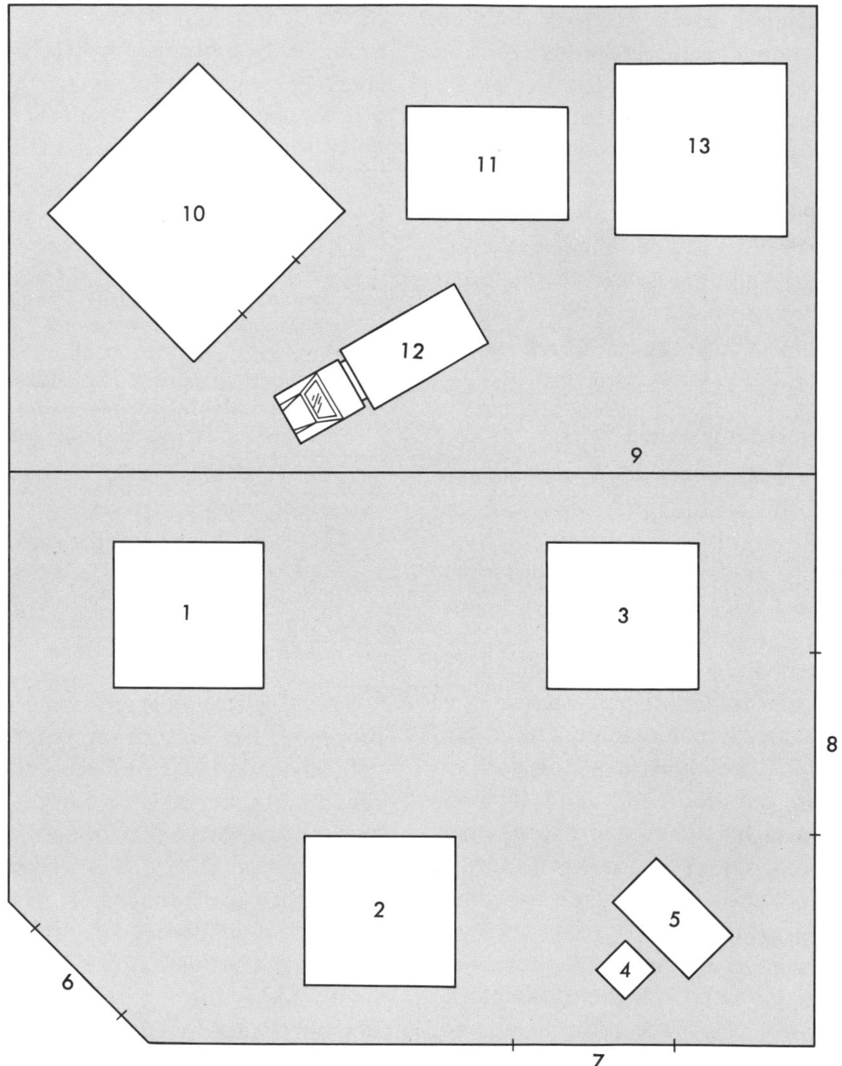

Figure 3.7*a*. In the Barker, Dembo, and Lewin frustration experiment, children are first allowed a period of free play in an area containing *1*, square of paper with child's chair, teddy bear, doll, cup, small truck and trailer, saucer, teapot, ironing board and iron, and telephone receiver; *2*, square of paper with box of crayons and two pieces of writing paper; *3*, square of paper with motor boat, sail boat, duck, frog, and fishing pole; *4*, the experimenter's chair; *5*, the experimenter's table; *6*, observation screen; *7*, entrance door; *8*, window; *9*, partition functioning as a wall. After a time the partition (9) is lifted, and the children are exposed to *10*, toy house with doll, chair, teddy bear, bed, ironing board, iron, telephone, stove with cooking utensils, cupboard, electric lights, curtain, and carpet; *11*, tea table with tea set; *12*, large truck and trailer; *13*, lake with real water containing an island with lighthouse, wharf, ferry boat, small boats, fishes, ducks, and frogs. Later the children are called back into the first area, and *9* becomes a transparent partition that permits *10* to *13* to be seen but not approached.

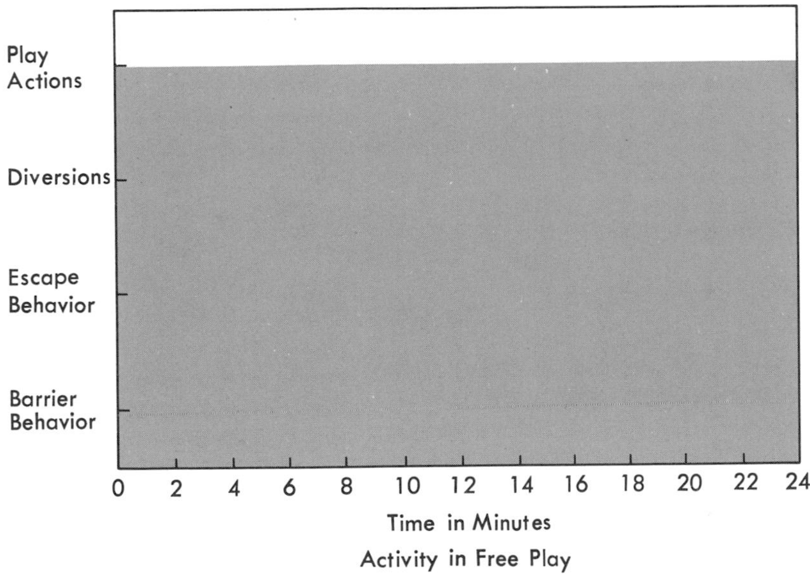

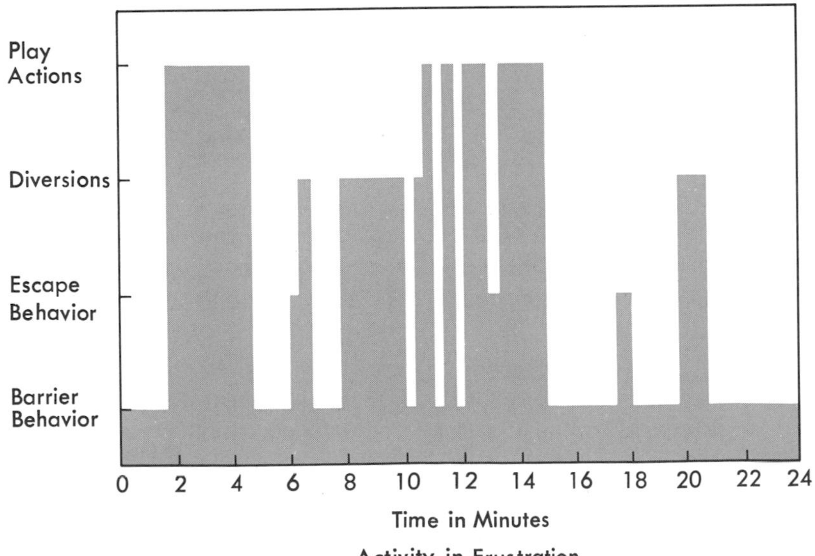

Figure 3.7*b*. Charts of the behavior patterns of one child during the free play and the frustration (or last) situation. *Barrier behavior* is behavior related to the barrier, or partition between the two areas. From *University of Iowa Studies: Studies in Child Welfare*, 1941, Vol. 18, No. 1.

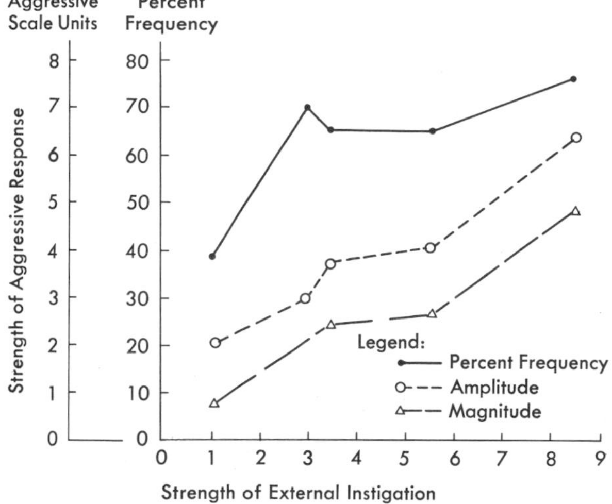

Figure 3.8 Strength of the mean aggressive response, measured by the percentage of frequency and by amplitude and magnitude as a function of the strength of external instigation. From Graham *et al.* (1951).

ondly, the identification of frustration itself is not easy. Karl Menninger, a severe critic of the frustration-aggression hypothesis, commented that "anyone who has had his toe stepped on, which is certainly not a frustration, knows how inadequate such a formula is" (Menninger, 1942). But Berkowitz has pointed out that it is far from clear that anyone suffering this kind of incident will react with aggression. If the stepped-on toe produces some blow to the victim's sense of self-esteem, or interferes with something he was doing, it would fit the frustration-aggression hypothesis, as it would if it was seen as a deliberate attack upon the victim's security and hence a frustration of his security needs. The measurement of these variables in any given case is exceedingly difficult, and it is not possible to accept Menninger's criticism as crucial to the general validity of the frustration-aggression hypothesis.

One of the earliest studies stemming from this hypothesis was reported by Miller and Bugelski (see Dollard *et al.*, 1939), who asked subjects to work with partners. The partner, however, was a confederate of the experimenter and did his share of the work in an ineffective and disruptive manner. As a result, the real subjects made many self-deprecatory remarks and showed lower self-esteem scores on a personality scale. These results were interpreted as showing that frustration produced aggression directed towards the self rather than the frustrating partner. Similar evidence of inward-turned aggression has been provided by studies from the World War II Office of Strategic Services (1948) and by Lindzey and Riecken (1951). Evidence of externally directed aggression has been provided by a few studies. Graham *et al.* (1951), for example, presented a list of incomplete sentences to a group of adolescent subjects. Each sentence began with a phrase indicating frustration, like "He hit me, so I. . . ." These partial sentences were grouped according to how much frustration they implied, and responses to them were rated for the amount of aggression they revealed. The general hypothesis, of course, was that the more frustrating the sentence, the more aggression would be revealed in the response. Figure 3.8 shows the general conformity of the results to the hypothesis.

In yet another study, Sears *et al.* (1940) imposed strong frustrations upon a group of men who thought they were subjects in an investigation of fatigue. The men, all habitual smokers, were required to stay awake all night and were not permitted to smoke. The experimenters also imposed arbitrary restraints on activity, conversation, and other ways of passing the time and even promised a meal that was never provided. All the men manifested aggression toward the experimenters to the extent that drawings made by one of the subjects showed violent and murderous themes.

Many other studies have been conducted along similar lines, and their findings have generally been that aggression follows frustration. Even so, Miller (1941) modified the somewhat extreme position of the original hypothesis to recognize that there are other, nonaggressive consequences of frustration. Moreover, several studies have failed to find aggression following frustration (for example, Pastore, 1950, 1952; Zander, 1944). Pastore observed that frustration was most likely to lead to aggression when the subject felt it was arbitrary rather than inevitable. For example, more aggressive reactions resulted from a situation in which the subject is told, "You are waiting for a bus at a marked bus stop and the driver intentionally passes you by," than from one in which the subject is waiting for a bus which turns out to be on its way to the garage.

The reaction a person has to a frustrating situation clearly depends very much on his previous learning concerning such situations and the means by which aggression can be expressed. Let us examine this now.

Learning aggression and its inhibition. In a general sense, aggressive behavior is disapproved in Western society. The prevailing philosophy expressed in this culture is that personal differences should be settled by discussion and negotiation, without violence or coercion. Like all such principles, this one is applied in practice only with certain modifications. Aggression against parents and figures of authority, against very weak or helpless persons or animals, and against the unintentional frustrator is particularly unacceptable. Among males, at any rate, aggression towards a peer of the same sex is often tolerated. In defense of society, it is even honored, and in defense of the individual in limited cases is approved or tolerated. It may be acceptable to attack an adult who is damaging your property deliberately, but it is not generally acceptable to attack the same adult if he is simply taunting you verbally. Society not only provides a scale of permissible targets and occasions of aggression; it also provides a scale of acceptable expressions of aggression for any given situation. The probability that any frustration will elicit an aggressive response towards a given target is subject to considerable personal control as a result of our having individually absorbed these social scales with their constraints.

Under some individual conditions, as well as in theoretical defense of society, it is not only permissible but desirable for a victim to display retaliatory aggression against an attacker. Male children are especially subject to fairly consistent social pressure from both peers and parents to maintain vigorous and courageous physical defense against attackers, even though this idea runs counter to the philosophy of negotiation and nonviolence. Cowardice is often operationally defined by the norms of our society as the refusal to manifest *justified aggression*. Thus, the small boy who must learn not to attack his smaller brother when the latter hits him must also learn to fight back when a neighborhood boy does the same thing. In the latter event, he not only will be safe from punishment, but is likely to be praised for his manliness.

Clearly then, the individual must learn some careful discriminations between who may and who may not be attacked, and under what circumstances. The form of these discriminations may vary enormously with factors like the social class to which the child belongs and the individual standards and values of his parents.

There are many contradictions even within social class lines. Ours is essentially a middle-class society, for example, but some middle-class parents are very punitive towards their children's aggression, while others, either from fear that restricting "natural aggression" by punishment will harm a child's personality development or on the general principle that children should not be punished, refuse to punish aggression altogether. Children from the second kind of family still learn to discriminate, however, between permissible and unacceptable aggressions, but the discriminations are taught them by subtler means than simple punishment.

Whatever the teaching method, individuals develop characteristic degrees of readiness to respond to specific situations with aggression; we may therefore usefully look upon "hostility" or "aggressiveness" as a personality trait with characteristics that are mainly determined by prior learning experiences. Some aspects of aggressiveness or hostility may also be determined by biological factors, but these will not be discussed here.

The interaction of aggressive personality and aggressive behavior is nicely illustrated in a study by Weatherley (1962), who assumed that women whose mothers had permitted aggression would have more aggressive personalities than those whose mothers had punished it. Classifying 100 college women on this basis, he subjected them to various humiliating and neutral experimental situations and found that those with permissive mothers responded more aggressively to humiliating conditions, while both personality types reacted in the same way to the neutral situation. The aggressive personality trait only affected behavior, in other words, under *circumstances* which were distressing.

In general, it seems clear that circumstances are the most critical determinants of whether and how aggression appears. Worchel (1957) and Reiser *et al.* (1955), for example, have shown that frustrated subjects are more likely to express aggression against a student than a faculty member and against an enlisted man than an officer in the army. Thibaut and Riecken (1955) found similar results in a study whose subjects were army officers interacting with experimenters disguised as officers of higher or lower rank than themselves. The experimenters frustrated the subject, who was later called on to assess the experimenter. The amount of hostility expressed about higher-status experimenters was lower than that directed at lower-status ones.

Taken as a whole, present knowledge of aggression can be summed up as follows: (1) Prior punishment for aggressive behavior regulates aggression: the more the punishment, the less the aggression. The individual's history of punishment is likely to depend on his social class, sex, and culture. (2) Aggression is more likely to be inhibited in the presence of potentially punishing targets (figures of high status or authority) than of nonthreatening ones. (3) Frustration will elicit nonaggressive responses if the environment does not contain sufficient cues for aggression. (4) The form of an aggressive response will itself depend upon the cues present for the performance of an aggressive act.

The measurement of aggression. The development of scales to measure tendencies toward aggression is even less advanced than comparable work for anxiety. The major measures of hostility are the Buss-Durkee Inventory and the Rosenzweig Picture Frustration Test.

Buss and Durkee (1957) derived scales for several different features of aggressive behavior from seventy-five true-false items which they compiled into a questionnaire. Analysis of responses showed that the test indicated two major factors of aggression. One is called *emotional hostility*;

it is characterized by resentment, suspicion, and negativism. The second is *overt aggression* and is characterized by verbal hostility, indirect hostility, and irritability. These characteristics are not interrelated in quite the same way for women, where negativism is more closely correlated with *overt hostility* than with *emotional hostility*.

Rosenzweig's Picture Frustration Test (Rosenzweig, 1945; Rosenzweig *et al.*, 1946, 1947) is a cartoon technique for studying aggressive verbal responses to frustration. The pictures show a person in a frustrating situation and a comic-strip balloon space in which the subject writes his own verbal response (see Figure 3.9).

I'm very sorry we splashed your clothing just now though we tried hard to avoid the puddle.

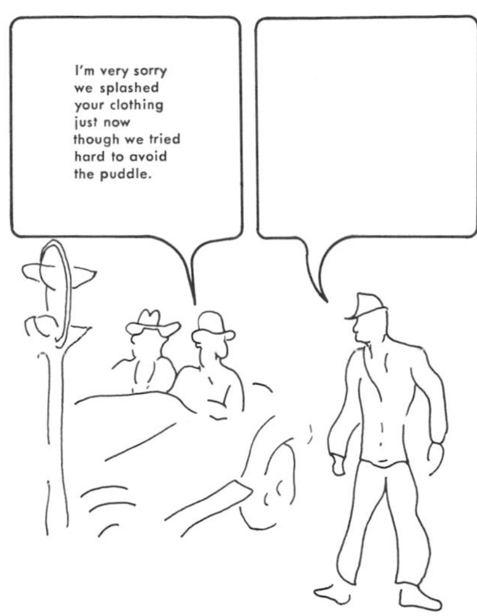

Figure 3.9 Drawing used to elicit verbal responses to frustration. The subject completes the reply to be made by the pedestrian by filling in the bland "balloon." Reproduced by permission from the Rosenzweig P-F Study, Adult Form, copyright 1948.

The test was devised to study both *ego-blocking* frustrations, where some obstacle directly frustratcs the subject, and *superego-blocking* frustrations, in which some charge, accusation, or incrimination serves to frustrate the subject. Responses to these situations are scored in three categories: *extrapunitive,* in which aggression is directed at the environment; *intropunitive,* in which the subject turns aggression against himself; and *impunitive,* in which the subject's response is not aggressive at all.

Generally speaking, neither the Buss-Durkee Inventory nor the Picture Frustration Test has shown much evidence of validity in the relatively little research that has been reported. Satisfactory means of assessing aggression are still sadly lacking.

Dependency

Our discussion of central human motives so far has concerned needs of an essentially negative kind. Anxiety, guilt, and aggression are all unpleasant consequences of fearful and distressing situations. Psychologists have also long been interested in positive motivations that lead people to seek each other's company, to turn to others for help, and to subordinate their own needs and desires in order to give help to others. There is no one accepted technical term to describe all of these motives, like *altruism, affection,* or *dependency,* but they may all be considered forms of *affiliative* motivation. Among them, the most important one may be *dependency,* for it appears earliest in life and may be the basis for the development of all the rest. It has been the subject of more psychological theorizing and empirical research than any other affiliative motive.

In general, dependency means the need to have other people solve one's problems, provide security, and assist in the fulfillment of other needs. Rotter (1954) has formally defined it as "the need to *have another person or group of people prevent frustration or punishment and . . . provide for the satisfaction of other needs*" (p. 132). Cofer and Appley (1964) define dependency as "*behavior that elicits aid, assistance, comfort, etc. from others*" (p. 741).

Guilford (1959) summarizes the outcome of several empirical studies which identify a dimension of personality called *self-reliance* versus *dependence*. This dimension is technically considered a *bipolar factor*, which means that its two ends are opposites that mutually exclude each other. The self-reliance pole of the dimension includes being dependable, that is, scrupulous in discharging one's obligations, depending upon one's own judgment, not craving attention or approval, not going to others for aid or advice, not being willingly submissive, and not expecting to be waited on (p. 440).

As we can see, there is considerable overlap in the definitions of dependency, but their common central core is the idea of seeking help from others, whether to fulfill some positive need or to gain protection against some aversive event. And the actual characteristics of dependent people all appear to be opposites of the attributes that Guilford has found related to self-reliance.

One aspect of dependency that distinguishes it from other major motives is the fact that it has no independent goal of its own. To be dependent means to turn to another person for assistance in gaining *some other goal*, like escaping danger or getting food. In other words, dependent behavior is a technique for obtaining other goal objects. In the case of other learned motives, behaviors originally established as means of reaching a specific goal may develop independence of their original goal and themselves operate as motivators of behavior. One may originally learn to work for money in order to buy food, for example, but getting money may later become its own motive. Dependency, however, cannot occur in the absence of some other motive—when a person turns to others for help, there is something he wants help with.

For this reason, it makes sense to say that we can only be sure a dependency motive is operating when the act of seeking assistance from others seems less economical than solving the problems by oneself would be. If it takes less time, or energy, or whatever to solve a problem alone than to get help with it, and a person seeks help anyhow, then the fact that he takes the trouble to do so must mean that *being helped* is itself of value to him, quite apart from the ostensible goal towards which he is being helped.

As a practical matter, it is not always possible to ascertain directly the degree to which being helped is of value to a person. One can *infer* dependency, however, by assuming that every culture and every individual situation has a norm of dependency and that dependent motivation is revealed whenever a person's behavior exceeds those norms. In America, for example, an adult is not considered dependent if he seeks professional help from a lawyer or physician, but he is considered dependent if he constantly asks others to decide what color necktie to wear, what to order in a restaurant, and so forth. Our assessment of dependency, therefore, tends to be relative to the individual situation and the expectations of the society.

The actual measurement of dependency is complicated not only by its relativistic aspects, but also by the fact that some current workers on this problem tend to include things that go beyond the definition of dependency, even though they are correlated with it. It has been argued, for example, that dependent people are likely to be unusually obedient to rules and regulations laid down by others, and obedience is often used as a correlative measure of dependency. But this expansion creates problems; many people obey rules because they feel that the general social welfare demands obedience, and many people break rules, not in a spirit of independence, but because they are hostile or aggressive. By including obedience among the measures of dependency, we introduce some variance that makes them less effective predictors of help-seeking behavior. Another example of this kind of inference is the argument that because dependent people are more likely than others to be homesick living away from home, preference for living at home versus, say, institutional living can be used as a measure of dependency. Such inferences are reasonable in their own right, but if they are confused with the help-seeking behavior which defines dependency, they make its measurement unnecessarily difficult.

Dependency measures, for the most part, have been verbal devices, especially projective techniques. Of these, the Rotter Sentence Completion method (Rotter and Rafferty, 1950) and the Thematic Apperception Test (Murray, 1943) have had most attention. Fitzgerald (1958) used them with special scoring methods and in combination with interviews and sociometric measures, to assess the dependency motives of male college students in eleven areas of concern, like school, home, girl friends, and so forth. Because in this attempt the projective devices were quite uncorrelated with each other and with the other measures (partly because they were contaminated with non-help-seeking items), Renner *et al.* (1962) conducted another investigation, like Fitzgerald's but using better scoring criteria. This time, by studying college students of both sexes and taking dependency ratings from the subjects themselves and also from their dormitory mates, a few small but statistically significant relationships were obtained between Sentence Completion scores and dependency ratings.

Other studies have served to further improve the Sentence Completion for the measurement of dependency. They have shown, for example, that dependent female prisoners tend to volunteer more as experimental subjects than independent ones (Maher and Repucci, 1964) and that dependent college students tend to seek more help with a problem-solving task than independent ones (Maher and Hedwig, 1958). At the same time, these and other studies have indicated that the concept of dependency is quite complicated and that it may include such traits as the willingness to be dominated by others, which strictly speaking is not part of the help-seeking notion. Because the motive of dependency seems so central to personality dynamics, considerable effort is currently being expended on investigating it, and further clarification of both the construct and its measurement can be expected.

Affiliation

Although dependency has been described as an affiliative motive, the need for affiliation (*n Affiliation*) is a motive in its own right. This concept was introduced into modern psychological literature by Henry Murray (1938), and the major work on it has so far been done by his students. Shipley and Veroff (1952) define *n Affiliation* as a desire for the recovery, maintenance, or attainment of a friendly or loving relationship. Following McClelland *et al.* (1953), they envisage this need as having two components, one with an approach and the other with an avoidance aspect. The approach aspect consists of seeking affiliation because the affiliative relationship is a pleasant stimulus; the avoidance component is the seeking of affiliation because rejection is a painful stimulus.

The need for affiliation is measured primarily by using special scoring procedures for the Thematic Apperception Test. Shipley and Veroff (1952) have established a manual for it in which high- or low-affiliation imagery is scored whenever the story includes a statement of concern about (1) being rejected or "jilted," (2) loneliness or lack of friends, (3) physical departure of a friend or loved one, including death, (4) psychological separation, such as quarreling with a friend, (5) unrequited love or friendship, or (6) reparation or penance to preserve a relationship. Examples of stories showing high and low *n Affiliation* are:

> Here are two old college friends who are meeting at a class reunion. They are glad to recognize each other as they were feeling a little lonely in the crowd of people, many of whom were unfamiliar to them. They shake hands and discuss old times and mutual friends. As the meeting comes to a close, they are making plans to get together more often and not to let the friendship fade away. (High *n Affiliation.*)

> A father is talking to his son, who has not done the chores for which he gets a weekly allowance. The father is pointing out that the son has his duties to do, just as adults have. The son decides to try to do better next time. (Low *n Affiliation.*)

Atkinson *et al.* (1954) used this scoring system to study the stories of subjects whose affiliation needs were aroused by conditions where being liked and accepted by others was considered important. Control subjects were given the thematic cards, or pictures to be described, under classroom conditions. Affiliation scores of the aroused group were significantly higher than those of the control subjects.

Atkinson and Walker (1956) later used the same kind of arousal and control conditions to compare subjects with high and low *n Affiliation* scores on a recognition task involving pictures of faces presented at rapid speeds. Those high in *n Affiliation* identified faces more readily than those with low scores did, and they did so most effectively in the aroused condition.

Apart from the above considerations, the desire to affiliate appears to depend both on one's birth order and the degree of situational anxiety that one experiences. When, under conditions relatively free of anxiety, first-born and only children are compared to later-born children with respect to their desire to be with others, no differences emerge. When first-born and only children are made anxious (as when they are waiting for a painful injection), however, they tend to prefer to wait with others, that is, to affiliate. Later-born children show no such inclination (Schachter, 1959).

The systematic study of positive social motives is a good deal more recent than the study of avoidant motivation. Until recently, too, biological measures for studying these motive states were unavailable, and we were entirely dependent on verbal, generally projective devices or on indices derived from small behavior samples. By and large, the progress of an area of inquiry depends on its access to good measuring instruments, and it is clear that dependency and affiliation are motives that will continue to require research development for many years.

Achievement and Competence

The need for achievement (*n Achievement*) has received more attention from psychologists than most social motives have. McClelland *et al.* (1949) initiated a series of studies on the need to achieve, originally without defining it very specifically. Taking the term itself from

Henry Murray (1938), they cited Sear's comment (1942) on its meaning:

> There are many names for this learned drive: pride, craving for superiority, ego-impulse, self-esteem, self-approval, self-assertion; but these terms represent different emphases or different terminological systems, not fundamentally different concepts. Common to all is the notion that the feeling of success depends upon gratification of this drive, and failure results from its frustration. (P. 236.)

Since then, students of achievement have regarded *competition against a standard of excellence* as the basic process in achievement motivation.

Measurement of this motive has depended heavily (although not exclusively) upon the Thematic Apperception Test (TAT). The subject composes stories to describe the TAT pictures, and the stories are recorded and scored for the presence of certain characteristics, including: (1) *achievement imagery*, that is, references to competition with a standard of excellence, such as unique accomplishment in the arts, long-term preparation for a career, or specific attempts to achieve a concrete goal; (2) *instrumental activity*, or indication that any characters in the story are engaged in activity intended to reach the goal; (3) *anticipatory goal states*, or anticipation by someone in the story of success or failure in reaching the goal; (4) *obstacles or blocks*, that is, the appearance in the story of any frustration or difficulty that might create obstacles to attainment of the goal (obstacles may be within the person himself, like lack of ability or education, or in the environment, like unforseeable catastrophes). This scoring system assumes, like the use of thematic productions itself, that motive states are reflected in fantasy. It also hopefully assumes that when the motive is aroused by some external stimulus, the fantasy technique will indicate a stronger motive state.

The technique is reliable in the sense that judges tend to agree on the way a story should be scored, but subjects do not remain very consistent with themselves if they take the test again after several weeks. It is therefore difficult to know how dependable the interpretations of any given test result are. Within these limits, the TAT does have some power to differentiate subjects who respond in a relaxed situation (non-achievement arousing) from those whose achievement needs are stimulated by tasks described to them as measures of ability. Under such conditions, the aroused groups produce higher TAT achievement scores.

Need for achievement and fear of failure. The relationships between achievement needs and other motives are not always straightforward. McClelland and Liberman (1949), for example, presented a series of words tachistoscopically to subjects; some of the words were related to achievement, while others were either neutral or concerned security needs. Subjects with high need for achievement recognized positive achievement (success) words fastest, but the poorest recognition of negative achievement (failure) words came from subjects medium in achievement needs. This suggests that achievement needs of medium strength may be based more on a fear of failure than on a hope for success.

Another aspect of the element of fear in achievement motivation is seen in a study of risk taking by children (McClelland, 1958). Children participating in a ring-toss game were permitted to stand as near to the peg as they wished or as far away as six or seven feet. Standing closer naturally raised the chances of success, but it also lowered the standard of achievement the child set for himself. Children with high need of achievement preferred medium risks (20 to 50 inches from the peg) while children with low need of achievement, though they mostly took the medium-risk choice, chose the low- and high-risk positions more often than the other children did. The aspiration level of the person with high achievement need seems to be a compromise between the desire for success, which would move him to take no risks, and the fact that success without risk is unsatisfying.

Competence. White (1959) has suggested that much of human behavior ordinarily called "exploratory drive," "curiosity," or "play," is really the basis of a need for competence. The competence motive is fulfilled, he says, when the individual gains mastery over the environment in any way, however limited. A child's development of simple skills and an adult's learning to hit a golf ball or perform surgery are intrinsically satisfying because they are means of mastering the environment. Success or failure in this sense is absolute, since one can be judged in terms of how much he has *actually* gained control of the environment rather than in terms of his ability to do something better than others can.

There has not been much research on the competence motive, but Kohn (1965) has recently reported studying a very similar problem, that of intellectual motivation. He suggests that it is possible to identify a motive for intellectual competence, which he describes as a

> positive affective reaction to problem-solving activity and to the successful solution of problems. . . . Such an affective reaction could render intellectual activity . . . reinforcing quite apart from the operation of extrinsic reinforcers like prestige, money, or social approval. (P. 21.)

He has reported preliminary efforts to develop a simple projective measure of this motive; it seems reliable and appears to be correlated with persistence in trying to solve insoluble puzzles.

The motives that have been discussed here are only a sample of those that have attracted scientific attention. They are probably all major motives that dominate wide ranges of human behavior, but they are far from the only ones. Space does not permit us to consider the many other motives that have been investigated, but it is hoped that the general methods of investigation will be clear from the examples given here.

MOTIVES IN CONFLICT

The discussion so far has dealt only with the effects of single motives on behavior. But people are really much more complicated than that implies, and much of their behavior results from the interaction of two or more motives operating at the same time. Behavior is rarely under the control of a single powerful motive, and much of it consists of momentary resolutions of conflicts between motives. Patterns of motivational conflict and their effects upon behavior will concern us in this section.

Types of Conflict

When a motive state leads to behavior that has been punished in the past, the individual is put in conflict because the very response elicited by the motive is one that experience has taught him not to make. This is called a *response-produced* conflict. A child who has been rebuked for hitting other children, for example, learns to control himself when he feels a fight coming on. But if he is then relentlessly taunted and provoked by another child, he is in conflict. He is faced with the incompatible motives of hostility and fear, and both of these arise from his own responses.

Another kind of conflict arises when a

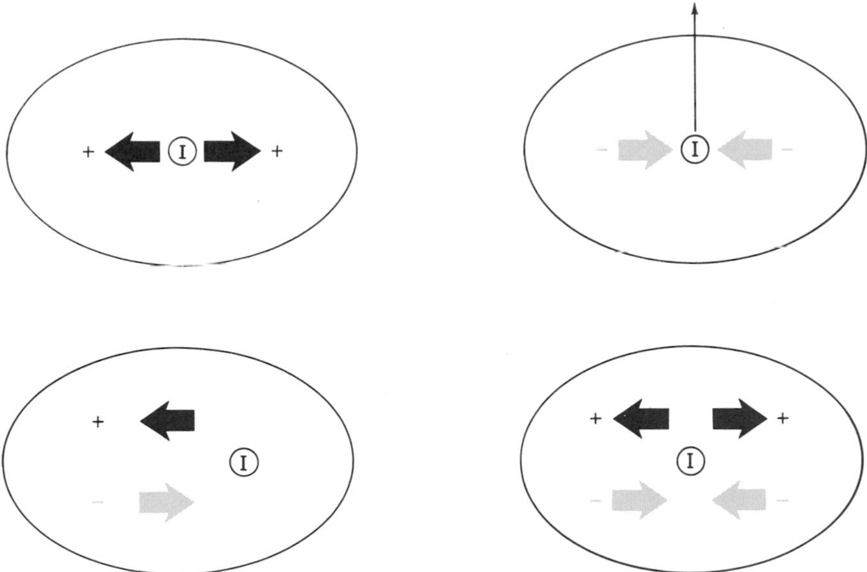

Figure 3.10 Classic Lewinian conflict paradigms: *a*, approach-approach; *b*, avoidance-avoidance; *c*, approach-avoidance; *d*, double approach-avoidance.

single stimulus has been associated with both reward and punishment. This is called *stimulus-produced* conflict. For the college student with high academic aspirations, for example, exams offer simultaneously a chance for distinction and praise and the risk of failure and embarrassment. When this kind of conflict is intense, it can be activated by the mere presence of such related stimuli as books or classrooms.

Both these conflicts are instances of a general type called *approach-avoidance* conflict, in which the twin components of past punishment (leading to anxiety and avoidance) and past reward (leading to an approach response) produce an emotional deadlock. There are two other general types of conflict: *avoidance-avoidance* conflict, where two unpleasant alternatives exist, as in "Shall I suffer the toothache or the dentist?" and *approach-approach* conflict, in which two attractive alternatives exist, as in "Johnny, which toy do you choose?" (see Figure 3.10).

The types of conflict we have identified here are largely hypothetical because most of the important conflicts people face are complex developments of these simple models. Often they are *double* approach-avoidance situations. Thus, a man who is considering marriage has two choices, each with both attractive and aversive attributes. Shall he marry, gaining a wife (good) but giving up his bachelor pad (bad)? Or shall he stay single, keeping his freedom (good) but risking loneliness and other difficulties (bad)? Because the alternative goals in such conflicts are not very clearly positive or negative, their resolution is a complicated matter. If all the variables involved remain unchanged, there is no reason to expect the conflict to be resolved at all. The individual may vacillate between one course of action and another for a long period of time. The very state of conflict is itself unpleasant, however, and there may come a point where virtually any choice will seem better than the tension of indeci-

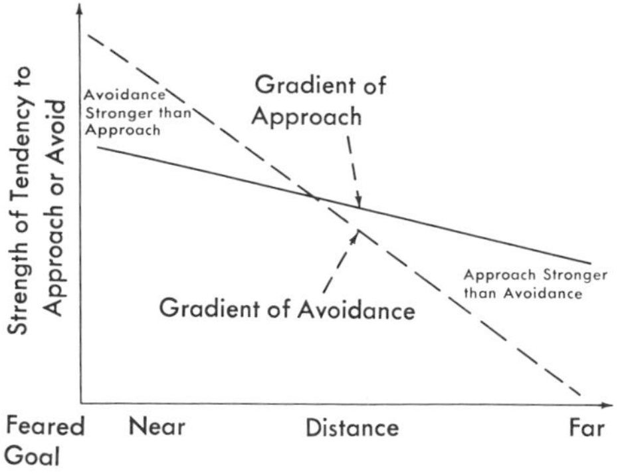

Figure 3.11 Simple graphic representation of an approach-avoidance conflict. The tendency to approach is the stronger of the two tendencies far from the goal, while the tendency to avoid is the stronger of the two near to the goal. Therefore, when far from the goal, the subject should tend to approach part way and then stop; when near to it, he should tend to retreat part way and then stop. In short, he should tend to remain in the region where the two gradients intersect. From Neal E. Miller, "Experimental Studies of Conflict," in *Personality and the Behavior Disorders*, edited by J. McV. Hunt, copyright 1944 The Ronald Press Company, New York.

sion. At such a point, the alternative closest at hand may be acted on and the conflict resolved. The indecisive bridegroom, tending toward the negative side about marriage, may break off the engagement, go abroad, or take some other relatively irrevocable step to eliminate his own indecision.

Determinants of Conflict

The mere presence of two competing motives does not produce a conflict unless the motives are relatively equal in strength. A person who has high motivation for academic success and little history of academic failure, for example, may not feel much anxiety about exams. The two competing motives, in his case, have very different intensities; for conflict to arise, the motives must have intensities within competitive range of each other.

This brings us to the problem of how to measure the strength of the competing motives which underlie conflict. Such things as distance from the goal (in either space or time), the likelihood and extent of punishment or reward that goes with either choice, and the intensity of motivation towards either goal are all important determinants of changes in the strength and probability of any response. Manipulating these determinants changes the equilibrium between socially derived motives, thereby instigating, intensifying, and resolving conflict.

Distance from the Goal

The most detailed work on the determinants of conflict and its resolution is that of Neal Miller (1959). Basing his research on the earlier work of Hull (1932), Miller has developed several postulates for predicting approach-avoidance conflict behavior. He used the concept of a *gradient* of approach or avoidance to describe the changing intensity of the tendency to continue approaching or avoiding a goal as one comes closer to it (see Figure 3.11). Miller's postulates state that the tendency to approach a desired goal increases as one nears it, and the tendency to avoid a feared goal similarly increases as one nears it. The avoidance tendency increases more rapidly than the approach tendency, moreover, and both vary with the strength of the underlying motives. This model of gradients has been largely developed and demonstrated in laboratory experiments with animals, and it appears to have very wide application for interpreting various important human response patterns, including displacement in psychotherapy (Murray and Berkun, 1955), the development of neurotic behavior (Phillips, 1956), and achievement activity (McClelland *et al.*, 1953).

Miller attempts to explain why the avoidance tendency increases faster than the approach tendency as a characteristic difference between biological and learned drives (motives). Maher (1964) points out that this model, developed with lower organisms, is not adequate for explaining some important kinds of human conflict. Miller's assumptions would not explain how conflicts arise for such situations as need for achievement versus fear of failure, desire for excitement versus fear of injury (as in sport parachute jumping or high diving), or any of the conflicts of social motives that we see every day.

Distance and time. Physical space between a subject and a goal is comparable to the more common human situation in which *time* lies between the subject and the goal. The man waiting in a hospital bed for surgery is separated from the event by time rather than by space, and his tension increases as the time grows shorter. The combat soldier waiting to attack at H hour becomes increasingly tense as time moves on, even though his spatial distance from the enemy does not change. While the spatial analogue is very useful in laboratory studies of conflict, we must be careful about generalizing from it to behaviors in which the time dimension is central, for the perception of time differs in some important ways from that of space.

In its simplest form, a person's movement towards a fixed object in space is accompanied by regular perceptual changes. The perspective and apparent size of the object change, and the visibility of details improves. Such systematic changes in vision are directly related to distance and tell the person continuously how near he is to the goal. The mere passage of time, however, does not of itself provide such information unless a clock is directly visible or the individual is able to observe some other rhythmically occurring event. When these cues are absent, many other variables enter the situation; monotony, the threat of punishment, or the promise of reward at the end of the time interval, all significantly affect the judgment of time's passage (Wallace and Rabin, 1960).

Despite these differences, there has not been much research specifically relating conflict to the time dimension. One animal study has been reported by Rigby (1954), who developed an ingenious apparatus delivering reward and punishment to a rat where time instead of space was the governing variable. He concluded that separate time-dictated gradients of approach and avoidance could be identified that are quite similar to each other in all important respects.

Epstein (1962) has reported the various indices of conflict in sport parachute jumpers from several days before their first jump through the day of the first jump. Their motives in conflict presumably are the positive attractions of excitement and prestige versus the fear of injury or death. The changes in the subjects' own estimates of how strong their approach and avoidant motives are on the day of the jump are especially interesting. The general shape of these gradients is roughly the same; there is some slight crossing at two points, and the approach gradient resumes dominance at the point just before the parachutist jumps (Figure 3.12). In this study, Epstein also observed the existence of a psychological "point of *commitment*," beyond which the parachutist no longer feels free to decide not to jump even though he can physically do so until the moment that he is actually falling. Once he stands out on the step ready to jump, he seems to feel that he now has no option but to do so. In this sense, the conflict is over, even though the goal, speaking narrowly, has not been reached. This observation is important because it shows that the conditions for conflict exist even when escape is possible. This is always true of spatial conflicts, for the subject can always turn

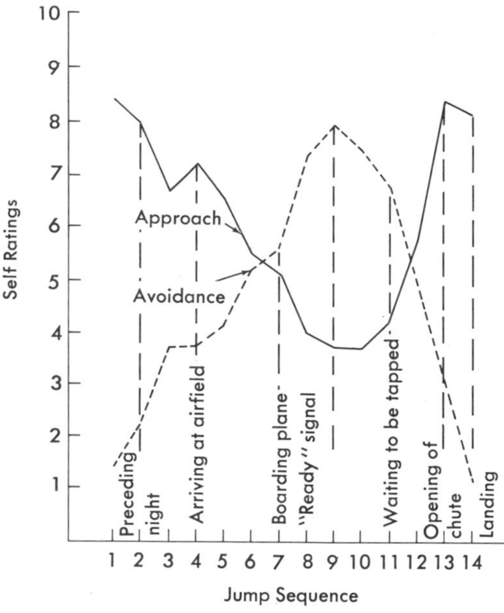

Figure 3.12 Self-ratings of approach and avoidance as a function of the sequence of events leading to and following a jump. Reprinted from S. Epstein, "The measurement of drive and conflict in humans: Theory and experiment," in M. W. Jones (ed.): *Nebraska Symposium on Motivation* by permission of the University of Nebraska Press, © 1962.

around and retreat from the goal. Escape from a temporal conflict, however, may become progressively less possible with the passage of time. The reluctant bridegroom may bow out of his impending mariage early in the engagement with little loss of face, but it becomes increasingly difficult to do so as the wedding date approaches.

Among parachutists, passing the point of commitment means that the approach motive is again dominant and that the fear motive has either decreased or been temporarily "inhibited." Some evidence of inhibition is suggested by the fact that many novice jumpers do not continue with the sport after the first or second jump. Also, Epstein obtained some indications of greater anxiety, including the occurrence of anxiety dreams, some time *after* the first jump than *before* it.

Further evidence for the value of a "point of commitment" concept comes from a study of temporal conflict in children (Maher *et al.*, 1964). In a choice situation, the subject was free to alternate between two goal routes. Various periods of time were allowed him in this experiment, and records were made of the length of time the child typically oscillated between the alternative choices. Typically, the oscillation tended to last a stable fraction of the total time—roughly until one-third of the time period had passed. Once the child had passed this point, he rarely showed any further indecision, suggesting that this point represented a psychological "point of no return" (Figure 3.13). Here again, there is a reappearance of dominance by the approach response rather than the increasing dominance of the avoidance response we would expect from the simple transposition of Miller's model of spatial conflict.

It is quite clear that we still have only a very limited understanding of the relationship of temporal distance to the strength of conflicting motives. The data suggest, however, that principles gained from the study of laboratory animals moving *in space* do not apply in the same way to the behavior of humans in a complex social environment.

Conflict and Punished Responses

Much human behavior is modified by the reward and punishment of responses made *in the presence* of a goal regardless of the subject's actual proximity to it. A child may be punished severely for sex play with a sibling but rewarded for affection towards the same sibling. Proximity to the sibling is irrelevant to the contingencies involved. By the same token, the child may be encouraged to be aggressive (to "stand up for himself") in deal-

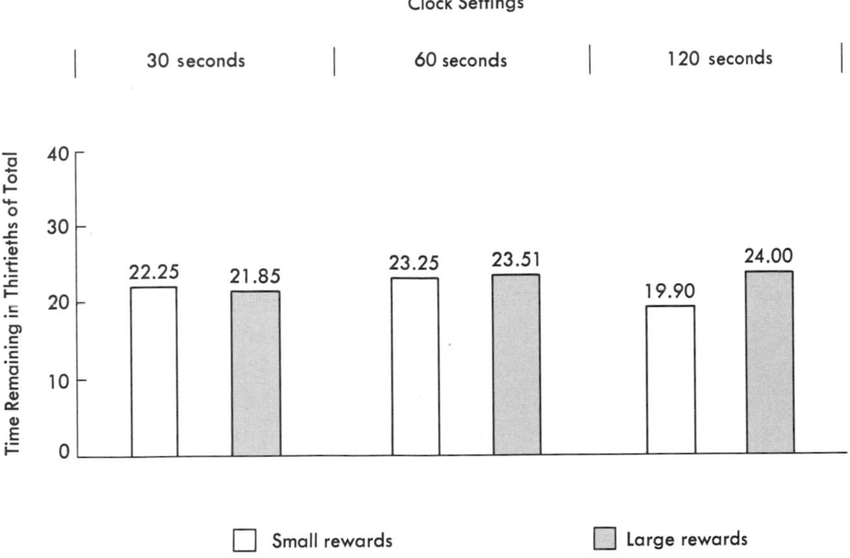

Figure 3.13 Relative stability of equilibrium points in temporal conflicts regardless of time base. Data from several experiments combined.

ing with neighborhood children but punished for aggression towards his brothers or sisters. The child must learn many other such discriminations in order to be "socialized," and thus he develops refined and graduated approach and avoidance responses to specific stimuli.

Under normal circumstances, the formative pattern of punishments and rewards is consistent across similar situations. The child is unlikely to receive punishment and reward repeatedly for *exactly* the same behavior occurring in the presence of the same stimulus. In this important respect, human beings acquire response patterns under conditions quite unlike those in which the rat is both shocked and fed repeatedly for making the same running response to the end of the same alley. If we did have completely systematic schedules of consequences for various responses, human conflict might be predictably engendered under four conditions: (1) Conflict would arise when a stimulus has some characteristics of two other stimuli, one of which is associated with punishment of the evoked response and the other with its reward. The child who is punished for fighting his siblings but rewarded for fighting the boy next door may thus be conflicted when a schoolmate enters his home as a house guest. (2) Conflict would arise when the required response possesses attributes of both a rewarded and a punished response. The man who must authorize necessary but dangerous surgery for his wife may be conflicted by the punitive and protective elements which are both present in his behavior. (3) Conflict would arise when internal stimuli evoke an approach response that is stronger than the avoidant response first developed. Sexual motivation during adolescence provides stronger stimuli towards sexual activity than was the case when infantile sexual curiosity was originally punished. (4) Finally, conflict would arise with a change in the punishment-reward contingencies, which often accompanies a change of environment. Such conflicts are typical of the problems encountered by some immigrants in adapting to a new culture. Adjusting to military service, or on a milder scale, to college, provides further instances of such conflict.

Biological Accompaniments of Conflict

A state of conflict is generally accompanied by certain biological changes, usually in the direction of increased arousal. Moss and Edwards (1964) instructed subjects to obey certain simple commands ("Close your eyes") and measured vasoconstriction of blood vessels during the response. The subject was then instructed *not* to make the response when commanded to do so. Under these conditions, vasoconstriction levels increased, evidently as a consequence of the conflict induced by the competing instructions.

Johnson (1963) examined the effects of conflict produced by difficult discrimination. Metronome signals were presented to warn subjects of a forthcoming electric shock, which they could avoid by a finger movement. A fast metronome beat (144 counts per minute) signalled shock, while a slow beat (60 counts per minute) meant no shock was coming. The two signals were brought closer together in rate of clicking until it became difficult to discriminate between them. For one group of subjects, the discrimination was made impossible. These conflictful conditions produced significant increases in heart rate and palmar sweat (over and above the effect of the shocks themselves), confirming that the conflict itself raises the level of arousal.

Similar findings had been reported previously by Berlyne (1960), who studied the effect of nonpunishing conflict upon the galvanic skin response (GSR), and found it greater under intense conflict than under low conflict. In his investigation, the variables of novelty, surprise, intensity, and distance from the stimulus were all controlled and therefore had no effect on the results. It is safe to conclude that conflict increases arousal beyond the increase resulting from the individual stimulus conditions.

Behavioral Consequences of Conflict

Returning to the approach-avoidance model of conflict discussed earlier, a state of conflict exists most clearly at the point where two gradients intersect, that is where the tendency to make an approach response equals the tendency to avoid. Students of conflict behavior in animals have observed that in this situation a pattern of behavior develops that includes elements of both responses: the animal advances and retreats in an oscillating fashion just as, in the study of temporal conflict mentioned above, the child typically oscillated between one choice and the other. If the tendencies to make the incompatible responses were really equal, then the equilibrium might never be disturbed nor the conflict solved. But such states of tense equilibrium are themselves arousing, as we have just seen, and the subject commonly engages in additional responses whose chief function seems to be to end the unpleasant state aroused by the conflict itself. The rat in a typical approach-avoidance apparatus, for example, will take any opportunity to get out of it. This behavior has sometimes been termed "leaving the field." Of itself, it resolves only those conflicts engendered by a specific environmental situation. Where the stimulus for approach is internal, however, and where the avoidance drive is conditioned to the approach response, simple environmental changes will not resolve conflicts. Most human conflicts are established around whole classes of objects and of responses rather than around very specific stimuli. Children are punished for being "aggressive," which encompasses a wide range of responses. They are rewarded for "doing well," which can include anything from making a good school record to being voted most popular member of the class. Leaving the field thus offers no practical solution for many human conflicts.

Temporary Solutions to Conflict

Among the kinds of response aimed at handling conflict, one type at least is prophylactic; that is, it handles conflict by preventing it from occurring. This response appears to consist of *avoiding* observation of the cues which arouse conflict. Avoidance may develop in the form of (1) not talking or thinking about topics that are related to the conflict, (2) forgetting past events surrounding the conflict, and (3) avoiding places or social situations where the cues for conflict are likely to occur.

An interesting demonstration of this phenomenon was reported by E. J. Murray (1959) in a study of the effect of sleep deprivation on fantasy stories. Subjects were military personnel deprived of sleep for 86 hours and subjected to considerable implicit pressure to stay awake. During the ordeal, they were shown three pictures that mildly, moderately, and strongly suggested sleep themes. Control subjects who were not put under pressure to stay awake produced sleep fantasies in direct relationship to the strength of suggestion of the cards, but the experimental subjects clearly avoided sleep topics. The conflict between wanting to sleep and the pressure to stay awake led to avoidance of thoughts or even words related to sleeping, which might increase the conflict.

Repression. Actively avoiding past events by forgetting them is called *repression,* and it has been a major topic of psychological concern since Freud's early studies of neurosis began leading him to the formulation of psychoanalytic theory. There has been so much formal investigation of repression, and it is so critical to understanding the development of neurotic disorders, that it would be improper to pretend either to review the literature or to adequately discuss its clinical significance here. The latter will be a subject of repeated concern throughout this book, especially in the third section. For the former, it is sufficient to state that repression appears to be a means of inhibiting conflict-arousing thoughts. To the extent that it is complete, there is some evidence that it successfully prevents conflict, but partial repression permits disruptive conflictful cues to disturb the individual's equanimity (Bobbitt, 1958).

When the stimuli that produce conflict are in the external environment, the individual may not only avoid words and thoughts relevant to them, but may even physically avoid some places related to them. If he has successfully repressed thoughts about the dangerous topics, his avoidance of certain places or persons may seem inexplicable to him. Whenever he is in a particular location, he becomes anxious without knowing why. Under these circumstances, he develops irrational fears called "phobias," whose main effect is to keep him away from the place or object in question. Phobias will be discussed at some length in Chapter 10.

Displacement. The concept of *displacement* is particularly important in conflicts. It is used in two ways. When a person inhibits a response to one stimulus and makes it to another similar stimulus, the response is said to be displaced. The executive who cannot express anger to his superior but yells at his secretary illustrates this idea, which is called *response displacement.* A second use of the word refers to *substitute activity* following the inhibition of a normally dominant response. Students of animal behavior have noted, for example, that when an intruder threatens the territory of the male stickleback fish, even though no

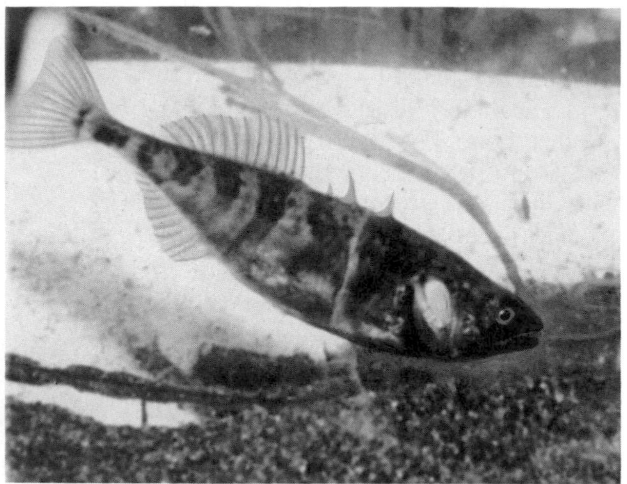

Figure 3.14 Stickleback digging a nest. Photo © Richard Guppy from National Audubon.

fighting begins until the enemy actually enters the defender's territory, the defending fish often digs a nest in the sand while waiting—a completely irrelevant response in these circumstances (see Figure 3.14).

Both forms of displacement can be explained by a common principle. In a state of conflict, the individual is aroused to act, but he has cues for both approach and avoidance responses. As long as the dominant response is inhibited, however, then any other response to any other local stimulus is likely to occur. The stickleback digs a nest because he is in a high state of arousal, and some of the stimuli for nest building are present. If, by chance, one of the local stimuli has a past history of evoking the inhibited response, then it will appear. The unfortunate employee who receives her boss's displaced wrath is thus victimized because the boss commonly responds to his subordinates with anger.

In a complex analysis of response displacement, Murray and Berkun (1955) have extended Miller's concept of approach and avoidance gradients to include not only distance from the goal, but stimulus similarity on any dimension. They assume that when a stimulus has acquired both approach and avoidance properties, then any new stimulus that is partially similar to it will elicit the same approach and avoidance response tendencies somewhat more weakly. In their view, the decline of response strength with decreasing similarity is more marked for avoidance than for approach tendencies. Starting from a stimulus situation where avoidance tendency is higher than approach, stimuli of decreasing similarity will ultimately weaken the avoidance tendency until it falls below the approach level, which has been declining at a slower rate. At this point, the approach response emerges—appearing as a displaced response to a new stimulus that is partially similar to an old one. Such displaced responses solve the original conflict by eliminating the dynamic equilibrium between competing tendencies.

Adaptive Solutions to Conflict

The solutions to conflict we have been discussing fail to solve it permanently. When the right stimulus conditions recur, the conflict reappears in full force. Permanent solutions demand one of two alternatives. Either the least desirable tendency must be weakened to the point where it never again equals the more desirable one, or the desirable one must be increased to a level exceeding the strongest undesirable tendency. Insofar as arousal level depends on the strengths of the conflicting motives, the latter solution (increasing the desirable response) is likely to produce more intense arousal than the former (weakening the undesirable response). Generally speaking, it is preferable to extinguish the avoidance component, at least where it involves irrational fears, but this is difficult because it requires the subject to remain close to the feared stimulus without making the avoidance response.

Response displacement provides one clue to a method of successfully extinguishing avoidance. By presenting the individual with a stimulus only slightly similar to the conflict-arousing stimulus, it is possible simultaneously to elicit the approach response and to achieve some extinction of the avoidance response. After some experience in this situation, the person may then be exposed to a stimulus more like the original because the avoidance tendency has been weakened by the displaced approach response of the first stage. In this sense, psychotherapy may be viewed as a situation in which, for example, the extinction of interpersonal conflict in relation to one's parents may be achieved by first extinguishing such conflicts towards a somewhat similar stimulus—the therapist. There are specific techniques of therapy which rely on the deliberate presentation of stimuli varying in similarity to the source of people's fears; some of these will be discussed in Chapter 15.

In some conflicts, a person may not have the ability to make a successful approach response, and in this case reducing avoidance tendencies solves nothing. A student caught between a strong need for achievement and a great fear of failure may simply lack the intellectual ability needed to achieve very much. Removing his fear of failure may therefore be impossible and, in any case, would not enable him to perform adequately. In this situation, nothing will solve the conflict except to find an alternative goal which is within the capacities of the individual, such as a career which does not demand great intellectual ability.

We have considered the essential elements in the establishment of conflicts of motive and the consequences of conflict states. We distinguished several kinds of conflict (approach-avoidance, approach-approach, and avoidance-avoidance) and enumerated some important determinants of them, using Miller's postulates in particular as a basis for analyzing how conflicts operate and the various means by which they are resolved. Conflict of motives, more than anything else, arouses people to cope with themselves and their environments by discovering new means of dealing with them. In this sense, conflict is largely the basis for the development of most positive abnormalities. But conflict can also produce disruptions of such strength in people's lives that their ability to cope with things is reduced rather than increased, and in this sense, it serves as the basis for many negative abnormalities as well. In either case, we cannot understand how people integrate the multitude of motives that are within them and that are imposed upon them by the outside world without understanding the nature of conflict.

THE INTEGRATION OF MOTIVES IN PERSONALITY

So far we have not studied in detail more than two motives interacting conflictfully. But human beings living in a social world are subject to such a constant pattern of motive arousal that the single or twofold cases we have considered so far fail to convey the true complexity of human behavior. The dynamics of behavior are expressed most elegantly in the various means by which people integrate their different motives to order the world intelligently and more or less systematically gratify their own needs.

Cognitive Styles

The process by which a person categorizes and organizes his perceptions of the environment is called cognitive style. Although the term refers specifically to the modes of *thinking* that are most characteristic of an individual, the general purpose of cognitive styles is the imposition of order upon the otherwise confusing panorama of events that impinge upon the person and that would otherwise demand multiple and confusing responses.

One of the most thoroughly studied cognitive styles is called *rigidity*, which for our purposes, may be defined as the tendency to persist in a single response even when doing so fails to elicit the reinforcements that would follow other responses. Military commanders in World War I, for example, persisted in frontal infantry attacks upon enemy trenches long after the advent of the machine gun had made this tactic suicidal. Despite tremendous losses for no gains, the tactic continued to be used for years with little sign that the responsible commanders were trying to find better approaches to battle.

Many individuals behave in just this way, seemingly unaware that the situation to which they continue to give the same response has changed in some important respect so that the response is no longer appropriate. Such perceptual tactics involve a tendency to oversimplify the environment, to ignore important differences, and to fail to make necessary discriminations.

Major work on this kind of personality structure has been performed by Frenkel-Brunswik (1949) and by Adorno *et al.* (1950), who have used the term "intolerance of ambiguity" to describe the psychological state underlying rigidity. They discovered relationships between rigid personality and authoritarian parental discipline in the home. Such authoritarianism is marked by a tendency of parents to resolve all issues in terms of black or white, good or bad. Children in such homes may be discouraged from doubting or being indecisive by punishment for ambiguity in their own behavior, which reinforces the tendency to make oversimplified responses to multifaceted situations.

While many studies have aimed at discovering the motivational antecedents of rigidity, our main interest in this pattern is that it serves to reduce the contradictory signals the environment ordinarily presents. Simplification by ignoring things that would disturb ordered perception is one pattern of integration.

A somewhat similar concept has been called *cognitive complexity*. Most work on it has stemmed from the ideas of George Kelly (1955), and the results closely parallel the work on rigidity. Kelly has developed a theory of personality which is chiefly concerned with the conceptualizing or categorizing habits of the individual. By means of a technique called the Role Construct Repertory Test, it is possible to identify different dimensions along which a person can classify or "construe" other people. Cognitively complex people use many different dimensions, while the cognitively simple use only a few. Studies have shown that cognitively simple people tend to assume that other people feel the same way they do and to omit conflicting or contradictory items from memory.

Another approach to the problem of how people resolve contradictions is the theory of *cognitive dissonance* of Leon Festinger (1957). It argues that receiving incongruous or dissonant information creates tension in the individual which he must reduce. It is dissonant for a man who considers himself efficient to find that he is forgetting appointments, or for a man who thinks he is financially shrewd to find that he has made a bad bargain. Whenever dissonance occurs—and in a complex environment this happens fairly often—the individual seeks new information that will reduce the dissonance. A man who, having considered and rejected one model of car, has bought another may seek confirmation of his wisdom by listening selectively to positive information (like advertisements) about the car he chose and to negative information (such as another owner's complaints) about the one he rejected. This is called *postdecision dissonance.*

The general principle of dissonance reduction is equally applicable to many other situations. Some investigators have claimed, for example, that when an individual strongly expects an unpleasant event to happen and is given the choice of enduring it or avoiding it, he may choose to endure it rather than risk having his expectations violated (Aronson *et al.,* 1963). In general, the dissonance principle asserts that people behave and perceive things in ways that confirm their strongly held expectations—even unpleasant ones. As with rigidity, the internal consistency of behavior is maintained by a technique of selective perception and seeking of information.

Cognitive Control

Klein (1954) has studied the role of cognitive control in the integration of behavior by using a device called the Stroop Test as the means of evaluating people's degree of control (Stroop, 1935). The Stroop Test is a series of names of colors printed in colors other than the one the word represents (see Plate 2). The word *blue,* for example, is printed in red. In this test, the subject must read the *color* of the ink, *not* the *word;* for the word *blue,* he must say "red," inhibiting the strong tendency most people have to read the word as it is written. Individuals who were least subject to the interference of the words were compared with people showing high interference on a task that required them, while themselves thirsty, to estimate the size of a thirst-relevant object, such as a Coke or a glass of beer. Ordinarily, when a drive is deprived, people overestimate the size of drive-related objects. In this situation, however, the high interference group underestimated the size of the test object, and the low interference group overestimated it. Low interference may result from focusing attention on the central stimulus and excluding other stimulation from awareness, which might in turn lead to an overemphasis on the attributes of the central stimulus. The process governing these results is not known, but the phenomenon illustrates clearly that the effective consequences of a motive are considerably modified by the perceptual style of the subject.

Even here, integration of behavior is evidently achieved by selectively attending and not attending to various aspects of the environment. The mechanisms that control attention are vital for governing the way in which organized behavior flows from the combination of motivational stimuli that continually impinge upon us. There is good reason to think that serious behavioral pathology ensues from the breakdown of attention mechanisms and that much psychotic behavior may be traced to just such difficulties. Perceptual habits effectively modify motivated behavior, but how such habits are established is far from clear.

SUMMARY

In this chapter, we have examined some of the definitions and classifications of human and animal motives, keeping human behavior at the center of our concern. The directive and energizing functions of motivation have been discussed along with their consequences for a variety of behaviors, and some of the most important human motives, both biological and socially learned, have been studied with particular attention to problems of measurement connected with them. Although each motive state described has its own peculiarities, we have also examined the common features of all motives in terms of arousal and inhibition.

From these issues, we have given detailed consideration to the problems of motives in conflict, and finally we have examined briefly some of the general perceptual and cognitive processes by means of which the person organizes and integrates his behavior.

GLOSSARY

ACTIVATION—see AROUSAL.

ADAPTATION—reduction in strength of response upon repeated presentation of a stimulus; getting used to a stimulus.

ADRENAL CORTEX—the thin outer layer of the adrenal gland.

ADRENALINE (EPINEPHRINE)—a hormone secreted by the adrenal gland that increases arousal.

ACTH (ADRENOCORTICOTROPIC HORMONE)—a hormone secreted by the pituitary gland.

AFFECT—a generic term for feeling, emotion, mood, temperament, and so on.

AFFILIATION MOTIVE (*n Affiliation*)—a desire for the recovery, maintenance, or attainment of a friendly or loving relationship.

AGGRESSION—behavior intended to injure or distress another person.

AMBIGUITY, INTOLERANCE OF—the psychological state believed to underlie rigidity; a tendency to oversimplify the environment, ignore important differences, and fail to make necessary discriminations.

ANDROGEN—a hormone, secreted in both sexes but more abundantly in the male, that influences the development of the male characteristics, structural and behavioral.

APHAGIA—undereating.

APPROACH-APPROACH CONFLICT—conflict resulting from the existence of two attractive alternatives.

APPROACH-AVOIDANCE CONFLICT—conflict produced by the fact that a particular goal is at once both attractive and aversive.

AROUSAL—internal or external state of increased bodily activity.

AROUSAL THRESHOLD—the amount of stimulation required to produce arousal.

AUTONOMIC LABILITY SCORE—an organism's physiological response to stress, relative to the resting rate of the same parameter.

AUTONOMIC NERVOUS SYSTEM—a major division of the nervous system, concerned chiefly with the regulation of the glands and internal muscles.

AUTONOMIC RESPONSE SPECIFICITY—the tendency of individuals to respond with maximal autonomic activation always in the same physiological system regardless of the nature of the arousal stimulus.

AUTONOMIC TENSION SCORE—the absolute change in a parameter that indicates an organism's physiological response to stress.

AVOIDANCE-AVOIDANCE CONFLICT—conflict resulting from the existence of two unpleasant alternatives.

AVOIDANCE BEHAVIOR—a response or a sequence of responses designed to prevent the occurrence of anticipated pain.

AVOIDANCE CONDITIONING—the process of learning a response that prevents the appearance of a noxious stimulus; usually a signal indicates that the noxious stimulus is coming, and a response must be learned and performed to avoid the stimulus.

BIOLOGICAL MOTIVE—a motive which arises from the biological nature of the individual.

BIOSOCIAL MOTIVE—a learned motive in which biological variables play a relatively minor part.

BIPOLAR FACTOR—a factor that has two opposite and mutually exclusive extremes; black and white are polar events in the factor of color.

BUSS-DURKEE INVENTORY—a scale that measures hostility.

CATECHOLAMINE—a class of chemical substances produced by the adrenal medulla and elevated in the body during physiological stress.

CEREBRAL CORTEX—the surface layer of gray matter of the brain.

COGNITION—a generic term for any process whereby an organism becomes aware of an object; it includes perceiving, recognizing, conceiving, judging, and reasoning.

COGNITIVE COMPLEXITY—the relative

amount of different dimensions a person uses to categorize objects and things.

COGNITIVE CONTROL—the direction and degree to which attention is focused and deployed.

COGNITIVE DISSONANCE, THEORY OF—a theory that describes how people resolve contradictory evidence; it holds that receiving information which is incompatible with one's prior commitment or position creates psychological tension which the individual must reduce.

COGNITIVE STYLE—the manner in which a person categorizes and organizes his perceptions of the environment to avoid having to make multiple and confusing responses.

COMPETENCE MOTIVE—a motivational state inferred from the organism's attempt to gain mastery over the environment.

CONCURRENT VALIDITY—the correlation between a given measure and one already known to assess a particular state.

CONDITIONING—the learning of a particular response as a consequence of exposure to specific stimuli which either elicit or reward it.

CONFLICT—the state in which two or more incompatible motives are aroused at the same time.

CONGENITAL ANALGESIA—a disorder whose victims are completely insensitive to pain from birth.

CONSCIENCE—see SUPEREGO.

CONSTRUCT VALIDITY—a measure is said to have construct validity to the extent that it predicts or is correlated with behaviors that are theoretically relevant to it; for example, a test designed to measure anxiety will have construct validity if neurotic persons score higher on it than non-neurotics.

CONSUMMATORY RESPONSE—the particular act that achieves the goal in a motivated behavior sequence.

CONTINUUM—a scale such that between any two values, it is always possible to have a third value.

CORTICOID SUBSTANCES—substances produced by the adrenal cortex, whose major function seems to involve the regulation of inflammatory reactions to infection or wounds.

DENIAL—a defense mechanism whereby a person refuses to accept the truth of a negative evaluation of himself or of something he values.

DEPENDENCY MOTIVE—the motivation that leads a person to turn to others for help.

DISCRIMINATION—the ability to recognize and react differently to different objects or stimuli.

DISPLACEMENT—propensity to respond to a stimulus other than the dominant one that occurs when conflict causes the response to the dominant stimulus to be inhibited.

DRIVE—see NEED.

DYNAMICS—the complex of forces which make behavior a moving, constantly changing phenomenon.

EEG (ELECTROENCEPHALOGRAPH)—an instrument for measuring electrical activity on the surface of the brain.

EOSINOPHILS—a type of blood cell that is reduced during physiological stress.

EQUILIBRIUM—a condition in which opposing forces are balanced.

ESCAPE BEHAVIOR—a response that removes the sufferer from pain.

EXACERBATION—the process of making more violent or severe.

EXPLORATORY DRIVE—curiosity.

EXTINCTION—progressive elimination of the conditioned response by withholding the rewards or reinforcements which usually follow it.

EXTRAPUNITIVE RESPONSE—aggression directed towards the environment.

FANTASY—daydreaming; creating mental images, which often are determined by needs and wishes.

FIXATION—as used here, repetition of an ineffective technique to secure a frustrated goal.

FRUSTRATION—anything that interferes with goal-directed behavior.

FRUSTRATION-AGGRESSION HYPOTHESIS—the hypothesis that frustration always leads to aggression and that the presence of aggression is always indicative of frustration.

FUNDAMENTAL DISTRESS—specific fears of the human newborn which do not appear to have been conditioned to pain.

GOAL—that which brings a behavior sequence to an end.

GOAL REGRESSION—reversion to a goal that was preferred at an earlier stage of development.

GRADIENT—the change in the magnitude of a variable as it progresses in a specified direction.

GUILT—the subjective feelings that result

from doing something that is forbidden, or from the failure to perform some act to which one is obligated (see Chapter 4).

HOSTILITY—a motivational state that may lead to aggressive behavior.

HYPERPHAGIA—overeating.

HYPOTHALAMUS—part of the brain that is thought to take part in the control of hunger and other autonomic responses.

IMPUNITIVE RESPONSE—a response to frustration that is not aggressive, but rather condones what has occurred.

INHIBITION—prevention of a response, even though the stimuli that normally elicit the response are present.

INNERVATION—the excitation of a muscle or gland by a nerve.

INPUT EVENT—events that are antecedent to a response and often subject to laboratory manipulation.

INSTRUMENTAL-ACT REGRESSION—shifting to earlier immature techniques to secure the frustrated goal.

INSTRUMENTAL RESPONSE—an act which precedes consummation and makes it possible.

INTELLECTUAL MOTIVE—a motive for intellectual competence.

INTRAPUNITIVE RESPONSE—aggression directed to the self.

MECHOLYL—a drug that causes a rapid short-term drop in blood pressure; Mecholyl is often used in physiological studies of anxiety.

MMPI (MINNESOTA MULTIPHASIC PERSONALITY INVENTORY)—a personality questionnaire used primarily for assessing psychopathology.

NORADRENALINE (NOREPINEPHRINE)—a substance secreted by the adrenal medulla which produces the kind of body reactions that characterize the anxious state.

ORIENTING RESPONSE—the response of paying attention in the direction of a stimulus.

OUTPUT EVENTS—events that follow a response and that change as a result of input changes.

PATHOLOGICAL GUILT—a severe type of guilt that is reflected in persons who seem to be seeking punishment.

PITUITARY-ADRENAL AXIS—a major biological system that reacts to threatening situations or stress: the pituitary gland secretes a hormone that activates the adrenal gland, which then secretes other substances that are crucial for the body's defense against harm and infection.

POINT OF COMMITMENT—the point of no return in an approach-avoidance conflict.

POLYGRAPH—an instrument for recording autonomic changes related to arousal; colloquially known as the lie detector.

POSTDECISION DISSONANCE—a state of "intellectual discomfort" that arises after a decision has been made and that results in a special preference for information that supports the chosen alternative.

PROJECTIVE TEST—a relatively unstructured test in which a person is asked to respond imaginatively to inkblots, clouds, cartoons, vague pictures, play materials, and such.

PROPHYLACTIC RESPONSE—a response aimed at handling conflict by preventing it from occurring.

PSYCHOTHERAPY—the use of any psychological technique in the treatment of mental disorder or maladjustment.

REINFORCEMENT—anything that increases the probability that a given response will continue to follow a given stimulus.

REPRESSION—the exclusion of ideas, memories, or feelings from awareness, commonly because they provoke anxiety.

RESPONSE DISPLACEMENT—see DISPLACEMENT.

RESPONSE-PRODUCED CONFLICT—a conflict that occurs when a response that was punished in the past is currently elicited by a particular motive.

RETICULAR ACTIVATING SYSTEM—a brain structure presumed to function somewhat like a "switchboard"; it is responsible for activating the cerebral cortex or screening out stimuli so that a response does not occur.

RIGIDITY—the tendency to persist in a single response even when doing so is unrewarding; the relative inability to alter actions in accord with changing conditions.

ROLE CONSTRUCT REPERTORY TEST—a technique used to identify the dimensions along which a person classifies other people.

RORSCHACH TEST—a projective test using inkblots.

ROSENZWEIG PICTURE FRUSTRATION TEST—a projective test for measuring aggressive responses to frustration.

ROTTER SENTENCE COMPLETION—a projective test for such motives as dependency.

SCHEMATIC MODEL—a model that is intended to show the essential relationships between concepts.

SECONDARY INHIBITOR—any stimulus which has been associated with the action of a specific inhibitor and thereby acquires inhibitory power of its own.

SELF-RELIANCE—the ability to depend on one's own judgment and efforts without craving attention or approval or going to others for aid or advice.

SPECIFIC INHIBITOR—an inhibitor that has the power to reduce distress regardless of the situation that generated it—for example, nonnutritive sucking in the newborn.

STIMULUS-PRODUCED CONFLICT—conflict that arises when a single stimulus has been associated with both reward and punishment.

STROOP TEST—a technique for evaluating a person's degree of cognitive control.

SUPEREGO—in Freudian theory, one of the three major dynamic systems of personality, representing the learned and internalized moral demands of parents and society.

TAYLOR MAS (MANIFEST ANXIETY SCALE)—a questionnaire that measures general anxiety.

TELEMETRY—as used in this chapter, a process whereby autonomic bodily changes are measured from a distance.

THEMATIC APPERCEPTION TEST—a projective test, devised by H. A. Murray, for measuring a variety of motives.

THEMATIC TEST—any test in which the subject tells a story.

TRAUMA—any experience that inflicts damage upon the organism.

VICARIOUS LEARNING—learning without direct experience, such as by reading or imitation.

REFERENCES

Adorno, T. W., E. Frenkel-Brunswik, D. Levinson, and R. N. Sanford. *The authoritarian personality*. New York: Harper & Row Publishers, 1950.

Aronson, E., J. M. Carlsmith, and J. M. Darley. The effects of expectancy on volunteering for an unpleasant experience. *Journal of Abnormal and Social Psychology*, 1963, **66,** 220–224.

Atkinson, J. W., R. W. Heyns, and J. Veroff. The effect of experimental arousal of the affiliation motive on thematic apperception. *Journal of Abnormal and Social Psychology*, 1954, **49,** 405–410.

——— and D. C. McClelland. The projective expression of needs: The effect of different intensities of the hunger drive on thematic apperception. *Journal of Experimental Psychology*, 1948, **38,** 643–658.

——— and E. L. Walker. The affiliation motive and perceptual sensitivity to faces. *Journal of Abnormal and Social Psychology*, 1956, **53,** 38–41.

Ax, A. F. The physiological differentiation between fear and anger in humans. *Psychosomatic Medicine*, 1953, **15,** 433–442.

Bash, K. W. An investigation into a possible organic basis for the hunger drive. *Journal of Comparative and Physiological Psychology*, 1939, **28,** 109–135.

Beach, F. A. Effects of cortical lesions upon the copulatory behavior of male rats. *Journal of Comparative and Physiological Psychology*, 1940, **29,** 193–239.

———. Effects of injury to the cerebral cortex upon the display of masculine and feminine mating behavior by female rats. *Journal of Comparative and Physiological Psychology*, 1943, **36,** 169–198.

Berkowitz, L. *Aggression: A social psychological analysis*. New York: McGraw-Hill, Inc., 1962.

Berlyne, D. *Conflict, arousal and curiosity*. New York: McGraw-Hill, Inc., 1960.

Bindra, D. *Motivation: A systematic reinterpretation*. New York: The Ronald Press Company, 1959.

———, A. L. Paterson, and J. Strzelecki. On the relation between anxiety and conditioning. *Canadian Journal of Psychology*, 1955, **9,** 1–6.

Bobbitt, Ruth A. The repression hypothesis studied in a situation of hypnotically induced conflict. *Journal of Abnormal and Social Psychology*, 1958, **56,** 204–212.

Brobeck, J. R. Neural regulation of food intake. *Annals of the New York Academy of Science*, 1955, **63,** 44–55.

Buss, A. H., and A. Durkee. An inventory for assessing different kinds of hostility. *Journal of Consulting Psychology*, 1957, **21,** 343–349.

Byrne, D. Repression-sensitization as a dimension of personality. In B. Maher (ed.), *Progress on experimental personality research*, Vol. I. New York: Academic Press, Inc., 1966.

Cameron, D. E. Autonomy in anxiety. *Psychiatric Quarterly,* 1944, **18,** 53–60.

Carlson, A. J. *The control of hunger in health and disease.* Chicago: University of Chicago Press, 1916.

Clark, R. A. The projective measurement of experimentally induced sexual motivation. *Journal of Experimental Psychology,* 1952, **44,** 391–399.

———. The effects of sexual motivation on fantasy. In D. C. McClelland (ed.), *Studies in motivation.* New York: Appleton-Century-Crofts, 1955.

Cofer, C. N., and M. H. Appley. *Motivation: Theory and research.* New York: John Wiley & Sons, Inc., 1964.

Dollard, J., L. Doob, N. Miller, O. Mowrer, and R. Sears. *Frustration and aggression.* New Haven, Conn.: Yale University Press, 1939.

Ehrenfreund, D. The relationship between weight loss during deprivation and food consumption. *Journal of Comparative and Physiological Psychology,* 1959, **52,** 123.

Epstein, S. The measurement of drive and conflict in humans. In M. R. Jones (ed.), *Nebraska symposium on motivation, 1962.* Lincoln, Neb.: University of Nebraska Press, 1962.

Festinger, L. *A theory of cognitive dissonance.* New York: Harper & Row, Publishers, 1957.

Fitzgerald, B. J. Some relationships among projective test, interview, and sociometric measures of dependent behavior. *Journal of Abnormal and Social Psychology,* 1958, **56,** 199–203.

Ford, C. S., and F. A. Beach. *Patterns of sexual behavior.* New York: Harper & Row, Publishers, 1951.

Frenkel-Brunswik, E. Distortion of reality in perception and in social outlook. *American Psychologist,* 1949, **4,** 253.

Funkenstein, D. H. The physiology of fear and anger. *Scientific American,* 1955, **192,** 74–80.

Graham, F. X., W. A. Charwat, A. S. Honig, and P. C. Weltz. Aggression as a function of the attack and the attacker. *Journal of Abnormal and Social Psychology,* 1951, **46,** 512–520.

Guilford, J. P. *Personality.* New York: McGraw-Hill, Inc., 1959.

Hall, J. F. The relationship between external stimulation, food deprivation, and activity. *Journal of Comparative and Physiological Psychology,* 1956, **49,** 339–341.

——— and P. V. Hanford. Activity as a function of a restricted feeding schedule. *Journal of Comparative and Physiological Psychology,* 1954, **47,** 362–363.

Hendrick, I. Facts and theories of psychoanalysis. New York: Alfred A. Knopf, Inc., 1934.

Hill, W. F. Learning theory and the acquisition of values. *Psychological Review,* 1960, 67, 317–331.

Hull, C. L. The goal gradient hypothesis and maze learning. *Psychological Review,* 1932, **39,** 25–43.

Irwin, O. C. The distribution of the amount of mobility in young infants between two nursing periods. *Journal of Comparative and Physiological Psychology,* 1932, **14,** 428–445.

———. Changes in activity between two feeding periods. In W. Dennis (ed.), *Readings in child psychology.* Englewood Cliffs, N.J.: Prentice-Hall, Inc., 1963.

Jasper, H. In H. Jasper, *et al.* (eds.), *Reticular formation of the brain.* Boston: Little, Brown & Company, 1958.

Johnson, H. J. Decision making, conflict, and physiological arousal. *Journal of Abnormal and Social Psychology,* 1963, **67,** 114–124.

Kaelbling, R., F. A. King, K. Achenbach, R. Branson, and B. Pasamanick. Reliability of autonomic responses. *Psychological Reports,* 1960, 6, 143–163.

Kelly, G. A. *The psychology of personal constructs.* New York: W. W. Norton & Company, Inc., 1955.

Kessen, W., and G. Mandler. Anxiety, pain and the inhibition of distress. *Psychological Review,* 1961, **68,** 396–404.

Kinsey, A. C., W. B. Pomeroy, and C. E. Martin. *Sexual behavior in the human male.* Philadelphia: W. B. Saunders Company, 1948.

———, ———, ———, and P. H. Gebhard. *Sexual behavior in the human female.* Philadelphia: W. B. Saunders Company, 1953.

Klein, G. S. Need and regulation. In M. R. Jones (ed.), *Nebraska symposium on motivation, 1954.* Lincoln, Neb.: University of Nebraska Press, 1954.

Kohn, P. M. Serendipity on the move: Towards a measure of intellectual motivation. *Canadian Psychologist,* 1965, **6,** 20–31.

Korchin, S. J., and H. A. Heath. Somatic experience in the anxiety state: Some sex and personality correlates of "autonomic feedback." *Journal of Consulting Psychology*, 1961, **25**, 398–404.

Lacey, J. I. Individual differences in somatic response patterns. *Journal of Comparative and Physiological Psychology*, 1950, **43**, 338–350.

———, D. E. Bateman, and R. Van Lehn. Autonomic response specificity. *Psychosomatic Medicine*, 1953, **15**, 10–21.

Lawrence, D. H., and W. A. Mason. Food intake in the rat as a function of deprivation intervals and feeding rhythms. *Journal of Comparative and Physiological Psychology*, 1955, **48**, 267–271.

Lazarus, R. S., C. W. Eriksen, and C. P. Fonda. Personality dynamics and auditory perceptual recognition. *Journal of Personality*, 1951, **19**, 471–482.

———, H. Yousem, and D. Arenberg. Hunger and perception. *Journal of Personality*, 1953, **21**, 312–328.

Lindsley, D. B. Psychophysiology and motivation. In M. R. Jones (ed.), *Nebraska symposium on motivation*. Lincoln, Neb.: University of Nebraska Press, 1957, pp. 44–105.

Lindzey, G., and H. V. Riecken. Inducing frustration in adult subjects. *Journal of Consulting Psychology*, 1951, **15**, 18–23.

Maher, B. A. The application of the approach avoidance conflict model to social behavior. *Journal of Conflict Resolution*, 1964, **8**, 287–291.

——— and E. Hedwig. Unpublished data. Northwestern University, 1958.

——— and N. D. Repucci. Unpublished data. Harvard University, 1964.

———, N. Weisstein, and K. Sylva. The determinant of oscillation points in a temporal decision conflict. *Psychonomic Science*, 1964, **1**, 13–14.

Malmo, R. B. Anxiety and behavioral arousal. *Psychological Review*, 1957, **64**, 276–287.

———. Activation: A neuropsychological dimension. *Psychological Review*, 1959, **66**, 367–386.

Mayer, J., and N. W. Bates. Blood glucose and food intake in normal and hypophysectomized, alloxan treated rats. *American Journal of Physiology*, 1952, **168**, 812–819.

McClelland, D. C. Risk taking in children with high and low need for achievement. In J. W. Atkinson (ed.), *Motives in fantasy, action and society*. Princeton, N.J.: D. Van Nostrand Company, Inc., 1958.

———, J. W. Atkinson, R. A. Clark, and E. L. Lowell. *The achievement motive*. New York: Appleton-Century-Crofts, 1953.

———, R. A. Clark, T. B. Roby, and J. W. Atkinson. The projective expression of needs: IV. The effect of the need for achievement on thematic apperception. *Journal of Experimental Psychology*, 1949, **39**, 242–255.

———, ———, ———, and ———. The effect of the need for achievement on thematic apperception. In J. W. Atkinson (ed.), *Motives in fantasy, action and society*. Princeton, N.J.: D. Van Nostrand Company, Inc., 1958.

———, and A. M. Liberman. The effect of need for achievement on the recognition of need related words. *Journal of Personality*, 1949, **18**, 236–251.

Menaker, T. Conflict about drinking in alcoholics. Unpublished doctoral dissertation, Harvard University, 1964.

Menninger, K. *Love against hate*. New York: Harcourt, Brace & World, Inc., 1942.

Miller, N. E. The frustration-aggression hypothesis. *Psychological Review*, 1941, **38**, 337–342.

———. Liberalization of basic S-R concepts: Extensions to conflict behavior, motivation and social learning. In S. Koch (ed.), *Psychology: A study of a science*, Vol. 2. New York: McGraw-Hill, Inc., 1959.

Money, J. Sex hormones and other variables in human eroticism. In W. C. Young (ed.), *Sex and internal secretions*, Ed. 3. Baltimore: The Williams & Wilkins Company, 1961.

Morgan, C. T., and J. T. Morgan. Studies in hunger: II. The relation of gastric denervation and dietary sugar to the effect of insulin upon food intake in the rat. *Journal of Genetic Psychology*, 1940, **57**, 153–163.

Moskowitz, M. J. Running-wheel activity in the white rat as a function of combined food and water deprivation. *Journal of Comparative and Physiological Psychology*, 1959, **52**, 621–625.

Moss, T., and A. E. Edwards. Conflict vs. conditioning: Effects upon peripheral vascular activity. *Psychosomatic Medicine*, 1964, **26**, 267–273.

Murray, E. J. Conflict and repression during sleep deprivation. *Journal of Abnormal and Social Psychology*, 1959, **59**, 95–101.

——— and M. M. Berkun. Displacement as a function of conflict. *Journal of Abnormal and Social Psychology*, 1955, **51**, 47–56.

Murray, H. A. *Explorations in personality*. New York: Oxford University Press, 1938.

———. *Thematic Apperception Test manual*. Cambridge, Mass.: Harvard University Press, 1943.

Office of Strategic Services Assessment Staff. *Assessment of men*. New York: Holt, Rinehart & Winston, 1948.

Otto, D. Correlates of religious and death concern. Unpublished honor thesis. Harvard College, 1963.

Pastore, N. A neglected factor in the frustration-aggression hypothesis: A comment. *Journal of Psychology*, 1950, **29**, 271–279.

———. The role of arbitrariness on the frustration-aggression hypothesis. *Journal of Abnormal and Social Psychology*, 1952, **47**, 728–731.

Phillips, E. L. *Psychotherapy: A modern theory and practice*. Englewood Cliffs, N.J.: Prentice-Hall, Inc., 1956.

Quigley, J. P. The role of the digestive tract in regulating the ingestion of food (from the regulation of hunger and appetite). *Annals of the New York Academy of Science*, 1955, **63**, 6–14.

Reiser, M. F., R. B. Reeves, and J. Armington. Effects of variations in laboratory procedures and experiments on ballistocardiogram, blood pressure and heart rate in healthy young men. *Psychosomatic Medicine*, 1955, **17**, 185–199.

Renner, K. E., B. A. Maher, and D. T. Campbell. The validity of a method for scoring sentence completion responses for anxiety, dependency and hostility. *Journal of Applied Psychology*, 1962, **46**, 285–290.

Rigby, W. K. Approach and avoidance gradients and conflict behavior in a predominantly temporal situation. *Journal of Comparative and Physiological Psychology*, 1954, **47**, 83–89.

Rosenzweig, S. The picture-association method and its application in a study of reactions to frustration. *Journal of Personality*, 1945, **14**, 3–23.

———, H. S. Clarke, M. S. Garfield, and A. Lehndorff. Scoring samples for the Rosenzweig picture frustration study. *Journal of Psychology*, 1946, **21**, 45–72.

———, E. E. Fleming, and H. J. Clarke. Revised scoring manual for the Rosenzweig picture frustration study. *Journal of Psychology*, 1947, **24**, 165–208.

Rotter, J. B. *Social learning and clinical psychology*. Englewood Cliffs, N.J.: Prentice-Hall, Inc., 1954.

——— and J. E. Rafferty. *The Rotter incomplete sentences blank*. New York: The Psychological Corporation, 1950.

Runquist, W. N., and L. E. Ross. The relation between physiological measures of emotionality and performance in eyelid conditioning. *Journal of Experimental Psychology*, 1959, **57**, 329–332.

Sarason, I. G. Empirical findings and theoretical problems in the use of anxiety scales. *Psychological Bulletin*, 1960, **57**, 403–415.

Schachter, S. *The psychology of affiliation*. Stanford, Calif.: Stanford University Press, 1959.

——— and B. Latané. Crime, cognition, and the autonomic nervous system. In D. Levine (ed.), *Nebraska symposium on motivation, 1964*. Lincoln, Neb.: University of Nebraska Press, 1964.

——— and J. E. Singer. Cognitive, social and physiological determinants of emotional state. *Psychological Review*, 1962, **69**, 379–399.

Schnore, L. F. Satellites and suburbs. *Social Forces*, 1957, **36**, 121–127.

Sears, R. R. Success and failure: A study of motility. In Q. McNemar and M. A. Merrill (eds.), *Studies in personality*. New York: McGraw-Hill, Inc., 1942.

———, C. I. Hovland, and N. E. Miller. Minor studies of aggression: 1. Measurement of aggressive behavior. *Journal of Psychology*, 1940, **9**, 275–295.

———, E. Maccoby, and H. Levin. *Patterns of child rearing*. New York: Harper & Row, Publishers, 1957.

Shipley, T. E., Jr., and J. Veroff. A projective measure of need for affiliation. *Journal of Experimental Psychology*, 1952, **43**, 349–356.

Siegel, P. S., and M. Steinberg. Activity level as a function of hunger. *Journal of Comparative and Physiological Psychology*, 1949, **42**, 413–416.

Solomon, R. L., and L. C. Wynne. Traumatic avoidance learning: Acquisition in normal dogs. *Psychological Monographs*, 1953, **67**, 1–19 (Whole No. 354).

Stroop, J. R. Studies of interference in serial verbal reactions. *Journal of Experimental Psychology*, 1935, **18**, 643–661.

Stunkard, A. J., and H. G. Wolff. Correlation of arteriovenous glucose differences, gastric hunger contractions and the experience of hunger in man. *Federation Procedures*, 1954, **13**, 147.

——— and ———. Studies in the physiology of hunger: I. The effect of intravenous administration of glucose on gastric hunger contractions in man. *Journal of Clinical Investigation*, 1956, **35**, 354–363.

Taylor, Janet A. Drive theory and manifest anxiety. *Psychological Bulletin*, 1956, **53**, 303–320.

Thibaut, J. W., and H. W. Riecken. Authoritarianism, status, and the communication of aggression. *Human Relations*, 1955, **8**, 95–120.

Treichler, F. R. The relationship between deprivation weight loss and two activity measures. Unpublished Ph.D. dissertation, Pennsylvania State University, 1960.

Tsang, Y. C. Hunger motivation in gastrectomized rats. *Journal of Abnormal and Physiological Psychology*, 1938, **26**, 1–17.

Veroff, J. Development and validation of a projective measure of power motivation. *Journal of Abnormal and Social Psychology*, 1957, **54**, 1–8.

Wallace, M., and A. I. Rabin. Temporal experience. *Psychological Bulletin*, 1960, **57**, 213–236.

Wangensteen, O. H., and A. J. Carlson. Hunger sensations in a patient after total gastrectomy. *Proceedings of the Society of Experimental Biology*, 1931, **28**, 545–547.

Weatherley, D. Maternal permissiveness toward aggression and subsequent TAT aggression. *Journal of Abnormal and Social Psychology*, 1962, **65**, 1–5.

Wenger, M. A. Professor Boring's robot becomes emotional. *American Psychologist*, 1948, **3**, 339.

White, R. W. Motivation reconsidered: The concept of competence. *Psychological Review*, 1959, **66**, 297–333.

Worchel, P. Catharsis and the relief of hostility. *Journal of Abnormal and Social Psychology*, 1957, **55**, 238–243.

Young, P. T. *Motivation and emotion*. New York: John Wiley & Sons, Inc., 1961.

Zander, A. F. A study of experimental frustration. *Psychological Monographs: General and Applied*, 1944, **56**, No. 3 (Whole No. 256).

SUGGESTED READINGS

1. Adorno, T. A., E. Frenkel-Brunswik, D. Levinson, and R. N. Sanford. *The authoritarian personality*. New York: Harper & Row, Publishers, 1950. A classic investigation into prejudiced attitudes and behavior that has resulted in considerable research on authoritarianism. Although recent data have changed our views on the measurement of authoritarianism, this monograph remains of considerable interest.
2. Berkowitz, L. *Aggression: A social psychological analysis*. New York: McGraw-Hill, Inc., 1962. A penetrating examination of the literature in this area that concludes with an integrative theoretical analysis.
3. Cofer, C. N., and M. H. Appley. *Motivation: Theory and research*. New York: John Wiley & Sons, Inc., 1964. A comprehensive survey and analysis of theory and research in motivation.
4. Dollard, J., L. Doob, N. E. Miller, O. Mowrer, and R. Sears. *Frustration and aggression*. New Haven, Conn.: Yale University Press, 1939. On the basis of an interpretation of both psychoanalytic and learning theories, the authors argue that frustration always brings aggression. The universality of the thesis is now disproved, but the argument remains interesting for those many occasions when frustration and aggression *are* linked.
5. Magoun, H. W. *The waking brain*. Springfield, Ill.: Charles C Thomas, Publisher, 1963. Perhaps the clearest exposition of the functions of the reticular activating system and arousal.
6. Maher, B. A. *Principles of psychopathology*. New York: McGraw-Hill, Inc., 1966. A treatment in greater detail of the principles and research described here and their implications for understanding negative psychological abnormalities.

7. McClelland, D. C., J. W. Atkinson, R. A. Clark, and E. L. Lowell. *The achievement motive*. New York: Appleton-Century-Crofts, 1953. A report of the early research on the achievement motive. Both McClelland and Atkinson have gone on to extend the relevance of this motive to a variety of settings.
8. Murray, H. A. *Explorations in personality*. New York: Oxford University Press, 1938. A seminal treatise on psychological needs and situational demands that continues to retain its influence on modern theory and research.
9. Schachter, S., and J. E. Singer. Cognitive, social and physiological determinants of emotional state. *Psychological Review*, 1962, **69**, 379–399. The main theoretical paper on the view that emotion is a joint function of unlabeled arousal and cognition. An important contribution for students who are interested in the relations between psychological and physiological functioning.
10. White, R. W. Motivation reconsidered: The concept of competence. *Psychological Review*, 1959, **66**, 297–333. The author argues persuasively for a motive to deal effectively with reality, to be competent.

4

Personality Development

JEROME KAGAN

It is as hard to get an unambiguous definition of personality as it is to get definitive results in an experiment on extrasensory perception. Definitions of personality are open-end and tentative; they rarely specify a limited set of responses or traits. Cattell (1950) regards personality as "that which permits the prediction of what a person will do in a given situation." For him, it is a set of terms that allows us to explain a particular person's behavior. Lazarus (1961) defines personality as the organization of behavioral dispositions within the person. His definition is more widely accepted because it not only deals with the characteristics people display, but also notes that these characteristics have different strengths in relation to each other. *Personality* refers, then, to the hierarchy of behaviors a person is capable of and to the relationships among these behaviors. Let us illustrate this definition with two simplified personality profiles. Imagine two men, Peter and Jack, each with only three major motives: the desire for recognition from others, aggression toward others, and the desire for approval or acceptance. For Peter, the recognition and aggression motives are both very strong, and the approval motive is relatively weak. For Jack, the desire for approval is strongest, the aggression motive moderate, and the desire for recognition weakest of the three. Peter would appear ambitious and status seeking to others, and his seeking of recognition would have an aggressive flavor. He would rarely be concerned with pleasing others. Jack, on the other hand, would usually be conforming and concerned with the opinions of others, although he would occasionally exhibit a flash of rebellion or sarcasm. Both men are influenced by all three motives, but they have different personalities because the strengths of these motives

Preparation of this report was supported, in part, by Research Grant MH 8792 from the National Institute of Mental Health, United States Public Health Service.

and the relationships among them are different in each man.

DEFINITION OF PERSONALITY TRAITS

Most psychologists agree that if a trait or behavior pattern is to be considered an aspect of personality, it should be stable over time and place. A personality trait or variable, in other words, is a specific disposition that an individual tends to display in different situations and over relatively long periods of time. An important third requirement, however, is that there be clear and dramatic differences among people in the frequency and intensity of the disposition in question. If a class of behaviors is to be regarded as a personality variable, it should display considerable variability when it is measured in a large group of people. The tendency to use the article *the* before nouns, for example, shows stability over time and consistency across situations, but it is not a personality trait because it varies only minimally among people. Loudness or intensity of voice, however, can be viewed as a personality trait because it is stable over time and place and shows considerable variability among individuals. An incredibly large number of response tendencies meet these criteria of stability and high variability.

THE ROLE OF THEORY

The particular personality variables studied most intensively during the past three decades have been determined by three dominant interests among social scientists: psychoanalytic theory, social learning theory, and a statistical technique for studying behavior called "factor analysis." Psychoanalytic and social learning theories have called attention to the motives behind behavior, especially sexuality, hostility, and dependency; to anxiety and the defenses people make against it; and to imitation of others as a means of learning personality dispositions. The empirical investigations based on these points of view have used overt behavior, interview responses, and verbal interpretations of ambiguous stimuli as the main sources of information from which to infer motives, anxieties, and defenses (see Chapter 3).

Factor analysis has mostly relied on written replies to questionnaires or on slight variations of this method. This procedure yields a different kind of information from observations of overt behavior or interview judgments, and scientists who use this approach are consequently concerned with a different set of variables. Factor analysis has been used to study modes of interpersonal behavior like introversion-extraversion, people's awareness of their emotions and feelings, and finally, the degree of influence of motives like dependency, hostility, and sexuality.

Some aspects of personality have been studied extensively because of their particular importance to psychiatry and to the general well-being of society. These include traits bearing on mental health, as evidenced by technical names such as "psychopathy," "neuroticism," "depression." One of the best known personality questionnaires, the Minnesota Multiphasic Personality Inventory, measures different facets of an individual's total personality in relation to the clinical conditions listed above.

The most recent work in personality discusses behavior in the areas of thinking and problem solving. The investigators at this new frontier insist that these behaviors are legitimately personality variables because they display substantial variation among people, stability over time, consistency across situations, and theoretically at least, linkage to motives, anxieties, and defenses. These behaviors include type of conceptual categorization of familiar and unfamiliar stimuli, quality of performance in complex perceptual discrimination tasks, and speed of decision in problem situations requiring a choice of one of several answers. The study of conceptual dispositions may eventually form a bridge between the areas of personality and thinking, two domains of psychological research that previously had little overlap in procedures or terminology. Some investigators, for example, have found that extremely active boys make intellectual decisions faster than inactive boys do, suggesting that personality traits are related to intellectual ones.

A WORKING VOCABULARY AND SET OF ASSUMPTIONS

Most of the responses discussed so far concern adult functioning, and most studies of personality traits have been concerned with interrelationships among a number of well-established responses. This chapter deals, however, with developing patterns of interrelationships, rather than with these relationships in their mature form. Since psychologists disagree among themselves as to the areas of behavior that are most critical in adult functioning, the developmental psychologist has a doubly difficult task. He not only must understand how the adult's personality was formed, but he also must decide which responses deserve emphasis so that he can study those behavior dimensions developmentally. In the present discussion, the working vocabulary and basic assumptions to be presented deal with five major constructs or ideas: motives, standards, affects, defenses, and overt instrumental acts.

Motives and Their Characteristics

A motive is defined here as a wish for a specific class of events. The desired events can be external (that is, in the environment) or internal, in the form of cognitions (images, thoughts, associations, and feelings). All motives have a primary cognitive component because a wish is a mental act or cognition; therefore, infants, who have not developed imagery or language, do not have motives, as we use the word here. Hunger, thirst, and pain avoidance, which were called biological motives in the previous chapter, will here be regarded as *needs*; they can be gratified only through the occurrence of specific external events.

Motives wax and wane in intensity, for the attainment of the desired event temporarily reduces the intensity of the wish. Latent motives become active when a person recognizes a discrepancy between his desires and reality. To illustrate, children have different intensities of hostile motivation. Some have a great potential for hatred; others very little. We say that the motive is latent when the child is not thinking about wanting to hurt someone or to make someone unhappy. The motive becomes active, however, if the child is frustrated or attacked. Now he may wish to make his attacker cry, and there is a discrepancy between what he desires and reality. The extent of that discrepancy determines the intensity of his hostile motivation.

The major motives that develop during the first dozen years are:

1. Desire for physical expressions of affection.
2. Desire that certain people show they value the child and regard him positively.
3. Desire for instrumental aid from others.
4. Desire to destroy someone; the desire to perceive that someone is unhappy or hurt.
5. Desire to dominate others, to control the behavior of others.
6. Desire for genital stimulation.
7. Desire to be similar to a model.

8. Desire to determine one's own actions autonomously and to be free of coercive control from others.
9. Desire to reduce anxiety.
10. Desire to be competent at selected tasks.
11. Desire to act in maximal congruence with established standards.

Standards

A standard is an evaluation of the appropriateness of a response, belief, motive, or affect. People attempt to develop and maintain belief systems about the self that are maximally congruent with attributes that are widely regarded as "good" and to renounce and avoid attributes regarded as "bad." The bases for the evaluation "good" or "bad" are culturally derived. The Western community considers it good to be valued by others, to be attractive to others, to have the necessary instrumental skills and competencies to deal with selected problems, to possess the attributes and skills considered appropriate for one's sex, to be rational and coherent, to be independent and responsible, and to avoid overt behaviors or preoccupation with thoughts prohibited by the primary reference group (for example, anger, sexuality).

As a child grows up, he gradually learns the standards of the world around him. Some of these standards are learned as the simple consequence of reward and punishment, but others, such as standards of physical attractiveness, are evidently learned through sheer repetition by someone the child respects and loves until he is led to believe in them. To the young child the environment appears unordered and unpredictable. He does not always know what to expect or what is expected of him, and he searches for rules by which to evaluate his behaviors, thoughts, and feelings. The standards learned during the first seven or eight years derive, in large measure, from the communications about behavior and attributes that are most frequently presented to him by his family and friends. If parents remind their son, "Don't cry, don't cry," a half dozen times a day, every day, their words eventually have a permanent impact on the child's evaluation of crying.

The most significant standards are summary ideas of how a person should think, feel, and behave, and these standards together compose the child's ego ideal, that is, the way he would ideally like to be. The formation of the ego ideal involves the process of identification, which will be discussed later. When the child feels that his thoughts or behaviors do not agree with the standards of his ego ideal, he becomes motivated to do something about the disagreement. Thus, there are two major kinds of motives in the child: (1) desire for a specific class of activity, such as genital stimulation, or physical expression of affection or approval, and (2) desire for a feeling of increased congruence with a standard.

It is important to recognize that the same overt behavior can result from either a desire for a specific event or a desire for increased congruence with a standard. For example, a man's display of verbal aggression to his wife can be motivated by a desire to see his wife unhappy (hostile motive) or by his desire to increase his congruence with a standard that says, "A masculine husband should be aggressive toward his wife." Many classes of behavior that appear similar may actually serve different motives.

Affects

Affect or emotion is extremely difficult to define and still harder to measure. A differentiation should be made, moreover, between the excited states of the infant and the emotions of the older child who possesses language. Words like *depression, grief, anger,* and *excitement* are really descriptions of a complex stimulus pattern made up of physiological events, cognitive components (wishes, beliefs, standards), and classification of the external context in which the person finds himself. It is nonsense to suppose that an infant can experience disgust, pride, or guilt. The infant has not had the experiences necessary to the development of those feelings and does not have the language labels to designate them. The infant's crying and thrashing, which are often called emotional, are usually a direct consequence of internal discomfort. The crying of a ten-year-old, however, is typically not linked to any specific pattern of internal physiological stimulation. More often it is a function of the predicament the child is in and the implicit label he gives this predicament: "Someone hit me"; "I'm afraid"; "I'm hurt"; "I have no friends." These cognitive components, together with the pattern of stimulation from muscles and viscera, elicit an overt response that is called "emotion." We shall use the word *affect* as a general term to designate a psychological state in which some form of *labeling* of context and internal stimulation occurs. We shall use terms like "hungry," "cold," "pained," "startled," "sleepy," and "irritable" for states in the infant that produce behavior that adults regard as "emotional."

People can have as many affects as there are words to label combinations of internal states, cognitions, and external contexts. As William James (1890) has written, "There is no limit to the number of possible different emotions which may exist, and why the emotions of different individuals may vary indefinitely." The primary component of an affect is a perceived change in the intensity and quality of the mosaic of internal stimulation from muscles and viscera, and specific affects are linked to differing intensities, as different sounds are tuned to different locations on the basilar membrane of the ear. Some theorists believe that intensity depends upon *level of arousal* or *level of activation*; the reticular formation and related central nervous system structures play a major role in this process (see Chapter 3).

Grief, sadness, depression, apathy, and lassitude are characterized by low levels of arousal, in which the person perceives the internal level of stimulation *as less intense* than is customary. The level to which he is accustomed is called his "adaptation level." Excitement, rage, joy, fear, and anxiety are characterized by perception of increased arousal. The absolute level of activity of central nervous system structures, muscle action potentials, or heart rate is not a faithful index of the degree to which a person is experiencing an affect, however; affect may occur whenever a person recognizes a change in intensity of internal stimulation from what he regards as normal for him.

The language label the individual applies to his state is a secondary component of affect. The label chosen depends on (1) the direction of the change he notices in arousal, (2) the content of the images and thoughts he is having when the change in arousal is perceived, and (3) the immediate contextual situation. A perception of lowered arousal combined with thoughts about missing one's sweetheart on the part of one in the physical context of a strange hotel room is likely to be labeled *depression or loneliness*. The same level and quality of arousal, combined with thoughts about the hard day at the office on the part of one who is taking the late bus home at 7:30 P.M., is likely to be labeled *fatigue*.

Schachter and Singer (1962) have demonstrated that after an injection of adrenalin, which raises the perceived arousal level, the specific label the individual applied to his feelings depended on the situation he was in and the thoughts he was having. An aroused person will regard himself as angry or happy depending on the situational context. A child presumably learns specific affect labels as a result of informal tutoring by the social environment. A mother sees her child laughing and remarks, "You sure are happy today"; or she tells her six-year-old who is stamping his feet in protest, "Do not show your anger to your mother."

Infants under six months apparently experience only two major arousal levels: one resulting from unpleasant and one from pleasant events. Displeasure from pain, hunger, cold, or sudden changes in level of external stimulation increases arousal level. The child's main reactions to it are crying and motor activity. The affect of *pleasure* is characterized by lowered internal arousal occurring when pain is being reduced, hunger or thirst is being gratified, or certain forms of tactile stimulation, such as stroking, are being experienced. The behavioral reactions to pleasure are smiling, postural quiescence, and relaxation.

During the second half of the first year the simple relation between pleasure-displeasure and level of arousal disappears. The process of learning enters the picture. In the first place, pleasurable experiences become associated with increased level of arousal. The child smiles, laughs, and thrashes when he is tickled, spoken to, or given mild surprises (as in a peek-a-boo game). We say the child is excited. Further, behavioral signs of displeasure can occur not only with high arousal and pain, but also when the child anticipates a painful experience, when a perceptual expectancy is violated (for example, although he expects to see his mother come in the door, a strange man enters instead), or when he is separated from his mother. Crying and motor activity are the reactions to these conditions also, but each involves some prior learning. An expectancy must be learned before it can be violated.

Another development during the latter half of the first year is the emergence of *rage*. Rage is characterized by an increase in arousal level when the infant loses a goal object, wants a goal object he can see but not reach, or is bodily restrained. The familiar behavioral reactions of crying and motor activity during rage often differ in form and intensity from the crying of pain or fear.

These four arousal situations, *pain, pleasure, rage,* and *excitement,* may be the foundation for the more finely differentiated affects of anxiety, distress, sadness, anger, elation, joy, grief, apathy, disgust, shame, and guilt. These affects are attached to specific cue complexes by the child's social environment, which labels his affect for him, points out his behavior in a specific situation, and tells him he is feeling a certain way. Thus a recognition of change in internal arousal, in imagery, thoughts, and associated cognitive components, and in environmental context are linked together and given a name.

As the child grows, his overt *behavior* comes increasingly under the control of the *name* he gives this stimulus complex and becomes less strongly tied to the level or quality of internal arousal he perceives. The ten-year-old considers himself happy because he is in a particular situation (for example, watching a funny movie), perceiving a certain quality of arousal. Once thinking he is "happy," he is more likely to laugh than if he had not primed himself by labeling his state at the moment. The one-year-old infant laughs as a result of direct changes in arousal level and external contexts without the intervention of mental labels for the situation.

Fear, anxiety, shame, guilt, rage, anger, happiness, sadness, excitement, joy, loneliness, and pain are primary affects for members of Western civilization because the words for them are typically used to label arousal changes in different contexts, and specific behavioral reactions to them are learned.

This list closely resembles the list of eight primary affects proposed by Tomkins (1962) and Tomkins and McCarter (1964), who postulate that each affect is associated with distinct facial responses in such a way that the feedback from these facial muscular patterns is necessary for the affect to be felt. Their eight affects are: (1) interest—excitement, (2) enjoyment—joy, (3) surprise—startle, (4) distress—anguish, (5) fear—terror, (6) shame—humiliation, (7) contempt—disgust, and (8) anger—rage. The selection of these particular affects is largely determined by the fact that they are associated with different facial reactions, whereas the list I propose is based more on the cognitions linked to the internal changes. The differences in these lists imply a difference of opinion about where the focus of affect lies. At all events, cross-cultural data suggest that words for anxiety, joy, sadness, and anger exist universally, and it seems likely that the same core of affects is common to all societies of men.

Sources of anxiety. The unpleasant affects center around the elusive experience of anxiety. Everyone learns anxiety as a reaction to various cues that combine internal stimuli, cognitions, and external events. Formally, anxiety is an anticipatory cognitive response, which means that after a stimulus—either a thought or an external event—has become attached to the mosaic of fearsome stimulation in a context, it becomes capable of eliciting an anticipation of the feared event. The anticipation of the feared event is the state of anxiety. The major sources of children's anxiety are: (1) anticipation of loss of nurturance or affection, (2) anticipation of physical harm, and (3) recognition of incongruity between the child's own standard and his current attitude or behavior. Refinements and subtle combinations of these three classes of anxiety make up the unpleasant affects of helplessness, guilt, and shame, which appear during the preschool and early school years. As we saw in Chapter 3, intensive empirical effort and thoughtful concern have still yielded no firm agreement on a valid method of measuring the universal human experience of anxiety. Anxiety can be defined physiologically as an unpleasant emotional state usually characterized by a perception of increased motility of the gastrointestinal tract ("butterflies in the stomach," or diarrhea), increased heart rate, palmar sweating, shivering, flushing, and muscular contractions. Anxiety often has a cognitive component too, which consists of the anticipation of an unwanted event. In some cases, the child is not clearly aware of what is frightening him, but is nevertheless anxious because of anticipated physical harm, loss of affection or nurture, or recognition of incongruity with a standard.

The anxiety resulting from recognition of discrepancy with a standard is called "shame" if the child expects censure from others and "guilt" if the source of censure is internal. These two processes will be considered in more detail later in the chapter.

Defenses

Anxiety generates its own special reactions, and responses that act to reduce and control it are given the name of defenses. A detailed discussion of defenses is presented in Chapter 10. For our purposes, it is sufficient to note that the child develops both behavioral and conceptual defenses against anxiety. The overt reaction of *withdrawal* from an anxiety-arousing situation is one effective defense. The four-year-old who hides his face in his mother's lap when a stranger enters graphically illustrates defense by withdrawal. Refusal to go to school the morning of a test and running from the nursery after an embarrassment are other instances of withdrawal that are common during the preschool and early school years.

The cognitive analogues of behavioral withdrawal from an anxiety-arousing object include attempts to remove anxiety-arousing thoughts by the mechanisms of *repression, denial,* or *projection.*

Substitution of goals is another common defense among older children and adults. This defense is elicited when reaching a desirable goal is blocked by practical obstacles or inhibited by anxiety. In such cases the child often selects a substitute goal. A boy who is incompetent at athletics and feels alienated from his peers may select a substitute activity to prove his competence and to maintain congruence with his standards for masculinity. Finally, the defense of intellectual analysis—the attempt to mitigate anxiety through intellectual understanding of it—begins to occur in the schoolchild and becomes a strong habit during adolescence.

Overt Instrumental Acts

So far we have discussed motives, standards, affects, and defenses. All these categories refer to cognitive or to affective behavior—that is, to thoughts or feelings. Another class of behavior consists of acts performed to support the other four categories. We refer to these as instrumental acts. A child will learn a behavior that is instrumental in gratifying his motives and increasing congruence with his standards. Urgent pleas for affection, studying algebra until midnight, or stealing money are instrumental responses aimed at obtaining desired goals or maintaining congruence with standards, the same act often serving more than one purpose at a time. A girl's request for help from a teacher can gratify a concrete need for aid, a desire to display behavior that is congruent with the feminine sex role standard, or a dependent wish to obtain attention, or it can gratify all of these.

Motives, standards, affects, defenses, and *instrumental acts* constitute the basic vocabulary needed to describe and interpret the development of the behaviors responsible for personality differences among adolescents and adults. It is especially important to examine the behaviors of preschool and school-age children because some motives—for example, hostility, affection, anxieties, and defenses—have their primitive beginnings during the first three years of life. The responses developing during this time determine the child's future receptivity to experience in much the way that the setting of a radio tuner determines what signals of what frequencies will be received. Some periods of development are more critical than others for certain purposes, it seems, and a consideration of these periods and of the responses associated with each is a major aspect of this chapter.

CRITICAL PERIODS

The term "critical period" is borrowed from biology. It refers to the fact that some environmental events have maximal influence on development during a certain time period and negligible effects before or after that time. The critical period of an environmental element is its era of maximum effect. Transplanting part of a recently fertilized egg, for example, will have one effect during the early hours after fertilization and a very different effect forty-eight hours later. Castration of a male rat during the first five days after birth may dispose him towards female patterns of mating behavior at adulthood, but castration after the fifth day has little influence on mating behavior

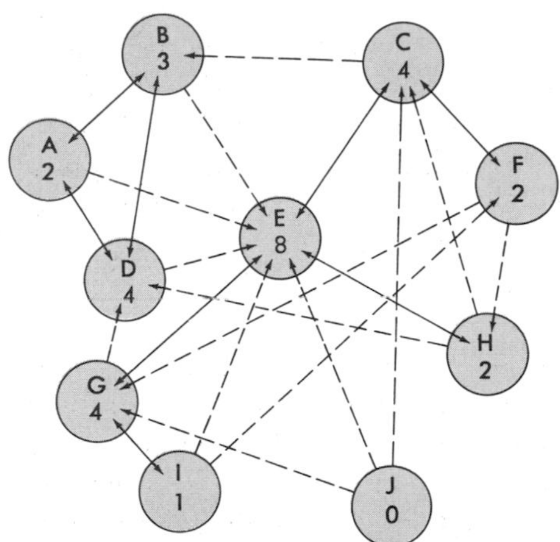

Figure 4.1 Sociogram of a group of workmen. Each person, represented here by a letter, was asked to vote for the three men most desired as working companions. Numbers represent votes. Thus *E* received 8 and *J* received no votes. Solid lines represent mutual choices. *A* and *B*, for example, voted for each other. Broken lines indicate one-way choices. *J*, for instance, voted for *E*, *G*, and *C*, but they did not select him. The person voted for by most (that is, *E*) is designated in sociometric research as a "star." *J*, on the other hand, is an "isolate." From N. R. F. Maier, *Psychology in Industry*, Ed. 2, Houghton Mifflin, 1955, p. 130.

in adulthood (Young *et al.*, 1964). Apparently, the loss of testicular androgens (male hormones) in rats due to castration has a major effect on future behavioral development only if it occurs during the first five days of postnatal life.

Critical-period phenomena in biology typically involve changes in a particular organ or physiological process. When the term is applied to psychological development, it refers to a particular response system—to either overt acts, affects, standards, motives, or defenses. The phrase *critical period* does not necessarily imply genetic unfolding of innate response tendencies. Rather it implies that each of the major behaviors, affects, standards, and defenses of the adult usually begins to grow during its own specific time period of maximal growth. The idea of the critical period suggests that, in a graph of psychological development where each curve represents a different response system, the rate at which a response is acquired, and consequently the age during which its slope is maximal, will differ for different responses (Figure 4.1). To postulate a critical period for language development is equivalent to stating that there is a period, say from two to six years, during which the rate of acquisition of language skills is most rapid and that modifications in the environment during this four-year span will have a maximal facilitating or debilitating effect on the quality of the child's language at maturity.

The rest of this chapter delineates the major critical periods, the salient responses associated with each one, and the environmental events that seem to be most influential in shaping the final response. Major attention will be directed to the motives, anxieties, standards, and defenses mentioned earlier.

Critical Period I: Birth to Eighteen Months

The major responses a child acquires during the first year and a half include: (1) the association of pleasure with the adult who cares for him—that is, an appreciation of the value of a human caretaker, (2) an anticipation of nurture when he feels discomfort, and (3) a feeling of anxiety at separation from mother or violations of perceptual expectations. Behaviors that indicate the development of these responses include the social smile, which appears during the first half year of life; crying and signs of anxiety about strangers, appearing in the second half year of life; signs of separation anxiety between twelve and eighteen months; and general interest in other people as evidenced by laughing, visual following, reciprocal play, and a variety of vocalizations. The environmental conditions on which these responses depend include the regularity of the care and nurture given the infant, especially the interval between onset of pain in the infant and the administration of nurture by the mother, the frequency of physical contact, and the frequency of vocalizations addressed to the child. The most critical element concerning environmental events in the first eighteen months is the balance between pain and pleasure in the infant's interactions with human caretakers; this defines *the nature of the infant's relationship* with the adults who minister to his needs.

We do not yet understand in detail how these responses are acquired. It is currently believed that the regular simultaneous occurrence of hunger, cold, or other form of discomfort, on the one hand, and the appearance of a nurturant caretaker, on the other, teach the infant to *anticipate the presence of a caretaker when he is in discomfort*. The caretaker in turn becomes associated with need satisfaction and thereby acquires reward value, so that his presence becomes a desirable goal. Finally, the initiation of vocal and facial play with the infant stimulates him to emit vocalizations and smiles to human agents. Rheingold (1956) has demonstrated that social responses to humans can be increased by increasing social contact. Smiling, frowning, and other social movements of the face, moreover, if they are reinforced by the adult who originally interacts with the infant, will be used with a complete stranger. Brackbill (1958) demonstrated that smiling can be increased by the simple reward of picking the child up and extinguished just as easily by failure to administer the reward. Infants raised in impersonal institutional surroundings vocalize, smile, and cry less frequently than family-reared infants, which supports the contention that interaction with humans provides both incentive and reinforcement for these responses (Provence and Lipton, 1962; Dennis, 1960).

Showing anxiety to a strange face by crying, motor activity, and withdrawal is common during the second half of the first year. Anxiety to strangers is less frequent in institutionalized than in family-reared infants, indicating that a close relationship to one caretaker may be a necessary condition for it. This anxiety illustrates how violations of expected perceptions elicit anxiety in the infant. By eight months of age, the child has built up a stable image of his mother's face. When a new face appears, he begins to scan it expecting to verify his mother's countenance. When further study belies this expectation, he is frightened and cries. Almost any stimulus pattern in which novel components appear in a familiar context violates the child's expectancy and may frighten him.

The child who does not receive regular care from one or two caretakers—either out of conscious neglect or because he lives in an impersonal and understaffed institution—learns a different set of behaviors to discomforts like hunger, thirst, and cold than the infant who receives regular nurture. If he is often uncomfortable without being attended to, the infant usually discovers ways to reduce the gnawing discomfort from within. He may bang his head, rock back and forth, pull his hair, or go to sleep. Each of these responses assuages temporarily the discomfort from hunger, cold, a rash, or pinprick. This infant does not learn to expect a helpful human in time of pain and fear, but learns to soothingly stimulate his own body or to withdraw into sleep—primitive versions of behaviors that signify severe psychopathology at age six.

In sum, expecting nurture from human agents, associating positive, pleasant feelings with adults, and displaying facial and vocal reactions to adults are primary dispositions acquired during the first eighteen months. This eighteen-month period is critical because the absence of a regularly nurturant caretaker may lead the child to habitually turn his attention too much toward his own body and to withdraw from the social environment when he experiences discomfort and anxiety.

Biologically Based Differences in Infancy

The last dccade has witnessed a healthy antidote to the *tabula rasa* bias that dominated psychology from 1920 to 1950 (see Chapter 2). Recent studies of infants indicate dramatic early differences among them on several dimensions. Some of the differences at two or three months of age may be transient and of little influence on later development, but some of the dimensions that differentiate infants during the first half year may direct important developmental processes.

Vigor of activity. Intensity of motor activity is one of the most striking characteristics that differentiates young infants. Some move their arms and legs with great force, others with little vigor; some infants cry lustily, others weakly and shallowly; some bang objects together or strike their cribs with force, others lightly. The vigorous infant will probably get into more mischief than the more placid one and, as a result, be punished more often. At the same time, the vigorous child is more likely to conquer frustrations that block attainment of goals because he has the strength to remove them and the disposition to strike out motorically.

Threshold for attention to external stimulus. Infants also differ in the amount of stimulation necessary to attract their attention. Some infants appear to recognize slight changes in visual or auditory stimuli; others require greater changes before they will attend. The threshold of attention has sometimes been called "perceptual sensitivity."

Rate of processing stimulation. A third difference is the rate at which infants become "bored" with an activity or a new stimulus. Some will play with a simple toy or push a cradle gym steadily for ten or fifteen minutes without any apparent loss of interest. Others have much shorter interest spans. They will play with an object for thirty or forty seconds, then shift to a new toy or a new sound or sight. They may return to the original object later, but they typically do not spend long periods involved with a particular object or stimulus. Be wary, however, of concluding that these infants will still be "distractible" when they are in the second grade. The distractibility of the eight-year-old and the rapid stimulus processing of the six-month-old are probably only superficially similar, and each is the result of different forces.

Irritability threshold. A fourth biological difference is the ease with which crying is elicited and the ease with which the child is mollified. Some infants become irritable at slight provocation, while others do not cry unless pain and discomfort are relatively great.

It is interesting, in this connection, that some infants typically begin to fret for a half minute and then stop spontaneously, as though they possessed internal mechanisms that brake the build-up of extreme discomfort. Other infants begin to cry, and in a matter of minutes are bellowing with rage, the crying increasing until it reaches maximum intensity. These infants seem to lack the capacity to inhibit tantrums; once fretting begins, the reaction must carry to completion.

It is easy to imagine how differently these two infants would affect the same mother. The hyperirritable infant is more likely to vex a parent, to provoke more punishment, to elicit less affection and, as a result, to experience a very different pattern of social reinforcements than the more placid child.

These behaviors comprise the most obvious dimensions of difference among young infants during the first critical period. It is not yet possible to state the exact relationship among these attributes, but it seems clear, in any case, that *unlearned* behavioral dispositions are present at birth. Some of these, moreover, are stable over time and facilitate or impede the acquisition of particular motives, anxieties, and instrumental acts, either directly or as an indirect result of the special reactions they evoke in the person caring for the child.

Anxiety and Symptoms of the First Critical Period

There are three major sources of anxiety during the first eighteen months of life: pain, separation from the primary caretaker, and violations of the child's expectancies. The latter may be responsible for the phenomenon of anxiety to strangers because, in the child's initial scanning of a human face, he expects to see his mother's countenance, and that expectancy is violated by a stranger's appearance. This phenomenon shows the fallacy of the widespread myth among many parents and social scientists that signs of anxiety are always indicators of psychopathology. If anxiety to strangers is facilitated by a close relationship with one caretaker, then it is not necessarily a sign of nascent pathology.

Some of the common anxiety symptoms during the first year are vomiting, irregular feeding patterns, irregular sleeping, and chronic crying without apparent provocation. These symptoms appear to be influenced both by basic biological characteristics of the child and the consistency of the nurture he receives.

Critical Period II: Eighteen Months to Three Years

The onset of the second critical period is heralded by three developments—the ability to locomote, the ability to use language, and the imposition by the parents of the first socialization demands. As the child masters crawling, walking, and running, he becomes capable of having an instrumental effect upon objects around him. He can grasp a toy that catches his attention rather than cry for his mother to bring it to him. He can reach for cookies, push open doors, crawl around obstacles, and climb up and down chairs. The two-year-old is learning some vital things during this era of unrestrained locomotion, especially that he is capable of obtaining desirable goals and of overcoming frustrations. He is actually practicing the responses that accomplish these ends and is learning instrumental effectiveness through the coordination of large and fine motor movements.

The emergence of language is the second salient characteristic of this period. The child learns the meaning of *no* and *yes*, the intent of requests, demands, and prohibitions, and the connection between a word and its referent (as "look at the *dog*," "drink the *milk*," "see the *moon*").

Finally, parents begin making socialization demands during the second and third years. During the second year, most mothers begin to impose constraints over bowel and bladder control and over exploration. In both instances, the child is required to inhibit a complex response that is strongly motivated and has been practiced for a long time. After twelve months of debonair response to the internal stimuli that signal defecation, the child must suddenly learn to interrupt this natural response sequence and to prevent defecation from occurring. He must also learn to restrain his desposition to pull out drawers, wander aimlessly down the street, or rock fragile vases on their precarious bases.

Learning Inhibitions

The mechanism by which the child learns these inhibitions is not completely clear, but at least two kinds of processes seem to be involved, *punitive* training and *incentive* training.

Punitive training teaches inhibitions by creating *anxiety over commission of the prohibited act.* Precisely how this occurs is not completely understood; apparently, the mother elicits anxiety in the child through physical punishment and gestures that threaten the withdrawal of nurture. The sequence seems to work as follows:

Urge to defecate ⟶ Response of defecation ⟶ Imposition of punishment ⟶ Anxiety over free defecation

If these events occur close together, the anxiety response eventually moves forward in the temporal sequence until it is elicited by the very stimuli that signal defecation. The naturally prepotent response to anxiety, evidently, is temporary inhibition of the elicited response. The child might then signal his need to defecate, using postural or language signs, or he might even go to the bathroom, if he could walk and knew the connection between defecation and that room in the house. If the anxiety is based primarily on anticipated loss of nurture, however, rather than only on punishment, an extra cognitive component must have been established prior to the socialization training. The child must have had previous experiences in which the caretaker threatened to withdraw nurture. Two-year-olds are probably conceptually mature enough to make this association.

Separation Anxiety

One of the developmental bench marks of the second year is *separation anxiety;* its appearance indicates that the child of eighteen months has learned to expect displeasure if the caretaker leaves. Separation anxiety typically begins at ten or eleven months and increases in intensity until fourteen months; it is characterized by extreme upset and crying when the child sees his mother leave him or is separated from her for a long time. In a recent experiment at the Fels Institute, thirteen-month-old children initially played happily with toys while their mothers sat in a corner of the room. After fifteen minutes, the children were placed behind a transparent barrier with mother and toys on the other side. Some children fretted but only occasionally and moderately. After five minutes behind the barrier, each child watched his mother leave the room; almost instantly, most children began to cry with strong fear.

Bowlby (1960) has suggested that separation anxiety during the second year signifies that the mother or surrogate has acquired sufficient reward value that her absence is extremely painful. The child's previously most excruciating experiences of pain probably occurred when the mother was absent. The child became hungry, for example, in the mother's absence and associated the discomfort and anxiety of his hunger with her absence. Watching her leave could then become a signal for anxiety because of the link between her absence and pain. Learning this complex association would depend on a mother-infant interaction in which the mother was typically nurturant and the child grew to expect nurture, so that he could regard her absence as a distinctly new event. If no regularly nurturant relationship with an adult had been established, however, the mother's presence would not have acquired reward value. No strong bond would have been established between pain anxiety and awareness of mother's absence, and separation anxiety consequently would be minimal. The complete absence of separation anxiety in a fourteen-month-old child might therefore reflect a minimally nurturant bond between caretaker and infant. Even such a young child is mature enough, it seems, to have learned anxiety to cues signaling potential loss of maternal nurture. Like the anxiety over punishment, this fear can also become anticipatory, disrupt the natural and automatic defecation sequence, and produce inhibition of the defecatory reflex.

The Requirements for Learning Inhibition

The greater the child's awareness of what his parents want, the more easily inhibition training will proceed. If the child has an idea of the desired response and the appropriate place to evacuate, these cognitive links will come to mind simultaneously with the anxiety over defecation and will facilitate successful inhibition. The optimal conditions for learning inhibition of evacuation are: (1) a nurturant relation between caretaker and child such that anxiety over loss of nurture and disapproval can be effective incentives for learning, (2) verbal instructions telling the child what he should do, like "hold yourself in," and (3) sufficient symbolic maturity for the child to understand what is required of him. Inhibition of spontaneous evacuation is usually the first instance of inhibition learning and, as such, has special importance in the developmental history of the child. For some children, it is the first time the perception of mother as a source of pleasure becomes modified by elements of anxiety. Toilet training assumes psychological importance, therefore, because it is often the first major socialization demand. Freud was correct in postulating the significance of toilet training but his reason, that the anal area was an erogenous zone, ignored the important social training connected with it.

Anxiety caused by punishment, disapproval, or loss of nurture is not the only basis for learning to inhibit spontaneous evacuation. Three *incentive* mechanisms may also foster this inhibition: identification, imitation, and simple reward. Identification is the process by which a child tries to make himself similar to his parents. In order to strengthen his identification with them, he might try to learn proper toilet habits. This notion is speculative, however, because the desire to be like his parent is usually not strong during the second year of life and does not become strong until around four years of age.

The child might spontaneously imitate the parents' toilet habits just as he imitates them when he picks up daddy's pipe or applies mother's lipstick. But for imitation to take place, the child must have the opportunity to see the adult action that is to be copied. Evacuation is not a public act, and many parents close the bathroom door behind them, so the child does not have any clear model of the behavior he is to imitate. Moreover, it hardly seems likely that the eighteen-month-old would associate the sight of a parent going to the bathroom with his own need to evacuate.

Finally, the child might learn to inhibit evacuation by being rewarded for successful inhibition, but it is not easy to explain why any inhibition would occur in the first place. It is theoretically possible for a child to become trained through consistent reward of inhibition every time he goes to the toilet. In practice, however, most parents find it extremely difficult to refrain from a punitive statement or action when the child has an accident, which makes it likely that anxiety over physical *punishment* or *disapproval* is always involved to some degree in the acquisition of proper toilet habits.

We have been using toilet training as an illustration for explaining the possible mechanisms of inhibition learning. Inhibitions on unrestrained exploration or destruction of property are presumably learned in a similar manner. The parent punishes the prohibited response, interposing anxiety between the stimuli to exploration or destruction and the prohibited actions themselves. The major difference between the socialization of defecation and of exploration lies in the distinctiveness of the original stimuli that trigger the prohibited sequence. The cues for defecation are internal, intense, and relatively distinct, while the stimuli that incite exploration are *external* and less distinct. If the child were punished for pulling the pots from the kitchen cabinet, this inhibition might not be extended to the stimulus of a bedroom closet, and he would then have to be taught to inhibit this exploration by means of a new punishment sequence. Learning to inhibit exploration probably takes more time and is less successful than learning to inhibit evacuation because the original cues are less distinct and more frequent throughout the day. The urge to defecate ordinarily occurs only once or twice daily, but the urge to explore can be aroused a hundred times a day by virtually every interesting object around. Since the parent cannot be present to punish each "dangerous" exploration, there are many opportunities for a learned anxiety reaction to exploration to be extinguished.

Consequences of Overly Severe Toilet Training

Since intense anxiety can accompany the toilet training regimen, other anxiety-based responses can be established also during the six- to twelve-month period when training is practiced with the greatest vigor. Some of them have undesirable consequences that may last into adolescence and adulthood and may be viewed as indirect results of overly severe bowel and bladder training, that is, training by punitive procedures that generate strong anxiety. The immediate negative consequences are (1) hostility and fear toward the training agent, usually the mother, (2) anxiety over sexual thoughts and behavior, (3) anxiety over dirt and disarray, (4) acquisition of the self-labels "dirty" and "bad," and (5) inhibition of permissible spontaneous expression. Each of these responses will be considered separately.

Generation of hostility and fear. A mother who is overly punitive or threatening in her training will become a signal for anxiety arousal in the child. Excessive punishment of toilet accidents, moreover, will generate urges to resist maternal coercion and to express aggression toward the parent by pushing, kicking, or biting, or by direct verbal attacks on the parent. Less direct methods of expressing hostility mostly involve resistance to the training itself, often expressed by refusal to evacuate while sitting in the bathroom. Sometimes the mother will sit with the child for half an hour and, finally exasperated, remove him, only to watch in horror while he immediately urinates or evacuates on the floor. The mother is likely to reveal her upset at this event and thereby gratify the child's hostile motives, reinforcing his resistant disposition.

Anxiety over sexuality. The second possible outcome of severely punitive toilet training involves sexual functioning. The three-year-old does not clearly distinguish the act of evacuation from the organs involved or from the products. He tends to use the same simple words for all of them, generalizing among them, so the anxiety associated with the acts or products of elimination spreads to the genital organs as well. The proximity of the external genitals, urethra and anus guarantees that anxiety over evacuation and elimination will generalize to sexual functioning when the seven-year-old learns words for genital stimulation. If the strong anxiety linked to the genitals persists into adolescence, it may give rise to serious conflict over sexual behavior. The close semantic link between bowel and bladder functions and genital-sexual ones was demonstrated in an interview study with mothers by Sears *et al.* (1957), who found that middle-class mothers could not keep the topics of sex training and toilet training separate. The questions were separate, but the mothers' answers were not. "When we were discussing modesty standards (actually referring to sex and nudity), mothers would describe their efforts to train their children not to unrinate outdoors" (pp. 107—108). In the minds of many mothers and in the minds of children, there is an intimate association between urination and evacuation, on the one hand, and exposure of genitals and sex modesty on the other. It is not surprising that the anxieties associated with these areas support each other.

Anxiety over dirt and disarray. A feeling of discomfort aroused by bodily dirt is easily generalized to dirt everywhere in the child's environment. If the mother tells the child, "You are dirty," every time he soils his pants or gets his clothes dirty, and if she punishes him too, anxiety will become attached to the word *dirty* and, in time, to dirty fingers, dirty rooms, dirty floors. One defensive response he may develop to relieve the anxiety is to remove and avoid dirt compulsively, and to abhor any kind of disarray. This may give rise in adulthood to the compulsive neuroses described in detail in Chapter 10.

Anxiety over self-concept. Calling the child dirty each time he soils should affect his self-concept because the parent's reactions toward the child and their verbal evaluations of him are the basic sources of his attitudes toward himself. Repetition of the charge, "You are dirty, smelly, naughty," persuades the child to believe these accusations because he is prone to view his parents as omniscient. He will learn during the preschool years that people avoid dirty objects, and his behavior may begin to reflect his expectation that people will avoid him.

Learning inhibition of impulsive responses. The essential characteristic of toilet training is that it teaches inhibition. The child learns to inhibit a response that seeks expression by using a complex cue containing elements of anxiety. Neurophysiologists recently have shown new interest in studying neurophysiological inhibition, and psychologists have begun corresponding studies of choice and decision making and of response inhibition. Psychological theorizing during the last forty years has been concerned primarily with how organisms learn and maintain new responses. The more recent theoretical concern with inhibition and choice asks a different question: How is an organism with such a large number of response possibilities able to inhibit irrelevant responses and to select one correct alternative from an array of so many possible behaviors?

Inhibiting responses to strong cues, such as the internal stimuli to evacuation, is a major component of socialization and is regarded, therefore, as a mature disposition. If this tendency gains too much strength too quickly, however, it may lead to generalization of the tendency to inhibit responding whenever anxiety is experienced, even if the elicited response is a good one. The inhibition of a disposition to explore a new object because of anxiety is a possible consequence of fearful and tense experiences in toilet training; inhibition of all aggressive or sexual behavior may be another consequence.

Research on Toilet Training

There are many research reports on the effect of parental socialization practices on the child's behavior, but most studies are methodologically fragile and subject to multiple interpretations. A brief summary of some of the most relevant work follows.

Psychologists generally agree that training should be delayed until the child is conceptually and motorically prepared for it. He should be able to sit up comfortably by himself and to understand simple communications about the task required of him. This suggests that easy learning of bowel and bladder control is not possible until the child is well into his second year. Sears *et al.* (1957), in their interview study of over 300 mothers, found that the majority initiated bowel training between nine and fourteen months and completed it at approximately a year and a half. Mothers who started bowel training later, however, trained the child in less time than those who started earlier; training was accomplished with most ease when initiated after twenty months of age.

Mothers' attitudes toward toilet training are related to their attitudes toward other behaviors that have to be socialized. Severity in toilet training tends to be accompanied by strict demands in the areas of table manners, orderliness, making noise, school achievement, obedience, and aggression to parents. Mothers who practiced harsh toilet training also strictly forbade masturbation or social sex play. Sears *et al.* write:

> We get the impression of a rather pervasive quality of strictness in the mothers who are most severe in toilet training. They seem to have been seeking to achieve more mature standards of conduct at a faster pace than other mothers. They had more of a tendency to drive rather than to lead their children and they used a more punitive kind of discipline. (Pp. 121–122.)

The clinical literature is marbled with studies showing that early and severe toilet training is correlated with future mental illness. There are several obvious flaws in these kinds of correlational studies, however. First, mothers who are strict in toilet training tend to be severe and punitive in other things. The mother's general punitiveness may be critical, therefore, rather than her specific toilet-training practices. Second, the child who had difficulty learning to inhibit bowel evacuation for whatever reasons might invite more punishment and hostility from the mother, and the continuing friction between the child's resistance and mother's insistence could create the conditions necessary for the development of symptoms. Thus, even if the empirical associations are valid, their interpretations are still equivocal.

The second critical period is witness to four major developments: (1) locomotor and perceptual motor coordinations that permit the child to actively influence his environment, (2) inhibition of responses that are strongly motivated, (3) the capacity to feel anxiety over the threatened loss of parental nurturance, and (4) speech and comprehension of language.

The response processes surrounding toilet training have received emphasis in this section because they provide a good model of early socialization, whether of exploration, toileting, destruction of property, or genital manipulation. The core sequence

Stimulus to an action ⟶ Anxiety ⟶ Inhibition of a prohibited act

is repeated many times during the first decade of life and establishes the inhibitions which the culture deems necessary for social maturity.

Critical Period III: Age Three to Six Years

The preschool years are marked by dramatic development of individual behavior differences and a weakening of the mother's exclusive influence on the child as his interactions with father and siblings increase. Moreover, the acquisition of new beliefs and action, which previously had been determined solely by patterns of reward and punishment, is now fostered by a powerful new motive—the desire to be like a model. This motive pushes the child to imitate his parents and siblings and adds an entirely new dimension to the socialization process. Finally, the child's thinking ability matures rapidly during this three-year interval, and he begins to evaluative himself and others in terms of good-bad, strong-weak, fast-slow, and masculine-feminine.

Seven major responses are established during this period: (1) identification with parents, (2) acceptance of standards for sex-typed behaviors and a beginning awareness of sex roles, (3) motivation to develop skills, (4) guilt, (5) formation of defenses against anxiety and guilt, (6) characteristic means of expressing dependency and aggression, and (7) beginning development of an active or passive orientation towards others.

Identification

The concept of identification is somewhat controversial. Some people find it useless for explaining anything about human development, and even those who regard the concept as fruitful disagree on its definition and measurement. Since Freud's original discussion of identification (Freud, 1925), contemporary writers have presented searching analyses and suggested significant modifications of this idea (Bronfenbrenner, 1960; Kagan, 1958; Lynn, 1959; Maccoby, 1959; Mowrer, 1950*a*; Parsons, 1955; Sanford, 1955; Sears, 1957; Whiting, 1960). A major disagreement revolves around the question: To what events or processes does *identification* refer? It has been applied to overt behavior, to a motive system (the need to identify with someone), to the process by which behaviors are acquired, and finally, to a belief about the self.

Kagan (1958) has defined identification as an individual's belief that he possesses some of the attributes of a revered model (for example, parents, siblings, relatives, peers, fictional figures). We say that a child identifies with adult figures who he thinks command desirable resources and, as a result of these identifications, he shares vicariously in the joys and sorrows of his models. A six-year-old boy feels proud as he watches his father defeat a rival in tennis or his brother hit a winning home run. A young girl feels the elation of being "grown up" as she puts on her mother's apron and attempts to bake a pie. A ten-year-old feels ashamed when the police arrest his father or commit his mother to a mental institution. In each of these examples, the child is behaving as if he possessed some of the characteristics of an older person he admires and wants to emulate. The proud boy feels as if he himself had won the tennis match; the girl behaves as though she herself had mother's culinary skills as she prepares to bake a pie; and the ten-year-old feels as though he, and not the parent, had been arrested or "sent away." The term *identification* is used here to mean all vicarious sharing in the affective states of one's models.

There appear to be four fundamental psychological processes whose interactions comprise identification: (1) The individual believes that he and a model share some significant attributes, particularly that some of the desirable characteristics of the model are also his. (2) The individual vicariously experiences emotional reactions that the model might himself be feeling in the situation or that correspond to the situation the model is in. The pride a child feels as he watches his father give a speech is such a vicarious reaction. (3) The individual wants to acquire those attributes of the model that he perceives as desirable and to achieve the positive goals he believes the model possesses. The child perceives adults, especially his parents, to be stronger and wiser than himself, to have special privileges, and to have access to desirable goals. His perception that the model commands these things makes him want to be like the model in order to have them for himself. (4) The individual tends to adopt and practice the attitudes, values, and behaviors of a model.

These four processes combine to yield two causal sequences. First, if the child believes that he shares attributes with the model (1), he will then experience vicarious reactions that correspond to what happens to the model (2). The pairing of these two events defines the *feeling* of identification. This does not imply anything about the child's behavior or the imitation of attributes displayed by the model. A second causal sequence involves the last two variables. If the subject wants to have the desirable attributes and goals of the model (3), he will tend to adopt the model's behaviors and attributes (4). These processes generally interact; if the child adopts attributes of a model because he desires to attain those goals, he will then perceive that he shares *more* attributes with the model and, as a result, will experience vicarious reactions appropriate to the model. The very imitation of models implies that the child shares vicarious affect with them.

The child may perceive his similarity to the model either through adoption of the model's attributes or from communications informing him that he shares similarities with the model. To be sure, the child is initially given some fundamental similarities to his parents, including surname; affects such as anger, joy, and disgust; and physical similarities like color of eyes, skin, and hair and special skin markings. As a result of these many congruences, the typical six-year-old believes that he is more similar to his parents, specifically the parent of his sex, than he is to any other adult.

The idea that a child shares the feelings of a model with whom he identifies has not been thoroughly demonstrated as yet, though common sense and common observation both suggest, for example, that children ordinarily favor their own parents if they are in conflict with a strange adult. At least one experimental study shows, moreover, that in such a contest contrived in the laboratory, children displayed not only overt signs of pleasure and the like when their parents bested strangers, but covert physiological ones as well: the heartbeats of the children varied with the progress of the contest, increasing most when their parents succeeded and the stranger failed. (Kagan and Phillips, 1964).

Motivation to command the model's goals and adopt his attributes. The desirability of a model depends on his nurture of the child, his command of desired goals, especially power over the child and other adults, his competence at tasks the child regards as important, and others' acceptance of him. If these conditions are met and the child perceives some initial similarity between himself and the model, he will begin to adopt and practice some of the model's behaviors. The child's desire to command the goals of the model leads him to imitate the model because he assumes that if he possessed some of the same external characteristics, he might also possess the model's desirable psychological properties—power, affection from others, and competence. In effect, the child behaves as if he believed that objects that look alike on the outside have similar internal properties. Thus, the greater the overlap of external similarities between himself and the model, the greater the hope that he will possess the model's power, competence, and affection—the intangible qualities he wishes to command. The desire for those qualities leads him to adopt the model's external characteristics. Each time he imitates the model, he perceives an increased similarity to him. This perception strengthens the possibility that he possesses the model's covert characteristics and allows him to share in the positive affects of the model. The more desirable the model, the greater the degree to which the child will strive to adopt his attributes, and the child, in turn, will perceive still more similarity to the model, which promotes still more intensive vicarious reactions in the child. At its fullest strength, the process of identification involves all of these basic processes.

Identification and behavioral development. The processes surrounding identification and imitation of a model are as influential in determining behavioral differences among children as are rewards and punishments. The lower class child who is rewarded for studying and punished for failure in school, but whose parents do not display any personal interest in the acquisition of knowledge, will not be as motivated to master school tasks as the middle-class child whose parents display an active interest in these matters. Children attribute special value to behaviors practiced by models. One major reason for the poor academic performance of lower class children is not their parent's failure to reward perseverance in school but their failure to provide a model for learning. Patterns of aggressive, dependent, and sexual behavior similarly assume different strengths in the child's behavioral repertoire in accord with the responses displayed by the models the child has chosen for identification. When the reinforcement pattern (of reward and punishment) is congruent with the model's overt behavior, as when a mother rewards dependency in her daughter and is herself dependent, these two major socializing forces acting in concert make it likely that the girl will be dependent. When the reinforcement and identification conditions act antagonistically, however, the behavioral outcome is less certain, as when a mother rewards independence and punishes dependence, but is herself excessively dependent upon her husband and friends. Similarly, if a father rewards aggression in his son but is not himself aggressive, the frequency and style of aggressive behavior in the son are difficult to predict. Consistency between the behavior rewarded and the model's own behavior is more common than inconsistency because parents are prone to reward implicitly those behaviors they themselves manifest most frequently.

Theories of modeling. The fact that children imitate behavior they have observed in adults even without encouragement of rewards and punishments is not disputed, but there is serious disagreement about the interpretation of this phenomenon. Bronfenbrenner (1960) thinks there is no generalized motive in the child to become like one or the other parent. Among those who think there is we find three overlapping but distinct positions. Maccoby (1959) and Bandura (1962) discuss the adoption of role behaviors and the conditions under which the child rehearses covertly or displays the behavior of a model to whom he has been exposed. Both authors dislike the term *identification.* Maccoby suggests that frequency of exposure to the model's behavior and amount of power the model commands are the two major determinants of the child's imitative behavior. Bandura treats imitation and identification as synonymous. He suggests that mere exposure to behavior displayed by a model is a sufficient condition for learning it. My position suggests that if the model were not desirable, imitation would be minimal. Bandura acknowledges that any condition that will increase the attention paid to the model, which would occur under conditions of Maccoby's and Kagan's theories alike, *increases* the probability that the person will learn the model's behavior. But such conditions alone could not be enough for imitative learning, or else Bandura would have to attribute the masculine behavior of six-year-old boys to forces *other* than imitation or role practice simply because they have been more exposed to women than to men. Bandura might contend that the masculine behavior of young boys is primarily the result of the parents' reward for such behavior. I believe that a boy's behavior results more from his attempt to increase his similarity to father in order to strengthen his identification with him.

Mowrer (1950*a*) emphasizes the love relation between child and model and suggests that the child imitates the model's behavior because the latter has acquired reward value by nurturing the child. The boy presumably adopts father's interest in cars, for example, because this activity has been made attractive by its link to a nurturant adult. Practicing the behavior is motivated by the desire to reproduce a valued response. Mowrer's view suggests that, under ordinary circumstances, the child will adopt the behavior of its most nurturant parent.

Sanford (1955) has offered a different and more restricted definition of identification. He suggests that the term be used only for instances in which a person's self-esteem is threatened by a model. Under these circumstances the person takes on, as a fancied means of defense, the behavior of the threatening model. Sanford urges that identification should only be invoked to refer to such a "maladaptive crisis reaction" (p. 112). He would not consider most "imitation" related to his concept of identification.

Two final theorists, Parsons (1955) and Whiting (1960), are somewhat closer to the position presented here. They favor the term *identification* and suggest that the degree to which the model commands desirable goals is a critical determinant of adoption of his behavior. They also believe that vicarious sharing in the positive goals of the model is an important part of identification.

Many theorists acknowledge the relevance of the model's power as a factor in the extent to which identification, imitation, or role practice occur, but few place much stress on whether the child feels some initial similarity to the model. If the child felt he possessed *no* attributes in common with the model, however, he would doubt his ability to share vicariously in the model's goals, that is to obtain an identification with the model. As a result, he would not strive to increase his behavioral similarity to the model. There is clinical evidence, for example, that sons with excessively powerful and competent fathers fail to identify with them. One explanation of this failure may be that the boy perceives in himself no major similarity to his father; they may differ in body build, in expression of anger, joy, or sadness, and in occurrence of failure at tasks. When the child lacks even minimal similarity to the parent, he may be discouraged from attempting to establish an identification and consequently will not strive to adopt the model's characteristics.

Children do not imitate every person to whom they are exposed, of course, not even every person with power. Moreover, vicarious sharing in the affective states of a model seems related to role practice, which in turn appears to depend on degree of perceived similarity. A Negro child is apt to feel less sadness when a powerful Caucasian boy in his class is hurt than when the same misfortune befalls a less privileged Negro peer 100 miles away.

Research on identification and imitation. Studies of the correlates of similarity between a model and a child are subject to multiple interpretations. Not all imitation is motivated by the desire to be like a model, and not all behavioral similarities between a model and a child are based completely on either imitation or identification. Some studies lend support to these relationships, however.

One study (Mussen and Distler, 1959) suggests that a nurturant relation between father and son is important in the formation of identification. Kindergarten boys were given a test to assess their degree of masculine interests. The ten most masculine and ten least masculine boys were tested in a doll-play situation. The doll-play themes of the masculine boys showed more perception of the father as nurturant and powerful than did the themes of the nonmasculine boys. Identification with the father is facilitated when the child sees him as nurturant and powerful vis-à-vis the mother.

Bandura *et al.* (1962, 1963*a* and *b*) have done ingenious work on imitation by young children. Typically, they place nursery school children in laboratory situations with a variety of adult models. The experimenters manipulate the amount of reward, power, or nurture the model possesses or receives, and the models display unique postural, motor, and verbal responses. The child's imitation of the various models is then observed. The results of these studies suggest that the more rewarding the model is to the child, the greater the child's imitation of him.

Children are more likely to imitate an adult who is in a power role *dispensing* prizes than one who himself *receives* desired objects from a nurturant, powerful adult. In one experiment (Bandura *et al.*, 1963*a*), preschool children were exposed to male or female adults who variously dispensed or received desirable objects. Then problem tasks were given, and the adults displayed unique responses. One, for example, would pick up a special colored cap, place it upon his head at an odd angle, and make strange sounds and movements. After this the models left the room and the child was asked to perform the same tasks. The child's tendency to imitate the models' unique responses was assessed. The model who dispensed the desirable objects was imitated much more than the one who received these prizes. Moreover, the male in the power position (of giving) was imitated much more than the female in the same role. Finally, preschool boys who received gifts from a female in a situation where an adult male was ignored tended to imitate the ignored male rather than the female because, they said, they felt sorry for him. Evidently, not only the power of the model but also his sex influences the child's imitation. Bandura suggests that the critical determinants of who and what the child imitates are the people and responses that *attract his attention.* He argues that the reason a model's power increases imitation of him is that "power behavior" attracts the child's attention. Since attention in turn is based partly on the psychological needs of the child, it seems likely that power, affection, and competence—each of which is a major motive for the child—are attributes of the model that will increase imitation. Adults who command the goals that gratify these needs would be "attended to" by the child. This essay adds one more factor in stating that the act of imitation is not merely an end in itself but a means to a more critical goal, namely, to permit the child to feel enough like a model that he can share vicariously in the model's goals.

One final question remains, namely: What determines exactly which responses of the model the child is likely to imitate? No precise answer can be made at this time, but it seems reasonable to guess that the child will imitate behaviors that seem to him instrumental in attaining desirable goals and serve to *distinguish* the the model from other people.

Self-labels as a consequence of identification. Identification is important not only for the sculpting of overt behavior but also for self-definition, that is, development of the self-concept. The child labels himself as good or bad, strong or weak, big or small, smart or dumb, and these self-appellations influence his behavior. The child's self-evaluations on these scales are determined, in part, by his social experience and correspond somewhat to his history of social encounters, including things like his ability to defeat a rival, demonstrate his strength, or achieve good grades. But he is also prone to label himself in accord with the model he feels most similar to. The boy who is identified with his intelligent father begins to regard himself as intelligent; a girl who is identified with a beautiful mother views herself as attractive. Negative self-evaluations can be similarly established if a model's attributes are undesirable. A child's belief that he shares basic similarities with a negatively valued parent, or that he is hateful, mean, aggressive, disturbed, unintelligent, unpopular, or incapable of warmth or affection are all conditions that later dispose him toward psychopathology.

Since the child does not want to possess these undesirable attributes, one would think he would resist these negative beliefs about himself. On the other hand, the child believes that if he shares some attributes with a model, he will experience vicariously the affects and events that occur to the model, and a five-year-old is confronted with the fact that he is more similar to his parent than to any other adult he knows. They share the same surname and often the same features. Moreover, people tell the child that he resembles a particular parent. In effect, then, he must develop some minimal identification with the parents regardless of how undesirable they are. As the child begins to recognize the negative qualities of the parental model, he also begins to believe that some of these qualities are inevitable parts of his own personality.

Sex Typing

Sex typing refers to the tendency of a culture to encourage different behaviors for boys and girls and to establish different attributes as desirable for each sex. The child learns these values between three and ten years of age, and although sex typing is most pronounced during the school years, the process begins during the preschool period.

The concept of sex typing and its close relatives, sex role and sex role identification, have been studied considerably during the last decade, but it has surprisingly not been popular among psychologists, for the behavioral differences between the sexes are public and have an ancient and transcultural heritage. Sociology and anthropology have not been as neglectful of this concept; more than a quarter of a century ago, Linton (1936) wrote, "The division and ascription of statuses with relation to sex seems to be basic in all social systems. All societies prescribe different attitudes and activities to men and to women."

The different standards of behavior for boys and girls are called "sex roles." A *standard*, you recall, is a belief about the appropriateness of a related set of attributes or responses, like overt acts, attitudes, wishes, and feelings. The feeling of deviating from a standard causes anxiety. Many standards of behavior are equally salient for boys and girls, but sex role standards dictate the adoption of different responses by boys and girls. They are important because of their influence on a broad band of behaviors.

Sex role standards are learned associations between a class of personal attributes, on the one hand, and the concepts of male and female, on the other. A sex role standard summarizes culturally approved characteristics for males and females. From about three to seven years of age, the child gradually comes to realize that people fall into the categories of boys or girls, men or women, fathers or mothers. The early assignment of people into these distinct classes is aided by a variety of cues including dress, bodily form and proportion, strength, distribution of hair, depth of voice, posture at the toilet, and characteristic behavior in the kitchen, the garage, or the back yard.

There are three kinds of masculine and feminine characteristics: (1) physical attributes, (2) overt behaviors, and (3) feelings, attitudes, motives, and beliefs—covert attributes. The characteristics that go with maleness and femaleness in our culture are not clearly crystallized in the mind of the six-year-old, of course, but there is considerable overlap between the standards of the first grader and those of the adult.

Physical attributes. Analyses of communications presentations of males and females and studies of preadolescent and adolescent youngsters show that American girls regard an attractive face, hairless body, a small frame, and moderate-sized breasts as the most desirable characteristics for a girl; boys regard height, large muscle mass, and facial and bodily hair as the most desirable physical characteristics for boys. A girl should be pretty and small; a boy, large and strong (Cobb, 1954; Frazier and Lisonbee, 1950; Harris, 1959; Jersild, 1952; Nash, 1958).

Overt behaviors. Society's differential standards of public behavior are not as clear as the standards for physical attributes, but they are strongly felt nonetheless. One important sex-typed behavior involves aggression. The standard requires girls and women to inhibit verbal and physical aggression but gives boys and men license and even encouragement to express aggression when attacked, threatened, or dominated by another male. Under the circumstances, naturally, males display more aggressive behavior than females at virtually all ages (Bandura *et al.*, 1961; Dawe, 1934; Hattwick, 1937; Maccoby and Wilson, 1957; Muste and Sharpe, 1947). The difference is also present in the make-believe themes children tell to dolls or about pictures (Bach, 1946, Pintler *et al.*, 1946; Sears, 1951; Whitehouse, 1949), and in their different perceptions of adult males and females; both boys and girls agree that the father is more aggressive than the mother (Emmerich, 1959; Kagan, 1958; Kagan *et al.*, 1961; Kagan and Lemkin, 1960). This perception of father as more dangerous also holds for many animals of both aggressive and nonaggressive species, like tigers, rabbits, alligators, and birds (Kagan *et al.*, 1961). Adults also regard men as more aggressive than women (Bennett and Cohen, 1959; Jenkins and Russell, 1958), and parents have different standards about aggression for their children, expecting more overt aggression from boys than from girls (Kohn, 1959; Sears *et al.*, 1957).

Another class of sex-typed overt behavior includes dependency, passivity, and conformity. Girls are allowed greater license to express these behaviors, whereas boys and men are pressured to inhibit them. The data on sex differences in passivity and dependency are less consistent than those for aggression, but dependency, conformity, and social passivity are generally reported for females more than for males at all ages (Crutchfield, 1955; Hovland & Janis, 1959; Kagan & Moss, 1962; Lindzey and Goldberg, 1953; McCandless *et al.*, 1961; Sanford *et al.*, 1943; Sears *et al.*, 1953). Moreover, affiliative and nurturant behaviors are generally regarded as more appropriate for females than for males, and most investigations reveal more frequent occurrence of affiliative and nurturant behavior and greater preoccupation with people and with harmonious interpersonal relations among girls than among boys (Goodenough, 1957; Hildreth, 1945; Honzik, 1951; Lansky *et al.*, 1961; Terman and Miles, 1936; Whitehouse, 1949; Winker, 1949).

Correspondingly, children view women as more nurturant than men, and adult women see themselves as more nurturant than their male counterparts (Bennett and Cohen, 1959). The circle is complete; both children and adults expect more dependency, passivity, and nurture from females and more aggression from males.

Additional sex-typed standards include the development of skill and interest in motor and mechanical tasks for boys (Kagan and Moss, 1962; Tyler, 1947) and an interest in clothes, dolls, and babies for girls (Honzik, 1951; Tyler, 1947).

During the adolescent and early adult years some derivatives of these sex-typed patterns are added to the sex role standard. For females, these include submissiveness to males, inhibition of overt signs of sexual desire, and cultivation of domestic skills (Douvan and Kaye, 1957; Harris, 1959). For males, independence, interpersonal dominance of men and women, initiation of sexual behavior, sexual conquests, competence at some skill, and acquisition of money and power become critical sex-typed behaviors (Bennett and Cohen, 1959; Child *et al.*, 1946; Douvan and Kaye, 1957; Harris, 1959; Jenkins and Russell, 1958; Kagan and Moss, 1962; Tuddenham, 1951; Walters *et al.*, 1957).

Game choices and sex-typed behavior standards. Young children choose games, toys, and fantasy heroes in keeping with the behavioral standards outlined above. The large body of research on children's game and toy preferences shows that boys choose objects related to sports, machines, aggression, speed, and power roles, whereas girls select games and objects associated with the kitchen and home, babies, personal attractiveness, and other fantasy roles like nurse or secretary in which they have a subordinate relation to a male. Knives, boats, planes, trucks, and cement mixers are regarded by school children as masculine; dolls, cribs, dishes, and nurses' equipment are considered feminine (Foster, 1930; Honzik, 1951; Rosenberg and Sutton-Smith, 1960; Vance and McCall, 1934).

There are also social class differences in the game choices of children. Rabban (1950) asked children from three to eight years old in middle- and working-class homes to select the toys they liked best. The choices of lower class boys and girls conformed more closely to traditional sex-typed standards than the choices of middle-class children did, suggesting that differentiation of sex roles is sharper in lower class families. This agrees with the finding that lower class mothers encourage sex typing more consistently than middle-class mothers (Kohn, 1959). Moreover, the difference in sex typing between the classes is greatest for girls (Rabban, 1950). Apparently the middle-class girl is much freer to express an interest in "masculine" toys and activities than the middle-class boy is in "feminine" things. This agrees with the finding that, among girls, there is a positive correlation between the educational level of the family and involvement in masculine activities (Kagan and Moss, 1962).

Feelings, attitudes, motives, and wishes. The *covert* attributes that are closely linked to the concept of *female* in our culture include the ability and desire to gratify a love object and to elicit sexual arousal in a male; to be a wife and mother and to give nurture to one's child and affection to a love object; and to feel emotion. For males, the primary covert attributes include a practical attitude towards problems; sexual prowess and the ability to gratify a love object; suppression of fear; and a capacity to control emotion under stress (Bennett and Cohen, 1959; Jenkins and Russell, 1958; Parsons, 1955). There are less systematic data about these covert attributes than about the overt behaviors listed earlier, but clinical studies (Bieber *et al.*, 1962) and self-ratings by adults (Bennett and

Cohen, 1959) support these statements.

In sum, females are supposed to inhibit aggression and the open display of sexual urges, to be passive with men, to be nurturant to others, to cultivate attractiveness, and to maintain an affective, socially poised, and friendly posture with others. Males are urged to be aggressive in face of attack, independent in problem situations, sexually aggressive, competent in tasks, in control of impulses, and suppressive of strong emotion, especially anxiety. Parsons (1955) dichotomizes social roles as *instrumental* or *expressive*; this is consistent with the attributes we have repectively labeled *masculine* and *feminine.*

This list may strike readers as old-fashioned, unrealistic, and unrepresentative of contemporary values because of the rapid rate at which sex role standards are changing in modern society. Even so, the data indicate that American children continue to believe that aggression, dominance, and independence are more appropriate for males and that passivity, nurture, and affect more appropriate for females (Parsons, 1948; Hartley, 1960). Hartley writes:

> In response to those who are overly concerned about the effect of apparent recent sex role changes . . . from the child's point of view, there are no changes; he sees only the picture as it appears in his time and this picture shows remarkably little change from traditional values. (P. 91.)

Sex Role Identity

A sex role standard is a belief shared by the members of the culture about the proper characteristics of males and females. But the abstract ideal of male or female, as viewed by the culture, is never exactly the same as any real person's idea of his own masculinity or femininity. Such concepts depend largely on how much an individual believes he possesses sex-typed traits. *The degree to which a person regards himself as masculine or feminine is called his sex role identity.* This belief is one component of the complex interlocking set of beliefs which make up a person's *self-concept* or *personal identity.* For most people, sex role identity is an especially important part of their self-concept, one to which they cannot declare indifference and on which they often evaluate themselves.

The degree of matching between the sex role standards of the culture and an individual's assessment of his own sex role identity partly answers the question, "How masculine (or feminine) am I?" Sex role identity is not completely conscious, however; meeting the culture's sex role standards does not guarantee the integrity of one's sex role identity. A man who *acts* masculine in terms of the standards does not necessarily feel that he *is* highly masculine. It is probably impossible, on the other hand, for a man with none of the culturally approved sex-typed behaviors to regard himself as highly masculine. Possession of some sex-typed traits, in other words, is necessary but not sufficient for a firm sex role identity.

Unfortunately, there is little empirical information that tells how a child establishes sex role identity. The discussion that follows must therefore be limited to speculation and conjecture. At least three kinds of experiences determine how much a child regards himself as masculine or feminine: (1) differential identifications with parents, older siblings, and special peers, (2) acquisition of the traits that define masculinity or femininity, and (3) perception of how much other people regard him as masculine or feminine.

Identification. One important consequence of a boy's feeling of identification with his father is the attempt to take on the father's characteristics. Each time he successfully imitates an *overt* behavior or attitude of the father, he perceives an increased similarity to him, which strengthens his belief that he possesses some of the father's *covert* characteristics. *One of these covert attributes is the self-label of masculinity.* A strong identification with the parent of the same sex at seven years of age thus facilitates the development of a similar sex role identity.

The sex-typed behavior of the parent is then critical in the sex role identity of the child. The father with masculine interests may foster a quite different identity than one who is passive, nonaggressive, withdrawn, and uninterested in athletics or machines. The boy with a nurturant and competent father who does not display masculine sex-typed behaviors will confront the societal standard for masculinity when he enters school. Since his overt behavior is likely to be less sex-typed than that of his peers, he will soon perceive a sharp discrepancy between his attributes and those of other boys. He may be accused of being a "sissy" and may conclude from all this that he is less masculine than others and therefore somehow inferior to them.

The child who has identified with a masculine father does not experience this dissonance on starting school. His sex role identity is supported not only by his identification with the masculine father, but also by the perceived similarity between himself and the standard for masculinity displayed by his peers.

The process is similar for the girl. If she identifies with a mother who displays traditionally feminine behavior, she should be submissive with boys, inhibit aggression, cultivate personal attractiveness, and be interested in domestic activities. The girl identified with a mother who does not manifest traditional feminine attributes is not likely to adopt a feminine sex role and may begin to question her femininity and adequacy when she confronts the values of the peer group and perhaps the accusation that she is a "tomboy."

Children who have minimal identifications with their parent of the same sex may adopt the sex role behavior of peers, siblings, or relatives as a basis for an appropriate sex role identity. But a weak identification with the parent of their sex may prevent the child from developing the confidence to master many sex-typed skills. The strength of the child's identification with this parent and the parent's actual sex-typed behaviors must both be assessed in order to predict the strength of the child's sex role identity.

Acquiring sex-typed attributes. The acquisition of desirable sex-typed attributes also helps formulate the child's sex role identity. The boy who learns to be dominant with peers, sexually aggressive with girls, or competent on the athletic field begins to regard himself as masculine. The girl who becomes popular with boys, socially poised with adults, or capable of giving nurturance labels herself feminine. The strength of a sex role identity can be considered a function of the discrepancy between the personal inventory an individual makes of his own sex-typed attributes in relation to the ideal attributes prescribed by the culture. The more he acquires culturally approved attributes, the smaller is this discrepancy; these acquisitions can therefore produce favorable modifications in the self-label. The opposite effect is also possible; loss of traits or skills that are parts of a person's masculine or feminine self-image can widen the gap between actual ideal and attributes and make a sex role identity more vulnerable.

Perceptions by others of sex role identity. The third set of events that influences a sex role identity is experience with other people whose opinions alter one's self-label. This is closely related to the acquisition of sex-typed skills discussed above, because people's perceptions of our attributes are important bases on which we evaluate what those attributes are worth.

If men and women react toward Bill as though he were dominant and strong, the discrepancy between Bill's model of masculinity and self-concept will be small. Similarly, if a girl continually hears praises of her attractiveness, her self-concept will shape itself accordingly and the self-ideal discrepancy will be reduced. Neither the experience of gaining sex-typed skills nor favorable impressions from others seems to be as important to sex role identity as is identification with parents, which forms the main foundation for this development. Still, acquisition of sex-typed skills and experiences congruent with sex role are each influential to some degree in determining how much an individual labels himself as masculine or feminine; it is the sum of these three processes that finally produces sex role identity.

Overt sex-typed behaviors. The learning of sex role behaviors, like sex role identity, is facilitated by the desire to identify with a model. Other motives influence this learning, too, especially desire for affection and acceptance from parents and peers and anxiety about rejection by significant others. Most parents punish aggression and sexuality more consistently in daughters than in sons and passivity, dependency, and fear more consistently in sons than in daughters (Aberle and Naegale, 1952; Kohn, 1959; Sears *et al.*, 1957). Moreover, the fact that most children feel that their parents want them to adopt sex role attributes (Fauls and Smith, 1956) predisposes them to shun inappropriate sex-typed activities in favor of behavior that is congruent with sex role standards. If a child's parent of the same sex displayed sex-appropriate behavior, however, but the parent of the opposite sex did not reward, or even punished, the child for those attributes, he would be ambivalent and conflicted over whether or not to display sex role behavior (see the discussion of conflict in Chapter 3). To predict accurately the occurrence of sex role behavior, one must assess (1) the degree of identification with the parent of the same sex; (2) the degree and kind of sex-typed behavior displayed by each parent; and (3) the pattern of rewards issued by each parent.

It is of interest to note that masculine and feminine sex-typed responses require different *amounts* of reaction from other people in order to be learned. It is almost impossible for a girl to decide whether she is attractive, poised, or socially passive without continued interaction and feedback from the social environment. Girls are forced to depend upon people and to court their acceptance in order to gain the experiences that help to establish sex-typed behaviors. The critical significance for girls of adult and peer acceptance probably contributes to the conformity and concern with social desirability, which is typically greater among females than males (Crutchfield, 1955; Hovland and Janis, 1959).

Boys, on the other hand, develop many important sex-typed behaviors while alone. Masculine skills often involve *solitary* mastery, the achievement of which the boy can assess without having the reactions of others. Gross motor or mechanical skills are chief among such activities. The ten-year-old boy shooting baskets in his backyard or fixing his bicycle, for example, receives assurance from these solitary endeavors that he is acquiring masculine attributes. Independence of the attitudes and opinions of others, moreover, which implies relative independence of their wishes, is itself a sex-typed (masculine) trait. The typical boy, therefore, tries to suppress his anxiety over social rejection because showing it is not considered masculine in this culture.

The idea of sex role identification has some ambiguity, as we have seen, but it also has some value so long as the concepts *male* and *female* and the dimensions *maleness* and *femaleness* are basic to our language and culture.

The four-year-old child has already divided the world into male and female people and is concerned with the differences between them. By the time he is seven, he is committed to molding his behavior according to the cultural standards for his biological sex and he shows uneasiness, anxiety, and even anger about behaving in ways regarded as characteristic of the opposite sex. The epithet "sissy" to a boy or "tomboy" to a girl arouses strong negative feelings. The desire to behave in accordance with sex role standards extends far beyond an interest in sports for boys and cooking for girls into many important domains of behavior, including school work, sexual behavior, and vocational choice, and has a strong and continuous effect on behavior over the course of development and into adulthood.

Guilt, Shame, Fear, and Conscience

Guilt first emerges during the preschool years. This development is significant because guilt represents a new level of conceptual functioning in which the child recognizes that his behavior has deviated from some established standard and inhibits a response because of this deviation as such rather than because of anxiety over anticipated punishment or disapproval from another person. The internalized standards that underlie guilt become referees for final approval or veto over beliefs and behaviors. It is fortunate that this is the case, for socialization of the child would be exceedingly difficult if the only incentives for inhibition of asocial acts were external, like fear of reprisal or desire for nurture. The desire to avoid the unpleasant feeling of guilt within the self replaces the desire to avoid rejection or punishment from other people. Guilt, shame, and fear, each of which is derived from anxiety, are each possible consequences of deviation from a standard; which actually occurs depends on the specific standard in question, the nature of the deviation, and the degree to which fear of external reprisal is involved.

How is a standard learned? Several different mechanisms seem to be involved in learning a standard. As indicated earlier, the child may learn to value a specific act or belief because it increases his similarity to a desired model; identification is thus one source of new standards.

A second source is equally fundamental. One of the universal, yet neglected facts of human, and even primate, functioning is that the organism extracts from experience certain firm expectations of what is and of what will be. The observation that chimpanzees become upset at the sight of a mutilated chimp or human form led Hebb (1946) to postulate that every encounter with a stimulus pattern helps to fix in mind a rigid expectation of that stimulus pattern. Violation of an important part of that expected pattern, such as a head with no body, elicits fear, while the pattern itself becomes a standard. A four-year-old child who has been exposed repeatedly, twenty times a week for several years, to verbal descriptions of how he should behave, like "Wash your hands" and "Do not yell at your mother," eventually "hardens" cognitively and accepts these statements as the proper ways to act. (This process may also be the means by which he learns a stable expectancy of "what dogs (or anything else) are like." Continued exposure plus the assignment of the verbal label "dog" lead to a fixed expectancy about behavior as well as about appearance. Discrepancies from that expectation are liable to elicit anxiety, just as behavior that is discrepant from a standard is liable to do.

A third set of conditions that gives rise to a standard involves anxiety over expected punishment. The child is punished for stealing, for example, and the reasons for the punishment are told to him before, during, or after it is administered. The child then criticizes himself, and his intentions to inhibit the transgression become covert rehearsals of inhibition. The next time he is tempted to transgress, thoughts of this situation are aroused and lead, in turn, to associations with the previous punishment and anxiety and to expression of the standard, "Don't steal."

Recent empirical evidence suggests that the timing of the punishment is important. Aronfreed (1964) has suggested that if the behavior desired from the child is a "self-critical" response like "I am bad; I stole it," then punishment should be administered before the parent tells the child the reason for it. He found that school-age girls were most likely to be self critical if adults first punished them and *then* verbalized a sentence which they would adopt as their own self-critical response. If these findings from an artificial laboratory situation can be generalized to more naturalistic contexts, as Aronfreed suggests, it appears that the optimal conditions for the establishment of self-critical remarks in a child is a sequence of first punishment and then verbal reproach, rather than one of first telling the child about the violation and then punishing him.

This suggestion is reasonable in that the punishment experience forces the child's attention to the adult and causes him to question the reason for the punishment. Thus, the child is most attentive and receptive to learning a self-critical remark when the verbal rationale follows the punishment. Aronfreed, however, assumes that the self-critical remark is learned as a result of the anxiety reduction that occurs at the termination of punishment. He also wisely differentiates between learning a self-critical comment and learning to inhibit a particular act. A self-critical comment may be taught by the sequence indicated, but it does not always predict behavior inhibition.

Although self-criticism and inhibition are not the same thing as a standard (one can have a standard and never verbalize a self-critical remark or inhibit an action), these data suggest that the timing of punishment is an important element in the process of forming standards.

A final source of acquisition of standards is the socializing agent, usually the mother, once she has acquired reward value through her nurture so that her words, deeds, and values share this reward value. Mowrer (1950*b*) has argued that one motive for the infant's spontaneous vocalizations is the desire to produce stimuli that have acquired reward value. The sounds are "sweet music" because they symbolize the mother's sounds, which have reward value. One could argue similarly that statements such as, "Do not lie," "Do not hit" can acquire reward value and their practice, like the practice of vocalizations, can be a source of reward.

How much each of these four processes contribute to the learning of standards is a problem that is being investigated with vigor. Regardless of the mechanisms, however, the child does learn verbalizations that evaluate things on a good-bad dimension, and he experiences unpleasant affect when he recognizes that his thoughts or actions are not congruent with the standards that are classified as "good."

The acquisition of standards and the capacity for guilt require considerable conceptual maturity. The first sign of the development of standards appears around two years of age, but consistent standards and anxiety about deviation usually do not appear until three or four years of age.

Guilt and shame. The differences between guilt and shame have provoked many essays. At one level, the dichotomy is superficial and arbitrary, for unpleasant affect following transgression is characteristic of both. A popular distinction between them hangs on the relative importance of *anxiety about reprisal* by an external agent. The child is said to be ashamed when he feels that *other* people disapprove of him, usually for something wrong he has done. Guilt, on the other hand, does not involve the expectation of reprisal from others. The child is said to feel guilt when he has violated a standard of his own; the source of reprisal then is self-criticism. Shame probably appears first developmentally, for the learning of standards is nourished by social acceptance.

The order in which specific standards are established during the early years is not known in detail but wise conjecture is possible. The first standards probably concern toilet habits, for the three-year-old feels shame, and perhaps the four-year-old feels guilt if he soils or is enuretic. The next class of standards to appear depends on the specific family experiences of the child. Standards concerning anger, interpersonal aggression, destruction, dependence, crying, masturbation, and sexual exhibitionism all start to be established simultaneously or close together.

The last standards to appear during the preschool period revolve around sex-typed attributes and task competence. The former standard has already been considered. Standards of competence evolve from behavior which can be seen in many five-year-olds. The child may cry if he loses a competitive game; he may throw down parts of a puzzle that he cannot fit together successfully; he may withdraw sheepishly from a task he cannot master. From these experiences, the child learns to recognize a level of performance toward which he can appropriately strive, that is, a standard. Dependence, aggression, sexuality, competence, sex typing, and bowel and bladder control are the six major areas around which standards are developing during the period from three to six years of age.

The role of language in the emergence of standards. One determinant of how fast standards are established is the extent to which relevant behaviors and associated affects are given unambiguous verbal descriptions. Hostile feelings and thoughts are most often given verbal tags by the social environment. Because aggressive postures and behaviors are public, parents are sensitized to them and often respond to the child's pouting, foot stamping, or verbal barbs by remarking, "Don't be angry" or "Stop being so mad." In addition, parents display signs of their own anger that are labeled as such by others. The child's feelings of sexual excitement, urges for mastery, or feelings of dependence or helplessness are less often labeled by the adult community. Thus, one expects earlier emergence of standards for aggression and anger than for dependency, sexuality, and mastery.

Defenses against anxiety, shame, and guilt. During the first two to three years of life, anxiety results almost exclusively from separation from the caretaker and violation of expectations. The child has two main reactions to these events: crying and behavioral withdrawal. The preschool years are witness to three new major sources of anxiety: loss or withdrawal of nurture, physical harm, and shame or guilt over violating standards; some psychologists call the latter *conflict-produced anxiety*. The child who thinks about masturbating, for example, may experience anxiety from the conflict between a standard that forbids genital manipulation and a wish that urges it. This opposition of a standard and a wish is the essence of conflict. The anxiety is a *result* and not the *cause* of the conflict.

The child's defensive apparatus matures during the preschool period, and he shows five early forms of defense aimed at reducing anxiety: behavioral withdrawal, regression, denial, repression, and projection. These will be discussed in more detail in Chapter 10, but they are presented here in their developmental context.

The most frequently used defense of preschool children is direct avoidance or flight (behavioral withdrawal). The child will hide his eyes or run to his room when a stranger enters the house; he will refuse to approach a group of strange children despite his desire to play with them; he will retreat from a jungle gym if he doubts his ability to climb it. The withdrawal temporarily removes the child from the feared situation, but since the tendency to withdraw is strengthened each time it is practiced, it is very likely to be used again in future stressful situations.

Regression is the reappearance of a response that was characteristic of an earlier phase of development. Thumb-sucking and bed-wetting are regressive acts in children who have previously stopped this behavior. The child who regresses is probably attempting to withdraw from a current anxiety-arousing situation to a less anxious state characteristic of his earlier years. Sustained regressive behavior is most frequent when a new baby is brought into the home: the older child often adopts infantile behaviors. Some of the behaviors that have been called regressive in this connection may be the result of a partial identification with the infant intended to gain desired goals which the older child thinks the infant commands.

Denial and repression are the cognitive counterparts of physical withdrawal. Withdrawal occurs when the child is confronted directly with a threatening situation and must either face it or flee. More frequently, however, the source of anxiety is a *thought*. Since the child cannot run from it, he attempts to attenuate the anxiety it provokes through the defenses of *denial* or *repression*. By means of denial, the child convinces himself that an anxiety-arousing situation or event is not true. The child who has been openly rejected by his mother and has recognized her hostility uses denial by insisting that his mother is kind and loving. Some children who feel rejected by their natural parents may seek solace by denying that these people are their parents. The child then insists that he is adopted and that his true parents love him.

When repression is used as a defense, the child blocks out the frightening event by removing it completely from awareness. Repression is neither a refusal to remember an event nor a denial of its reality. In repression, the child has no awareness of the anxiety-arousing thought or event and seems to have forgotten it. In denial, the meaning of the thought or event is denied, but its substantive nature is retained in consciousness.

Projection means attributing an anxiety-arousing thought or action to another, when it really applies to oneself. The five-year-old frequently projects hostility and blame for his own misdeeds onto others. The child may bump into an adult while running after a playmate. He projects the blame onto the playmate by telling the adult, "He made me chase him. If he hadn't made me chase him, I wouldn't have bumped into you."

These conceptual additions to the mentality of the four-year-old are successful in reducing anxiety and therefore become habits. There is probably some relationship between the type of defense chosen and the specific source of anxiety, but it is not yet clear. Hostile feelings are most likely to be projected onto others, it seems, while sexual thoughts are more likely to be repressed. Anxiety over physical harm most often leads to behavioral withdrawal.

Symptoms of the preschool child. The preschool years are witness to a broad new array of symptoms of psychological disorder. The term *symptom* has a three-part definition. It is a response that is regarded as (1) socially undesirable; (2) statistically deviant, that is unconventional; and (3) the product of anxiety and conflict. Symptoms appear to follow some developmental scheme, for there are tentative indications that each occurs most often during a specific developmental period, though their causes, at least during the preschool years, tend to be disguised. The major symptoms of this period are phobias (fears), temper tantrums, mutism, soiling or enuresis, extreme aggression to peers, headaches, vomiting, and constipation.

It is generally assumed that extreme anxiety over physical harm or guilt over violation of a standard can elicit some of the phobias and extreme fears manifested by preschool children. In many cases, a child's guilt makes him think of reprisal, and he develops a phobia for any situation or person that is linked with the agent of possible reprisal. Thus, the preschool child may develop irrational fears of driving in an automobile, going to a particular store, approaching a certain person, playing with specific toys, leaving the house, or almost anything else.

Symptomatic temper tantrums, soiling, and enuresis can be the result of years of harsh socialization practices or extreme rejection during the first years of life. Moreover, the arrival of a new sibling when the first child is four years old can provoke him to hostility towards both sibling and parent and to other acts whose aim is to generate unhappiness in the caretaker.

Dependent, Aggressive, Sexual, and Mastery Behavior in the Preschool Child

The following sections discuss some of the antecedents and correlates of four major classes of behavior. They emphasize behavior rather than motives because, as we have seen in the previous chapter, it is not easy to infer motives from behavior. The activation of a motive in a two-year-old leads immediately to behavior aimed at gratifying it. Two-year-olds have not learned to delay or inhibit gratification of any strong need. The five-year-old has learned that he must delay gratification of many desires and must inhibit certain acts. Fear of rejection, guilt, and identification needs motivate most of this inhibition. The *absence* of dependent or aggressive behavior, therefore, is no proof that the child's dependent or aggressive motivation is low, for this absence may only signify that such behavior is strongly inhibited.

The emergence of sexual behavior. During the preschool period, many children discover that touching their genitals produces pleasant sensations; most children practice some form of self-stimulation during these years. In one study (Sears *et al.*, 1957), about half of a group of 379 mothers reported observing sex play in their children. Because many mothers are reluctant to report this information and many children are hesitant to explore their genitals openly, these figures are only conservative estimates of the frequency of genital play in young children. Genital stimulation is pleasant, and so the child's interest in this area increases to a point where he also becomes interested in the genitals of others—siblings, parents, and peers. Curiosity about the sexual anatomy of others is often punished and thus leads to anxiety. According to Sears *et al.* (1957), only 5 percent of the mothers in their study reported complete permissiveness about masturbation, and less than 15 percent permitted the child to run about the house naked. Thinking about the genitals thus elicits the anticipation both of uniquely pleasant sensations and of anxiety. This combination of pleasure and moderate anxiety produces heightened preoccupation with this area.

The child's interest in sexual matters is fostered by another motive having little to do with sexuality, that is curiosity. He is curious about many things in his environment and naturally about the anatomical differences between the sexes as well. The objective differences between boys and girls are important to the child, and his desire to know about his environment, combined with his sexual interests, results in a continuing concern with the genitals. It is important to realize that the preschool child's preoccupation and anxiety are centered on the genital *organs* and not on the *actions* we label sexual behavior. However, the anxiety that is attached to the genitals and their sensations will become attached to sexual acts when the child is older and recognizes the close relation among the genitals, sexual excitement, and sexual behavior.

Hostility and aggression. The child's tendency to display overt aggression is determined by the intensity of his desire to hurt others, the degree to which the environment instigates or inhibits hostility, the strength of the link between anger and aggression, and the amount of anxiety, guilt, and inhibition he associates with overt aggression.

There are many incentives to anger in the preschool child. Restriction of autonomy, deprivation of goals, and punishment typically elicit resentment and rage against the frustrating agent. Moreover, the annoying intrusion of siblings and the suspicion that they are more loved than he can elicit anger at both sibling and parent. The child is disposed to express his anger by hurting the resented agent, destroying his property, striking him, or verbally attacking him.

Three aspects of an aggressive response should be separated: (1) the form of the response, (2) the object to whom the aggression is directed, and (3) the child's awareness of the hostile intent of his actions.

One child may soil to express anger at his mother but be completely unaware of the resentment that provoked the soiling. Another may be painfully aware of his strong anger and show undisguised verbal aggression but nothing else. The different conditions that lead one child to soil, a second to yell, and a third to strangle a stray cat are as significant as the fact that all three responses are regarded by psychologists and psychiatrists as aggressive actions. Aggressive behavior can assume three major forms: physical or verbal competition, resistance or disobedience to someone's wishes, and destruction of property. Each of these acts can be directed at the true source of the anger or can be displaced onto a substitute person or object. Investigations of aggressive behavior in the preschool child have focused mainly on verbal aggression to parents and peers, disobedience and resistance to adults, and aggressive stories told in laboratory situations. The results of many investigations suggest the following tentative statements.

For boys, both minimal punishment and extreme physical punishment of aggression tend to be associated with frequent aggressive behavior. Minimal punishment is more closely associated with aggression against parents and extreme punishment with aggression toward peers. The reasons for these relations are not clear. The relationship between parental punishment and aggressive behavior in the girl is somewhat simpler. In general, the greater the punishment for aggression, the less aggression she displays to parents or peers. This sex difference in the relation of punishment to aggression—curvilinear for boys and linear for girls—is a result, in part, of differential sex typing for aggressive behavior. The models girls choose for emulation are usually nonaggressive, and most girls possess a standard that calls for the inhibition of aggression. Girls, in short, place greater inhibition upon aggressive behavior, and a girl's exposure to an aggressive model is less influential than a boy's is (Bandura *et al.*, 1963*b*). It is possible, finally, that constitutional differences favoring vigorous motor activity in boys contribute in some way to the striking sex difference in aggressive behavior. Further studies on this issue are necessary.

Dependency. Dependency refers to many responses that appear to have a similar intent: to obtain *aid, affection,* or *praise* from another person. Unfortunately, assessment of intent from an overt act is difficult and fallible, but it is clear that aggressive, sexual, or dependent behaviors can each serve many different purposes; that is, phenotypically similar acts can have different psychological significance.

With respect to dependency, in particular, it is possible for different wishes to elicit requests for aid or for affection. As with aggression, the desire to meet a sex role standard can provoke dependent behavior. Many young girls "play dependent" and seek nurture and praise because it gratifies their desire to be feminine. The term "dependent behavior" reflects a cultural bias, and the Western definition of dependency is probably not applicable to all cultures. Walters and Parke (1964) observe that:

> One may argue that a child learns a variety of responses such as asking for help and soliciting approval that may or may not be regarded as dependent according to the circumstances in which they occur and the value system within which his behavior is judged.

Dependent preschool behavior includes seeking help with problems, requesting assurance, clinging to adults, showing reluctance to be separated from adults, and soliciting affection and praise. Mothers generally begin to encourage more independent, self-reliant behavior during the preschool period and become increasingly impatient when the child behaves dependently. By the time the child is five years old, most mothers expect him not to ask for help with dressing, toileting, and solving minor problems. The development of independence and self-reliance are usually rewarded by the mother. The five-year-old has strong tendencies favoring both independence and dependence, and he displays both behaviors. Children who show alternately independent and dependent behavior in nursery school settings seem to be more conflicted about dependency than those who consistently act more one way or the other (Beller, 1955, 1959).

One would expect that a mother who always rewarded and rarely punished dependency would produce a highly dependent child and that children reared in a very rejecting environment during their earliest years may not behave dependently because dependent behavior is not rewarded. Empirical research tends to support these expectations. In the absence of maternal nurture during the first three years of life, children show minimal dependent behavior (Spitz and Wolff, 1946). However, these children grow up in environments that are extremely rejecting and not representative of the average American family. In two other studies (Sears *et al.*, 1957; Kagan and Moss, 1962) with more representative groups of mothers, consistent reward of dependency or inconsistent punishment of it were each associated with a high degree of dependent behavior in the child. Maternal acceptance did not necessarily foster dependency, however, for if the mother valued and rewarded *independence*, the child showed it more.

Some research on dependency has involved the relationship between arousal of dependent motives and how much the child will subsequently work for praise and social approval on a simple task like placing marbles in a hole. These experiments (Gewirtz and Baer, 1958; Walters and Ray, 1960) indicate that isolating preschool children for a short time makes them more persistent on simple tasks where the reward for performance is social approval. Evidently the short isolation elicited anxiety about loss of nurture and motivated attempts to gain adult reassurance. After a thorough review of the literature on dependent behavior in preschool children, Walters concludes:

> The withholding of rewards will increase susceptibility to social influence provided that dependency habits are already strongly established in the frustrated person's response repertoires and the testing situation is conducive to the manifestation of dependency behavior. In contrast, the presentation of aversive stimuli serves to reduce the incidence of dependency behavior unless rewards are also intermittently provided. (Walters and Parke, 1964.)

There are many parallels between the development of dependent and aggressive behavior. Both involve a clash between the desire for expression and a standard that dictates their inhibition. The child desires to be helped or to express his anger but fears punishment, loss of love, or violation of internal standards. Parental reward of these behaviors tends to increase their occurrence; consistent parental punishment usually decreases their occurrence; and inconsistent reward and punishment lead to high frequency of occurrence.

It should be noted finally that there are important sex differences in the degree to which anxiety is attached to each of these behaviors. Girls are more conflicted about aggression, and boys are more conflicted about dependency.

Mastery. Mastery is generally defined as an overt attempt to improve proficiency at a nonsocial task. There is no logical reason why social poise, fighting ability, ability to attract a partner of the opposite sex, or development of beauty should not be regarded as mastery responses, but the term conventionally refers to skills involving objects, intellectual skills, and some forms of gross motor coordination, rather than to attributes involved directly in interpersonal relations.

The fundamental motive for the child's attempts at mastery is a critical issue that is still being debated. Twenty years ago this behavior was believed to serve the motives of dependency, recognition, or aggression. It was assumed that the child mastered school subjects in order to attain the praise of his parents; the boy practiced football to obtain recognition from his peers or in the service of competitive or hostile motives. Thus, mastery behavior was viewed as a derivative response produced by more fundamental motives. Current theorists are more prone to view mastery as a basic motive in its own right. White (1959) has been a vigorous spokesman for this position; he postulates a motive of *effectance*, which is a desire to perfect one's skills. The possibility that dependence, aggression, or recognition needs help to provoke mastery is not eliminated, but another basis for mastery behavior is also suggested.

There is clearly arbitrariness in deciding what behaviors are related to mastery. Virtually any response can be perfected, and not all such achievements necessarily serve the same motives equally well. Psychologists must develop more sophisticated constructs in the area of mastery, and a wise direction seems to be a double classification of behavior based on the *specific response skill* and the *major intent* of the mastery behavior (social recognition, mastery for its own sake, sex role congruence, competition with others, power motivation, or desire for approval).

There are sex differences in overt mastery attempts of intellectual tasks; boys are more likely to choose difficult problems than girls. In one study, young children were allowed to complete a first puzzle given them but were made to fail a second one. The children were then asked whether they wanted to try to finish the puzzle they had failed or to attempt the easier one again. Among preschool children, there were no striking sex differences in response. With increasing age, however, boys showed a greater tendency than girls to return to the failed puzzle (Crandall and Rabson, 1960).

Mastery of intellectual and academic skills is one of the most stable aspects of a child's personality. Girls who are motivated to acquire knowledge and perfect skills during preschool years tend to retain this motivation during adolescence and early adulthood (Kagan and Moss, 1962). Two factors seem to be important in facilitating mastery: the amount of reward given by the parent and the degree to which the parent of the same sex is an effective model for mastery. For example, mothers who encourage walking and talking during the first three years of life had children whose mastery level in school was higher than that of children whose mothers were less encouraging. This effect was more dramatic for girls than for boys, perhaps because of the greater identification of girl with mother (Kagan and Moss, 1962; Moss and Kagan, 1958). Finally, attempts at mastery are not subject to many prohibitions for either sex, and there is apt to be a close relationship between the preschool child's attempts in this area and his basic motivations.

Peer Interaction in the Preschool Years

The child does not respond socially to other children his own age until he is well into his third year, and even then interactions are brief and typically nonreciprocal. The three-year-old usually plays alone or parallel with another child. There is minimal cooperative effort and minimal capacity to play games that have rules to which each player must conform. Socially dominant and socially passive children form two rather clear groups, much clearer than can be seen in a group of seven-year-olds where many children display a mixture of dominance and withdrawal. There is imitation of one child by another. If one child runs his tricycle, several children are likely to follow. Hearty laughter on the part of one child can spread quickly through the group.

In a nursery school situation, most four-year-olds work alone with clay, painting, block building, or gross motor play. Others sit and watch, passively studying the group. A third group follows the adults visually or remains closely attached to them, searching their faces for cues of approval and disapproval. In most groups of middle-class children, physical aggression is rare and sex-typed play of stereotyped masculine or feminine role models is not yet a dominant behavior. Most of the children spend time in gross motor activity with tricycle, jungle gyms, running, skipping, and large block building or else practice fine motor and artistic skills. The changes between the third and fifth year include increased social interaction with a peer and more cooperative play. Solitary withdrawal and "watching others" decrease markedly. There is an increase, with age, in the percentage of children that exhibit competitive behavior or make competitive remarks. In one study, (Greenberg, 1932), two-year-olds did not compete and made only undirected movements toward materials. Competitive responses began between the ages of three and four and became much more intense between the ages of four and six, when grabbing material from another child and making self-flattering remarks increased. This behavior was associated with a diminished tendency to give materials to a peer or to help a peer. In another study (Leuba, 1933), thirty-two children were observed putting pegs into a pegboard, first working individually and later paired with another child performing the same task. The two-year-olds seemed to be primarily interested in the play material, and their behavior was unaffected by the presence of other children. The three- and four-year-olds exhibited a variety of responses, including rivalry, and their work performance increased. Among the four- and six-year-olds, the desire to surpass a peer was strong, and seemed to be a dominant motive.

There are dramatic individual variations in the tendency to compete during the preschool years, and there is a general tendency for children from democratic and permissive homes to be more competitive than those from more restrictive homes. Sex and socioeconomic status are also related to competitive relationships among preschool children. In one study (McKee and Leader, 1955), three- and four-year-old children of different age, sex, and socioeconomic background were brought in pairs to a playroom where there were two piles of blocks. The children's competitive and aggressive responses were recorded. As expected, there was more competition among the older than among the younger children. Moreover, the lower middle-class children competed more than those from the upper middle-class group, and boys competed more than girls.

The preschool years are witness to a flowering of motives and behavior systems that are linked with differing degrees of anxiety and inhibition. The desires for genital stimulation, nurture, aid, affection, and mastery of a skill and the wish to hurt or injure another are active components of the motive structure of a six-year-old. Since the school situation poses important socialization tasks for the child, it is critical that he emerge from the chrysalis of the preschool period with a conceptual maturity and a mosaic of defenses against anxiety that are capable of dealing with the stressful demands of the extrafamilial environment.

Critical Period IV: Six to Ten Years

It is generally acknowledged that there is a dramatic change among Western children both in overt behavior and in the form and quality of cognitive products between six and ten years of age. The popular explanation of these changes relates them to the varied experiences associated with school. But since many cultures institute formal changes in responsibilities and expectations for task mastery between the sixth and eighth year of life, fundamental psychological changes may transpire during these years which may provoke many cultures to institutionalize the mastery of specific skills and attributes.

This discussion is confined to the fouth critical period among children of the Western community. The critical responses established at this time include (1) learning new attitudes regarding intellectual mastery, including anticipation of success, fear of failure, standards of competence, and the development of relationships to the adult teacher, (2) learning an active social orientation with peers, (3) crystallization of attitudes toward the self with the peer group as the primary reference group, (4) learning differential anxiety and guilt over aggression, sexuality, and dependency, (5) the firmer establishment of particular defenses against anxiety, (6) practicing sex role standards and the crystallization of a sex role identity, and (7) the development of standards of rational thought and behavior, autonomy, honesty, and responsibility.

The major psychological dimensions along which adults differ can be discerned in close to mature form by the time the child is ten years old. Motives for power, competence, hostility, affection, acceptance, recognition, and sexuality are hierarchically organized in different patterns. The primary standards for sex role behavior, rational judgments, autonomy of action, honesty, and responsibility are exercising their influence on behavior. The major sources of anxiety have been learned, and preferred defensive reactions to anxiety have become more automatic and predictable. Moreover, the early school years produce complex psychological symptoms that intrude into the child's functioning, including extreme fearfulness, as in phobias or nightmares; somatic disturbances of psychological origin, like ulcerative colitis, asthma, headaches, repeated vomiting, and skin disturbances; stereotyped and repetitive rituals, like hand-washing, postures at bedtime, and obsessional thoughts; and motor tics, like blinking of the eyes or twitching of the face.

The early school years provide a fairly faithful preview of the child's behavior during the next ten to fifteen years and, therefore, are a good period to institute prophylactic procedures with children who display early signs of pathology.

The School Situation

For most children, school entrance marks the first continuous separation from mother for a large part of the day. The school situation presents the six-year-old with a new adult he must obey and whose approval he is expected to court. This adult requires him to learn and practice responses that are not initially rewarding. The school's major responsibilities are to develop (1) the desire to master intellectual skills, (2) a positive valuation of learning, and (3) the ability to persevere in problem solving and to formulate long range goals. The school also helps the child to establish peer relationships, and recently educators have decided that improving the quality of peer relations is part of the pedagogical enterprise.

In almost every instance, the child's first teacher is a woman who offers assistance to him, praises good behavior and punishes bad, and nurtures him when he is anxious. The teacher's grooming, attitudes, and actions are generally similar to those of the child's mother, especially if teacher and mother are both from the same social class. Many children view the teacher as a substitute mother. Therefore, the motives, attitudes, and acts that the child displays to his own mother are likely to be repeated for the teacher. Since mothers are generally viewed by young children as more nurturant and less fearsome than fathers, there are advantages to having a woman as the child's first adult contact in school.

However, there might be some gain, especially for boys, if the first teachers were men. The typical six-year-old boy is establishing an identification with his father and other male models, and his attempts to become more similar to adult males increase his tendencies to rebel against the mother and to deemphasize the power and competence of adult females. The frequent mischievous behavior of first- and second-grade boys suggests that they are less anxious than girls about potential rejection by the female teacher. The fact that academic retardation and conduct problems are more frequent among boys than girls in the first five years of school suggests also that boys enter school with greater resistance to its restraints than girls do. This resistance might be less if the teacher were a man. Finally, boys might associate the act of acquiring knowledge more with masculinity if their elementary teachers were men instead of women, since the sex role associated with an activity depends primarily on the sex of the person who normally performs it. Cooking, sewing, and caring for children are feminine because women typically do them. Repairing fences, mowing the lawn, and fishing are masculine because men do them. Since elementary school classes are conducted by women, young children tend to view schoolwork as more feminine than masculine and, therefore, more appropriate for girls than for boys. This attitude may increase girls' motivation to master reading and spelling, but it may also inhibit deep involvement for some boys.

The main things to be learned during the first five years of school are reading, arithmetic, spelling, and the social habits and attitudes that are valued in this culture. The teacher's values are typically middle class; she rewards neatness, obedience, cooperation, and cleanliness, and punishes waste, lack of responsibility, lying, aggressiveness, and eccentricity. Children of middle-class and well educated parents are more highly motivated and perform better in the primary grades than children of lower class and less educated parents. The reasons for this social class difference are well known. School success is more important in the upper middle class than in the lower classes. The middle-class child recognizes that the career to which he aspires depends heavily on the acquisition of academic skills. Moreover, middle-class parents encourage their children to work hard in school and to develop an interest in intellectual hobbies in the home. Finally, the child of a doctor, lawyer, or architect sees his father read books or journals and display a personal interest in intellectual problems. Middle-class parents act as models who not only reward mastery of intellectual tasks but also display an active involvement in intellectual mastery that indicates to the child that they value these goals.

The attitude of peers is important in the child's desire to master academic skills because motivation for scholastic success can be strengthened or reduced by the values of the peer group. In many middle-class groups, scholastic success is highly valued by the children. In a number of studies of middle-class children, the better students were the most popular children. Lower class, and particularly slum, children do not value scholastic achievement as much, and popularity among peers is not enhanced by school success. Davis points out that the middle-class child learns a socially adaptive fear of getting poor school grades, of being aggressive toward the teacher, of fighting, of cursing, and of having early sex relations; the slum child learns to fear quite different social acts. His gang teaches him to fear being "taken in" by the teacher and of being "a softie" with her. To take homework seriously may be a disgrace. Instead of boasting of good marks in school, one conceals them (Davis, 1948).

The Role of Intelligence

A child's intelligence test score (his IQ), his social class, and his grades in school are all positively related to each other. The personality correlates of school success, like persistence, nonaggression, and responsible behavior, are also similar to the correlates of IQ. Children who show large increases in IQ score during the early school years tend to persist in school, obtain good grades, and to care about intellectual achievement. Thus, the amount of increase in IQ is a rough index of the child's desire to master academic skills.

The correlation between a child's IQ score at age six and his score at age ten is about + 0.70, suggesting that some children show significant changes in intelligence test score between these ages. Investigations at the Fels Research Institute have revealed some provocative correlates of increase in IQ score (Sontag *et al.*, 1958). The subjects were 140 boys and girls for whom annual IQ scores and behavioral observations were available from the preschool years through early adolescence. Some children's IQ scores remained stable, others decreased, and still others increased. Twice as many boys as girls showed major increases in IQ, while more girls declined in IQ. The children who increased in IQ, in contrast to those who decreased, were more independent, more competitive, and more verbally aggressive.

The child's IQ score depends partly on his desire to master and improve his problem-solving skills, which is related in turn to parental encouragement and modeling. The mothers of a group of Fels children were rated on the degree to which they encouraged their children to talk and to walk during the first three years of life (Kagan and Moss, 1962). There was a positive relation, among girls, between maternal encouragement of early progress and the amount of IQ increase the girl showed during the years six to ten. The correlation for boys was also positive, but lower. This sex difference may be a function of the girl's identification with her mother. A mother's concern with intellectual mastery may have a greater effect upon her daughter than her son, an interpretation supported by the fact that mother's education is a better predictor of girls' than of boys' IQ scores at three, six, and ten years of age.

In another study, twenty boys and twenty girls from the first three grades were given a variety of tests and were also observed in a free play situation. Their parents were extensively interviewed. Girls who showed an intense interest in intellectual activities during free play had parents who encouraged intellectual mastery (Crandall *et al.*, unpublished ms.). This relation was positive but lower for the boys. Another study implicated the role of the father in the development of mastery in young boys. Forty boys, nine to eleven years of age, were divided into two groups: those who told many and those who told few achievement stories. An investigator visited the home of each boy and asked him to perform some problem tasks while the parents were watching. The boys who told many achievement stories performed more efficiently than those who told few stories (Rosen and D'Andrade, 1959). The behavior of both parents was observed while the child was performing. The mothers of high achievement boys tended to be more involved with their sons and more identified with them. They felt close to their sons, wanted them to be competent, and made demands for achievement, but affectionately. The fathers of these boys were not overly demanding and gave the boys autonomy and freedom of choice.

When the results of the many studies are considered, it appears that middle-class boys with mothers who are protective and affectionate and who encourage school achievement obtain the best grades in school. Girls who perform well in school, however, have mothers who are not overly affectionate and who encourage their daughters to be independent. The first five years of school furnish important clues to the child's later motivation for intellectual mastery; the child who does not develop strong motivation by early adolescence is not likely to change later.

Four factors appear crucial to intellectual mastery. The child's desire to master academic skills arises first largely from his desire to maintain a nurturant tie to parents who encourage this behavior and second from his identification with a parent who is an effective model for intellectual mastery. If a child is to be very much motivated toward intellectual mastery, he should see his parent as a nurturant and accepting person who values intellectual competence for himself. If the parent is rejecting, the child may not be eager to please him and may not be disposed to master academic tasks. Third, the greater the parental *emphasis* on intellectual mastery, the stronger the child's motivation will be. A final factor is the degree of autonomy fostered or restrictiveness imposed by the parent. An intellectually adequate but overpowering and autocratic parent may create serious feelings of inadequacy in the child, who is likely to develop the belief that he can never be as powerful or as competent as the parent, especially if the parent is of the same sex. Under such circumstances, the child may withdraw from intellectual challenges.

The Peer Group

The power of the peer group as a socialization agent is based on one primary incentive—acceptance. The values of the peer group conflict in some areas with those of parents and teachers, and its power in such conflicts is very great. There are two reasons for the influence of peers on a child's values. First, the peer group fosters rebellion against the socialization demands of the adult community. Peers promote sexual exploration and license aggressive play and venting of hostility. The child feels safer in expressing these prohibited acts with peers, and the peers function as a psychotherapeutic agent when he feels anxious about them. Second, the child trusts the group's evaluation and often mistrusts that of adults, whom he may see as either overly accepting or overly critical of him. In either case, he may feel that he is not able to obtain a faithful evaluation of his attributes from adults but believes in the essential validity and wisdom of peer evaluation, especially of his competence at diverse skills, his ability to dominate, his attractiveness, or his intelligence. The child is not able to arrive at any absolute judgment about the degree to which he possesses a specific trait, and he requires contact with others in order to assess it.

Many of the child's attitudes about himself are the product of his perceived rank in his peer group; his opinion of his verbal skills, for example, depends less on his absolute IQ than on his perceived rank among his age mates. Of two children, each with identical IQ scores, but one living in a town of 2000 and the other in a city of one million, the former is more likely to stand out among the brightest in his peer group. His expectancy of success with intellectual tasks will be greater than the city boy's, and his behavior when he is faced with difficult problems will be less anxious.

The role of the peer group as a matrix in which the child makes self-evaluations has not been sufficiently emphasized. This function is critical, and the child implicitly recognizes his dependence upon peers for his own evaluation. This dependence helps explain why peer acceptance is courted and rejection feared by most children.

Factors affecting peer acceptance. Since the child uses the peer group for self-evaluation, different consequences accrue to youngsters who are accepted or rejected by peers. It is important, therefore, to understand the factors that promote and militate against peer group acceptance. A popular technique of measuring peer acceptance asks children to name the classmates they like and dislike and to list the children who are friendly, smart, dominant, and so forth (see Figure 4.1). Each child in a camp cabin, for example, might be asked to name three children he would like to have as teammates or as visitors at his home. Bonney (1943) used this technique—called *sociometric*—to study the personality of popular and unpopular fourth-grade children. Classmates and teachers rated the most and least popular children on twenty variables. Popular children were rated much more socially aggressive and outgoing. They manifested one of two personality syndromes: the first was characterized by strong, aggressive traits such as leadership, enthusiasm, and active participation in events; the second involved a cheerful disposition and a friendly attitude toward others. There are, of course, sex differences in the traits that lead to peer acceptance (Bonney, 1943). Among first-grade girls, popularity is associated with a docile temperament. In the fifth grade, physical attractiveness and friendliness were more important. Among first-grade boys, physical prowess and daring were critical attributes, while fairness in play and leadership ability were more important among third-grade boys. Although the characteristics of popularity vary with age, they closely follow sex role standards.

The child's social class background is very important in determining his prestige among peers. Lower class children tend to have the poorest reputations among children of all social classes because they have less command of the personal resources that the wider community values. There is some interaction between social class and sex-typed traits with respect to popularity. Lower class boys respect two masculine types: the aggressive, belligerent boy and the outgoing sociable boy who is not necessarily aggressive. The effeminate boy who is conforming, passive, and not involved in masculine activities is always rejected. The lower class boy who does very well in school may also alienate himself from his peers. Lower class girls are willing to accept the verbally aggressive girl who shows a strong interest in boys and the friendly, pretty, and studious girl who is not necessarily a leader. A lower class girl can be a good student without alienating her friends. Middle-class boys accept those who are skilled in competitive games but are not blatantly aggressive. Friendliness and studiousness are also accepted. As in the lower class, the boy who is frightened, passive, and conforming is rejected. There is only one acceptable stereotype for middle-class girls: the attractive, friendly, and socially vivacious girl.

The child's status among his peers strongly affects the course of his socialization and contributes to his ability to exercise influence over others. In one investigation, eight groups of boys and eight groups of girls, aged eleven to fifteen, were studied in a summer camp (Polansky *et al.*, 1950). Observers recorded all interactions involving attempts to influence others. Children who had high status were aware of their position, felt more secure and accepted by the group, and were able to sway the behavior of others by both direct and indirect techniques.

Dominance and submissiveness with peers. The tendency to adopt a passive or a dominant approach to age mates is a remarkably stable disposition from age ten through adulthood, especially for females. Some children characteristically initiate communications with peers, suggest activities for the group, and resist pressure to conform to others. The passive child typically is quiet with peers and follows the suggestions of others. Activity and passivity are determined by many interacting forces, especially identification with a dominant or passive parent and the degree to which the child expects acceptance or rejection by his peers. The expectation of acceptance in turn depends on the degree to which the child believes he possesses the attributes that peers value, such as beauty, strength, skill, and verbal facility. Obviously, the child's *actual* body build and attractiveness are of critical importance. Finally, parental restriction of the child's autonomous behavior, that is, the degree to which the parent punishes attempts at domination and rewards submissiveness, also influences the child's posture with peers.

The Influence of Siblings

The psychological influence of younger siblings on the child's development is felt most keenly when the firstborn child is between four and eight years old, at which time the arrival of a new sibling is the greatest threat to him. The secondborn reciprocates by viewing the older sibling as an omnipotent and invulnerable competitor with special privileges and status. Each of the birth order positions thus carries with it some advantages and disadvantages.

The results of several studies suggest that firstborn and only children are subjected to more parental restrictions, greater acceleration, and more intense induction of guilt, while younger children in a family are handled more permissively but are likely to be dominated by older siblings. The firstborn child is likely to be more anxious over potential rejection by adults than are later born siblings, more likely to identify with adults, and more likely to view what happens to him as the product of his *own* efforts or mistakes. Firstborns adopt and practice the values of their parents with greater vigor than later born children, and a disproportionately high percentage of eminent men are firstborn or only children, perhaps because they respond more to the exalted aspirations parents often have for their children.

There are also disproportionately large numbers of firstborn children among the patients at child guidance clinics. This statistic may reflect the fact that firstborn children are more subject to anxiety, which accompanies the tendency to identify with and adopt the standards of their parents. However, this finding could also reflect the fact that mothers are more anxious and concerned with the development of their first than with their later born children and, therefore, more likely to bring that child to a clinic.

The most comprehensive study of the effect of siblings on behavioral development has been reported by Koch (1956*a* and *b*), who studied ordinal birth positions, sex, and spacing of siblings in 384 five- and six-year-olds from families with two children. The four types of sibling combinations—older boy-younger girl, older girl-younger boy, two girls, and two boys—were equally represented, and there were groups of siblings separated by one to two years, two to four years, and four to six years. Teachers observed and rated these children on a variety of behaviors. All the major variables—sex, ordinal birth position, and spacing—were associated with differences in the child's behavior.

The sex of the older sibling was one of the most important determinants of sex-typed behavior in the younger child. Girls with older brothers rather than older sisters were relatively more masculine in their behavior, that is more ambitious, more aggressive, and better on tests of intellectual ability. Boys with older sisters were less masculine than boys with older brothers. Evidently, the younger child identifies somewhat with the older sibling because the older is perceived to command desirable resources.

When ordinal position alone was considered, it was found that firstborn children had stronger and more consistent standards of honesty, responsibility, and aggression than did secondborns. However, the effect of ordinal position depended on the sex of the siblings and on spacing. When the siblings were the same sex and separated by less than two years, there were few behavioral differences between them. When they were four years apart and of opposite sex, behavioral differences were most marked. Koch concluded that a two- to four-year difference between siblings was most threatening to the older child. If the firstborn was three years old when the new baby arrived, he was most likely to become anxious over possible withdrawal of nurture. If the firstborn was only a year old, on the other hand, his self-image was still so diffuse that he probably did not regard the baby as a major threat to his bond with his mother and, therefore, not as a competitor for her affection. If the older child was eight when the new sibling arrived, he was already on the road to independence from his parents and was less threatened by the newcomer. In general, sex, ordinal position, and spacing all interact to influence the child's behavior.

Symptoms

During the preadolescent period, the complete range of adult symptoms can appear—psychosomatic symptoms such as ulcerative colitis or skin disorders, hysterias, nightmares, inhibition of skills, undisguised aggression, excessive social anxiety, tics, obsessions, rituals, and hallucinations. It seems best to group according to their presumed sources rather than their manifest similarities.

Anxiety over loss of parental nurturance. Anxiety over possible loss of parental acceptance disposes the child to conform excessively to parental demands and to feel intense guilt when a violation has been committed or even when he *thinks* about violating parental wishes and standards. Excessive conformity is a positive and often an effective way of bolstering the belief that the parents still value him, but it demands that the child inhibit his own wishes in order to reduce anxiety over potential loss of nurture. The guilt that results when such efforts fail may be signified by nightmares, ritualistic behaviors, or acts which seem intended to invite punishment. The intensity and exact source of guilt depend on the specific behaviors or thoughts involved. Hostile, aggressive, and sexual thoughts and behavior, selfishness, dishonesty, and regressions like crying or temper tantrums are the responses most heavily socialized from ages three to ten and are the primary sources of guilt during the early school years.

Reactions to guilt. There are two major responses to guilt feelings. One can be regarded as *restitutive* in intent: The child accepts the blame and behaves as though he should be punished for his misdemeanors. He is likely to make self-deprecatory statements, do things that will lead to punishment, or develop fears of death, illness, or mutilation. A typical example is that of an eleven-year-old girl who suddenly developed an intense fear of dying after accidentally choking on a piece of food. She was badly frightened by this experience and soon after told her parents that she had rabies and was going to die. She was talked out of the belief, but then became convinced that she had cancer. Psychological study of the child and the family revealed that socialization of hostile thoughts and aggressive behavior was unusually severe; there were constant verbal reminders of the wickedness of hostile feelings. The girl admitted strong resentment of her mother and younger siblings, but believed that she had no right to feel as she did and that she must be a bad girl to have these thoughts. The belief in imminent death appeared to be a direct consequence of her guilt over these hostile thoughts toward her family. There are less dramatic modes of self-punishment as well; performing poorly in school and inviting peers to be rejecting are less obvious manifestations of guilt-laden unhappiness in the child.

The second kind of reaction to guilt is *defensive*; it reduces guilt directly, usually by projecting the blame for the prohibited act onto others. It is not well understood why some children react this way while others take the self-punitive route; probably, however, the less intense the guilt, the more the child will attempt to minimize it through direct means. The most common direct defense against guilt is to blame the prohibited action on another person. The familiar cry of the accused six-year-old, "I didn't hit him and anyway he started it," is the clearest example of projecting guilt. Other common forms of this response include blaming school failure on the teacher, blaming peers for rejection. Finally, the child may try to reduce guilt through intellectual analysis, that is by rationalizing the transgression.

Existing research indicates that the parental milieu most conducive to guilt is one in which an affectionate relationship between parent and child has existed for several years and love withdrawal is the method of socialization. Under these conditions, the child values the mother's nurture and is made anxious and guilty at the thought of losing it.

Hostility to parents. A second attitude that generates symptoms in the preadolescent child is strong hostility to parents, the intent of which is to cause anxiety in them. The methods of expression depend, in part, on the models of aggressive behavior to which the child has been exposed. The most direct one is physical aggression toward the parents. Its purest form, homicide, is rare among young adolescents and virtually unknown among children under ten. Verbal aggression is the most common form of hostility during the early school years and, if not strongly punished, is an effective way for the child to quickly gratify his hostile feelings. The maladaptive responses that result from strong hostile wishes often occur when the child is not able to express his hostility verbally and is forced to use indirect means. The indirect strategies typically involve choosing a behavior that will cause anxiety without revealing the aggressive intent. There are not many responses that fit this requirement. Those that do are often frustrations of strong wishes the parent has for the child, for school success, honesty, social poise, and responsibility. By failing in school, violating parental standards for social conduct, or regression, the child elicits anger and emotional upset in the parent and thereby gratifies his own hostile wishes. The child is typically unaware of the intent of his actions and must himself suffer the realistic pain and anxiety that accompanies school failure or peer rejection.

Sexual feelings. A third class of symptoms is generated by desires for physical affection from the parent of the opposite sex and recognition of the pleasant quality of genital stimulation. For many children, anxiety is a constant accompaniment to these wishes and to their gratification.

The desire for heterosexual affection finds its clearest expression in the contrast between the ready conformity of young girls to the requests of adult males and the resistance they show to the demands of adult females. This preferential conformity to the adult of the opposite sex is less clear in boys because of their general reluctance to appear passive and conforming to *any* adult.

The behavioral signs of high sexual anxiety are quite dramatic. The phobic avoidance of children of the opposite sex and the strict partitioning of group play by sex is one evidence of the anxiety felt over close contact between the sexes during the preadolescent years. The sudden resistance a daughter shows to her father over dressing is another sign of this anxiety. At age five, she may readily dress and undress in his presence. At ten, she insists on closed doors and blushingly demands that the father leave the room when she dresses or prepares for bed. Moreover, anxiety over masturbation, like anxiety over aggression, can lead to nightmares, obsessive rituals, and self-punitive procedures.

The appearance of tics may also be related to sexual anxiety. Some of the more common tics are eye blinking, rolling of the lips, movement of the muscles of the lower face, and jerky movements of the fingers or wrists.

A final source of conflict derives from the pressures the schoolchild feels to conform to the standards for sex-typed behaviors. Some of these conflicts are described in the section on the preschool years. During the school years, conflict over violating male sex role standards often leads boys to inhibit any display of emotion or of passivity, both of which are considered inappropriate to a masculine ego ideal. For girls, withdrawal from competitive intellectual efforts, especially in mathematics and the sciences, can be a result of anxiety over female sex role standards.

This discussion of symptoms in the school age child suggests the value of delineating symptoms by origin or cause rather than by content or manifest form. Failure in school can be either the product of strong hostility to a parent or the self-punitive act of an eight-year-old. A nightmare can stem, for example, from guilt over hostile feelings to a sibling or from anxiety over sexual fantasies toward a parent. The school years are characterized by maximal socialization of aggression, sexuality, dependency, and sex-typed standards. The nine-year-old experiences conflict in all these domains, for sexual and aggressive thoughts rise to consciousness daily. As a result, some preadolescents develop symptoms in association with them.

THE ROLE OF PARENTAL PRACTICES

This chapter has thus far described the major classes of responses learned during the first decade of life. These are responsible for the dramatic individual differences in behavior noted in most ten-year-olds. However, there has been no systematic discussion of the parental behaviors and attitudes that give direction to these responses. Parents are the major sources of frustration, joy, pleasure, or anger for the child and thus are the major agents governing psychological development. Parents are at the top of a hierarchy of influences that includes siblings, peers, teachers, and the public media, in that order. This hierarchy corresponds roughly to the temporal order in which these things become important in the child's life. Parents and siblings exert their influence early, peers and teachers during the early school years; the public media have their maximal effect just before and during early adolescence. The modes of influence are somewhat dissimilar among them, though direct and vicarious reward and punishment and modeling continue to provide the mechanisms for all of them. If parental nurture, acceptance, and praise are valued, as they usually are, selected responses will be established and maintained because parental nurture acts as a reward. The early vocalizations and primitive speech of the two- and three-year-old are accompanied by peals of praise and recognition by adults. These rewarding reactions from adults act as incentives to develop more language. The six-year-old is praised for tying his shoes, picking up his fork correctly, or learning his multiplication tables, and this praise strengthens these accomplishments. Punishment is a second method of effecting changes in behavior. Whether from spanking, scolding, threatened rejection, or deprivation of goals, the anxiety generated by punishment usually leads to inhibition of the undesirable response and often to substitution of another act. Inhibition of evacuation, aggression, or masturbation is controlled, in part, by the anxiety attached to the stimuli originally arousing them. Finally, the modeling process associated with identification molds the child's behavior.

Parents, teachers, and peers act in all three capacities for they all reward, punish, and act as models. Public media like books, movies, and TV exert influence primarily through the modeling process, and their influence is often underestimated. In sum, the behavior during infancy is molded by nurture and affection; punishment is added to the recipe during the second and third years; and modeling assumes salience during the fourth and fifth years.

The influence of the mother. The aspects of the mother's behavior that are most salient to the child are not completely clear, and a differentiation must be made between concrete behaviors, such as spanking, scolding, or kissing and abstractions like *rejection* or *acceptance*. The acts that define maternal rejection differ for different cultural groups. Mothers in the isolated rural areas of northern Norway rarely talk to their children and move them around like shoes out of place. An American psychologist would call this same behavior in a middle-class Chicago mother rejection, but it may not be indicative of rejection in a rural Norwegian mother. Basically, rejection is an *attitude* of dislike and hostility toward the child, and it is not obvious which *behaviors* should be regarded as the best indicators of that attitude. Neglect of the child's needs for food, warmth, or comfort, open and direct criticism, and expressions of rage at the child are reasonable indicators of a rejecting attitude. But many mothers seldom express these behaviors in undisguised form. There is no general agreement on the more subtle indexes of a rejecting attitude.

It is generally assumed that rejection-hostility is one end of a dimension whose other pole is typically labeled acceptance-affection. Like rejection, acceptance is an attitude that finds expression in varied ways. Psychologists often assume, without sufficient reflection, that physical affection is the *sine qua non* of maternal acceptance. This is plausible, but probably incorrect. Some mothers may have difficulty initiating close physical contact with their children because affectional behavior arouses anxiety over sexual thoughts and feelings. Some mothers may be aware of strong hostile feelings toward the infant, and display intense physical affection in order to reduce their guilt and anxiety over this basic resentment. The mother's behavior is, at best, only an indirect guide to her attitudes. There is considerable slippage between her *attitude* and her *behavior*. Nonetheless, the idea that there is a dimension of parental rejection-acceptance has dominated empirical research in human development. Schaefer (1959) has analyzed the many variables that have been observed in the behavior of mothers and has concluded that the dimension of love (acceptance) versus hostility (rejection) is a fundamental fact of maternal behavior. It is possible, however, that the conceptual heritage of Western psychologists has demanded this result. Our prose and poetry, much older than empirical work in the social sciences, speak as if the dimension of love versus rejection were real, and this attribute is typically the first one people evaluate when they watch a parent and child interact.

Schaefer's studies reveal a second factor in parent-child relations called the control-autonomy dimension. This dimension is closer to concrete behavior than the acceptance-hostility continuum is. A controlling mother consistently punishes deviations from her standards, prevents the child's explorations of new areas, and punishes independence of action. The autonomy-giving mother—sometimes called the permissive mother—allows the child to express his idiosyncratic tendencies and does not punish his free exploration or assertions of independence. It is of interest to note that the mother's behavior on the hostility-acceptance continuum is more stable over long periods of time than it is on the control-autonomy continuum, perhaps because the degree to which a mother controls her child depends partly on how much he needs to be controlled. This is a feedback system in which the mother typically reacts to the child in a way that is guided both by her internalized ideal for him and by the child's behavior. Acceptance-hostility, on the other hand, appears to be a more permanent aspect of the mother's basic temperament.

More recently, Becker (1964) has suggested a refinement of Schaefer's model. Becker accepts the acceptance-rejection factor but suggests that Schaefer's control versus autonomy dimension should be divided into two relatively uncorrelated factors: (1) restrictiveness versus permissiveness, and (2) anxious emotional involvement versus calm detachment. Only further empirical work will determine whether it is profitable to divide the control-autonomy dimension in this way.

Numerous studies have attempted to relate these maternal dimensions to the child's behavior. Most of the investigations are cross sectional in design. They have used children between three and fifteen years of age, have used only parental interviews to assess maternal acceptance or restriction, and have rarely supplemented these data with direct observations of the mother.

Despite these methodological weaknesses, there is some degree of unanimity in the results. Children of hostile mothers are more likely to express aggression to peers, to develop psychosomatic symptoms, to regress in toilet training, and to become psychotic. Children of controlling-restrictive mothers are more likely to withdraw from stress or become excessively rebellious and to develop exaggerated fears and obsessive-compulsive symptoms. Restriction, unlike acceptance, is inversely correlated with level of maternal education and with social class. For this reason, the associations between restrictiveness and the child's behavior must be regarded with caution as they could be the consequence of social class.

Schaefer suggests that the acceptance-hostility and control-autonomy dimensions are uncorrelated and that mothers should be categorized into one of four types: accepting and controlling, accepting and autonomy giving, hostile and controlling, and hostile and autonomy giving. He suggests further that each of these four maternal types is linked to specific syndromes of disorder in the child. The antisocial child who displays his aggression directly is linked to a mother who is both rejecting and autonomy giving. It is implied that the rejection creates strong hostile feelings in the child and reduces his motivation to inhibit asocial behavior, while the permissive atmosphere implies that the child's aggressive behavior is not punished. The child who displays signs of excessive guilt, phobias, tics, obsessive thoughts, academic problems, or ulcerative colitis is presumed to have experienced the combination of acceptance and control. His mother would place excessive socialization demands upon her child, and the strongly nurturant tie would entice him to adopt her standards. An accepting mother creates excessive anxiety over loss of nurture in the child and a reluctance to violate maternal wishes.

The psychotic child is assumed to be the product of excessive rejection and extreme control. The rejection presumably creates feelings of self-hatred and strong hostility toward the mother. However, the control prevents the child from expressing his feelings and leads to fear of the prohibited behaviors. The combination of negative self-image, extreme guilt, and failure to learn how to retaliate could lead to serious and persistent withdrawal.

This scheme is admittedly oversimplified, for it neglects the influence of the father and the role of biological variables that might predispose the child toward particular pathological syndromes. It is a beginning, however, and has not been rejected out of hand because it has some counterparts in the empirical world.

Other maternal variables. Other maternal variables should be considered, for dimensions other than acceptance-hostility and restrictiveness-autonomy also affect the child's behavior. For example, little attention has been paid to the *degree of consistency* the parent displays in her behavior toward the child. Rejecting mothers are, of necessity, inconsistent in their ministration of nurture. Perhaps it is the behavioral inconsistency rather than only the hostile attitude that defines a rejecting maternal atmosphere. Similarly, the degree of verbal discipline and the offering of a rationale for discipline have been ignored. A mother who is restricting and arbitrary, in contrast to one who explains her restrictions, is apt to confuse the child and generate strong hostility. The coherence and rational quality of the mother's communications to the child are dimensions that also need further study.

Infancy is the time when the child is most helpless and maximally dependent upon the ministrations of the mother. This situation provides a setting for another variable that has been ignored, namely, the delay between the onset of need in the child, as evidenced by his crying, and the administration of some nurture that will reduce the need.

The behavior of the parent *as perceived by the child* is a variable of a different order. The parent is a model, and the attitudes and acts he or she exhibits are likely to be adopted by the child. When the parent's own behavior is consistent with his demands, the child is provided with a consistent context for socialization. The child is confronted with an inconsistent situation, on the other hand, when the parent speaks aggressively to the spouse, strikes the child and insults friends, but consistently punishes all such displays of aggression in the child. The effect of the parent as a *model* for aggression in the above situation is probably as critical as the *punishment* of aggressive behavior (Sears *et al.*, 1957).

The sleeper effect. The above discussion has assumed an immediate and continuous connection between the mother's behavior and the child's, but some maternal behaviors display a "sleeper" effect. A maternal practice early in life, say acceleration of the two-year-old child's intellectual skills, may have a more profound influence on his intellectual mastery at age ten than at any previous age. The Fels longitudinal investigation suggests that such sleeper effects are possible (Kagan and Moss, 1962). For example, a maternal tendency to be critical of one- to three-year-old daughters was highly predictive of adult mastery in these women, while a similar tendency during the preschool or early school years showed a negligible relationship to adult mastery behavior. Similarly, maternal protectiveness and nurture of the daughter during the first three years pre-figured a tendency toward withdrawal from stressful situations in adulthood, whereas protection during the preschool years showed no relationship to adult passivity under stress. One explanation for these results is that the reciprocal nature of the mother-child interaction changes with time. The child's ability to provoke relatively permanent changes in specific maternal reactions increases with age. A six-year-old is more likely to produce a major alteration in the mother's characteristic responses to him than the two-year-old is. The child's actions have the power to change the mother's behavior increasingly as he grows older.

The mother typically establishes expectations as to what her child should be like, that is, standards to which his behavior should conform. The greater the discrepancy between her expectations and her evaluation of the child, the more likely she is to exert pressure on him toward greater conformity with her expectations. The infant's personality is relatively unformed and the discrepancy between her standards and what she perceives in him is necessarily small. She sees the infant as she would like to see him, as an object primarily to be acted upon. Maternal behavior toward an infant, therefore, is not as influenced by the child's behavior as her behavior toward the ten-year-old is. A mother's concern with the intellectual development of her two-year-old is more likely to be an index of her own basic needs and values than is her concern with her ten-year-old daughter who is failing in school. Similarly, encouragement of independence, a critical attitude, or overprotectiveness toward a ten-year-old may be newly developed reactive measures to the child's dependence, rebelliousness, or fragile defenses respectively. It is possible that particular maternal practices, such as nurture, restrictiveness, and hostility, during the first three years provide the most sensitive index of the mother's basic attitudes toward the child and, perhaps, of her more lasting effect on his future behavior. The elucidation of such cause-effect sequences in development may require a long-term research design. A cross-sectional investigation of the relationship between maternal protection and passivity in a ten-year-old might yield a negligible association between these variables, but if the maternal behavior were repeatedly assessed after the child was three years old, a strong positive relation might emerge.

Certain classes of parent-child interaction variables are particularly susceptible to the sleeper effect. Maternal behavior that is likely to change over the first decade, such as show of affection, reward of dependency, and physical punitiveness, is more likely to display this effect than is behavior that tends to be stable, like mothers' attitudes toward sexuality or toward sex-typed traits. Furthermore, maternal reactions that are specific to the child's behavior during school years, such as concern with grades or punishment of overt aggression, may give misleading impressions of the general relations of maternal and child behavior.

SUMMARY

The major theme of this chapter has been that the five primary response systems—motives, standards, affects, defenses, and instrumental behaviors—are established at different periods in development. Although the ratio of ignorance to fact is high, and this chapter contains much conjecture, present knowledge does begin to give a picture of the psychological growth of the typical child and the approximate time of emergence of selected responses. However, there is considerably less information on the *mechanisms of that growth* and the *ways in which environmental events influence response organization.* This essay on psychological development is more descriptive than theoretical, and it closely resembles Jean Piaget's scheme of intellectual development (1928, 1950, 1952).

Present theories of cognitive and behavioral development, however, do not have the tight net of interlocking propositions that would permit us to make satisfying explanations of many important events. The constructs of identification, anxiety over loss of love, motives of power, autonomy, mastery, affection, hostility, and sexuality, and standards for sex roles have been treated speculatively in this chapter. The results of experiments done in the next two decades will be the judge of the utility of these ideas. Two conclusions seem reasonably safe at this time: (1) the behavioral profile of the ten-year-old is a fairly good predictor of the child's behavior a decade later, and (2) the timing of environmental rewards and punishments and the attributes of the child's models during the first decade are critical influences on behavior during adolescence and early adulthood. The importance attributed to *the timing* of environmental events makes long-term investigations mandatory if we are to gain detailed knowledge of development in the first 100 months.

GLOSSARY

ACCEPTANCE-HOSTILITY CONTINUUM—the dimension describing the range of "closeness" in interpersonal relations.

AFFECT—feeling, emotion.

AFFILIATIVE BEHAVIOR—aimed at establishing friendly and harmonious interpersonal relationships.

AGGRESSION—behavior *intended* to injure or distress another person.

ANXIETY—in this chapter, an unpleasant feeling state usually characterized by (the perception of) increased motility of the gastrointestinal tract, increased heart rate, sweating palms, shivering, flushing, and muscular contractions; the feeling state that occurs with anticipation of an unwanted event.

CONSCIENCE—the personal system of ethical values against which the individual judges his own and others' intentions and behaviors.

CONTROL-AUTONOMY DIMENSION—a continuum describing the amount of regulation the parent imposes on the child.

COVERT ATTRIBUTES—attributes that are not directly observable.

CRITICAL PERIOD—a time during which certain environmental events have maximal influence on behavior or development.

DENIAL—refusal to accept negative feelings about the self.

DEPENDENCY—reliance on others for the satisfaction of physical and psychological needs.

EFFECTANCE—a motive reflecting the desire to perfect one's skills.

EGO IDEAL—the way an individual would like to be.

ENURESIS—bed-wetting.

EROGENOUS—giving rise to sexual or erotic behavior or feeling.

EXPRESSIVE SOCIAL ROLE—according to Parsons (1955), the female social role, characterized by passivity, nurture, and affect.

GUILT—as used in this chapter, a form of anxiety created when a person recognizes that his *behavior* has deviated from some established (personal) standard; some writers, particularly psychoanalysts, feel that the *impulse* to deviate from a personal standard may also give rise to guilt.

IDENTIFICATION—the process by which a person comes to believe that he possesses some of the attributes of a revered model; it involves vicarious sharing in the affective states of the model (see Chapter 10).

INCENTIVE TRAINING—as used in this chapter, teaching processes that rely mainly on identification, imitation, and simple reward.

INDEPENDENCE—self-reliance.

INSTRUMENTAL SOCIAL ROLE—according to Parsons (1955), the male social role, characterized by aggression, dominance, and independence.

MASTERY BEHAVIOR—the attempt to improve proficiency at a task.

MODEL—an individual whose behavior is imitated by another.

MOTIVE—as used in this chapter, a wish for a specific class of events; usages of this term vary greatly (see Chapters 3, 9, 10 for other usages).

MUTISM—refusal to speak.

NASCENT PATHOLOGY—the earliest stage of pathology, or behavior in the process of becoming pathological.

NEUROPHYSIOLOGY—the branch of physiology dealing with the activity of the nervous system.

OVERT BEHAVIOR—observable, "gross" behavior (responses).

PASSIVITY—a general tendency on the part of an individual to let others be dominant in interpersonal relationships.

PERSONAL IDENTITY—see SELF-CONCEPT.

PERSONALITY—the hierarchy of behaviors of which a person is capable and the relationships among these behaviors; a set of terms that allows us to explain a particular person's behavior.

PHOBIA—abnormal anxiety or fear.

PROJECTION—the attribution of one's own traits, attitudes, or subjective processes to other people or groups.

PROPHYLACTIC—preventive.

PSYCHOPATHOLOGY—mental illness; negative psychological abnormalities.

PUNITIVE TRAINING—teaching inhibitions by creating anxiety over commission of prohibited acts, usually by means of threats or punishment.

REGRESSION—the return because of stress or frustration to early, immature modes of behavior, often with the general defensive purpose of evading the challenges and problems of maturity.

REINFORCEMENT—that which strengthens a response.

REPRESSION—the exclusion of psychological contents (for example, memories and feelings) from awareness, commonly because they provoke anxiety.

SELF-ESTEEM—the degree to which one psychologically values himself.

SEX ROLE BEHAVIOR—behavior identified as masculine (for example, dominance) or feminine (for example, passivity).

SEX ROLE IDENTITY—the degree to which a person regards himself as masculine or feminine.

SEX ROLE STANDARD—the sum of culturally approved characteristics of masculinity and femininity.

SEX-TYPED SKILLS—skills identified as being either masculine (such as sports) or feminine (such as housekeeping).

SEX-TYPED TRAIT—a behavioral trait identified as masculine (such as assertiveness) or feminine (such as nurturing).

SEX TYPING—the tendency for a culture to encourage different behaviors for boys and girls and to establish different attributes as desirable for each of the sexes.

SEXUAL EXHIBITIONISM—inappropriate exposure of sex organs.

SOCIALIZATION—the process whereby a person (especially a child) acquires sensitivity to social stimuli (especially the pressures and obligations of group life) and learns to get along with, and behave like, others in his culture or group.[1]

SOCIOMETRY—a technique for assessing the degree to which an individual is liked or respected by his peers.

SOMATIC DISTURBANCES—physical disorders.

VALUES—an abstract concept, often merely implicit, that defines for an individual or for a social unit what ends or means to an end are desirable.[1]

REFERENCES

Aberle, D. F., and K. D. Naegele. Middle-class father's occupational role and attitudes toward children. *American Journal of Orthopsychiatry*, 1952, **22**, 366–378.

Aronfreed, J. The origin of self criticism. *Psychological Review*, 1964, **71**, 193–218.

Bach, G. R. Father fantasies and father typing in father separated children. *Child Development*, 1946, **17**, 63–79.

Bandura, A. Social learning through imitation. In M. R. Jones (ed.), *Nebraska Symposium on Motivation*, Vol. X. Lincoln, Neb.: University of Nebraska Press, pp. 211–268.

———, Dorothea Ross, and Sheila A. Ross. Transmission of aggression through imitation of aggressive models. *Journal of Ab-*

[1] This definition is taken from H. B. English and Ava C. English, *A comprehensive dictionary of psychological and psychoanalytical terms*. New York: David McKay Company, Inc., 1958.

normal and Social Psychology, 1961, **63,** 575–582.

———, ———, and ———. A comparative test of the status envy, social power and secondary reinforcement theories of identification learning. *Journal of Abnormal and Social Psychology,* 1963*a,* **67,** 527–534.

———, ———, and ———. Vicarious reinforcement and imitative learning. *Journal of Abnormal and Social Psychology,* 1963*b,* **67,** 601–607.

Becker, W. C. Consequences of different kinds of parental discipline. In L. W. Hoffman and C. Hoffman (eds.), *Annual Review of Child Development.* New York: Russell Sage Foundation, 1964.

Beller, E. K. Dependency and independence in young children. *Journal of Genetic Psychology,* 1955, **87,** 25–35.

———. Exploratory studies of dependency. *Transactions of the New York Academy of Sciences,* 1959, **21,** 414–426.

Bennett, E. M., and L. R. Cohen. Men and women: Personality patterns and contrasts. *Genetic Psychology Monograph,* 1959, **59,** 101–155.

Bieber, I., *et al. Homosexuality.* New York: Basic Books, Inc., 1962.

Bonney, M. E. The constancy of sociometric scores and their relationship to teacher judgments of social success and to personality self-ratings. *Sociometry,* 1943, **6,** 409–424.

Bowlby, J. Separation anxiety. *International Journal of Psychoanalysis,* 1960, **41,** 89–113.

Brackbill, Yvonne. Extinction of the smiling response in infants as a function of reinforcement schedule. *Child Development,* 1958, **29,** 114–124.

Bronfenbrenner, U. Freudian theories of identification and their derivatives. *Child Development,* 1960, **31,** 15–40.

Child, I. L., E. H. Potter, and Estelle M. Levine. Children's textbooks and personality development: An exploration in the social psychology of education. *Psychological Monographs,* 1946, **60,** No. 3.

Cobb, H. V. Role wishes and general wishes of children and adolescents. *Child Development,* 1954, **25,** 161–171.

Crandall, V. J., W. Katkovsky, and Anne Preston. Parent behavior and children's achievement development. Unpublished.

———, and Alice Rabson. Children's repetition choices in an intellectual achievement situation following success and failure. *Journal of Genetic Psychology,* 1960, **97,** 161–168.

Crutchfield, R. S. Conformity and character. *American Psychologist,* 1955, **10,** 191–198.

Davis, A. *Social class influences upon learning.* Cambridge, Mass.: Harvard University Press, 1948.

Dawe, Helen C. An analysis of two hundred quarrels of preschool children. *Child Development,* 1934, **5,** 295–303.

Dennis, W. Causes of retardation among institutional children: Iran. *Journal of Genetic Psychology,* 1960, **96,** 47–59.

Douvan, E., and C. Kaye. *Adolescent girls.* Ann Arbor, Mich.: University of Michigan Press, 1957.

Emmerich, W. Parental identification in young children. *Genetic Psychology Monograph,* 1959, **60,** 257–308.

Fauls, L. B., and W. D. Smith. Sex role learning of five-year-olds. *Journal of Genetic Psychology,* 1956, **89,** 105–117.

Foster, J. C. Play activities of children in the first six grades. *Child Development,* 1930, **1,** 248–254.

Frazier, A., and Lisonbee, L. K. Adolescent concerns with physique. *School Review,* 1950, **58,** 397–405.

Freud, S. Mourning and melancholia. In *Collected Papers,* Vol. IV. London: Hogarth Press, Ltd., 1925, pp. 30–59.

Gewirtz, J. L., and D. M. Baer. The effects of brief social deprivation on behavior for a social reinforcer. *Journal of Abnormal and Social Psychology,* 1958, **56,** 49–56.

Goodenough, F. W. Interest in persons as an aspect of sex differences in the early years. *Genetic Psychology Monographs,* 1957, **55,** 287–323.

Greenberg, P. J. Competition in children and experimental studies. *American Journal of Psychology,* 1932, **44,** 221–249.

Harris, D. B. Sex differences in the life problems and interests of adolescents, 1935 and 1957. *Child Development,* 1959, **30,** 453–459.

Hartley, R. E. Children's concepts of male and female roles. *Merrill-Palmer Quarterly,* 1960, **6,** 83–91.

Hattwick, L. A. Sex differences in behavior of nursery school children. *Child Development,* 1937, **8,** 343–355.

Hebb, D. O. On the nature of fear. *Psychological Review,* 1946 **53,** 259–276.

Hildreth, G. The social interests of young

adolescents. *Child Development,* 1945, **16,** 119–121.

Honzik, Marjorie P. Sex differences in the occurrence of materials in the play construction of preadolescents. *Child Development,* 1951, **22,** 15–36.

Hovland, C. I., and I. L. Janis. (eds.). *Personality and persuasibility.* New Haven, Conn.: Yale University Press, 1959.

James, W. *The principles of psychology.* New York: Henry Holt & Co., 1890.

Jenkins, J. J., and W. A. Russell. An atlas of semantic profiles for 360 words. *American Journal of Psychology,* 1958, **71,** 688–699.

Jersild, A. T. *In search of self.* New York: Columbia University Press, 1952.

Kagan, J. The concept of identification. *Psychological Review,* 1958, **65,** 296–305.

———, B. Hosken, and S. Watson. The child's symbolic conceptualization of the parents. *Child Development,* 1961, **32,** 625–636.

——— and J. Lemkin. The child's differential perception of parental attributes. *Journal of Abnormal and Social Psychology,* 1960, **61,** 440–447.

——— and H. A. Moss. *Birth to maturity: A study in psychological development.* New York: John Wiley & Sons, Inc., 1962.

——— and W. Phillips. The measurement of identification. *Journal of Abnormal and Social Psychology,* 1964, **69,** 442–443.

Koch, H. L. Attitudes of children toward their peers as related to certain characteristics of their siblings. *Psychological Monographs,* 1956*a,* **70,** No. 426, 1–41.

———. Some emotional attitudes of the young child in relation to characteristics of his siblings, *Child Development.* 1956*b,* **27,** 393–426.

Kohn, M. L. Social class and parental values. *American Journal of Sociology,* 1959, **64,** 337–351.

Lansky, L. M., U. J. Crandall, J. Kagan, and C. T. Baker. Sex differences in aggression and its correlates in middle class adolescents. *Child Development,* 1961, **32,** 45–58.

Lazarus, R. S. *Adjustment and personality.* New York: McGraw-Hill, Inc., 1961.

Leuba, C. An experimental study in rivalry in young children. *Journal of Comparative Psychology,* 1933, **16,** 367–378.

Lindzey, G., and M. Goldberg. Motivational differences between males and females as measured by the Thematic Apperception Test. *Journal of Personality,* 1953, **22,** 101–117.

Linton, R. *The study of man: An introduction.* New York: Appleton-Century, 1936.

Lynn, D. G. A note on sex differences in the development of masculine and feminine identification. *Psychological Review,* 1959, **66,** 126–135.

Maccoby, Eleanor E. Role taking in childhood and its consequences for social learning. *Child Development,* 1959, **30,** 239–252.

——— and W. C. Wilson. Identification and observational learning from films. *Journal of Abnormal and Social Psychology,* 1957, **55,** 76–87.

McCandless, B. R., C. B. Bilous, and H. L. Bennett. Peer popularity and dependence on adults in preschool age socialization. *Child Development,* 1961, **32,** 511–518.

McKee, J. P., and S. B. Leader. Relationship of socioeconomic status to the competitive behavior of school children. *Child Development,* 1955, **25,** 135–142.

Mowrer, O. H. Identification: A link between learning theory and psychotherapy. In *Learning theory and personality dynamics.* New York: The Ronald Press Company, 1950*a.*

———. On the psychology of talking birds—a contribution to language and personality theory. In *Learning theory and personality dynamics.* New York: The Ronald Press Company, 1950*b.*

Mussen, P. H., and L. Distler. Masculinity: Identification and father-son relationships. *Journal of Abnormal and Social Psychology,* 1959, **59,** 350–356.

Muste, Myra J., and Doris F. Sharpe. Some influential factors in the determination of aggressive behavior in preschool children. *Child Development,* 1947, **18,** 11.

Nash, H. Assignment of gender to body regions. *Journal of Genetic Psychology,* 1958, **92,** 113–115.

Parsons, T. Age and sex in the social structure of the United States. In C. Kluckhohn and H. A. Murray (eds.), *Personality in nature, society and culture.* New York: Alfred A. Knopf, Inc., 1948, pp. 269–281.

———. Family structures and the socialization of the child in T. Parsons and R. F. Bales (eds.), *Family socialization and the interaction process.* New York: The Free Press of Glencoe, 1955.

Piaget, J. *Judgment and reasoning in the child.* London: Routledge & Kegen Paul Ltd., 1928.

———. *The psychology of intelligence.* New York: Harcourt, Brace & World, Inc., 1950.

———. *The origins of intelligence in children.* New York: International Universities Press, Inc., 1952.

Pintler, M. H., R. Phillips, and R. R. Sears. Sex differences in the projective doll play of preschool children. *Journal of Psychology,* 1946, **21,** 73–80.

Polansky, N., R. Lippitt, and F. Redl. An investigation of behavioral contagion in groups. *Human Relations,* 1950, **3,** 319–348.

Provence, Sally, and Rose C. Lipton. *Infants in institutions.* New York: International Universities Press, 1962.

Rabban, M. Sex-role identification in young children in two diverse social groups. *Genetic Psychology Monograph,* 1950, **42,** 81–158.

Rheingold, Harriet L. The modification of social responsiveness in institutional babies. *Monographs on Social Research in Child Development,* 1956, **21,** No. 2 (Serial No. 63).

Rosen, B. D., and R. D'Andrade. The psychosocial origins of achievement motivation. *Sociometry,* 1959, **22,** 185–218.

Rosenberg, B. C., and B. Sutton-Smith. A revised conception of masculine-feminine differences in play activity. *Journal of Genetic Psychology,* 1960, **96,** 165–170.

Sanford, R. N. The dynamics of identification. *Psychological Review,* 1955, **62,** 106–117.

——— *et al.* Physique, personality and scholarship: A cooperative study of school children. *Monograph of the Society for Research in Child Development,* 1943, **8,** No. 1.

Schachter, S., and J. E. Singer. Cognitive, social and physiological determinants of emotional state. *Psychological Review,* 1962, **69,** 379–399.

Schaefer, E. S. A circumplex model for maternal behavior. *Journal of Abnormal and Social Psychology,* 1959, **59,** 226–235.

Sears, Pauline S. Doll play aggression in normal young children: Influence of sex, age, sibling status, father's absence. *Psychological Monographs,* 1951, **65** (6).

Sears, R. R. Identification as a form of behavioral development. In D. B. Harris (ed.), *The concept of development.* Minneapolis: University of Minnesota Press, 1957, pp. 149–161.

———, E. E. Maccoby, and H. Levin. *Patterns of child rearing.* New York: Harper & Row, Publishers, 1957.

———, J. W. M. Whiting, V. Nowlis, and P. S. Sears. Some child-rearing antecedents of aggression and dependency in young children. *Genetic Psychology Monograph,* 1953, **47,** 135–236.

Sontag, L. W., C. T. Baker, and V. L. Nelson. Mental growth and personality: A longitudinal study. *Monographs on Social Research in Child Development,* 1958, **23,** No. 68.

Spitz, R. A., and Katherine M. Wolff. Anaclitic depression: An inquiry into the genesis of psychiatric conditions in early childhood. In A. Freud, W. Hoffer, and E. Glover (eds.), *The psychoanalytic study of the child,* Vol. II. New York: International Universities Press, 1946, pp. 313–342.

Terman, L. M., C. C. Miles, *et al. Sex and personality: Studies in masculinity and femininity.* New York: McGraw-Hill, Inc., 1936.

Tomkins, S. S. *Affect, imagery, consciousness,* Vol. I. New York: Springer Publishing Company, Inc., 1962.

——— and R. McCarter. What and where are the primary affects? Some evidence for a theory. *Perceptual and Motor Skills Monogr. Supple. 1, 18,* 119–158.

Tuddenham, R. D. Studies in reputation. III. Correlates of popularity among elementary school children. *Journal of Educational Psychology,* 1951, **42,** 257–276.

Tyler, Leona E. *The psychology of human differences.* New York: Appleton-Century, 1947.

Vance, T. F., and L. T. McCall. Children's preferences among play materials as determined by the method of paired comparisons of pictures. *Child Development,* 1934, **5,** 267–277.

Walters, J., Doris Pearce, and Lucille Dalms. Affectional and aggressive behavior of preschool children. *Child Development,* 1957, **28,** 15–26.

Walters, R. H., and R. D. Parke. Social motivation dependency and susceptibility to social influence. L. Berkowitz (ed.),

In *Advances in experimental social psychology,* Vol. I. New York: Academic Press, Inc., 1964, pp. 231–276.

———, E. Ray. Anxiety, social isolation, and reinforcer effectiveness, *Journal of Personality,* 1960, **28,** 358–367.

White, R. W. Motivation reconsidered: The concept of competence. *Psychological Review,* 1959, **66,** 297–333.

Whitehouse, Elizabeth. Norms for certain aspects of the Thematic Apperception Test on a group of nine and ten year old children. *Personality,* 1949, **1,** 12–15.

Whiting, J. W. M. Resource mediation and learning by identification. In I. Iscoe and H. W. Stevenson (eds.), *Personality development in children.* Austin, Tex.: University of Texas Press, 1960, pp. 112–126.

Winker, J. B. Age trends and sex differences in the wishes, identifications, activities and fears of children. *Child Development,* 1949, **20,** 191–200.

Young, W. C., R. W. Goy, and C. H. Phoenix. Hormones and sexual behavior. *Science,* 1964, **143,** 212–218.

SUGGESTED READINGS

1. Aronfreed, J. The origin of self criticism. *Psychological Review,* 1964, **71,** 193–218. A learning-theoretical analysis of guilt and self-criticism.
2. Freud, S. Mourning and melancholia. In *Collected papers,* Vol. IV, London: Hogarth Press, Ltd., 1929, pp. 30–59. (First published in 1917.) Freud's first description of the process of identification. He applied the concept to the understanding of depression, but it appeared even then to have broader implications. For later formulations see Freud's *Group psychology and the analysis of the ego* (New York: Liveright Publishing Corporation, 1921) and *The ego and the id* (London: Hogarth Press, Ltd., 1923). The relevance of identification to certain aspects of sex typing is described in "The passing of the Oedipus-complex," *Collected papers,* Vol. II, 1924, pp. 296–276.
3. Kagan, J. The concept of identification. *Psychological Review,* 1958, **65,** 296–305.

   A review of the literature on identification which concludes with the view that identification has a strong affective component.
4. Kagan, J., and H. A. Moss. *Birth to maturity: A study in psychological development.* New York: John Wiley & Sons, Inc., 1962.

   The results of a longitudinal study conducted at the Fels Institute are presented here. Children were examined shortly after birth and periodically thereafter. The data obtained at each time period were intercorrelated.
5. Mussen, P. H., J. J. Conger, and J. Kagan. *Child development and personality.* New York: Harper & Row Publishers, 1963. A comprehensive textbook on personality development largely from the point of view described in this chapter.
6. Sears, R. R., Eleanor E. Maccoby, and H. Levin. *Patterns of child rearing.* New York: Harper & Row Publishers, 1957. A systematic account of the effects of a variety of child-rearing practices.

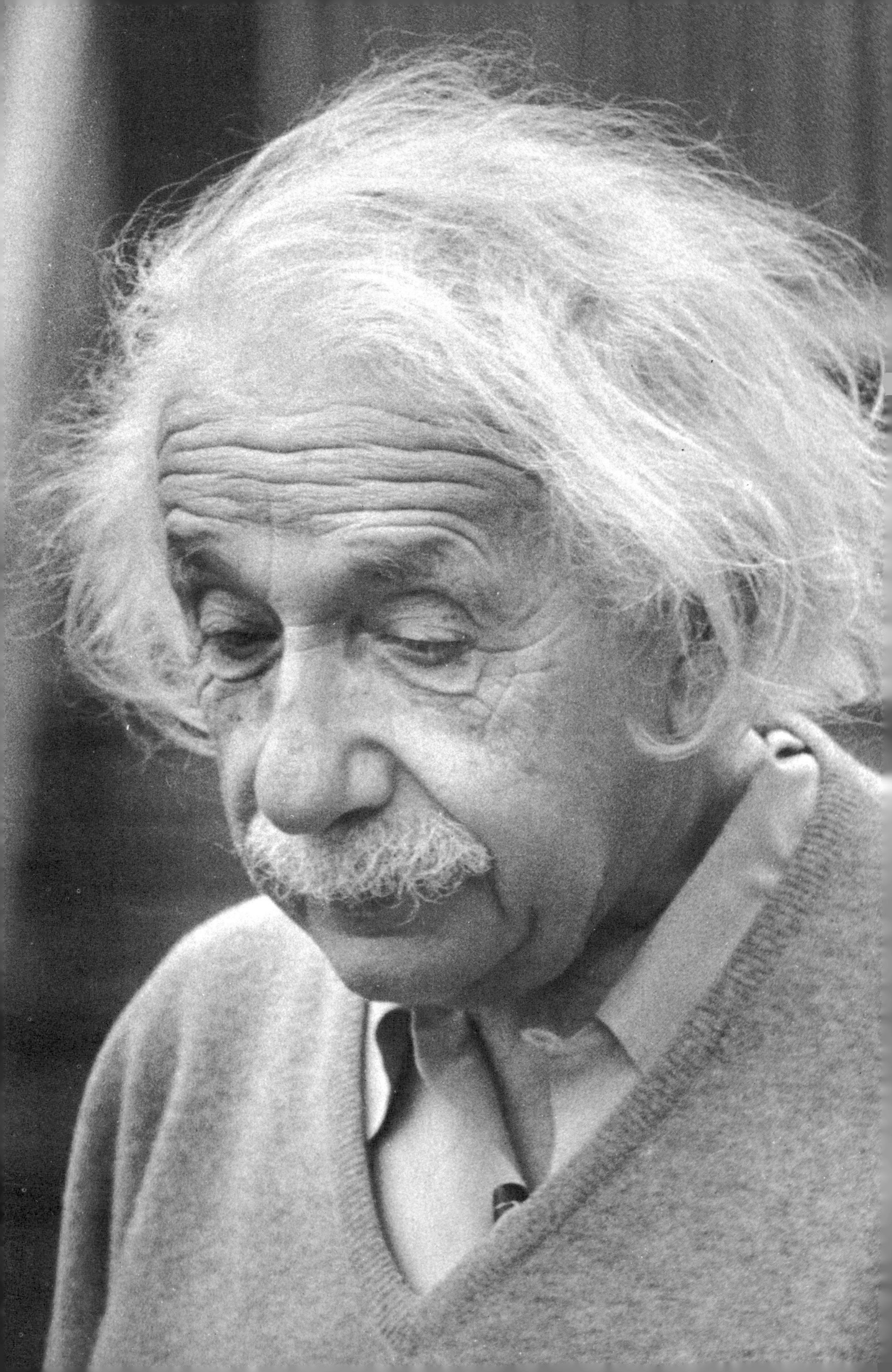

SECTION II

Positive Abnormalities

Albert Einstein. Photo © Ernst Haas, Magnum.

5 People at Midpoint: The Search for Normality

WILLARD A. MAINORD

When a person questions whether or not he is normal, he is really asking two different things: (1) Am I like most people? and (2) Am I neurotic? It may be possible to get an answer to the question about neurosis by going to some "expert" who has faith in his own evaluative techniques. Many psychological tests attempt to answer the question, and psychiatrists do, indeed, certify by a label the presence or absence of neurosis. If one told an expert he had turned down a position with a corporation that could satisfy all his ambitions because of an inexplicable fear of enclosed chambers that would not permit him to ride the elevator to and from the seventieth floor, where the corporation's executive offices were located, there is little doubt that he would be labeled neurotic. On the other hand, if a student notices some discomfort whenever he is required to take an elevator but does it anyway, he probably would not be called neurotic, but neither would he be likely to get an answer to the first question—nobody knows whether most people are a little frightened by elevators or not.

The absence of information is common in attempts to describe the average or typical man because the concept of normality has stubbornly resisted adequate definition. Before an idea can be scientifically investigated and described, it must be *defined.*

PROBLEMS OF DEFINITION

In arguments, we often say that something is "true by definition." That phrase reflects an often unnoticed fact, namely, that definitions are necessarily arbitrary. Logically, either all definitions are true or no definitions are true, depending upon how you look at them. A definition gives us a method of identifying an object or a function or a concept. If we follow the method, we will discover the same thing the writer of the definition saw, though our own examination may yield an even better method of identification than the first definition did. In that case, our definition will be more *useful*, though no more *true*, than the first definition.

Take, for example, the word *dog*. Webster says, among other things, that a dog is both domesticated and carnivorous. If that definition were taken literally, a lost puppy that became wild and developed an appetite for cherries, as a dog of my acquaintance did, would no longer be a dog, and the unquestioning believer in the utility of definitions would ignore this nonconformist in his search for a dog. On the other hand, the animals he would collect undoubtedly would be dogs. Thus, the definition could be thought of as both true and useful if the only concern were to obtain some dogs, but it would have no value if it were used to find all dogs, however true it might remain. The biologist, of course, has a more reliable definition than the dictionary, but he was able to formulate the better definition only because of special knowledge which makes it possible to identify dogs anatomically no matter how untamed they are and how peculiar their diets. But the dictionary was written for the nonspecialist, and it is a perfectly good source of definitions that are adequate when applied to the average or "normal" dog. The point is that definitions differ in their usefulness but not in their truthfulness.

Sometimes events are defined in terms of causation. For instance, static electricity is defined as the product which results from rubbing certain substances against each other, and the "better" of two teams is defined by the result of a contest. Some fundamentalist religious groups define social problems as the consequence of "turning away from God." With that definition, it seems reasonable to work for social reform by trying to change religious attitudes towards greater piety.

A useful definition is one which leads to fruitful investigations and descriptions, and ultimately, to solutions to problems. But we do not yet have a useful definition of normality, and any definition we use will probably have to be revised later. We do not have to wait, however, until all the knowledge is available to attempt to discover what the *typical* man is like. All we need is an arbitrary definition, hopefully a cogent one, to proceed with the investigation.

Although a definition is arbitrary, it need not be frivolous. It seems likely that a logically derived definition will have more utility than one whimsically plucked out of the air. Recognizing the problem, Mowrer, 1948) has contributed a now classical discussion of the nature of normality. We shall draw heavily upon his discussion and also cover some of the material in Chapter 1 again with a somewhat different emphasis.

Before psychology was significantly concerned with emotional adjustment, normality was a matter of statistics. Briefly, it referred to a selected range of measures whose center was the arithmetic average. Notice that we have used the word *average* without conveying any real meaning, as we have said nothing about any characteristic which would specify *the kinds* of measurements from which the average is to be obtained. The term *average* may be applied to anything from height to emotional adjustment, but is usually best restricted to one dimension at a time. Since average intelligence may be found in a man seven feet tall, the man may be called "average" if we are discussing intelligence only or extremely unaverage if we are discussing height only. The more measures taken, the more confusing the picture becomes if we want to make a generalization about him. Consider the following hypothetical case.

Without actually looking up the independent probabilities described in Chapter 1, let us examine some traits of John Doe. He is a male, and he had only 1 chance in 2 of arriving at that condition.

He is from the lower middle class; perhaps there is 1 chance in 3 of belonging to that portion of the population. He is married (3 chances in 4), and he is an adult (also 3 chances in 4). He has two children (1 chance in 5) and a job (9.5 in 10); he works as a painter (1 chance in 500). If we multiply these independent probabilities, it is evident that they are very unlikely to occur together. John Doe has literally dozens more attributes we could measure, but just from those mentioned already we can conclude that he has only 1 chance in 38,070 of being himself! We can also conclude that if we were able to describe anyone completely, we should find, as philosophers, novelists, lovers, and the authors of Chapter 2 have been saying all along, that each individual is a unique entity who cannot be duplicated anywhere. No individual, as a whole, is average; rather each person is almost a statistical impossibility.

Such a reaffirmation of individuality, however, leaves us with an even more difficult task if we are to find a workable definition of normality, especially since we want one that will be restricted to a single dimension.

Let us return to an examination of some of the problems involved in the statistical approach. Intelligence as measured by almost any of the well-standardized tests is an excellent example of the statistical approach in action. An IQ of 100 is average and, in that sense, normal. On the other hand, IQ's of 150 and 50 are equally unlikely and would have to be considered equally abnormal. But many people object to describing markedly different groups with the same adjective and so are unwilling to call both the dull and the bright abnormal. This objection, which is primarily an emotional one, probably results from attitudes built around another definition of *normal.*

Once it was assumed, somewhat arbitrarily, that emotional disturbance was a form of *disease,* it became inevitable that *medical* thinking should permeate both the conceptual scheme and the technical vocabularly of psychological troubles. From the medical point of view, the well-functioning organ is healthy and the malfunctioning one is unhealthy. If we use the words *normal* and *healthy* as synonyms, the normal state is obviously a desirable one. The concept has been carried over to emotional disturbance, and it has become customary to speak of psychotics and neurotics as abnormal and the rest of the population as normal. It is hardly surprising that people were unwilling to be considered abnormal when the word implied not only a difference from most people but a negative difference. It is not unusual for a person undergoing psychotherapy to express a desire to be "just a normal person like everyone else."

The search for the typical. The professionals in the field of mental health were not well satisfied with such usage as it was obvious that, whatever the nature of emotional maladjustment, it could not be clearly confined to "abnormal," here meaning atypical, people. The typical man, too, showed some evidence of sickness. If "abnormals" are located at one end of a sick-well continuum and "normals" at the other, we must say that the normal man is not sick at all and the typical man is not altogether well, since he fits in the middle. From such a framework, we run into difficulty. If the normal man can be identified only by the *absence* of sickness, we can say what he is *not* but we cannot describe him. Similarly, all that can be said about the typical man is that he is not unusually sick and has only mild symptoms. (From this, we could argue in turn that most people operate below peak efficiency, as mild symptoms may depress performances of some kinds, and that the typical sense of well-being is not as high as it might be.)

It became increasingly apparent that it was necessary to translate "well" into some more meaningful idea than "not sick." Initially, it seemed reasonable to define health as whatever was opposite to the symptoms that described the sick person, but this was not satisfactory because the logical opposite of undesirable behavior was not necessarily desirable. For instance, the manic patient is usually said to be *hyper*active, and the opposite of hyperactivity is *hypo*activity, a symptom of depression. One resolution of the problem was to conclude that "extremes" of any kind were unhealthy. This, however, left us in the awkward position of attributing extremely good performance to an undesirable condition—as Freud's concept of sublimation seems to do. If extremely good performance results from being ill, it seems reasonable to search for ways to acquire the illness! It soon became obvious that the ideal man was not merely the opposite of the sick one.

The search for an ideal type. In response to the situation, pleas for a description of the ideal man became ubiquitous (Jahoda, 1958), and attempts were soon forthcoming. Maslow (1954) perhaps produced the most ambitious effort along these lines. For him, the ideal man is "self-actualized." That is, he perceives the world accurately and is not "thrown" by what he sees; he accepts himself without much thinking, is typically spontaneous, and is intensely involved in solving problems; he enjoys privacy, is enthusiastic even about familiar things, and has close interpersonal relationships with other superior people. Maslow expands the description, but it can be seen already that the self-actualized man must be rare indeed. Maslow agrees. In his empirical research, he finds only a handful who meet his criteria. If Maslow's self-actualized man is equated with the ideal person at the "not sick" end of the sick-well continuum, what now can be said of the typical man at its center? Only that he is deficient in Maslow's attributes as well as mildly sick, as we said before. We still have nothing at all to say about his traits except what can be inferred from either the unwell or the ideal. But this approach to normality, based upon either the opposite of the mentally ill or upon the ideal man, necessarily leaves the average man still faceless.

Normality and misery. We have barely touched upon the kinds of approaches that try to say something about the condition of the normal man. Sometimes a satement acquires impressiveness merely because it remains alive. Thus, many people remember that Thoreau believed that "the mass of men lead lives of quiet desperation." *Life* magazine reports that a psychiatrist has drawn the professional conclusion that practically everyone is unhappy. In terms of our discussion up to this point, these observers would agree either that normal people are typically unhappy or that typical people are abnormal. And distressing as such conclusions may be, they are by no means necessarily the gloomiest.

Erich Fromm (1955), for instance, after examining the nature of most familiar societies, is impelled to conclude that they are so poorly designed to satisfy needs and potentialities of man that man must become insane in order to come to livable terms with an insane society. From Fromm's scheme of things, we can understand the unusual kind of hero in Joseph Heller's *Catch 22*, who "proves" that, in combat conditions, one has to be crazy to fly and is therefore disqualified from flying. Fromm's typical man is not only afraid to be free (1961), but his very fears keep him ignorant of the potentially inviting society that would emerge if the existing society did not demand delusional and self-destructive behavior in order for one to adjust and survive. The remedial task he proposes would be a gigantic one in which "therapy" would be necessary for an entire culture!

The psychoanalytic point of view offers little more in the way of comfort. Freud's typical man is driven by instincts, which, because they are callously ignored by a too demanding society, are psychologically buried (repressed). However, even repression is likely to lead to pain as the instincts will not be denied and society will punish their expression until the suffering individual finds methods of becoming his own punisher. Unless successfully rescued by psychotherapy, which may be financially impossible or almost interminable, the emotional cripple will continue to be beset by anxieties which are repeatedly aroused and which produce more repression to maintain makeshift defenses that are in constant need of repair. The energies expended upon defense rob the individual of much of his ability to extract satisfactions from the world. And as the most pessimistic clincher, because the sources of anxiety are buried, the typical man does not even have the knowledge which would make it possible for him to solve his problems in any rational manner. A most significant point for our argument is that, according to Freud, the important determiners of the typical man's adjustment are buried and invisible, so that we are again left with very little to say in terms of some positive description.

This has not been a comprehensive survey of the conceptual schemes which offer descriptions of the average man. However, the approaches mentioned are representative in their implicit agreement not only that the typical man is rather unhappy but also that he should be exposed to a variety of remedial measures. This consensus does not, however, agree with a comparatively recent study based upon questionnaire-interview methods (Srole, 1962). A large and presumably representative sample of Americans reported themselves to be, at worst, "pretty happy." But even this more optimistic estimate shares with other opinions the common inability to *describe* the average man.

To sum up the points of view we have been examining, we find that "Everyman" is to some degree pictured in two kinds of statements: (1) Statements based on the conviction that the average man shares many characteristics of the emotionally disturbed. These are milder versions of statements used to describe individuals who have had clinical attention. (2) Statements based on hypothetical ideal types whose emotional well-being depends on assets found in insufficient quantities in the average person. In either case, it should be noted that the statements are not derived from a study of representative men but instead are inferences drawn from atypical samples. Under the circumstances, it is not surprising that there is little to be found in psychology or psychiatry about the concerns that are most important to the average man himself. By what means might the mass of mankind achieve a greater sense of satisfaction? It is impossible to say unless we can cogently argue that we have some good idea of what the average man is like. Emotionally and behaviorally it is still unfortunately safe to say that John Doe has yet to be found. It is ironic to reflect upon the fact that we know more about the average man's sexual behavior (Kinsey, 1948) than we do about—let us say—his choice of a profession. This is true in spite of the common belief that it is practically impossible to overcome social prejudices sufficiently to investigate sexual behavior.

Most people who write about normality are completely willing to abandon any attempt at a statistical definition. But such wholesale desertion may be premature. There may be other possibilities in this approach that have yet to be examined. Let us return to the nature of people at midpoint by assuming that the average is normal, knowing full well that there are a number of pitfalls and difficulties to be surmounted.

Statistical Normality As a Social Concept

We have already shown that if all the multitude of measurable characteristics were actually included in our consideration, we would be forced to conclude that each individual is impossible to duplicate. Having accepted that premise, we might then, along with Allport (1937), decide that individuality must be the starting point of personality description. To make the same point somewhat differently, we might study a man systematically until we could formulate some laws of behavior that apply, as far as we know, *only to him*. This process could be repeated until we have found a representative sample of individuals. If then, when we look at our results, we find some individual behavior patterns repeated time and time again, we might believe we have discovered some universal laws of human behavior.

Theoretically, there is no reason why such an approach should not eventually pay off, but the intensive study of any one man could easily exhaust the lifetime of an investigator, and a collection of many such studies would be a frightening prospect in terms of size alone. White's *Lives in Progress* (1952) is an eloquent example of what can be done with extensive study of only three individuals. After reading it, one may feel that he now knows three previously anonymous people rather well. Nonetheless, he still will be able to say very little about the average man.

Many psychologists embrace a point of view derived from "operant" learning and based on the conviction that all behavior changes resulting from experience can be explained by the consequences associated with them. Many of these investigators believe it is possible to discover universal laws by examining a few individuals or even only one. Their arguments are often compelling, but their techniques only define the potentialities of the average man and explain how behavior change comes about. In other words, the operant approach may tell us much about how the average man becomes what he is, but it can tell us nothing at all about what he is. Understanding the learning process does not reveal *why* certain things have been learned, but only *how* they were learned. If the average man is to be known, we must have a method of determining what as well as how he learns.

We must also keep in mind that the average man is an abstraction which can only be drawn from observations of many individuals. Our task here is to define this abstraction as usefully as possible. The normal man is average, but average at what?

In recent years, another group of behavioral scientists has adopted a point of view which is usually called "social learning." The premise on which it rests can be boiled down to this: In our society, the basic biological needs are typically satisfied so efficiently that they no longer serve as significant sources of learning, maintaining, or modifying behavior. Rather, people are more commonly motivated by, bedeviled by, and rewarded by the consequences of social behavior. The apparent exception to the rule—sexuality—turns out really to be no exception at all. Biological outlets for the sex drive are routinely available, but the social requirements for reaching them result in conflicting demands which have to be resolved. What seems to be a problem of meeting biological needs turns out to be a problem of social complications. If we can accept the notion that all significant adjustment problems can be approached by examining social processes, we should expect to discover methods of value not only for understanding the average man but also for the control of emotional disorders.

If a social definition of the average man seems reasonable enough to merit further exploration, there are at least two reasons why we might prefer to study groups of subjects rather than individuals. First, social processes involve social situations which, by definition, require two or more participants. Second, if the crucial factors in personality are social factors, the relevant variables are much more likely to be found in group situations than in an individual's report of his social responses.

Having accepted the restrictions of a social definition, we find ourselves considering different variables from many of those customarily employed in other approaches to normality. We cannot explain behavior in terms of motivation, if indeed we ever could. As indicated in Chapter 3, we necessarily have to infer motivation from measurements of observed behavior. For instance, there is no real difference between saying that "Joe eats twice as much as most people" and "Joe sure has a terrific appetite," except that the first statement is testable and the second is not. We have no way to measure the strength of an appetite other than by observing eating. Similar concepts all refer to essentially private experience and thus are at least one step removed from social data. Any individual response taken by itself will confront us with the same difficulty, as we can never be sure if an individual response is self-generated or socially generated. We might resolve the difficulty, however, if we form our basic abstractions, not around an individual's behavior, but around the collective social response to him. Normality then becomes a matter of how much an individual elicits social responses that are similar to the social responses elicited by others. The total social response is composed of the positive and negative responses which the person elicits from others; these can

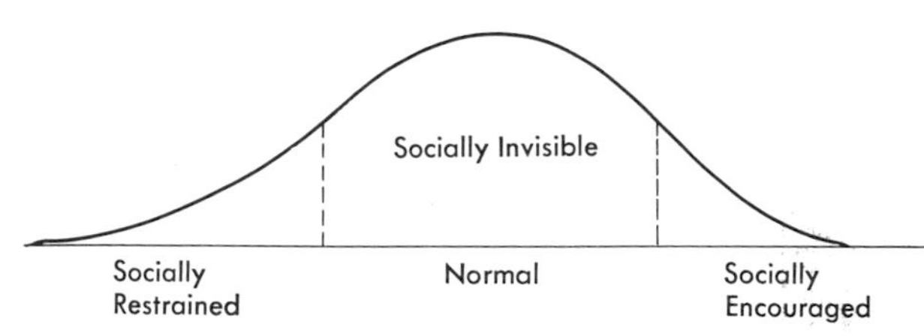

Figure 5.1 Social types based on responses elicited from others.

be added up to yield a net surplus, deficit, or zero.

In discussing other approaches to normality, we have repeatedly observed that the average man stubbornly remains invisible. This seemed a somewhat troublesome conclusion as the hope was always that some approach would make it possible to describe the normal man. It may have been that his invisibility was not necessarily a defect of the various systems, but simply the most representative description that could be made of the normal man.

Suppose we construct a continuum running from one extreme, which we shall call "socially restricted," to an opposite extreme, called "socially abetted" (see Figure 5.1). If individuals are located on such a scale, we place at the socially restricted end persons like those found in penitentaries or mental hospitals who are forced by society into some kind of particularly confining situation. At the other end of the scale, we locate those elected to high office, those proffered power and material rewards, and others who are urged and helped to expand their activities because of the overall approval of the society. In both of these categories we find people who are *socially visible*. They behave in ways that attract attention and concern from some of the sources of social power. But in the middle of the continuum is found the great majority of mankind whose total behaviors hardly impel society to respond at all. These are the members of a category we shall call "social invisibility," and it is that very invisibility which is the defining characteristic of the normal man. Jones *et al.* (1961) offer pertinent experimental findings indicating that "a person who conforms to salient social expectations reveals little about his basic and distinguishing characteristics." In any social framework, a statistical definition of normality as seen from modal behaviors would have to be based upon conformity, which, by definition, is the most common mode. Thus the findings of Jones *et al.* could be restated to agree with our point: "a person who conforms (and most persons do) reveals little about his distinguishing and basic characteristics (is invisible)."

If invisibility is the base line, several interesting and possibly useful conclusions can be drawn. It is not difficult to see that, of all the many behaviors likely to be observed in any man, only a comparatively few have enough social impact to cause society to forcibly confine him. The same conclusion can be drawn about the other end of the scale: very few behaviors result in any formal action by society for the benefit of one man. The remaining and vastly greater number of acts in a person's repertoire elicit little or no response from society and are methods of behaving normally. With this definition of normality, we can then say that *there are infinitely more ways to be normal than abnormal.* Thus, we can at once insist that each individual is an absolutely unique entity and yet that most of us are normal. This notion is analogous to a testing situation. If a group of students is given a test comprised of 100 true-false items, there is absolutely only one set of answers that will yield a score of 100 and only one set that will yield a score of 0. But because a score of 50 can be achieved by any number of combinations of answers, there are literally thousands of ways of scoring precisely in the middle. To continue the analogy, we are suggesting that the individual is constantly taking social tests and that society, the author and grader of the test, is indifferent to the enormous variety of responses which place his scores in the middle of the range.

With the proposed definition, we have the advantages for scientific purposes of being able to identify—albeit by exclusion—the actual individual who can be said to be normal. We can learn something about him merely by means of a guideline to where he may be found. Once he is found, other characteristics may be teased out.

The Unique but Unnoticeable Man

It is now possible to say two things about the normal man: he is unique and at the same time he is socially invisible. If this approach to normality is to be useful, however, it must be shown that we can reasonably account for the coexistence of uniqueness and invisibility. To do so, it will first be necessary to examine the process by which an individual acquires his social standards.

In a democratic society (and probably in all societies), collective man, represented by social institutions, has repeatedly exhibited more skill at specifying what may *not* be done than at specifying what should be. This is not surprising if, as seems to be the case, most people are made uncomfortable by similar kinds of things but are gratified by a myriad of different rewards. Consensus is easy to obtain about the undesirability of murder or theft, for instance, because practically everyone can agree that he would not want to be the victim of a murderer or a thief. Once everyone agrees, it is a short step to formally prohibiting the undesirable behavior. On the other hand, any attempt to get a consensus about positive behaviors is almost impossible unless

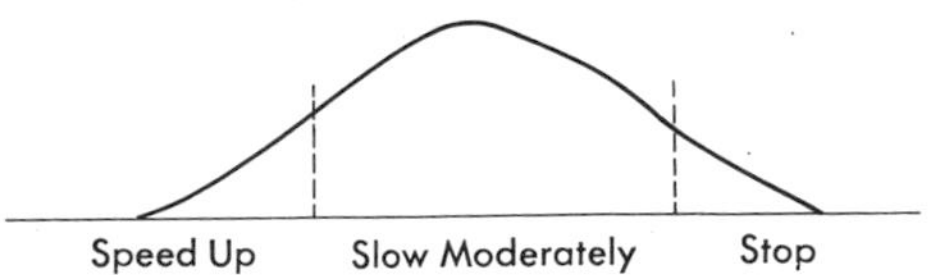

Figure 5.2 Driver behavior at unmarked intersection.

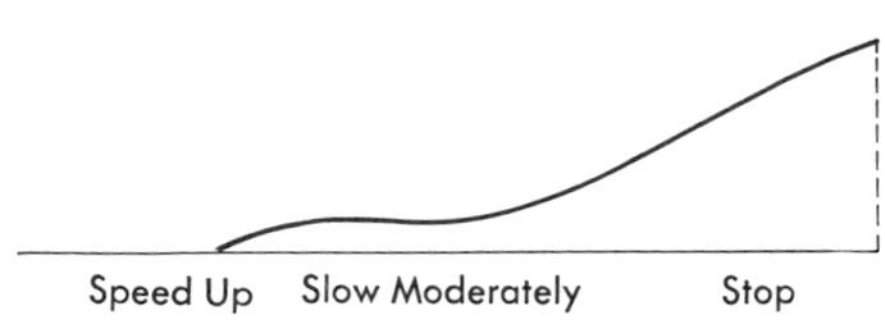

Figure 5.3 Driver behavior at intersection marked with STOP sign.

the different points of vicw are lumped under a broadly encompassing abstraction. The difficulty is so pervasive that even when consensus is reached, it often seems necessary to resort to prohibitions (or proscriptions) in order to make the directive concrete enough to enforce. As a current and vivid example, the 1965 Civil Rights Act was designed to provide the Negro in particular with "equal rights"—an abstraction of great complexity. As a practical matter, much of the new code is devoted, not to discussing the principle, but to spelling out what people must *not* do to violate those rights.

The net result of such a situation is that society is much more concrete, specific, and consistent when *pro*scribing than when *pre*scribing. Thus, if we selected almost any ten people at random, we could be rather certain that they all would have avoided breaking most of the common prohibitions, but we would be unable to find many common positive behaviors among them beyond those which supply the biological necessities. Consider the individual who is in a position to steal money if only he were willing to break the rules. Most people will not steal in such situations, but most people would like to have more money. Probably all of our randomly selected group would refrain from stealing, but the behaviors they would use to acquire more money would vary widely across the group.

Figures 5.2 and 5.3 graphically illustrate what happens to the distribution of behaviors when social regulation is introduced into a previously less structured situation, such as drivers passing through an unmarked intersection. As illustrated in Figure 5.2, most people slow down to some degree, and a very few either stop completely or increase speed markedly. Now if a STOP sign is added to the same intersection, we get the dramatically different curve shown in Figure 2.3. Instead of a symmetrical distribution tapering off on each side of the most common behavior, the curve is now asymmetrical: it tapers off on only one side of the mode and stops abruptly at the other. These two curves represent the two classes of social responses that are our immediate concern. The proscription, that is the STOP sign, is very specific in nature and elicits a great degree of conformity, but the unmarked intersection is more ambiguous and elicits a wider range of behaviors. Even if the drivers entering the unmarked intersection have a common goal, such as "driving cautiously," several different responses may accord with that end. Some might argue that they were driving cautiously inasmuch as they carefully looked in both directions to see that it was safe to maintain their speed. Certainly slowing down or actually stopping are attempts to be careful. It might even be argued that speeding up was justified because it permitted one to clear the intersection before an oncoming car approached. All these drivers would subscribe to the statement that they were driving cautiously even though there was wide divergence in their behaviors. On the other hand, if a STOP sign is present, it is no longer possible to defend any behavior as legal other than stopping. If interpretations differ, so will behaviors, but differing interpretations become less possible with unambiguous proscriptions like STOP signs.

One of the commoner questions about the average man has to do with the degree to which he is a conformist. Conformity to social norms has been suggested here as an identifying trait of the normal personality. In this sense, the constructive rebel *would* be called abnormal. (Are you willing to maintain that George Washington and the Founding Fathers were abnormal?) But more cogently it is also obvious that, no matter how the mass of men is examined, it is not possible to predict many common positive actions from common environments or common situations. We shall offer the conclusion that, insofar as proscriptions are involved, the average man is indeed a conformist, but in other respects he certainly is not. Because observing proscriptions attracts no attention, social invisibility is partly a function of observing the rules which leave the social body undisturbed.

An individual learns not to break the rules by experiencing the unpleasant consequences of breaking them. This kind of learning is called avoidance learning; its opposite, approach learning, occurs by experiencing the pleasant consequences of an act. It has been repeatedly demonstrated (Sheffield and Temmer, 1950), that avoidance learning is much more stable than approach learning. In common sense terms, avoidance learning persists because a person who consistently avoids a once dangerous object never has the opportunity of learning if the object is now safe. On the other hand, because approach learning involves contact with the goal, if the goal stops rewarding the learner, he will modify his response. Since conformity is a function of proscriptions, that is of avoidance learning, it is extremely stable and often persists even after the proscriptions are lifted. Thus it is possible for a child raised as a teetotaler to maintain that alcohol is unconditionally bad even though he has never personally experienced it and even though he may be surrounded by people who drink with control and with apparent enjoyment. Similarly, the oldster who condemns the younger generation may do so because he fails to realize that the proscriptions enforced in his own youth have been repealed.

If conformity can only be expected when a behavior is a function of unpleasant consequences, nonconformity, that is great individual differences, can be expected whenever there are alternative routes to a goal.

We have already touched upon one reason for this: the abstract nature of most socially desirable goals invites translation into a multiplicity of behaviors. But there is a simpler reason. Much of what is learned evolves from accidental encounters with attractive objects. If any event or object is encountered with enough frequency and with pleasant consequences, it will become a goal, but many potential goals never become part of a given person's experience and thus have no impact upon his style of life. It must be difficult for the illiterate to understand the passion of the bookworm.

In a society that is reasonably consistent in its prohibitions, the average person needs to spend very little time in the sterile process of simply avoiding things. With energies largely expended in the service of widely different goals, it is not at all mysterious that people vary markedly in their behaviors and still are not conspicuous. Any organized society has to allow for such divergencies if it is to be both stable and free. If divergency is expected, then it is the norm and does not in itself arouse attention. Thus nonconformity and social invisibility can be maintained at the same time, and frequent changes in behavior do not necessarily attract social attention. As a person adopts and abandons inconspicuous behaviors and combines them with other inconspicuous activities, the net social impact is the same. There is thus no social necessity to maintain a single style of life in order to be treated as normal.

Our list of statements about the average man is growing. We can now say that he is: (1) invisible, (2) unique, (3) conforming with respect to social prohibitions, (4) resistant to relaxation of prohibitions, (5) nonconforming in the service of positive goals, and (6) flexible in his behavioral modes within the limitations of the prohibitions. Men are understandably concerned with specific problems of existence and adjustment. The next section explores this view of normality in relation to some problems of importance in our daily lives.

THE PROBLEMS OF NORMALITY

Nonconformity

Social invisibility can be maintained by refraining from breaking prohibitions. On the other hand, it is obvious to almost any observer that people often do break social regulations and still escape significant social pressure or exposure. The Kinsey reports, for example, dramatically revealed widespread discrepancies between legal and social standards of sexual conduct and the actual behaviors of most individuals. In the first report, according to their own statements, over 90 percent of males would have served some time in jail for illegal sexual behavior had they been detected and were the laws strictly enforced (Kinsey *et al.*, 1948). If the report is pursued carefully, it becomes apparent that much forbidden sexual behavior was socially tolerated only because it was undetected. The Hartshorne and May studies (1928) indicate that honesty is dependent upon the situation and much less likely to be practiced if a person believes his cheating will not be observed by those in power. The evidence leads to the conclusion that much rule breaking is typical of the normal man but that it is done in such a way as to remain undetected. Since his invisibility is usually maintained, he must have developed some skill in evading scrutiny in situations where exposure might bring social retaliation.

Without damning or praising him, we are advancing the proposition that the normal man is, at times, dishonest and that the degree of his dishonesty depends on the degree of rule breaking and the price he fears would be extracted if his indulgences were made public. This conclusion is in direct opposition to an older approach to the problem of normality which argued that the normal man and the moral man were identical. When no stable agreements could be reached as to exactly what "moral" was, and when it was observed that seemingly moral men were not exempt from psychopathology, the moral definition crumbled, particularly under the attacks of Freud and his followers. For our purposes, moral standards are most important for understanding normality because it seems almost inevitable that discomfort must be associated with a fear of exposure if social regulations have been defied and might well be a crucial factor in the use of evasive devices to ward off social discovery. Mowrer (1961) argues that it is excessive reliance upon such defensive devices which leads the normal individual toward a neurotic or psychotic adjustment that perhaps ends with the social restriction of the mental hospital. Without considering the extreme of psychosis, however, we can examine discomfort associated with rule breaking as a source of problems in normal adjustment.

Techniques of nonconformist adjustment. A paradise dependent upon continual and consistent deception was enjoyed by Alec Guinness in the movie, *Captain's Paradise*. The Captain had two wives—one at each end of the ship's itinerary—but was quite complacent about his bigamy because he thought he had a foolproof system of concealing his behavior from anyone who might make trouble for him. As he had maintained his arrangement for a long time, he had evidence from experience to support his view. The plot illustrates one simple device that should be successful for comfortable rule breaking: *if it is done with foresight and skill, it might be possible to "commit the perfect crime."* But the evaded standards have to be those of society rather than the personal ones of the nonconformist if he is to avoid subjective discomfort. Persistent rule breaking increases the likelihood of exposure, of course, and if that should occur, it might no longer be possible to maintain internal comfort by any means. Further, it would be surprising if many people were skillful enough to justify confident expectations of never being found out.

A more common method, *finding a compatible society where deception is unnecessary*, is often used by the practicing homosexual. In many of our larger cities colonies of homosexuals have been allowed to construct their own subculture undisturbed by legal authorities as long as the taboo activities are kept within the colony. Inasmuch as one's secret homosexual activities are known to at least one other person, his partner, the homosexual in a heterosexual environment can never be completely sure that he will not be exposed. As long as he remains active, then, he should be plagued by discomfort. But if he practices the same behaviors in one of the homosexual colonies, there would be no need for secrecy and the source of discomfort would be eliminated.

Social invisibility, it should be reemphasized, is most easily maintained by following the model behaviors of the reference culture. As Mowrer (1961) has analyzed the problem, the homosexual who carries on his activities secretly is likely to end up breaking rules in a psychotic manner and to find himself in a mental hospital. If the homosexual carries out his activities openly in a heterosexual environment, he will either be jailed, or if homosexuality is seen as a mental disease, confined to a mental hospital. Ironically, either overt or covert defiance can in this case lead to the same ultimate restriction. *For the normal man, unfavorable visibility can arise either from open defiance, or by a more complicated process, from hidden defiance.*

Two more methods of rule breaking which might lead to a comparatively comfortable adjustment are illustrated in extreme form by the argument—apparently based on overwhelming evidence—that a rich man is never punished as much as a poor man for the same crime. One of the operating rules of our society seems to be that by convincing others that he is of great value, an individual accrues a kind of *social credit*: he can expect unusual latitude if he misbehaves and is likely either to go unpunished or to be let off with a mild slap on the wrist. Hollander (1965) has obtained evidence that tends to support the point. Briefly, he found that if an individual first exhibits *conformity and competence*, he can then not only maintain acceptance if he begins to be a nonconformer but can also attract followers who will expect and prefer nonconformity from him. The same principle actually leads to two processes which permit nonconformity without extracting the price of continued discomfort. The first process—that of *forgiveness without idolatry*—is illustrated by the well-known politician who sacrificed his chance for higher office by obtaining a divorce to marry a woman who had also been recently divorced. We might assume that he suffered some emotional loss from his diminished political power and prospects, but such a loss might be counterbalanced or outweighed by the emotional gain from his new marriage. In any case, he suffered no social penalties that interfered with his current powers.

The second process is exemplified by the extremely popular movie star who flagrantly flouts the usual conventions and not only continues to be successful as a movie star but attracts an even larger flock of adorers, many of whom emulate his behavior. In this case, the individual has managed to change the rules of invisibility so that an excess of *negative* visibility is canceled by his *positive* visibility. If the nonconformist only cares about those who approve of him and is unconcerned with those who disapprove, rule breaking should be a cource of some pleasure rather than of discomfort. However, the same behavior would lead to discomfort if the disapprovers happened to be important sources of social reinforcement for him.

The normal man, then, does break rules, but if he does so openly, he exposes himself to pressures that lead to abnormality—either positive or negative. Normality may be maintained either by transgressing secretly or by properly timing forbidden behaviors so that they become temporarily or even permanently modish. If the individual is willing to be open, he may pay a price for being conspicuous or, if he has in some way achieved leadership status, he may actually modify the rules of acceptability and increase his own prestige. The college student usually pays a price for visible nonconformity because he seldom has much social credit with the important sources of power. Inevitably, people of college age question established social regulations and often experimentally violate some of the rules. Consequently we should expect that their lack of social credit would make much distress inevitable through the experimental period. Perhaps this is one reason for the storminess of adolescence, which has been of so much concern to the observers of our society. For example, adolescents and early adults are the most active sexual performers, but in our society there are no socially approved avenues of gratification open to them. Secrecy, the commonest method of maintaining invisibility about one's sex life, is somewhat precarious as the individual has to trust others to maintain secrecy and also has to utilize whatever physical setting happens to be available. It is hardly surprising that the student complaining of emotional distress is likely to focus upon problems of sexuality as the cause. In the case of collegiate sexuality, the rules of the institution are often such that even one open violation is enough to bring expulsion from the campus, again demonstrating that visibility, whether positive or negative, draws corresponding social pressure.

The Sense of Well-being

Happiness or fulfillment or self-actualization are difficult terms to define precisely even though almost everyone agrees about some of their approximate meanings; an emotional state subjectively defines happiness well enough for most of us. We also tend to agree that an overall sense of well-being is a desirable goal, even one of prime importance. Many books promise formulae for happiness, but as we have already seen, there are still many reasons to believe that the average man feels a need for more reliable methods of enhancing his emotional state.

Logically, it would seem that current emotionality is partly a function of past, especially recent, experience and partly a function of expectations. These are correlated because expectations depend on learning, and "learning" is one way of saying "past experience."

Goldstein (1962) has summarized a series of studies, many of which help shed light upon the relationship between anticipation and subsequent feelings. If, for instance, an individual expects something to be *very* unpleasant and then discovers that it is only *slightly* unpleasant, the net result is a feeling of euphoria—an increased sense of well-being. Conversely, if a pleasant expectation is not met, the result is a tendency toward depression. As an individual is constantly experiencing and anticipating, we can see that simply going through a day subjects everyone to a variety of mood-modifying encounters. The individual who anticipates accurately would be neither pleasantly nor unpleasantly surprised and would be maximally equipped to cope with impending situations. The person whose anticipations are often inaccurate would be less able to cope successfully and would thus have a diminished sense of well-being. In our social framework, it would be extremely important then for an individual to be as accurate as possible in anticipating the nature of critical social situations.

We have said little so far about the anticipations of the normal man, but if we can examine the typical situation, we may be able to infer some of his typical anticipations and their relationship to coping and thus to "happiness."

Positive and negative life styles. If we remember that the average man is skilled in observing prohibitions but not so skilled in abstract goal attainment, we should expect that many of his past attempts to move forward were unsuccessful. If he then anticipates that new efforts will be useless, he may well respond to anticipated failures by restricting himself to goal-achieving routes that have previously been successful and have the merit of proven safety. (The drop-out, for instance?) Under such circumstances, the average man could hardly anticipate any significant improvement in his way of life because he would be doing nothing to change it. Such a pessimistic point of view would cancel ways to strike out in new directions, thus circularly insuring that there would indeed be no significant improvement in his way of life, at least not through his own efforts. Such a person might be one of those who live in "quiet desperation." The individual with such a dour set of anticipations might nevertheless be lucky and experience more pleasant surprises than most people and so might benefit psychologically from them. But any sense of well-being so dependent upon the unexpected makes the achievement of happiness a matter of sheer chance.

What all this means is that the normal man has a history of limited success, which leaves him with a limited number of common competencies that help to determine the regularities of daily routine from which he must derive whatever subjective satisfaction he can. As for changing himself or his circumstances, the average man tends to "play it safe"—a phrase that helps us understand the common individual who persists in following the same routine while simultaneously expressing overall dissatisfaction with his way of life.

If an individual had a consistent history of success in encountering new and difficult situations, increments in status and other social rewards would be recurrently associated with the challenge of new activities. Then, again by a perfectly straightforward learning process, a behavior pattern would be developed leading repeatedly to challenge and to novelty. Such a pattern followed long enough with continued success would lead to widespread competencies culminating in a positive abnormality. These might be the kinds of people who continue driving toward success even after it seems that they already "have everything."

The argument can be reduced to a sentence: A *sense of well-being is largely a function of competence.* It must be emphasized that reversing the statement would not be correct. A common complaint of the college student is that his grades are poor because he is unhappy. But it is probably more true that he is unhappy at least partly because his grades are poor. While the two statements are not really contradictory, it is still a mistake to ascribe poor functioning to emotional dissatisfaction for the practical reason that nothing can be done about a feeling state directly. We have yet to discover any methods of improving mood which would be followed by improved behavior, but there are methods of improving behavior which are followed by a more satisfactory mood.

Observers are often bewildered by people with patterns of unsatisfactory behavior which are maintained tenaciously. Such people do not seem to learn from experience. We have already described one of the ways that such a life style might be evolved and maintained, and the point remains that it is precisely because the individual does learn from experience that he continues behaving as he does. The same point can be made by drawing upon some animal studies. It has been shown that a rat will seek out a mild electric shock if that shock has been presented consistently as a cue to some desired goal. It has also been shown that such discriminative cues can be chained so that one leads to another and so on until the final goal is achieved. A rat could be carefully and laboriously trained to traverse a long alley, let us say a mile long, getting a mild but uncomfortable shock every fifty feet, and he could be taught to persist if food and water were available at the end of the alley. If a rat does much thinking about things as he continues to work toward his reinforcing goal, he must also do a good deal of grumbling.

Human relationships, unfortunately, may sometimes involve discomfort and reward in just about the same proportions as the illustrative alley. When two people form an enduring relationship, it is unlikely that they will find themselves equally capable of manipulating each other—in more common language, equally capable of "getting their own ways." Gossip on the campus often involves something like, "I don't know why he keeps dating her; she treats him like a dog." The situation is probably analogous to the electrified alley in that perhaps an occasional physical intimacy serves as the "goody" in the goal box for the boy. When people deal with each other, they sometimes train each other to continued acceptance of unrewarding modes within the relationship.

The feeling tone of any person who has emotional needs in relation to other people depends on his skills not only in forming relationships but in shaping relationships so that he obtains social gratifications with reasonable reliability and frequency. When we talk about "society's response," we may actually be referring to only one other individual, because a given behavior may be evaluated by only one other person. The same social rules apply, but the smaller the group, the more rapid the social reaction.

Sources of social reinforcement. The sources of social reinforcement can be rather neatly divided into two groups. Much social evaluation is done *institutionally* through the school, the armed forces, the business world, or the church, and the method of reinforcement is usually impersonal—grades, promotions, raises in salary, and assignment to positions of leadership. The other main source of social reinforcement is the *personal responses* which indicate to us that we are approved of by some other human being. It may be possible to receive a lot of personal social reinforcement without public exposure, but it is decidedly not possible to receive much institutional reinforcement and at the same time remain unnoticed. In a sense, only the *un*ambitious can be both normal and happy.

We have been preparing the ground for the assertion that there is very little relationship between happiness and normality. We have been able to deduce some reasons to expect that happiness, defined as a greater than average sense of well-being, is correlated with social skills which can be directed toward individuals or institutions or both. We should therefore expect that the normal man will be happier than the mental patient, whose social skills are poor, but not so happy as people who are recipients of conspicuous social approval. Even so, inasmuch as the stream of events is constantly changing, anyone's mood level should be in a near constant state of flux. And inasmuch as the abnormals on the negative end of the scale have fewer alternatives for action, their range of mood changes may be rather small. This is another way of saying that, for them, the distance from comparative misery to complete misery is not very far. On the positive end of the normality scale, however, the possible range of action is very great, and socially abetted individuals can convincingly answer the question, "What have you got to lose?" with a wide range of possibilities. From such a framework, the suicide of a movie idol like Marilyn Monroe is not too surprising because successful people may be expected to demonstrate a wider range of emotionality than others do. To borrow again from Mowrer (1961), emotional discomfort indicates no abnormality of affect but is a perfectly normal response to the situation that produced it.

The student who wonders about his own normality because he has periods of emotional distress has been asking the wrong question. We can agree that he *is* normal, but we are still left with the problem of what can be done about his bleak moods.

Remedial Measures

One of the reasons for the continued search for a definition of normality has been the recognition that most of our methods of helping people with emotional problems have not, as yet, demonstrated any great effectiveness (Eysenck, 1960, 1961). If the base line of normality can be satisfactorily drawn, it should be possible to construct a set of concepts and hypotheses that would lead to different approaches to treating the problems of adjustment. This leads us to a discussion of counseling and psychotherapy, subjects you will pursue in much greater depth in Chapter 15.

From the framework of this chapter, it seems evident that, if emotional problems result both from social restriction following rule breaking and from a lack of social gratification, two classes of remedial measures will be called for. Social restrictions can only be overcome by giving up nonconformist behavior. Lack of social reinforcement, however, can only be changed by the acquisition of competence in forming and maintaining satisfactory human relationships or in achieving favorable institutional recognition, or both.

The field of remedial psychological manipulation traditionally has been divided into psychotherapy and counseling. There has been much argument about the differences between them, and some people maintain that they are the same thing. Psychotherapy might be the term applied to procedures appropriate for socially restricted people who need to eliminate socially noxious behavior from their repertoires. Counseling would be the term for procedures designed to enhance an overall sense of well-being. As we are using the terms, the typical mental patient would need first psychotherapy and then counseling; the mental patient might first achieve normality and then, just as many other normals, still be quite unhappy. Counseling procedures would not be applicable before normality was achieved because social restrictions block the avenues of reinforcement open to normals.

If a social-learning framework is employed, the adjustment problems investigated might involve somewhat different variables than those used in other approaches. The assumption of this method is always that the individual in difficulty behaves in some manner that elicits social responses which are, from his point of view, undesirable. Increased social effectiveness, moreover, is the important criterion for improvement, so remedial measures must be built around the identification of defects—removing them if they are socially noxious, or building or enhancing skills if the defects are *lacks* as opposed to *offenses*. Psychological evaluation becomes a matter of identifying the modes of offending society and the absences of usable skill and the intertwined relationships which help maintain a useless stability.

Honesty and adjustment. Not all social behaviors are equally crucial in problems of adjustment. Our problem is to identify the class of behaviors that is of most significance for analyzing and correcting unsatisfactory life styles. We have already suggested that behavior related to moral values is most likely to shed light upon the problem. If an individual has an odd hobby, like collecting pancakes, he may well be regarded as peculiar but should not be subjected to much social pressure. If, instead, he insists upon collecting *your* pancakes, it is likely that restrictions will be placed upon him.

Unless moral terms are made operational, they may lead to an impalpable mysticism whose benefits, if any, result from inspiration. Almost everyone agrees, for example, that it is good to be honest, but few agree as to precisely what is meant by honesty. Operationally it can be defined as following *known rules* as opposed to deliberately breaking rules or cheating. Armed with such a definition, it becomes possible to label honest and dishonest behaviors if you know the rules applicable to a situation.

Since making honesty operational does not in itself provide us with anything useful, we will cite an illustration from actual clinical experience. A strikingly good looking girl of college age sought help because, as she saw it, men were constantly trying to "take advantage" of her. The net result, she felt, was that she could not trust anyone and the prospects of marriage were dim, even though that was her goal in life—if only she could find someone she could depend upon. When questioned about her attempts to solve her problem, she revealed that she went out almost every night hoping each time to find someone trustworthy. She would know she had found the right one when she could go through several dates without a demand for sexual intimacy. To make sure of not being deceived, she found it necessary to be quite provocative in both manner and dress and to encourage preliminary intimacies so that she could be sure her date could be trusted when really aroused. She argues, logically enough, that anyone can be trusted who feels no strong urge. She was extremely bitter that her dates consistently flunked the test.

This young lady agreed that it was important to be honest. She also agreed that it would be fair to define honesty as "following the rules." Finally, she agreed that if an invitation is extended, the rules require that the inviter has committed himself if the invitation is accepted. The conclusion (not reached so quickly as here) was that she was inviting sexual intimacy and then cheating by refusing to participate. She finally understood that the lack of trustworthy men had resulted from her own dishonest representations. She reported some months later that it was amazing the number of nice men she had met.

It is necessary to oversimplify in order to make a quick point. All that can be emphasized here is that a distressed individual can easily take remedial measures if the problem is defined in terms of his own misbehaviors, but if it is defined in terms of others' misbehaviors, the suffering individual is left helpless.

The reader may already have noticed that *honesty* was defined here to encompass many behaviors often given some other label. It can be extended to cover other less obvious activities. Most people will agree that being truthful is part of being honest and that being truthful means not misleading someone else. With such a definition, merely being quiet can be dishonest if the information withheld would lead the listener to a more accurate conclusion. Such an encompassing and yet operational term can shed light upon many of the complaints that arise from difficulties in social living.

Responsibility and adjustment. Society's institutionalized responses are not always clear, but there are some general rules governing them. Most critics of the social scene agree that there is a positive relationship between income and social approval. A business is clearly expressing approval of an employee if it offers him great financial inducement not to resign. Productivity is also positively correlated with both income and social approval, as are things like popularity and leadership. The psychological variable that supplies the necessary and sufficient conditions for producing such delightful outcomes, if a person has enough talent and some measure of luck, is *responsibility*, which can be operationally defined as *open initiation, acceptance, and fulfillment of social contracts*. Social contracts here are the many agreements and commitments an individual makes to others and to institutions. The word "open" is an important qualifier, as some people enter implicit social contracts which are not enforced or enforceable because the terms are not mutually known. In our society, it seems generally true that the more an individual seeks and obtains responsibility (which he usually can do only if he has consistently demonstrated dependability), the greater his financial reward, total productivity, social power, and social respect are. Irresponsibility leads to a diminution of all of these.

A person who expresses dissatisfaction with his life often complains of not "getting anywhere," of "being in a rut," and of being forced to live in a cold and unfeeling society. If he can be induced to examine his plight in terms of his own responsibility for it, he may be able to find deficiencies in himself centering around his reluctance to initiate, accept, or meet his social contracts.

Conformity, integrity, and adjustment. Only Pollyanna would say that noble motivation and sincere effort always ensure success. This is not the best of all possible worlds, and there are other factors in emotional problems and their resolution.

If anything resembling conformity is suggested as having desirable properties, some critics quite correctly point out that complete conformity would ensure the social status quo, no matter how undesirable that might be. Fortunately there is room for variety and nonconformity in the way of life of the average man because conformity is sometimes not only a sterile but a destructive goal. If the individual finds himself in emotional difficulty because of a destructive social environment, he needs to find ways not only to withstand the pressure but also to change the social environment or escape from it.

Integrity is the moral concept that seems most useful in considering how to maintain an adequate style of life under the circumstances.[1] Integrity here means *an open espousal and appropriate action in the service of a controversial point of view with the clear knowledge that one is thereby risking social retaliation.* Integrity can be meaningful only in the face of social opposition—if there is no opposition, there are no risks to be run.

Bandura and Kupers (1964) have shown that people provide their own reinforcements to some degree; that is, they tend to pat themselves on the back. An individual can see when he has taken an unpopular stand at some risk to himself in an attempt to live up to his own ethical code. Under those circumstances, the satisfaction of being able to say that a real effort was made to be "right" rather than to be popular can be important. People constantly evaluate themselves whether they wish to or not, and one source of satisfaction can be found only in the exercise of integrity if self-evaluation is to function as a source of continued self-esteem. Integrity has still other uses.

Many members of society admire integrity when they see it and are often impelled either to reward it or to restrain disapproval of the cause it serves. The individual who takes visible risks in the service of his ideals commands, at the very least, grudging admiration from most people. People with a reputation for behaving with integrity often attract either collaborators or followers who are going to be new sources of social reinforcement. It may seem surprising how often a member of an oppositional and yet idealistic group seems to be consistently cheerful even though he is a common target for majority disapproval. If the immediate social circle is unusually approving, the net social reinforcement of his nonconformity may be even greater than it was before he incurred majority displeasure.

For the mental health worker, the tools for changing behavior as well as the content selected for manipulation will be radically different from the conventional ones of Chapter 15 if they are to be consistent with this approach to normality and well-being. Even the same behavior will be seen in a new light as it is analyzed as social rather than private. Let us consider, for example, the "ego defense mechanisms" which you have briefly encountered in Chapters 3 and 4 and will cover in detail in Chapter 10.

Repression is the most ubiquitous as well as the most fundamental of all the defensive mechanisms. It has been defined as a loss of memory which serves to reduce anxiety, but we shall see that the behavior involved can be cogently analyzed as serving another purpose. Repression, operationally speaking, can only be identified by noting a gap in someone's verbal report of past events. The observer finds the gap rather surprising because to him it is so conspicuous. We agree with Freud that all behavior serves a function, so we must attempt to find what possible functions might be served by this omission. It seems self-evident that an incomplete report could be misleading to the listener, and if the information

[1] Moralistic terms are unusual enough in scientific discourse to make it advisable to add a word of explanation. First, while moralistic terms are used here, no effort will be made to make moral judgments; the terms are used only descriptively. Second, moralistic terms are social terms spelling out rules by which people are supposed to deal with each other. As Haley (1963) has pointed out, we have not developed any very comprehensive or useful set of concepts by which to describe social behavior, and the language of morality makes available a number of terms that can usefully apply to the scientific study of important behaviors. We are defending here the utility of moral terms but not necessarily the values they represent.

omitted is crucial to an understanding of what really happened, such a report preserves secrecy. Repression and lying by omission would serve the same social function, and from our framework would not be classed as separate behaviors because there is no way to decide which is which.

However, a psychotherapist would have a different task, depending upon which theoretical structure he embraced. The worker who must grapple with repressions as unconscious defenses must use tools designed to lift them so that the individual can consciously cope with the previously unavailable materials. The position of the social-learning theorist might very well direct him to find methods of unreinforcing social deception or even of making it noxious so that such inaccuracy will be extinguished and accuracy perhaps enhanced. He would be assuming, of course, that increased accuracy is therapeutically helpful in problem solving and that inaccuracy is a source of social disapproval. The therapist's techniques, stated in nonpsychological language, would be to hold the individual responsible for the accuracy of the report; if the therapist were not averse to blunt language, he might demand that the patient "quit lying." It should be remembered that the therapist is not basically concerned with the "ultimate truth" of what people tell him but is trying to find an effective strategy that will lead his patient to more effective social living. In the case of repression, either exposing the nature of the hidden material or holding the individual responsible for all of the truth should constructively modify inaccurate reporting.

In general, the defense mechanisms acquire a different mien if they are restated in terms of social interactions. Projection, like repression, has a self-protective function, but in this case someone other than the patient is gratuitously described as possessing the patient's own undesirable characteristics. Projection is identified operationally by noting a surprising gap in an individual's self-description along with the discovery that the missing statements are being used to describe someone else. In social terms, not only is the listener being misled about the nature of the speaker but also about the nature of some third party. Practically speaking, the social mischief involved in the disorder has been compounded as it now implicates other possibly innocent parties. At a completely conscious level, it is clear that one effective social gambit gained by this device is to convince an evaluator that the speaker must be rated rather highly.

It is possible to go through any list of defense mechanisms and, by examining the social interactions implied, to see that such tactics have potential social utility. As long as it is possible to find such relationships between a person and his social environments, corrective measures can be more easily anchored to the sources of social reinforcement than to unknown factors hidden in the unconscious. Validity, of course, is more important than ease of operation, but the meagre scientific evidence we have indicates that validity is improved rather than decreased when psychotherapy focuses upon the directly observable. As you will see in detail in Chapter 15, psychotherapeutic programs have been devised which concentrate upon the processes of learning or social relating, or both. Preliminary reports of their results are encouraging.

Some students have questioned the general applicability of a socially based theory because societies are visibly different in many ways. The processes that we have been examining probably have great generality because all societies have rules, reinforcements, and punishments which are largely dependent upon social behavior. The rules may regulate different classes of behavior, the reinforcers may be unfamiliar, and the social sanctions may seem irrational, but the normal man will still be invisible, and only the abnormals will be the objects of much social action.

THE USES OF ETHICS AND THE CONCEPT OF MATURITY

We have asserted that the crucial factors in social living are found only by examining behaviors which are said to be of moral importance. If so, then ethical codes potentially have great value to the individual.

If a social environment is to be confronted effectively, an individual must have as many generalized modes of behavior as possible or else each new situation is going to require learning again the entire process of problem solving. Ethical codes are general guides to social living which prescribe certain kinds of behaviors for certain kinds of situations. People in interaction are always potentially in competition or conflict. A code of ethics is the most economical method of escaping from such encounters without stimulating social sanctions, and it often helps in actually gaining social approval.

We are not suggesting that all codes of ethics will do equally well. In a relatively diverse society such as our own, chaos would be inevitable if some codes of ethics made it a duty to punish people who have a different code, and the individual would suffer greatly. But insofar as a code of ethics efficiently prescribes acts that will be acceptable to others or that will elicit approval, the individual is spared much conflict in his continued day-to-day existence.

The normal man, by conforming to *pro*scriptions, removes social pressure by avoiding it in the first place, but because his *pre*scriptions are less well formulated, he ends up with fewer accurate guides to social reinforcement. For these, he must depend on his own *maturity*. Though this word is used with many different meanings, maturity as defined here means the formulation and observance of a code of ethics that provides reliable avenues for both social acceptance and self-approval. Maturity then would be found only in the *positively abnormal*. The individual's code might even be revolutionary for, as we have already seen, if acceptance is earned, the door is open to nonconformity. The individual who wishes to be a reformer would probably be unsuccessful unless he had first demonstrated that he was capable of meeting the demands of the system he wants to reform. With positive abnormality, we find society less likely to retaliate, more likely to encourage, and more likely to shift its own standards in the direction of those representing positive abnormality. With positive abnormality, we also find the most demanding codes of ethics. The apparent paradox is that the more personally demanding the code is, the more social freedom is to be obtained. The college student is greatly concerned with freedom, having had comparatively little, and sometimes demands it from society before he has placed any great demands upon himself. His demand seldom meets with conspicuous compliance. Later in life, if he has been lucky enough to have learned to demand much of himself, he may find that he is urged to exercise the freedom he previously believed he had to fight for. Of course, such outcomes are not inevitable, but the general principle remains: an individual who denies himself absolute freedom by a demanding code of ethics is in the best position to obtain maximum freedom.

In conclusion, the normal man must often live with chronic discontent because his ethical code too often is useful only for evading social retaliations. Such a code is deficient because it is a poor guide in the search for positive approval.

SUMMARY

(1) There are many more normal than abnormal patterns of living. (2) The normal man is socially invisible—that is, he typically arouses little notice in society and little social pressure pro or con. (3) Normal individuals, like everybody else, are each unique. (4) The normal man conforms to most social prohibitions and tends to continue to observe regulations that are no longer appropriate. (5) The normal man is a nonconformist in his methods of reaching positive goals. (6) The normal man often shifts behavioral modes if prohibitions are not involved and if his competencies can still be utilized. (7) The normal man defies some social regulations but has methods of keeping his defiance secret or otherwise evading the usual social sanctions. If he is unable to evade scrutiny or to evade the sanction, he pays the price of losing some of his social power or prestige. (8) The normal man has available some devices that enable him to maintain his emotional comfort even after flouting a social regulation, but other devices which are effective in evading social displeasure also tend to diminish his sense of well-being. (9) Normality and happiness are not correlated. Happiness and social skills are correlated to some degree. (10) The normal man relies heavily upon a limited number of competencies and tends to perpetuate the satisfactions and discontent associated with the exercise of those competencies. (11) The normal man has a serviceable code of ethics which tends to be deficient in that it is poorly designed to enhance a sense of well-being. (12) The normal man differs from the abnormal man (at either end of the scale) only by the absence of conspicuous behavior in his repertoire; abnormal man, too, engages in countless inconspicuous acts.

The statements offered here in summary are all derived from the idea that, in a social universe, the most important factors in shaping and maintaining behavior patterns are social and can best be evaluated in those terms. It is possible to examine most behavioral modes from other frameworks, but the questions that will be asked and the answers given will be much different from those derived from a social base line.

Normals do not share to any significant degree the behaviors that are indices of abnormality, but normals and abnormals alike share in the great pool of normal behaviors. So, we can conclude, the abnormal is much more like the normal than the normal is like the abnormal.

GLOSSARY

ADJUSTMENT—the degree to which an individual maintains harmonious relationships with his environment, including his ability to resolve conflicts and gratify needs.

APPROACH LEARNING—learning to behave in a particular way in order to gain rewards.

AVERAGE—technically, any one of several measures of central tendency (such as mean, median, and mode); loosely, typical, ordinary.

AVOIDANCE LEARNING—learning to behave in a particular way in order to avoid unpleasant consequences.

BASE LINE—starting point.

BEHAVIORAL REPERTOIRE—all the behaviors possible for a given individual.

CAUSATION—as used here, a method of defining events in terms of the events that produced them.

CODE OF ETHICS (ETHICAL CODE)—general guide to social living which prescribes certain kinds of behaviors for certain kinds of situations.

CONCEPTUAL SCHEME—as used here, a theory or framework against which events can be understood.

CONFORMITY—obedience to the required or implied patterns or standards of behavior.

COUNSELING—advising designed to enhance an overall sense of well-being.

EGO DEFENSE MECHANISMS—psychological processes, usually unconscious, that neutralize the potentially upsetting impact of threatening events or ideas by distorting reality in significant ways.

ETHICAL CODE—see CODE OF ETHICS.

EUPHORIA—an emotional state of extreme well-being.

GOAL—that which is sought; the object, tangible or intangible, that behavior is directed toward.

HETEROSEXUAL—one who is sexually interested in persons of the opposite sex.

HOMOSEXUAL—one who is sexually interested in persons of the same sex.

HYPERACTIVE—overactive.

HYPOACTIVE—underactive.

IMPLICIT—understood without being directly stated.

INDEPENDENT PROBABILITY—the likelihood that an event will occur independently of the occurrence of other events.

INFERENCE—a judgment based on other judgments, not on direct observation.

INTEGRITY—as used here, the open espousal of and appropriate action for, a controversial point of view with the knowledge that this activity may invite social retaliation.

MANIC—behaving impulsively, with violent and uncontrollable motor activity.

MATURITY—as used in this chapter, the formulation and observance of a code of ethics that provides reliable avenues for self-approval and social acceptance.

MODAL BEHAVIOR—the ways in which most people behave.

NEGATIVE LIFE STYLE—a style of living characterized by "playing it safe" and restricting oneself to techniques that have proven successful in the past; an inclination to avoid rather than approach.

NONCONFORMITY—failure to conform to a generally accepted pattern or standard of behavior.

NORMALITY—generally, that which is expected, routine, or ordinary; statistically, a frequency distribution characterized by the large central portion of a bell-shaped curve; moralistically, acceptability; psychologically, "invisibility."

OPERANT LEARNING—a form of learning wherein a response (usually one that "operates" on the environment) is likely to occur because it has been reinforced.

OPERATIONAL TERM—a quality that has been defined by the operations or procedures employed to achieve it.

PERSONALITY—the hierarchy of traits, modes of adjustment, and behaviors of which a person is capable; a set of terms that allows us to explain a particular person's behavior.

POSITIVE LIFE STYLE—a style of living characterized by seeking new challenges and goals and finding new ways to achieve; an inclination to approach rather than avoid.

PROJECTION—the attribution of one's own traits to other people or groups; the attributed traits are commonly those that are present in, but unacceptable to, the self.

PROSCRIPTION—an imposed restraint.

PSYCHOTHERAPY—the use of any psychological technique in the treatment of mental disorder or maladjustment.

REINFORCEMENT—that which strengthens a response.

REPRESSION—the exclusion of psychological contents (for example, memories, and feelings) from awareness, commonly because the contents provoke anxiety.

RESPONSIBILITY—operationally, open initiation, acceptance, and fulfillment of social contracts.

SELF-ACTUALIZATION—Maslow's term for self-fulfillment; development of one's potentialities.

SOCIAL CREDIT—a "social bank account" that permits one, because he has convinced others of his social value, to break a few rules.

SOCIAL INVISIBILITY—relative inability to compel society to respond to one's behaviors.

SOCIAL LEARNING—acquisition of social behaviors from observation of, and reinforcement by, others.

SOCIAL REINFORCEMENT—a reinforcement given by an institution or other people.

SOCIAL VISIBILITY—ability to attract attention and concern from others, particularly those who are perceived as socially powerful.

SOCIALLY ABETTED—term describing persons who have been proffered power and material rewards or urged and helped to expand their activities because of the overall approval of the society.

SOCIALLY RESTRICTED—term describing persons, such as those found in penitentiaries and mental hospitals, who are forced by society into social retirement.

SUBCULTURE—a group of individuals within a culture who share special characteristics at the same time that they share the major characteristics of the entire culture.

SUBLIMATION—the acceptance of substitute goals with a higher social utility than the original goals.

VALIDITY—generally, the degree to which a particular measure actually assesses what it purports to assess; also, the degree to which a theory has been empirically verified.

REFERENCES

Allport, G. W. *Personality*, New York: Holt, Rinehart & Winston, Inc., 1937.

Bandura, A., and Carol J. Kupers. Transmission of patterns of self-reinforcement through modeling. *Journal of Abnormal Psychology*, 1964, **60,** 1–9.

Eysenck, J. (ed.). *Behavior therapy and neuroses*. New York: Pergamon Press, Inc., 1960.

——— (ed.), *Handbook of abnormal psychology*. New York: Basic Books, Inc., 1961.

Fromm, E. *Escape from freedom*. New York: Holt, Rinehart & Winston, Inc., 1961.

———. *The sane society*. New York: Holt, Rinehart & Winston, Inc., 1955.

Goldstein, A. P. *Therapist-patient expectations in psychotherapy*. New York: Pergamon Press, Inc., 1962.

Haley, J. *Strategies of psychotherapy*. New York: Grune & Stratton, Inc., 1963.

Hartshorne, H., and M. A. May. *Studies in deceit*. New York: Crowell-Collier and Macmillan, Inc., 1928.

Hollander, E. P. Competence and conformity in the acceptance of influence. In I. D. Steiner and M. Fishbein (eds.), *Current studies in social psychology*. New York: Holt, Rinehart & Winston, Inc., 1965.

Jahoda, Marie. *Current concepts of positive mental health*. New York: Basic Books, Inc., 1958.

Jones, E., K. Davis, and K. Gergen. Role playing variations and their informational value for person perception. *Journal of Abnormal and Social Psychology*, 1961, **63,** 302–310.

Kinsey, A. C., W. B. Pomeroy, and C. E. Martin. *Sexual behavior in the human male*. Philadelphia: W. B. Saunders Company, 1948.

Maslow, A. H. *Motivation and personality*. New York: Harper & Row, Publishers, 1954.

Mowrer, O. H. *The crisis in psychiatry and religion*. Princeton, N.J.: D. Van Nostrand Company, Inc., 1961.

———. What is normal behavior? In Pennington and Berg (eds.), *An introduction to clinical psychology*. New York: The Ronald Press Company, 1948.

Sheffield, V., and H. Temmer. Relative resistance to extinction of escape training and avoidance training. *Journal of Experimental Psychology*, 1950, **40,** 287–298.

Srole, L. Mental health in the metropolis. In *The midtown Manhattan study*. New York: McGraw-Hill, Inc., 1962.

White, R. W. *Lives in progress*. New York: Holt, Rinehart & Winston, Inc., 1952.

SUGGESTED READINGS

1. Fromm, E. *The sane society*. New York: Holt, Rinehart & Winston, Inc., 1955. The best elaboration of Fromm's view that society deeply affects individual psychological performance. The requirements of a healthy society and consequences for its members are examined.
2. Jahoda, Marie. *Current concepts of positive mental health*. New York: Basic Books, Inc., 1958. A survey and integration of various theories and conceptions of mental health.
3. Maslow, A. H. *Motivation and personality*. New York: Harper & Row Publishers, 1954. An introduction to notions of self-actualization and a discussion of the organization of personality necessary for self-actualization.
4. Mowrer, O. H. *The crisis in psychiatry and religion*. Princeton, N.J.: D. Van Nostrand Company, Inc., 1961. A series of essays dealing with the problems of guilt and interpersonal honesty and their effects on personality.

6

W. ROSS ASHBY

CRAYTON C. WALKER

Genius

Louis "Satchmo" Armstrong, the famous entertainer, has been described in a popular magazine as "an authentic American genius." They write:

> It is a simple fact of jazz music, the only art form America ever wholly originated, that virtually all that is played today comes in some way from Louis Armstrong. . . . More than any other individual, it was Armstrong who took the raw spontaneous folk music of the honky tonks and street parades and, quite unconsciously, built it into a music beyond anything musicians had previously imagined. It was a spectacular outpouring of born, unschooled genius. (*Life*, p. 93.)

Few would be tempted to deny these words. Armstrong's status as entertainer and musician is easy to document. But, having agreed that he is a genius, what do we mean by it? What *kind* of genius is he exactly? How do we *know* that he is a genius? On careful examination, these apparently simple questions prove surprisingly difficult to answer. This fact is important for the student of abnormal psychology, for it suggests that we often use the word *genius* without fully understanding what we mean by it. We are, it seems, guided more by vague intuitions about its meaning than by our mastery of it. We are also guided by some old myths about the nature of genius which confound rather than clarify our thinking about it.

In this chapter, we shall discuss the old ideas briefly and then turn to a different way of approaching the subject of genius which makes use of recent findings in several fields. Our aim is not authoritatively to define, nor even to attempt to summarize very completely what has been written about "genius." We believe the beginning student is better exposed to an appreciation of the real complexity of the subject and to an approach to it that tends to keep important issues uppermost.

The older ideas of genius imply rather consistently if vaguely that geniuses achieve their results by the effortless exercise of supernatural powers. These ideas are sometimes stated plausibly, but they are also very misleading. We will see why this is so and how the situation can be more naturally described by considering the subject of genius from a point of view suggested by methods recently introduced by psychologists interested in problem-solving behavior, by communication engineers, and by computer scientists. These methods include the study of *artificial intelligence,* which is intelligent behavior in man-made things; a mathematical tool called *information theory,* basically a way of keeping account of causes and effects; and *automata theory,* the mathematical study of the behavior of robots. Fortunately, we need not go into the technical details of these methods to make clear that, taken together, they strongly suggest that the productions of genius *can* come about through "ordinary" means, and that, where ordinary means (such as the human brain) are used, there is no such thing as unbounded cleverness.

THE MYTHOLOGY OF GENIUS

The idea of genius has been around for a long time, and it is useful to look briefly at its history because common thinking on the subject is much influenced by the historic trend. The influence of history in this case means that much of what passes for common knowledge about genius is virtually mythology. In ancient Greece, for example, if a man showed unusual ability, and neither his parents nor his experience provided a visible explanation, the ability was "explained" as a gift from the gods. As a dictionary will show, supernatural powers such as guiding spirits and tutelary deities are important in the history of *genius.* Even today we show more than a vestige of these ideas when we say a man has a "gift" for some activity. If there is a gift, there must be a giver and, especially if the ability in question, the "gift," is clearly unusual, it is easy to think that the "giver" himself is exceptionally powerful, unusual, and supernatural—in other words, a supernatural deity.

Hand in hand with the idea that genius is a supernatural gift goes the idea that the productions of genius come more or less without effort. It is easy to conjure in our minds the picture of Newton watching an apple fall to the ground, muttering "so *that's* it" to himself, and then quickly writing out the law of gravity. That is the way geniuses work, we think.

Why do we continue to think along these lines in this naturalistic age? What makes it difficult to conceive of genius in some other way? There are at least two reasons. First, men of lesser accomplishments seem to think that the prodigious achievements of genius are quite unattainable by ordinary means. Second, each of us has passed through a stage in our own youth when we actually knew a person of immeasurable knowledge, who could solve all problems (how to open a door, even how to tie a shoelace) by merely turning her attention to it. Though we generally become disillusioned later, we all bear some remains of the idea that to the really clever, there is no such thing as an unsolvable problem.

Mixed in with these erroneous habits of thought are two fundamental objective errors in common thinking about genius. The first concerns *originality*—what it is, and how it is involved in genius. This error results from failure to grasp the true meaning of originality and what it implies. The second error concerns *how geniuses are identified.* Many people feel that it is easier than it really is to see who the great geniuses are, or at least who they have been in the past. This error stems from a misunderstanding of how and by whom selections of various kinds are made and how candidates for the genius category are selected by these processes. The two errors are widespread and well accepted. Taken together, the confusion they engender supports the mythological interpretation of genius by making it difficult to believe that there is anything factual about the subject. Let us begin our task of sorting out fact from fancy by discussing originality.

The meaning of originality. When we think about genius, one of the first characteristics that comes to mind is originality. For example, the article on Louis Armstrong says that his music is "beyond anything musicians had previously imagined," a clear reference to the newness of his contribution. It is not hard to understand why we think of geniuses as original. One reason is our habit of considering genius in relation to the supernatural; deities are often described as creative, and the other way around, acts of creation, and therefore of originality, are commonly thought to be mysterious, mystical, and supernatural. It is quite understandable that we associate genius with originality, given such preconceptions of what genius is. Indeed, it is so easy to think this way that we are often inclined to go further and let an extreme capacity for original thought *explain* genius. That is, we call originality the most important single factor in genius. Is originality *that* central? To judge this point, we had better examine the concept of originality more closely.

It is conceivable, of course, that originality *is* a supernatural thing, but as scientists, we are only interested in the natural characteristics of things and so must view the subject only from that perspective. First, what does "original" mean? When we say something or someone is "original," we are making a judgment about that thing or person. This point is more important than it appears at first. The dictionary (Webster's New World, 1962) does not mention our judgmental role at all, saying only that "original" has to do with "never having occurred before." This implies that there is some way of telling whether or not an event has previously occurred. But events do not come with signs around their necks announcing that fact, and since virtually nobody is really able to say that any event has *never* happened before, there simply is no final way to tell. In that sense, the dictionary definition is useless. It hints at a more practical definition, however, of which we can make good use: *an event is original if it has not been observed before.* This definition recognizes that situations in which originality is to be judged involve an observation and an observer. This is not to say that all difficulties in the use of the term now end. In fact, they have just begun, for now we must take into account the peculiarities of the observer. When he says that something is original, for example, does he mean that it was not observed "in the last ten minutes," or "in the last hour," or "in the last 200 years"? Does he mean "not observed by me," or "not observed by any member of this class" or "not observed by any professional psychologist"? And so forth.

What has been gained by this redefinition, despite the problems it creates, is two things. Our practical definition of originality greatly reduces the tendency to think of it as supernatural and, taking account of the observer, introduces early in our discussion one of the factors which makes genius a complex subject.

We are now looking on originality as a property of perceived events. How usual or natural a property is it? How can it be produced? The answer is simple. Originality can be found everywhere and is produced by a great variety of things. A rabbit hopping across a snow bank produces an original set of tracks, each human fingerprint is original in its pattern, every gun fires a bullet with a distinctive scoring, and so on. In short, originality can be produced routinely by rather ordinary processes, including very straightforward mechanical processes. This conclusion has not always been so obvious as it is now. Until recently, matter was regarded as fundamentally inert. Most writings before 1900 contrast the inertness of nonliving matter with the mobility and changeability of the living. According to these preconceptions, machinery, because it is made of nonliving, inert stuff, could hardly be expected to show any of the important attributes of live things. Today, with more knowledge of the atom, and especially with a conglomeration of "dead" copper and germanium known as the "general purpose computer," we are more aware that matter is not as inert as it might seem.

The scientist and psychologist of the nineteenth century was seriously misled about the nature of "machines." With only such simple machinery as the steam engine and the watch before him, he was led to generalizations that are today known to be untrue. One of these was the notion that no machine could produce new ways of behaving: a machine could do only what it was designed to do, which excludes the production of novelty. Today, the question is seen rather differently. An atomic physicist, for example, might say the exact opposite: since every physical event is made up of fine details that are not predictable from one instant to the next, it follows that every physical thing is *always* doing something new. This point of view is of no practical use to psychology, but it does bring to notice again the importance of the *observer*: whether or not something seems to produce novelty depends partly on the resources and methods of the observer. To one observer, the successive ticks of a watch may be mere repetition; to another, who records the finest details, no two ticks may be identical. By changing observers, we can thus, it appears, change the watch from a device which cannot show originality to one which can. Of course, we do not really change the *watch* at all, but only the situation in which originality is to be judged. Keep in mind, though, that as far as *originality* is concerned, this change is a very real change indeed.

But there is a deeper complication. Suppose we make a weather vane to show which way the wind is blowing and mount it on the roof. Later, when it points to the source of the wind, we may claim that it is doing what we designed it to do *and no more*. Here we are studying its behavior by classifying it in one of two groups: (1) pointing at the source of the wind or, (2) pointing elsewhere. But what if we had studied its behavior by allotting its state to one of four: (1) pointing north, (2) pointing east, (3) pointing south, (4) pointing west. When the vane is pointing east, its state is a result of the *combined* actions of the wind and the designer. So far as the specific north, east, south, or west direction is concerned, the designer has in fact *delegated* some of his control to the wind. This makes it possible that the wind may evoke ways of behaving that were not foreseen by the designer. In other words, the question of whether a machine can do more than its designer has put into it is not useful. The fact that a designer can delegate his control carries with it the implicit possibility that the consequences of the delegation may be quite outside his initial expectation so that, to him, the machine seems to show "originality."

An excursion into the meaning of originality can lead into deep and subtle matters; here, we need notice only that purely mechanical, nonvital processes can generate as much originality as is needed for any development of new behaviors.

All that is necessary is access to some physical activity that presumably includes all possible combinations and sequences of events. Well-shaken dice, for instance, are capable of producing all possible combinations of the numbers one to six if they are thrown enough. Were the number of dice increased and the dots replaced by, or coded into, musical notes, they would be capable of producing all possible musical sequences. Coded into letters and punctuation marks, they could produce every possible literary sequence (though it would take a while). The equally irregular and unpredictable movement of the individual electron, an important source of the so-called background noise in electrical devices, can also readily be used to generate a sequence as complete in its possibilities as that of the dice. Finally, the living brain can get access to similar physically active causes, which the neurons of the brain can then code completely enough to leave no combinations out. Once the highly dynamic nature of all matter is appreciated, the production of originality, of behavior that has not been seen before, is a matter of purely technical interest to engineers.

It is interesting to note that the production of originality is a small problem to those who have had experience in psychiatry. Nowhere are new ideas seen in such wild profusion as in a mental hospital. The patient in acute mania, for instance, may produce in a few minutes more witty quips than many normal people produce in a year and enough dazzingly original ideas for curing social troubles to keep sociologists busy for many years finding out whether they are really workable. Where the patient fails, of course, is in his inability to discriminate and select. The problem of how genius achieves its results lies here, not in emphasis on originality, but on the processes of discrimination and selection.

Performers and performance. On the face of it, some people are obviously more noteworthy than others, whether they are conspicuously benevolent or not. Yet the fact is that an outstanding performance is no guarantee that the performer is himself outstanding *in any way*. This point is important because geniuses are supposed to be outstanding people, and since we have only their performances to use in judging them, we must understand how we can be misled. Consider the well-publicized millionth person to cross a bridge. It is clear that this person's instant conspicuousness is totally unrelated to any outstanding personal characteristics. He is not necessarily more talented, interesting, or worthwhile than the motorist who followed him across the bridge. It is only due to *our* characteristics, our counting in decimals, our emphasis on great magnitudes, our likes and dislikes in news reporting that the millionth crossing, and hence this particular person, is noteworthy.

Now consider this more involved example. Suppose that 1024 people are playing roulette, each backing his guess—red or black—ten times in succession. If one of these people won all ten times, many people would probably declare him exceptional and ask him to reveal his method. Obviously such an attitude to him would be ridiculous, yet what exactly is wrong with it? Is he not selected, as one man in a thousand, by the objective fact of his success?

He is, in fact, selected by *us*, the bystanders at the casino. For, if + represents a right choice, and − a wrong choice, it is *we* who have decided that we will notice and exalt the man who guesses ++++++++++. In fact, the man who guessed −−−−−−−−−− is no less remarkable, nor is the man who guessed ++−−++−−++. In fact, the man who produced +−−++−++++ is exactly as remarkable, and so on for each of the 1024 arrangements of ten successes and failures. The reason for the choice of 1 from 1024, is not to be found by examining *the man.*

The error in reasoning in these two examples is obviously that the person whose performance we selected as outstanding is noteworthy only because of our interests, for these particular performances came about *completely* by chance—the performers themselves just "lucked out." Calling the *men* outstanding in these circumstances is an error because, when we say a person is "outstanding," we really mean that *he* is responsible for the performances observed. If the person is noteworthy only because of the judgment we bring to his performance rather than because of what he brings to its execution, there is little reason to call *him* outstanding, or to expect outstanding performance from him in the future.

In studying genius, therefore, we must distinguish carefully "lucking out" and succeeding by some deliberate and controlled means. If we recognize that to call someone outstanding is essentially to make a prediction that, other things being equal, he will produce outstanding performances in the future, then the basic test of whether methods or abilities are outstanding is clearly to see if their use leads to further outstanding performance. If the basic test cannot be conducted, we can do no more than use the information at hand to guess what *might* have happened if the test had been applied. Such second-guessing rarely permits the issue to be resolved to our complete satisfaction. Judgments about performances that occurred only once, about persons who have completed their careers, and about people long dead, are especially liable to this weakness, a fact that considerably complicates the study of the classic geniuses.

In the examples above, outstanding performances occurred by chance, through no fault or talent of the performers. But even when it is quite clear that the performer's role is significant and deliberate, we are still involved as observers in judging whether the performance is outstanding or not. And the reason why some performances are considered worthy of note is that we, as observers, are critically influenced by the context in which the events occur. In the study of genius, this gives us the problem of trying to understand whether even a man's controlled and deliberate performances got him recognized as a genius because they were wonderful in their own right or because they simply happened to be more suited to the exigencies of time and place, thus giving them more publicity value than somebody else's deeds, but not reflecting greater ability.

Suppose, for example, two equally able scientists, one a year older than the other, were quite independently to make the same important discovery at precisely the same age. That is, the discoveries are made a year apart, and the older man's discovery occurs first. In this case, greater fame would fall to the older scientist, and many people would interpret this as evidence that he was the better scientist. His relatively greater fame is actually due, of course, to factors entirely beyond his control, such as the world's greater interest in new discoveries and the date of his birthday. Here is another example. At the turn of the century, many young painters broke away from the conventional forms. Today, Picasso is outstanding. Should we now, as psychologists, examine Picasso for his peculiar characteristics, or should we, as sociologists, ask what peculiar features in Western civilization make it celebrate his genius above that of others? However real the powers which Picasso brings to his painting, the idea that he is a genius, in the sense that his work is necessarily better than that of his competitors, is promoted without considering our needs of today, which are not always related to artistic merit.

Even where men of undoubted talent are concerned, the degree of their preeminence, if not their work itself, can thus be due to luck. It is almost impossible in the case of the classic geniuses of the past to make allowance for the amount of their preeminence due to *our* selection. Isaac Newton, for instance, always thought of quantities as "flowing" from one value to the next—an ideal predisposition for one who was to attempt to establish a mathematical system which deals with such processes (the differential and integral calculus). How would he have fared at the beginning of this century, when physics needed a man who could think of systems in which everything changed by discrete jumps? The available facts suggest that we might not have noticed Newton in this setting. He was not infallible, after all. Although interested and active in chemistry since his childhood, for instance, "he made no striking discoveries [nor] enlarged the knowledge of chemical action" (Moore, 1924, p. 157). To take a very different example, Adolf Hitler had many extraordinary successes before 1942 and was often acclaimed a genius, especially by Germans. Later events showed that he was actually a man with one method that happened to be peculiarly appropriate to Europe at that time; when the method later became inappropriate, he could do nothing but persist in it. We need not stop to consider these questions further at this time. It is sufficient for our purposes to recognize the fallacies which threaten our interpretation of extraordinary events and of the abilities of the men involved in them.

To summarize the discussion of originality and outstandingness, we are arguing, first, that originality is *not* peculiar to genius. By itself, originality is not even special. Rabbits can be original, fingerprints can be original, machines can be original, even *people* can be original. Originality is not necessarily good or helpful. Valuable contributions involve something more: *selectivity*. Second, we must consider carefully the influence the observer exercises on the process which eventuates in someone's being called outstanding. The observer's influence is capable of introducing error in describing the performer. It can suggest that an ordinary performer is extraordinary, and that an outstanding man is *very* outstanding. Retrospective judgments are especially liable to these errors and may be very difficult to correct.

With all the warnings now behind us of how to mistakenly see genius where it is not and assign attributes to it that do not apply, we can turn to a more positive discussion of what genius is and how we can understand it in the light of modern knowledge.

GENIUS AND INFORMATION

Investigations into the nature of genius have traditionally been conducted by two study methods—genealogy and IQ-type measurements. In the 1800s for example, Sir Francis Galton (1869) studied the family trees of eminent men and found some reason to believe that eminence ran in families, though he did not dismiss the effect of environment (see Chapters 1 and 2). Lewis Terman *et al.* (1925), studying children with very high IQ's found that, popular ideas to the contrary, they were better adjusted than most. These kinds of studies have had some value, but it has been limited, chiefly because the definition of the factors that together make genius, and of the way they must go together to make it, is very complex. The approach to genius presented in this chapter makes use of a method designed for the precise purpose of understanding very complex relationships. It is called "information theory."

The meaning of information theory. Many people saw information theory, when it was first introduced, as a new mystery, a new metaphysic, almost a new philosophy. It is really none of these, however, but essentially simply a means of counting and comparing things, mostly counting causes and comparing them to the number of effects. The night of Paul Revere's famous ride, for example, once he had determined that the British could come by only one of two routes—land or sea—Mr. Revere only had to compare the number of routes to the number of signals to know that two signals were sufficient "cause" for him to spread the alarm. All the various aspects of information theory, no matter how complex they seem, have this counting and this comparison at their core.

When the counting is simple, as in the example above, the method hardly deserves a special name. But there are innumerable very complicated situations where ordinary methods of counting are not adequate, and it is for such events that some refined technical methods of counting are graced with the name "information theory."

The importance of these technical methods lies in the help they give to the scientist who is trying to relate, not one cause to one effect, but a great number of causes to a great number of effects and who finds that each set is so intricately connected within itself that he is unable to determine by simple counting how many distinct causes are at work or how many distinct effects are produced. By the 1940s, the need for a new technique had become great; up to that time science had primarily related one cause to one effect, disposing of each pair before it turned to the next. Today, when we want to study such complex systems as computers, societies, brains—in which many parts intricately interact—we often find that specific cause-and-effect pairs are of small interest compared to the quantitative relation between a large number of causes and a large number of effects. In dealing with complex things, it is often important to know, for example, whether just this group of causes *could* produce that group of effects.

It is in this way that information theory becomes relevant in processes of selection. It is a scientific axiom that every effect has its causes, and the scientist often finds himself trying to relate many causes and many effects; his study naturally leads him to the use of information theory.

The theorems of information theory are ultimately based on the axiom that *appropriate selection among effects depends on an equal amount of selection among causes*. Stated this way, the axiom sounds vague and metaphysical, but we understand it quickly enough if a situation seems to violate it, if, for example, a student were to give the correct answer on an examination before the question had been asked, or a computer were to give the correct answer before the program had been inserted.

Another way of stating this axiom is to say that, if you can demonstrate that selection has been accomplished in the physical world, this selection must have an identifiable cause in the physical world. The more general axiom that physical events have physical causes, whether we can identify them or not, underlies all of science. What information theory does is simply apply the more general axiom to a class of events that formerly was not studied much, namely events which show selection. As a primarily mathematical tool, information theory has wide applicability, enabling us to use it in the study of genius. It is useful because it makes available a number of theorems about what can and cannot be achieved in behavior processes that involve selection. We have already indicated that selection is crucial in outstanding performances; we now take up the question of the extent to which selection is basic to genius.

Genius and selection. Selection means choosing the elements in a situation which will contribute towards some definite goal. If selection is to be evaluated intelligently, it must serve a demonstrable goal; we can't, for example, have a marksman who hits the target five inches from the bull's-eye and then says that was exactly where he was aiming. In large part, genius can be identified by exceptional powers of appropriate selection.

If we consider the course of Johann Sebastian Bach's career of musical composition as he moved from infancy to adulthood, we can see the processes of selectivity increasingly at work; he moved from near random activity to the creative choices of precise sets which made him immortal. No genius at first, he spread ink on paper in a way that made no sense, much less notes. Later in childhood, he directed his pen to making staff and notes, his markings now showing appropriate selection to some degree. Still later, the selections would be even more precise as the notes, no longer distributed to yield a childish melody, would make his listeners say, "How exactly right that chord is!" In his mature works the selection Bach used, while it appears obvious, is not easy to demonstrate.

The stylistic self-consistency in all of Bach's major works is so great that it is hard to say what would happen today if, as a test, ten mediocre composers were asked to try to restore ten bars in an unfamiliar work of his. It seems likely, though, that one of two extremes would occur. Either the restored music would sound grossly inappropriate because the composers would not be able to imitate Bach's characteristic selections of notes, or it might sound exactly like Bach because his stylistic characteristics are so precisely harmonious and systematic that anybody who understands them can see how given small pieces would have to be constructed. In either case, Bach's genius is reflected in the brilliance of his ability to select one sequence of notes above another. And our indecision as to what test to apply to his music is largely the result of our not knowing exactly what it is we find admirable in Bach's music.

Newton showed his genius partly by his ability to select the *right* operations for constructing his mathematical system when most other mathematicians of his time were choosing the wrong ones. Michelangelo, in the Sistine Chapel, put the paint in just the right places and with just the right shades when most of his contemporaries would have put them otherwise and would have failed to achieve his marvellous effects. And the ordinary tests of "intelligence" are based on the same objective feature: various answers are possible, and that child scores highest who can make the greatest number of appropriate selections.

On an IQ test, *appropriate* means correct, but not so much in an objective sense as in the sense that it satisfies a decision made *in advance* (by the test makers) about which answers show high and which show low intelligence. In evaluating genius, it makes an enormous difference whether the criterion for appropriateness was decided *before* or *after* the critical performance has taken place. Suppose, for instance, we wish to evaluate two painters. One says, "I am an expert in exact geometrical perspective. I will paint a picture of shadows falling across a spiral staircase." If he does it well, he is showing good selection in how he handles his materials. The second painter then says, "I am an expert in so distorting geometrical perspective that I can make even an ordinary fence appear ghostlike." If he does this well, he too can claim good power of selection. Yet, had the pictures been exchanged, each painter would have been judged incompetent. Now contrast both of these with an artist who does not state his aim but just paints a picture with nongeometric perspective. Has he succeeded or failed? The question has no meaning in the absence of a declared goal. Succeeded or failed at what? Any statement made by a bystander about whether he likes the picture or not is a statement about himself, not about the painter's talent.

For the work of most of the geniuses in history, the relevant goal was well enough defined that the candidate's success can be judged objectively. In 1650, during Newton's time, many mathematicians were trying to explain Galileo's experimental findings concerning the speeds at which things fall by devising laws of motion which would make sense for planets and falling bodies alike. In Michelangelo's day, the technical problems of perspective, such as how to paint a person who has an arm extending directly toward the viewer were being widely discussed. The problems of realistically representing the human body in flat paintings were already largely set before Michelangelo attempted to solve them. The classic geniuses often showed their powers on already long-standing problems rather than on ones formed in consequence of what the "genius" produced.

Whether the criterion is decided before or after the performance itself is as critical for evaluating a genius as is the distinction, in experimentation, between selecting an event for testing *before* doing the experiment and paying attention to it after the fact only *because of* the outcome of the experiment. The latter is like the marksman's saying he really meant to miss the target all along. In our present consideration of genius, the separation is readily made because, as a practical matter, our definition of genius always involves the production of solutions to difficult but defined problems for which control and skilled direction *is* needed. The theorems of information theory are directly applicable to problems of this kind.

Once a goal is defined, information theory proposes what may seem a disarmingly trite axiom: *If the goal is difficult*, it says, *you will have to do a lot of work to reach it*. The technical propositions in which this idea is rigorously and mathematically stated are called Shannon's "tenth theorem" (Shannon and Weaver, 1959) and Ashby's "law of requisite variety" (Ashby, 1963). Ignoring technical details, the laws are simple. They say that, if the factors known to be able to influence a performance would scatter it all over an area, x, if they could, and if, despite this, the performance that actually occurs remains within a narrower area, y, then there must be something at work controlling the performance and producing the lessened scatter. That regulator, or guide, or selector, or genius which exerts this control is said to be processing information about the total situation in a quantity corresponding to the missing area of scatter, that is x minus y.

To illustrate, suppose that Michelangelo made one million brush strokes in painting the Sistine Chapel. Suppose also that, being highly skilled, at each brush stroke he selected one of the two best, so that where the average painter would have ranged over ten, Michelangelo would have regarded eight as inferior. At each brush stroke he would have been selecting appropriately in the intensity of one in five. Over the million brush strokes the intensity would have been one in $5^{1,000,000}$. The intensity of Michelangelo's selection can be likened to his picking out one painting from five-raised-to-the-one-millionth-power, which is a large number of paintings (roughly 1 followed by 699,000 zeroes). Since this number is approximately the same as $2^{2,320,000}$, the theorem says that Michelangelo must have processed at least 2,320,000 "bits" of information, in the units of information theory, to achieve the results he did. (The numbers used here may be wrong, but the logic of the argument is right.) He *must* have done so, according to the axiom, because appropriate selections can only be achieved if enough information is received and processed to make them happen. No matter how complex Michelangelo's brain, no matter how subtle his ideas, and no matter whether the physical processes involved are electrical, chemical, or whatever, the appropriateness of his selections would have had to be purchased with informational work.

If this were generally the case, as information theory suggests, it would mean that to achieve what they did the classic geniuses had to be, not just smart, but hard workers.

The labors of genius. The question of whether the classic geniuses actually performed the amount of information processing demanded by theory can hardly be answered accurately. Too many personal facts about them have been lost. Nevertheless, the records of their lives show that most of them devoted an enormous part of their energies to the activities that made them famous. Many of them paid attention to little else, ruminating on their problems alone or in company, awake or dreaming. According to one biographer, Michelangelo "lived like an ascetic and worked like a pack-mule" (Hulshard, 1899, p. 7). And in his own words, "I strain more than any man who ever lived, unhealthy and with great exhaustion; and yet I have the patience to arrive at the desired goal" (Clements, 1963, p. 45). Newton, asked how he solved so many problems, replied simply, "By always thinking about them." And despite the legend that he could grasp a subject like plane geometry at one swift glance (Newton is rumored to have discarded Euclid as "a trifling book" after looking at a few proofs) or that he was completely self-taught, he actually had extensive training in mathematics at Cambridge University under a superb teacher named Isaac Barrow. The mathematician Gauss expressed this same idea in a personal letter:

> Perhaps you remember . . . my complaints about a theorem which . . . had defied all my attempts. . . . This lack has spoiled for me everything else that I found; and for four years, a week has seldom passed when I would not have made one or another vain attempt to solve this problem—recently very lively again. But all brooding, all searching has been in vain. . . . Finally I succeeded several days ago. (Dunnington, 1955.)

Every week for four years, with "brooding" as well as searching—here is information processing on a grand scale! But the evidence that this hard work actually has been done is easily lost, which is probably why we associate genius with easy accomplishment. Gauss continues in his letter, "Nobody will have any idea of the long squeeze in which it placed me, when I someday lecture on the topic."

It is probably pointless to follow the classic geniuses much further. The facts themselves are disputable; they have been much distorted by controversy and are everywhere subject to the fallacy implicit when *we* do the selection. One more thing, however, is relevant here for which their experiences may be instructive. As important as hard work (extensive information processing) is, work alone cannot account for great achievements. Mere searching, of the type that writes out all possible symbols for ten pages and then looks to see if a theorem has appeared, is easily shown to demand more time than there is in a thousand lives, yet alone in one. How then does a genius produce many theorems in one lifetime?

Efficiency in processing information. When information theory was first applied to artificial intelligence, it was concerned mostly with whether a process was *possible* or not. It tended to overlook the question of the relative efficiency with which the possible could be accomplished. Many of the early processes used extremely inefficient methods, so that the critic often had good chance to feel they could never be practical. Today it is better appreciated that the efficiency of an information-handling process is a most important consideration.

The problem-solving method known as "trial and error" illustrates the point. (By the way, "trial and error" does not necessarily imply that trials are made at *random*. The search can be an ordered examination of the various possibilities.) Suppose we have a problem to solve, and the available information is sufficient only for a partial selection; that is, it will get us only part way to the solution. Then we are left with no further reason for choosing this route over that route, for further choice can be justified only if further information is obtained. What do we do? "Trial and error" is about the only avenue left to us. But "trial and error" has two quite different aspects. It can be regarded as a blind leap at the solution, as a systematic way of obtaining the information *on which alone further appropriate selection can be based.* It can be used, in other words, either more or less efficiently to help solve the problem.

Most of the classic geniuses made no secret of their dependence on abundant trials, many of which proved useless individually, yet most instructive in the long run. Thus Gauss, in the letter quoted, refers to "all my attempts," "one or another vain attempt," and "all brooding, all searching." The idea that the genius always goes directly to the answer is clearly mythical, but he may use trials more efficiently than others. An extremely *in*efficient method for writing a worthwhile book, for instance, is to fill 200 pages with random letters, to do this many times, and then to take the best of the stack. Scientists are just now beginning to understand the mechanics of efficiency and applying them to hardware problems in which computers are taught to prove theorems, play checkers and chess, and compose music. A few of their observations and results will illustrate how great the difference between the efficient and the inefficient methods can be.

One very old but very important method makes use of specific information about the goal. The reason it is a good method seems to be only recently well understood (Campbell, 1960). Suppose someone has to find a route between a point on longitude A and a point on longitude *M*, and there are twelve stages *B*, *C*, *D*, *E*, and so on, with routes branching into three at each stage (see Figure 6.1). The number of branch routes to be explored between the points is excessive. From A, three branches go towards *B*; from longitude *B*, nine branch routes (3^2) go towards *C*; from longitude C, twenty-seven routes (3^3) go towards *D*; and so forth. From the start at A until the precise destination along longitude *M*, there are 3^{12} or a total of over half a million branch routes to be searched. But if the goal is known and this information put to use, the search can be started from both ends to find a route with a common point in the middle. From each end to the middle, the search is now only six stages long, and the number of branches is 3^6, or 729. The two searches now require 1458 branches to be tried instead of over a half million. Using the known goal this way saves *over*

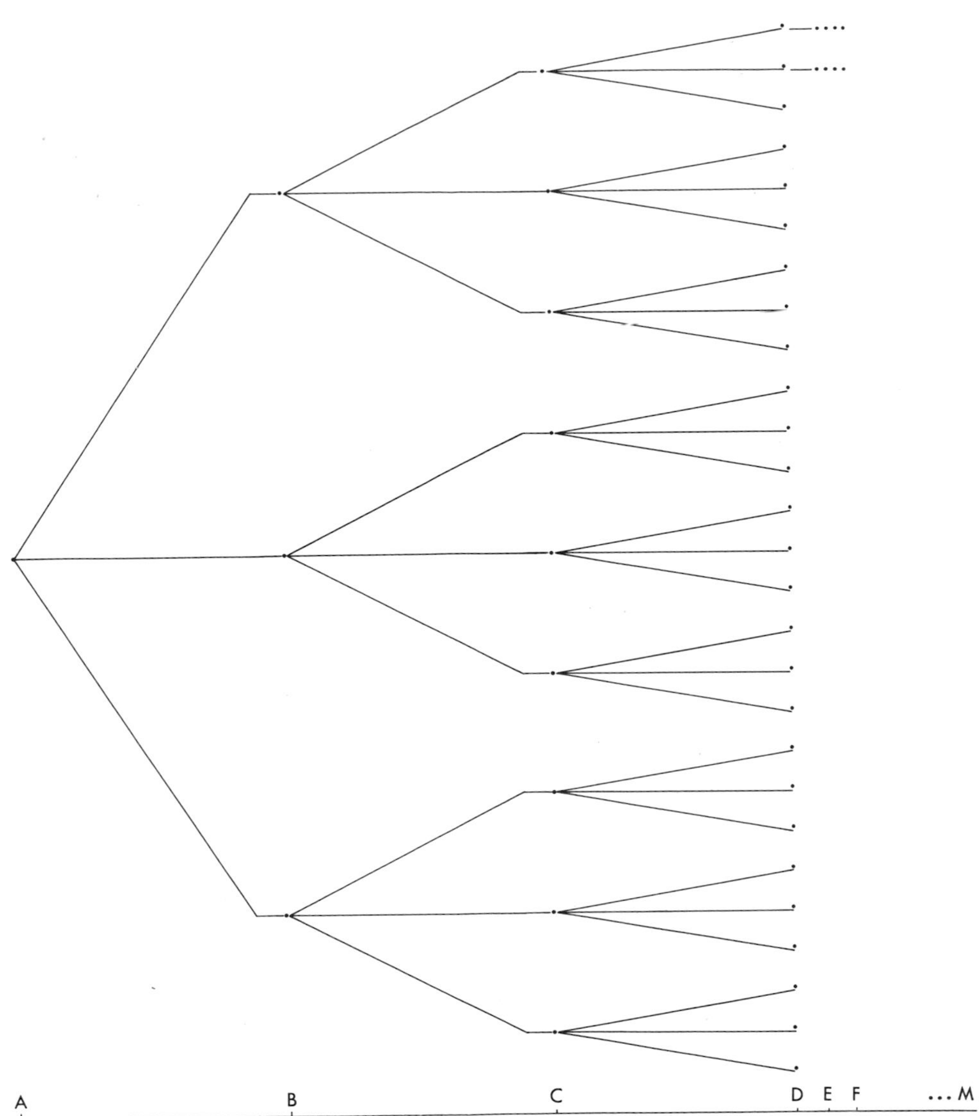

Figure 6.1 Branching routes from a point on A to a point on M.

350 times as much work as is necessary going one way from A to *M*. Working from both "ends" of the problem cuts the number of operations to roughly the square root of the original number required. Trying to go backwards from the goal may seem a little strange when the goal is the solution to a problem, so perhaps a concrete example will clarify matters. Suppose the goal is to land an operating instrument package on Mars. One way of approaching the problem is like going in one direction from A to *M*, searching all the branches: try all possible means of getting close to Mars, using all possible speeds and all known vehicles in all possible combinations, and see which one works. The second strategy considers *both ends* of the problem: to land operable instruments safely on Mars, we either must have the instrument package landing very slowly and softly, or we must build it tough enough to withstand the shock of a hard landing (branching alternatives). If we want a slow landing, we can use either parachutes or retro-rockets. If we use large parachutes, . . . and so forth. Here we are going backwards from the proposed landing on Mars, hoping to connect it with one of the alternative "paths" of search from Earth.

This theme can be pushed further. Suppose two intermediate subgoals happen to be known, at stages *E* and *I*. (In the Mars example, these might be "vehicle orbiting around Earth" and "vehicle orbiting around Mars.") There are now six search "trees," each two stages long, with nine branches in each tree. The whole process of finding a route from A to *M* now requires the testing of 6×3^2, or 54, routes. The method of working both ways, and of using subgoals, has cut the work to about $1/_{10{,}000}$ of what it was. The same principle applies regardless of the number of stages and branches, and regardless of whether the problem is a practical or a theoretical one. Newell *et al.* (1963), for example, discovered that the most efficient way to prove a theorem (finding an intellectual route connecting the axioms and known results at one end with the theorem at the other) is *not* to search deductively from axioms to theorem, going in the direction of the proof, but to search backwards from the theorem for any set of axioms and prior results that will justify it. What seems like the "natural" method, from axioms to theorem, they remark, is like looking for the needle in a haystack. The "reversed" method is like shaking a haystack and watching for the needle to fall out. These examples show the immensity of the range between efficient and inefficient methods of search by "trial and error." In the past, "search" has been judged usually in its most inefficient forms and has been found wanting as a method. But it can be very powerful when used efficiently.

Returning now to genius, we see that where there are many possibilities to be tried, searching extensively (working hard) will not accomplish much without searching efficiently. Presumably, the classic geniuses must have had remarkably efficient methods of search. This is the same, in essence, as saying they had remarkable *skills*. The question of how this efficiency of method comes about is precisely the same as that of how geniuses come to process more information than other people do. Nobody knows for sure. If we accept appropriate selection in high degree as the mark of genius, it is reasonable to believe that achievement of the high degree may be due to a basically better *method* of selection. Methods, of course, can be learned, but only after the information has come which would show the young aspirant the *better* ways to achieve appropriate selection. Life is usually too short for so extensive a study to be pursued by trial and error alone, and it seems likely that most geniuses who use better than ordinary methods for processing their information, do so for genetic or accidental, rather than for personally tested, reasons.

Genetics and genius. As indicated in Chapter 2, it is quite clear that genetic factors are critically important in intelligence, though much more is known about their contribution to intellectual defects than to parallel accomplishments. It seems quite clear, however, that genetic factors are also important in some kinds of favorably exceptional intellectual performance. The most dramatic illustration of this comes from so-called *idiots savants* (clever idiots), otherwise undistinguished, even feeble-minded people who can perform certain narrow intellectual tasks prodigiously well. Arithmetic abilities and feats of memory are the most common talents these people manifest, such as being able to do enormous long divisions or multiplications in their heads almost instantly or being able to recite exactly what day of the week January 23 fell on 100 years ago. Were it not for the narrowness and social uselessness of their skills, *idiots savants* would almost have to be called geniuses. The point to notice, in any case, is that some kind of genetic factor is the most reasonable explanation of their extreme skill. Since intelligence seems so clearly to be polygenically determined (see Chapter 2), it is quite plausible that either specific intellectually valuable information-processing methods or a predisposition to practice certain narrow tasks continually, both equivalent in their aid of exceptional performance, be inborn.

In a generally more positive vein, it is also well known that many of the classic geniuses appear at least to have had some similar genetically determined "methods." Many great writers had remarkable memories, among them Coleridge, Shelley, Goethe, and Freud. Here though, as in the case of the *idiot savant*, we must be careful not to go too far from the facts in thinking these talents are "inborn," for we have no assurance that practice did not also play an important part; but the fact of genetic differences among people is so clear that it would be unreasonable to say that the classic geniuses enjoyed *no* genetic advantages over their fellows. Furthermore, as Galton first showed, not only are many outstanding persons related, but often the talent within families is a rather specific one. The Bach family was active in music almost to the complete exclusion of other fields for at least seven generations; this is difficult to explain on grounds other than the genetic, even if we make allowances for family tradition and other cultural expectations (Brain, 1960).

The interesting question of what these very helpful inborn methods *are*, and how

Table 6.1
Estimated IQ's of Some Famous People[1]

Sir Francis Galton	200
John Stuart Mill	190
Johann W. von Goethe	185
Samuel Taylor Coleridge	175
Voltaire	170
Alexander Pope	160
William Pitt	160
Lord Tennyson	155
Sir Walter Scott	150
Mozart	150
Longfellow	150
Victor Hugo	150
Lord Byron	150
Thomas Jefferson	145
John Milton	145
Benjamin Franklin	145
Disraeli	145
Francis Bacon	145
James Watt	140
Rubens	140
Alexander Dumas	140
Napoleon Bonaparte	135
Charles Darwin	135
John Calvin	135
Edmund Burke	135

[1] As adapted from Catherine Morris Cox, *The Early Mental Traits of Three Hundred Geniuses,* Volume II, *Genetic Studies of Genius* with permission of the publishers (Stanford: Stanford University Press, 1926) by Norman Munn, in *Psychology: The Fundamentals of Human Adjustment*, Ed. 5 (Boston: Houghton Mifflin Company, 1966).

they are accomplished in the nervous system, must be left to future investigation, but we can make some plausible guesses about some kinds of genius, such as the composer of music. If we assume that music functions to arouse emotion, then someone in whom musical sounds evoke strong *feelings* may be peculiarly well endowed to "understand" music. If in addition, his own feelings can similarly arouse in him images of sounds, even an ordinary emotional life will provide him a rich source of sound variations. Assuming that he has a good ear for discriminating them and a good memory for reproducing them then, provided he gets good training, he can select efficiently among these many variations by exercising his emotional understanding of sounds in a critical way. Here we have at least the beginnings of musical genius.

The evidence from pedigree studies is not clearly on the side of inborn genius in all cases. Michaelangelo and Newton, in fact are two classic geniuses whose family backgrounds are totally unpredictive of either the direction of their interests or the height of their achievements. This does not rule out genetic factors, of course, but it does show that genetic "aids" can be subtle, and it suggests that environment may be of greater importance for the development of genius than is ordinarily assumed. But whether genotype or learning is critical to the faculties that a genius must have, there is no doubt that disciplined effort is critical to their expression. Whatever else may have been true of the physical or cultural backgrounds of the classical geniuses, what seems most characteristic is their profound dedication to their chosen fields of work.

Planning for Genius

Thus far, we have used the ideas and language of information theory to clarify the concept of genius, and have concluded from it that genius means a very high degree of appropriate selection in whatever area of achievement we are examining. If this is correct, we should be able to predict and perhaps control the occurrence of genius to a greater degree than ever before. Let us think of ourselves now as educators and consider what we need to do in order to plan for genius.

The first thing, of course, is to define concretely what it is we want to achieve (Sommerhoff, 1950). The need to do so might seem obvious, but there is actually some confusion of goals among educators; it is reflected in all the *nonspecific* goals that get specified as the aims of American education—like "originality," "creativity," or even "genius" itself. In such instances, society's real decision about what is original, creative, and ingenious is only made after the fact of accomplishment. You can only plan for facts, not after-the-facts; goals must therefore be specific accomplishments. If society cannot say what it wants, educators cannot plan to satisfy its wants.

In most respects, however, it is not hard to see what specific accomplishments would serve the interests of society and probably also be judged creative, original, and ingenious, and although these goals may in practice be difficult to achieve, their importance in theory is simple. Society wants, say, a solution to Fermat's Last Theorem, a symphony that would be more popular than Beethoven's Ninth, an efficient means of space travel, and so forth. These goals are clear and we can easily establish criteria to judge whether they have been achieved. The goals are not abstractions, however, anymore than are the criteria for judging them, and this is as it should be. The educator who says he wants to develop originality has probably not thought about the extremely original but useless productions of mental patients because it is not really originality that interests him, but selectivity. Educators train people in selectivity and discrimination rather than in the production of novelty as such.

Planning for genius starts with the definition of goals, but goals by themselves do not spell out the technology that is needed to achieve them. For this, the same general rules apply whether one is fostering genius in American children, in aborigines, or in a computer because the processes of selection, no matter how embodied, are bound by the same basic laws. The laws are stated accurately only in mathematical formulations, but as we have seen, they reduce to the need to process a large amount of information with relatively high efficiency. In the practical terms of education, this means *hard work* and *careful teaching*.

With the goal sufficiently well defined, nothing remains but work and luck (the unknown contributions of genetics, environment, and accident). The quantity of information implied by the total required acts of selection must be processed. Information that already exists must be absorbed; information that is lacking must be acquired. How it may be acquired is itself a selection problem to which the same laws apply again. Experimentation, which is basically trial and error, will probably be used to obtain the missing information for new problems.

Selection of the really rare demands processing of large quantities of information. A machine can work as long as it is plugged in, but a human being will process a lot of information about one topic only if he is strongly motivated and is obsessed, in the strict sense, by the topic. The use of all possible emotional and intellectual spurs is essential if the production of genius is to be pressed. Thus the second general rule, which follows definition of goals, is that the system, whether a computer or a child, must be taught to process the largest possible quantity of relevant information. Doing so requires efficient processing, and choosing the efficient method is itself an act of selection. If the subject or problem is really new, not only will the answer be unknown but also the method of investigation.

When all the specific useful training goals are totalled, it is clear that society needs a regular supply of geniuses rather than just occasional ones. At least, it constantly needs a large supply of *very* skilled people. Can this supply be assured? In a society such as ours, committed to letting people live largely as they choose, there probably is no *efficient* way of assuring the supply without restricting individual freedom. The only good alternative to controlling career choices, however, may be its virtual opposite: allowing the greatest possible freedom of education and career choice and the greatest possible opportunity to pursue them. This "method" assumes that society's benevolent indifferences, the accidents of heredity, and the individual's desires for achievement will somehow combine to produce the required number of skilled people. This is much the system we have now, in principle, but a great deal more needs to be done with it. Because our society is committed to individuals, the production of genius must be supported by the encouragement of individual efforts and by example, exhortation, and incentive.

The price of genius. As we have seen, the mechanics for fostering genius are: (1) defining the goal, (2) focusing the attention of as many children as possible, at the earliest age possible, on some subject. Let them work on the subject with the utmost intensity and with no time-wasting distractions. Some will probably come out geniuses. Of course, they may at the same time come out wrecks, for we are not dealing with hardware, and the artless application of these mechanics might lead to severe personality disorders like negativism or obsession, bizarre behavior, and perhaps even suicide. A discussion of the need for genius and how to plan for it must be balanced by a concern with the price that may be paid for genius.

As soon as one foregoes the romantic way of thinking about genius, he will discover that the classic geniuses were often unbalanced, narrow in their specilizations, and by definition, abnormal. Obviously, when we are using all our efforts to do one thing, we cannot be doing something else too, suggesting that the maximal use of one capacity must necessarily deprive other capacities of fulfillment. A price must be paid for genius, and the skill of the educator who fosters it is shown by how well he brings genius and its price into a suitable balance.

Seen in perspective, this is an interesting question from the point of view both of the individuals affected and of those interested in enhancing talent and its better use in society. There are two distinguishable installment payments involved in the price of genius: the cost of *becoming* a genius, and the cost of *being* a (recognized) genius. The first cost is that of exploiting an ability to the fullest; it means sacrificing other abilities. The second cost is the loss of social invisibility which comes with any abnormality, positive or negative (see Chapter 5). Neither of these costs are *necessarily* painful to the individual or to society.

In becoming distinguished men, for example, both Newton and Michelangelo showed an early inclination to concentrate on *their* interests and neglect other things, such as friends. The later lives of both men retained this reclusive air, but we should not jump to the conclusion that they were unhappy because of their lack of friends. It is difficult to tell how Newton felt about it; his solitary habits make him the despair of biographers. For Michelangelo though, we have more information; he said, "I have no friends of any kind, nor do I wish any, and I have not so much time that I can afford to waste it" (Clements, 1963, p. 114). *Was* Michelangelo unhappy because of the time he spent on his work? His letters do not sound as though they were written by an especially cheerful man, nor is his art gay and light. But this is no reason to think that he was a bitter, depressed, or wretched person either. If anything, it is probable, first of all, that Michelangelo did not value personal happiness as a glorious reason for being, if he ever thought about it at all and, secondly, that he was most genuinely happy when he was working. In any case, is it probable that he would have been happier as a merchant, a soldier, or an entertainer? The science of personality has not advanced to the point where we could answer these questions confidently even if the facts were clear. In speculating, though, we should remember that these intelligent men may have been doing what they preferred to do. It takes about ten years of playing tennis, some four to six hours a day, to build a championship game. The champion may realize that he has left many other things undone and may regret their omission, but he may be prouder still of the skill he has so laboriously developed. It is not stretching the imagination too far to think that Newton and Michelangelo may have made similar judgments.

This is not to say, on the other hand, that in exercising his talents the budding genius is happy with himself and a joy to those around him. Young Michelangelo's interests were a disappointment to his father, sculpting being then, as now, a socially suspect profession. Later on, his sarcastic speech and patronizing airs so enraged a fellow art student that the youth assaulted Michelangelo and broke his nose. Of Isaac Barrow, Newton's teacher and himself a distinguished intellect, it is said: "Endowed with a restless body and a vivid mind, he so plagued his teachers and was so troublesome at home that his father . . . prayed that if it pleased God to take away any of his children, he could best spare Isaac" (Moore, 1924, p. 3).

So it appears reasonable to guess that a young genius-to-be does not necessarily feel that the sacrifices he makes on behalf of his interests, while possibly dismaying his elders and drawing the ire and ridicule of his fellows, are unreasonably hurtful. The unhappiness of some geniuses, like Vincent Van Gogh, the Dutch painter who killed himself, writer Edgar Allen Poe, an alcoholic, and others, may be not so much the price of genius as the result of mismanaged lives. Such men as Charles Darwin, Albert Einstein, and Dante, after all, seem to have led relatively ordinary lives.

What about the cost of recognition itself? The unrecognized genius pays only the price of exercising his talent—and, if he has ambitions of eminence, of being unrecognized. The favorable recognition that is accorded positive abnormality has its price as well as its reward, but the subjective cost varies with the man. Michelangelo found fame could be vexing: "I am solicited so much that I can't take time out to eat" and again, "I cannot live under pressures from patrons, far less paint" (Clements, 1963, pp. 22, 19). On the other hand, Leonardo da Vinci, his contemporary and a man of wide accomplishment and decidedly different temperament, was apparently quite comfortable as a recognized genius. And Newton, exalted during his time as few men of intellect have ever been, moved without apparent regret from his university position into high public office.

The price of genius must be paid, but its costs to the man and to society depend on their peculiarities and cannot be predicted in any general way.

The limits of genius. Even a genius cannot do everything. As we saw in the previous section, his concentration on one activity necessarily detracts from the attention he can pay others. The question then arises as to just how much anyone, even a genius, *can* accomplish in his lifetime. Obviously, there must be some physical limit to what he can do without supernatural aid, despite the vague idea some people have that genius implies unlimited potential.

There is a very fundamental limit indeed. Using the ideas of information theory, the question of the genius's potential becomes one of how much information he can process. Bremermann (1962) has recently demonstrated that there is an absolute limit to what anything made of matter, whether mechanical, electronic, or neuronic, can do as a processor of information. The essentially simple argument goes as follows: Suppose a lump of matter is to compute, select, or otherwise process information. To do this, it must use energy, and its various energy states are represented by the various symbols involved in the computation. A light bulb, for example, might take on various brightnesses, each intensity of brightness being represented by a number or a letter. Because the process is taking place in matter, two physical laws can be used to give an upper limit to what happens. The first is Einstein's famous $E = MC^2$, which specifies the total amount of energy available if any given mass is totally transformed into energy. The process we are considering is therefore limited to the amount of energy that can be made available for it. The second physical law is the Heisenberg uncertainty principle, which sets a limit to how small the differences between energy levels can be and yet be detected at a given rate: very small differences cannot be detected very fast. Since the energy levels being used must be distinguishable from each other if each signals different information, the process is limited by this consideration as well. Putting the two laws together, it seems that the maximum rate at which each gram of matter can process information is 1.5×10^{47} bits per second. This number—15 followed by 46 zeroes—is called Bremermann's limit. Matter simply cannot handle information at a faster rate. It is a generous limit too, since it assumes that matter is entirely converted into energy than that the information is processed by a maximally efficient process.

Two facts here are especially worth notice. One is that Bremermann's limit rests on two of the most fundamental things known about matter, which suggests that it is quite dependable. The other is that although 10^{47} may at first seem a large number, it is extremely small if we consider the demands commonly made by problems in advanced information processing. For example, a thorough study of the game of chess would demand about 10^{1000} bits, with about 10^{150} being the lowest possible estimate. Using Bremermann's limit, if we were to assume that the whole earth, including its living matter, became one maximally efficient computer and that it were to work through all of geological time, it still could not process more than about 10^{73} bits—a negligible fraction of what the game actually requires. Thus no machine, and presumably no brain made of ordinary matter, can ever achieve a complete mastery of the game of chess. The practical attempt to foster genius should always include a quantitative estimate of its aims to give some assurance that it is not attempting the impossible.

The Imitation of Genius

This section might facetiously be titled "How To Be a Genius." Most readers of this chapter should be clearheaded enough to have some realistic idea of their chances of becoming true geniuses. In case of doubt, you could begin evaluating your possibilities by asking, "What do I spend most of my time doing?" If the lives of the classic geniuses are my guide, your answer will give some idea of the activities in which you have a chance of becoming proficient. Evidently, it is settled by early adulthood whether a person is interested in becoming a genius.

Most of us, of course, will not be geniuses, or close to it. But we can still improve our powers of appropriate selection and doing so can contribute very practically to our ability to perform well and to solve problems of all kinds. The title of this section is given humorously, but the content is not.

The first step in the solution of a problem is to *identify* it, that is to set up an explicit goal. The word *explicit* is important. The goal should be clear and accurate, and it should be *written down*. This avoids the easy vagueness about a goal that makes purposeful action toward it all but impossible.

Suppose you are faced with the examination question, "Discuss the fall of the Roman Empire." Surprising as it may seem at first, this is *not* the statement of *your goal*. This statement sets out what might be called the problem *area*. After all, there are scores of possible discussions of this topic. Your job is not to produce *all* these discussions, but to produce only *one* of them. The question is: Which? The immediate problem is to decide more exactly what *your* discussion is to be. A good way to begin is to examine the statement of the problem area one word at a time, using a sort of "free association" technique. Take the word "discuss." In the context of this particular course and this particular examination, does this word mean a ten- or a fifty-minute effort? Does it mean an emphasis on politics or on sociology? Will the instructor accept discussions in outline form? Should it be a discussion on the level that a high school senior would be able to follow, or should it be addressed to professional historians? Should the discussion be "open-end" or should it come to a definite conclusion? And so forth. Some of the answers to these questions make use of your knowledge of the historical facts. The answer to the question whether the discussion should have a "definite conclusion," for example, will depend on your evaluation of the factors involved in the fall of the Empire and perhaps of what the instructor's evaluation is. Notice that these questions are already starting a search leading "backwards," an important reason for using this technique.

Having tentatively answered your questions about the first word and having quickly written down these conclusions, you are ready for the next word: *the. The* fall? Was there only one fall, or were there several falls? Was there one *kind* of fall, or several kinds? And so forth. The next word is *fall.* Your "free" association to this word might go something as follows. If something falls it must have been "up" somewhere. In what sense was the Roman Empire "up?" If something falls, it may fall because it was pushed off a resting place. Does this apply to the Empire? Was it "pushed"? By what? Did it indeed have a resting place where it would have remained if the push had not come along? Or was the fall inevitable? And so forth.

This should give some idea of the process. Once the goal is set out in detail, nothing remains but to move toward it. But many students try to skip the important step of first defining the goal and instead try to answer the exam question by immediately writing down everything that comes to mind in connection with the problem area. In our experience, most students would do better if they used perhaps one fourth of their examination time defining the goal. This applies particularly to essay examinations.

On the other hand, there are situations in which the goal is given to you in a well-defined form and you just need to get there. In such cases, one can immediately begin "working from both ends." Even here though, some redefining of the goal may be helpful. For example, suppose the problem is, "Design a bridge to span a river 138 feet wide." An engineer might reach immediately for his slide rule to figure out a solution that uses cantilever spans. But he might have asked himself if a single rope held by a man on each bank would suffice. It is often good policy, even when the goal *seems* well defined, to go through a few of the steps of goal definition outlined above.

Time spent studying the goal is seldom wasted. Occasionally, it can lead to a dramatically helpful redefinition of the goal; in any case, it is vital to the "working backwards" search procedure which *should be used as a matter of routine.* (The interested reader might want to refer to Polya's writing (1945) on this topic.)

Before we leave the subject, we should consider two final points. First, originality *does* have a place in problem solution. In the search phase of problem solution, whether we are searching forwards or backward, originality is quite important to ensure that the search branches at each step are not unnecessarily restricted by prior expectations and habit; otherwise, possibly fruitful leads may go unexamined. How can originality be stimulated? The next time you have a difficult problem, try this. After you have defined the goal, try to unhinge your usual disciplined cast of thought. Try to think of the "wildest" solutions, or partial solutions, you can. Write these down without evaluating them in any way. When you have ten or fifteen of these uncensored attempts to solve the problem, *then* go back over them and pick out those that might be useful either to solve the problem outright, to get you closer to a solution, or to suggest subgoals or new goal definitions. This frame of mind was implicitly suggested in the discussion of setting up the goal, which is a problem in its own right and therefore uses the same general strategy as the main problem. You might recognize these suggestions for aiding originality as the technique of "brainstorming." The only difference is that brainstorming usually involves a group of people. There is no reason, however, why individuals cannot use it equally well, especially where its main value lies in keeping the task of producing originality separate from the task of selection.

Selectivity is our final point. Once a route from start to goal is found, it should be checked routinely to make sure it is a workable solution. As computer programmers put it, the final step in problem solution is "de-bugging." This phase should be expected and planned for: the column of figures should be added again; the essay should be reread; a model of the bridge should be built and tested. One does, of course, select during the search phase too; selection in the sense of checking should not be left to the end. However, even if great care is taken in selecting the intermediate steps, what may appear to be best there may not be best in the context of the final solution; therefore, the final solution itself must be scrutinized. This is particularly true when the problem is a new one.

The genius helps his own work by becoming familiar with a variety of similar problems, so that in many cases the "new" problem is to him really new only in minor details. He then appears to select the correct route at each step as if by magic. Actually, he has often made the selection in previous trial-and-error attempts with similar problems.

We end our discussion of genius with this postscript: this chapter is intended to provide a basis for both realistic appraisal and appreciation of exceptional intellectual accomplishment. The aim is not to "debunk" the classic geniuses or to disparage what they have done. On the contrary, the object is to indicate clearly what they *have* done. Many of the myths that need correction are things that have been said about genius by adoring but unappreciative people. The subject has long been obscured by the thought that the genius is an agent of the supernatural. Far from reflecting credit on the man, this judgment honors only the powers he is assumed to serve. A realistic understanding of genius is important; the world has not yet seen the end of accomplishment or of the need for it.

SUMMARY

The idea that the genius achieves what he does by exercising something like supernatural powers is very common and appealing. Recent work by scientists in several areas suggests that this idea is misleading and unnecessary and that the productions of genius may come about through the operation of ordinary processes. Two other common ideas about the nature of genius are that originality is its distinguishing mark and that it is obvious in any given case. Both of these ideas are likewise misleading. (1) Originality by itself is not crucial to genius. A machine, for example, can be original. In fact, the judgment of what is truly original depends entirely on the observer, not on the performer, which is why we can conclude that a machine, an animal, or anything else, *can* show originality. (2) The role of the observer is also important in deciding whether any particular performance is outstanding. In some cases, remarkable performances can come about without the performer's deliberately contributing anything very noteworthy at all. Even when it is clear that the performer's talent is involved, moreover, his performance may be over- or underrated, depending upon circumstances beyond his own control, such as the eccentricities by which an observer exercises his preferences. Since the term *genius* generally implies that a person's performance is outstanding, and since this judgment is so difficult to make, it is not at all self-evident who is and who is not a genius.

One factor that appears to lie at the heart of the subject of genius is *selectivity*. In large part, genius can be identified with a person's exceptional powers of appropriate selection. By "appropriate selection" we mean a selection that attains some defined goal. In judging the *appropriateness* of the selection, it is important to keep in mind that the goal should be specified in advance of the performance. If the goal comes into being after the performance is done, then there is no way of knowing whether the performance was selected sensibly (that is, ingeniously) or whether it occurred at random and just happened to serve some purpose.

Processes which involve appropriate selection can be helpfully described with the use of *information theory*. For such processes, information theory proposes a simple but important law: the more difficult the goal, the more work is required to attain it. This law in turn suggests that the classic geniuses were hard workers, and even a superficial acquaintance with their lives would seem to bear out this suggestion.

The classic geniuses probably did not rely on simple-minded kinds of trial-and-error searches to find the solutions to their problems. Although trial and error played a preeminent role in their work, they undoubtedly also used better than average *methods* of search. We are only now beginning to understand what the better methods are and why they are better.

In planning for genius, the first thing the educator must do is define as concretely as possible what is to be achieved. He must avoid vague goals, such as producing "well-educated" people. Such a term might well describe the finished product, but it does not greatly help to specify what is to be done in producing it. After the goals are defined, the next step is to so treat the system, be it a computer or a child, that the greatest possible quantity of relevant information is processed. The educator must also consider that requiring intensive concentration on the necessary activities may have some undesirable side effects, as the recognition of genius may also have. Such side effects, in many cases, are part of the cost of being (or being considered) a genius. They are not necessarily destructive, however, the genius is ordinarily *not* a madman.

Despite the vague idea some people have that the genius has unlimited potential, Bremermann's limit sets a bound on the amount of information that anything made of ordinary matter can process. As even the genius has only his brain and his tools to work with, he too can process only a limited amount of information. That the genius can do what he does despite these fundamental limitations makes his accomplishments all the more impressive.

GLOSSARY

ARTIFICIAL INTELLIGENCE—the "intelligent capacities" of man-made things, which are studied in an effort to understand genius.

ASHBY'S LAW OF REQUISITE VARIETY—see SHANNON'S TENTH THEOREM.

AUTOMATA THEORY—the mathematical study of the behavior of robots.

BIOGRAPHY STUDY METHOD—the method of studying genius by investigating the family trees of eminent men.

BIT—see information bit.

BRAINSTORMING—the use of "free association" to discover "wild" and "far out" solutions to a problem in order to produce useful and original alternative solutions.

BREMERMANN'S LIMIT—a law stating an absolute limit to the amount of information that can be processed at any given time (1.5×10^{47} bits per second by one gram of matter).

DISCRIMINATION—the process of detecting differences in objects.

EFFICIENCY (of information handling)—the skill involved in the use of a particular method for eliminating alternative solutions to a problem.

EXPLICIT GOAL DEFINITION—the exact identification of the problem for which a solution is required.

GENIUS—a person exhibiting creative or innovative ability of the highest order.

GENOTYPE—the sum total of the inherited characteristics of an individual (see Chapter 2).

IDIOT SAVANT (clever idiot)—a person of apparently low intelligence who can nevertheless perform certain narrow intellectual tasks, such as arithmetic computations, prodigiously well.

INFORMATION "BIT"—the unit of measure of amount of information; technically, the knowledge obtained by the removal of one-half of the possible solutions to a problem; thus, if there are only two alternative answers to a question, (such as "yes" or "no") the answer is said to contain one "bit" of information.

INFORMATION PROCESSING—the utilization of information, for example, the process of eliminating alternative solutions to a problem.

INFORMATION THEORY—a statistical means of counting and comparing alternatives in order to determine causes and effects.

IQ (INTELLIGENCE QUOTIENT)—the relation, expressed as a number, between a score obtained on a test designed to measure intelligence, and a person's chronological age.

NEURON—the individual nerve cell that is the fundamental unit of nerve transmission.

OBSESSION—an irrational, repetitive thought (see Chapter 10).

ORIGINALITY—an ability to produce something that has not been observed previously.

PEDIGREE STUDY—the method of studying family backgrounds to determine genetic causality.

SELECTIVITY—the ability to eliminate the relatively useless, and to locate the more useful, alternative solutions to a problem.

SELF-CONSISTENCY—the quality of having each element appropriately related to the other elements in a series.

SHANNON'S TENTH THEOREM—a mathematical statement about information processing that describes the selection of correct alternatives (and the rejection of faulty ones) in the course of solving a problem; it suggests that if the goal is difficult, one needs to do considerable work to attain it.

TRIAL AND ERROR—the method of problem solving that discards various alternative solutions until the proper one is found.

REFERENCES

Ashby, W. R. *An introduction to cybernetics.* New York: John Wiley & Sons, Inc., 1963.

Brain, R. *Some reflections on genius.* Philadelphia: J. B. Lippincott Company, 1960.

Bremermann, H. J. Optimization through evolution and recombination. In M. C. Yovits, G. T. Jacobi, and G. D. Goldstein (eds.), *Self-organizing systems 1962.* Washington, D.C.: Spartan Books, 1962, pp. 93–106.

Campbell, D. T. Blind variation and selective retention in creative thought as in other knowledge processes. *Psychological Review,* 1960, 67, 380–400.

Clements, R. J. *Michelangelo: A self-portrait.* Englewood Cliffs, N.J.: Prentice-Hall, Inc., 1963.

Dunnington, G. W. *Carl Friedrich Gauss: Titan of science.* New York: Exposition Press, Inc., 1955.

Galton, F. *Hereditary genius: An inquiry into its laws and consequences.* London: Macmillan & Co., Ltd., 1869.

Hulshard, E. *Little journeys to the homes of eminent painters.* New York: G. P. Putnam's Sons, 1899.

Life. April 15, 1966, pp. 93–116.

Moore, L. T. *Isaac Newton.* New York: Charles Scribner's Sons, 1924.

Newell, A., J. C. Shaw, and H. A. Simon. Empirical explorations with the logic theory machine: A case study in heuristics. In E. A. Feigenbaum and J. Feldman (eds.), *Computers and thought.* New York: McGraw-Hill, Inc., 1963.

Polya, F. *How to solve it.* Princeton, N.J.: Princeton University Press, 1945.

Shannon, C. E., and W. Weaver. *The mathematical theory of communication.* Urbana, Ill.: University of Illinois, 1959.

Sommerhoff, G. *Analytical biology*. New York: Oxford University Press, 1950.

Terman, L. M., *et al. Genetic studies of genius*. Vol. I. *Mental and physical traits of a thousand gifted children*. Stanford, Calif.: Stanford University Press, 1925.

SUGGESTED READINGS

1. Anastasi, Anne. *Differential psychology: Individual and group differences in behavior*. New York: Crowell-Collier and Macmillan, Inc., 1958, pp. 413–451. A presentation of several theories of genius—pathological, psychoanalytic, qualitative, and quantitative—and an evaluation of the relevant evidence bearing upon them. Attention is given to the methods for assessing genius and their relations to the various theories.
2. Galton, F. *Hereditary genius: An inquiry into its laws and consequences*. London: Macmillan & Co., Ltd., 1869. A classic treatise on eminence. Galton examines naturalistic data and demonstrates that the distribution of intelligence approximates the bell-shaped curve and that it is likely to be inherited.
3. Getzels, J. W., and P. W. Jackson. *Creativity and intelligence: Explorations with gifted students*. New York: John Wiley & Sons, Inc., 1962. An indication that, although intelligence is necessary for the development of creativity, other factors are also needed.
4. Gruber, H. E., G. Terrell, and M. Wertheimer. (eds.). *Contemporary approaches to creative thinking*. New York: Atherton Press, 1962. A symposium on the nature of creativity in a variety of contexts—among writers, physical scientists, philosophers, military men, and research workers.
5. Terman, L. M., and Melita H. Oden. In *Genetic studies of genius*, Vol. IV: *The gifted child grows up*. Stanford, Calif.: Stanford University Press, 1947. See comment with next entry.
6. Terman, L. M., and Melita H. Oden. In *Genetic studies of genius*, Vol. V: *The gifted group at mid-life*. Stanford, Calif.: Stanford University Press, 1959. Summaries of the researches of Lewis Terman and his associates into the origins, growth, and nurturing of genius that offer the best longitudinal data available on this problem.

7

Creativity

PHILIP W. JACKSON

SAMUEL MESSICK

The process by which ideas are born and new human products created is one of the most compelling topics within the purview of psychology. Indeed, long before the science of psychology existed, the mysteries of the creative act were the focus of speculation and wonder. It is impossible to present in a single chapter, or even in an entire book, the full history of thought with respect to the creative process. However, a brief summary of recent efforts to understand the sources and vicissitudes of creativity will be attempted here to provide the reader with a framework for viewing problems and progress in this field and to give him a background for the conception of creativity presented in this paper.

Parts of this paper appeared in an article entitled "The Person, the Product, and the Response: Conceptual Problems in the Assessment of Creativity," *Journal of Personality*, 1965, and are reprinted here with the kind permission of the editor of the journal and the Duke University Press. This work was partly supported by the National Institute of Mental Health, United States Public Health Service, under Research Grant M–4186.

RESEARCH EMPHASES IN THE STUDY OF CREATIVITY

Once Darwin had cast man in the perspective of his biological origins, systematic studies of creative excellence began to seek explanations of outstanding achievements less in terms of mystical inspiration, whether by the deity or the muse, and more in terms of naturalistic processes that could be captured in rational form. These attempts continued at a modest rate until suddenly, in the middle of this century, there was a dramatic upsurge of interest in the creative act and an explosion of empirical studies that over the past fifteen years have continuously altered the frontiers of our knowledge about the character of human invention. For purposes of a brief overview, research in creativity may be organized around six recurrent themes.

The Exceptionally Creative Person

Genius, as unusual creative ability is sometimes called, exists in every age, as do man's attempts to understand it. One of the earliest and best-known studies of outstanding persons was conducted by Francis Galton almost a century ago. As its title implies, Galton's *Hereditary Genius* (1870) expounds the thesis that there are genetic linkages among persons of unusual achievement in many different fields. He believed that the human race could be vastly improved through a program of artificial selection, and his studies of eminent men were undertaken in an effort to obtain support for this position. Although his work was influential when it first appeared, Galton's findings were marred by many methodological problems, which are described in Chapter 2. He completely ignored, for example, the contribution to eminence provided by advantaged environments and social privileges.

Rather than obtain superficial information about many famous people, as Galton did, some investigators have chosen to explore in depth the life history of a single person. One of the most famous of these case studies is Freud's *Leonardo da Vinci* (1948), in which the creative products of an adult are examined with reference to the childhood of the creator. Freud attempts to show how some of Leonardo's early experiences, particularly those with his mother, are mirrored in his most mature achievements, such as the famous *Mona Lisa*. The mystery of da Vinci's genius remains, but Freud's analysis enriches our understanding of how the personal history of the artist colors the content of his work.

Geniuses, by definition, are extremely rare. For the many reasons indicated in the preceding chapter they are also relatively inaccessible as subjects to students of the creative process. Accordingly, many investigators have turned to people whose talents, though unusual, are not of the rarest variety. In recent years, Anne Roe's studies of successful scientists (1952) provide a good example of this kind of research, as does MacKinnon's study of creative architects (1963). Roe (1952, 1953) asked groups of eminent biological, physical, and social scientists to give their family backgrounds and life histories and to submit to selected ability and projective tests. On the basis of these data, she concluded that successful scientists share several early background experiences that are important for their later development: they frequently came from families that placed a high value upon learning, for example, and were early exposed to demands for independence and to patterns of living that did not foster close personal ties. MacKinnon (1962, 1963) compared creative and noncreative architects on a wide variety of tasks and found the groups to differ on several dimensions of personality, interests, and values. In self-conception, for example, the creative architects described themselves as inventive, determined, independent, individualistic, enthusiastic, and industrious, while their less creative peers described themselves as responsible, sincere, reliable, dependable, clear thinking, tolerant, and understanding. The creative person, on the whole, appeared to be more open to experience from within and without and to exhibit a broad range of interests including many that are ordinarily considered feminine.

The Creative Process

The events that precede discovery have intrigued researchers for many years and continue to do so. In viewing the creative product as the end point of an evolutionary process, which may have taken anywhere from a few seconds to several years to unfold, many investigators have tried to describe the typical stages through which an idea passed on its way to being born. One of the best-known accounts of this gestation period is that of Wallas (1926), who argues that the formation of a thought could be divided into four characteristic stages: preparation, incubation, illumination, and verification. After outlining the typical life history of an idea, Wallas goes on to suggest practical ways by which thought processes might be consciously improved. In the same spirit as Chapter 6 (but for different contents) his suggestions treat the development of attitudes and work habits intended to increase the occurrence of seminal ideas and to capture them when they do appear.

A partial verification of Wallas' stages was provided by Patrick (1935, 1937), who studied the verbalizations of poets and artists as they produced poems and paintings under experimental conditions. Patrick also found that the thought processes of nonpoets and nonartists closely resembled those of the professional subjects, although, as might be expected, the products of the professionals were superior.

In recent years the act of discovery has been the focus of both empirical investigations and theoretical discourses. Bruner (1957, 1962), for example, has emphasized the importance of placing things in new perspectives—what he calls "combinatorial activity"—for producing "effective surprise," which he takes to be the hallmark of creativity. He particularly stresses the value of metaphorical combinations, in which diverse domains of experience are connected by symbol, metaphor, or image.

> Experience in literal terms is a categorizing, a placing in a syntax of concepts. Metaphoric combination leaps beyond systematic placement, explores connections that before were unsuspected. (1962, p. 6.)

Several other conceptions of creativity also stress this combinatorial basis. Mednick (1962), for example, defines creative thinking as "the forming of associative elements into new combinations which either meet specified requirements or are in some way useful." Koestler (1964), in one of the most ambitious theoretical analyses of recent years, views the creative act as the recognition of converging associations among previously unrelated dimensions of experience. He employs the term *bisociative* to describe the pattern of thought underlying creative synthesis. A classic example of this process is the well-known story of Archimedes' discovering that the volume of liquid displaced by an immersed object is equal to the volume of the object itself. The sudden conjoining of two lines of thought in Archimedes' mind—one having to do with the rise in level of bath water, the other having to do with the problem of calculating the volume of an irregularly shaped object—produced the shock of discovery that accompanies so many creative acts. Koestler elaborates on the details of this important process. A crucial part of his thesis, which is developed with great insight and clarity, grows out of his recognition that "discovery often means simply the uncovering of something which has always been there but was hidden from the eye by the blinkers of habit" (p. 108).

Creation and Mental Illness

For centuries a thin line between creativeness and madness has been noted, if not celebrated, in the single-minded absorption of the productive artist and the absent-minded disorganization of the "mad genius." The belief in the existence of a common basis for creative achievement and psychopathology was formalized near the turn of the century in Freud's sublimation theory of cultural evolution (1908, 1910, 1930). Freud held that creative products derived essentially from the resolution of neurotic conflicts over the expression of sexual desires. He invoked a mechanism called "sublimation" to describe the diversion of sexual impulses from sexual aims to new activities having social value. By means of this mechanism, he believed, the immense energy of the sexual instinct was diverted into creative activities, thereby spurring the cultural advancement of civilization. A classic model of this process, according to Freud, is the life and work of Leonardo da Vinci. In one of the most celebrated examples of psychoanalytic reasoning applied to a historical subject, Freud argues that the power of da Vinci's search for knowledge arose from the sublimation of his sexual interests.

Freud thus accounted for creative urges on largely negative grounds, as a by-product of defenses against the direct expression of unacceptable sexual wishes. This formulation was only halfheartedly embraced by other psychologists, however, many of whom felt that some kind of positive force was also necessary to account for creative strivings. Jung (1946), for example, talked about a "transcendent function" that governed the interaction of conscious and unconscious processes in the creative act and generally oriented the individual toward the realization of his potentialities. Kris (1952) held that although a gradual emergence from conflict plays a part in every process of creation, some conflict-free integrative powers are also required for creative communication. Goldstein (1939), Rogers (1959), and Maslow (1959) spoke of a drive or tendency toward "self-actualization" as the motivational basis for creative acts. Kubie (1958), and to some extent Schachtel (1959), felt that Freud's claim that creative products have neurotic roots is misleading. On the contrary, it is more likely the case that neurosis corrupts and distorts creativeness in every field. Indeed, to the extent that the artist is expressing a neurotic struggle, there is a danger that his product will convey primarily idiosyncratic meaning and thereby lose in social value.

The Growth of Creative Ability

Just as the creative act changes with time, the creative person does also. What happens to talented children? Do they become talented adults, or do their precocious abilities typically wither? Questions such as these require longitudinal studies, as indicated in Chapter 4. Clearly the most monumental of such studies is that begun in the late nineteen twenties by Lewis M. Terman (1925, 1930, 1947, 1954) and his associates. Terman's work, more than that of any other person, did much to destroy the myth of the inevitable decline of precocious talent. Indeed, the opposite was found. A thirty-year follow-up study of gifted children indicated that their initial superiority in physique, health, social adjustment, and moral character was generally maintained and that their early school achievement was matched by remarkable success in college and in their careers.

A different sort of developmental question, one that has become increasingly popular in recent years, concerns the gradual emergence of intellectual powers that might contribute to creative performance. How do cognitive processes evolve? Are children more imaginative than adults? How does the thinking of the very young differ from that of the mature adult? The work of Jean Piaget (1952, 1954; Flavell, 1963; Hunt, 1961) is most closely associated with questions of this type. Piaget's conceptions, derived from years of interviews with children, have done much to shape the form of research on human cognition. His observation, for example, that thinking processes develop through an invariant and universal sequence of stages highlights the need to evaluate even intellectual performance, let alone creative expression, in relation to the stage of cognitive organization.

Among recent work on developmental changes in creative ability, the studies of E. Paul Torrance (1962) and his students deserve special mention. Although he cautions against treating his data as normative, Torrance reports a drop in creative abilities at about the fourth grade level among the students he has tested. This decline is compensated for by later advances and does not show up on all tests of creative thinking. The ability to develop hypotheses about causality, for example, seems to improve steadily throughout the elementary school years.

Nurturing Creativity

To the extent that human abilities can change, the possibility of doing something to increase the likelihood of creative performance exists. Efforts towards this end are roughly of two kinds: First, there are attempts to encourage creative performance somewhat indirectly by providing a congenial environment for the creative person. Second, there are attempts to improve creative performance more directly and more systematically by providing training programs, "brainstorming" sessions, and the like.

Some of the earliest efforts to provide a conducive environment for creative performance are connected with the progressive education movement in this country, and they flow, in the main, from the writings of John Dewey. Hughes Mearns's (1925, 1929) descriptions of some of the experimental classes in the Lincoln School provide good examples of attempts to manipulate situational variables. In addition to using teaching methods that cut across the traditional subject-matter categories, Mearns and his fellow teachers tried to provide their students with rich opportunities for travel, a wide variety of extracurricular activities, and excellent reading materials. The outcome, as judged by Mearns's description of the students' work, was heightened creative expression for many youngsters.

More recently researchers have turned attention to aspects of the adult work environment that might be modified to increase creative production. Pelz (1963), for example, found that young scientists produced best when they acted closely with their administrative superiors but remained free to make their own decisions. Further examples are provided by Stein's analysis (1963) of research organizations that employ a high level professional staff. Organizations differ in their expectations of the researcher and in the institutional roles he must serve—scientist, professional, employee, and so forth—and these differences influence the opportunity for creative expression and, ultimately, the quality of the creative product.

Attempts to increase creative ability through direct training have become increasingly fashionable in certain industries, but the success of these efforts is more a matter of testimony than of empirical proof. There is some evidence (Maltzman, 1960) that performance on tests of originality or the production of uncommon responses increases after special kinds of training, but the meaning of such increases, in terms of the person's total creative potential, is difficult to ascertain.

General Creative Abilities

Studies of genius and persons of exceptional talent tend to leave the impression that creative abilities are dichotomously distributed, that the world is divided into the "haves" and the "have-nots." Yet, as should be quite clear from the preceding chapters, most human qualities are shared by most (if not all) people, so that possession becomes a matter of degree rather than of all or nothing. Many pioneering efforts in psychological measurement, such as those of James McK. Cattell and Alfred Binet, laid the groundwork for our present understanding of the distribution of intellectual abilities within the general population. Among present-day researchers, J. P. Guilford has probably done more than anyone to advance our knowledge of the complexity of human intellect and of the relation of creative abilities to the total range of human abilities. Guilford's factor analyses of aptitudes have led to the identification of several types of performance that are important for creative thinking. They have also led to the development of a model for the structure of intellect that points to several other cognitive abilities, as yet dimly understood, that are potentially of great relevance to creative production (Guilford, 1950, 1957, 1959, 1964).

THE CREATIVITY-INTELLIGENCE DISTINCTION

Although there are many ways to describe man's mental complexity—and particularly to depict his cognitive strengths—the two terms *intelligence* and *creativity* seem to have the greatest summary power. It is this concentration of meaning that explains the endurance of these two words in the layman's language and their continued use in professional discussions.

Typically, efforts to distinguish empirically between creativity and intelligence have concentrated on attempts to demonstrate that tests requiring the production of unusual responses involve somewhat different abilities than conventional tests of intelligence. But as Golann (1963) quite correctly points out in his review of studies of creativity,

> These data are in a sense arbitrary: intelligence is not performance on a test; creativity is more than test performance or being judged as creative. What is needed for the understanding of the relationship between creativity and intelligence is not only data at the correlational level, but conceptual reorganization as well. (P. 560.)

The controversy created by some of the recent research studies of creativity has focused attention on narrow, empirical aspects of the distinction between creativity and intelligence instead of on some of the unresolved conceptual problems. Consider, as an instance, the present practices for developing tests of creativity. In the main, intelligence has been measured by tests of vocabulary and quantitative reasoning, and creativity by tests of fluency and originality. The latter tests have been found to correlate only slightly with traditional IQ measures but to relate, instead, to several personal and social variables not typically associated with intelligence (Barron, 1955; Getzels and Jackson, 1962; Guilford, 1957; Mednick, 1962; Wallach and Kogan, 1965). Researchers have become excited, for example, over the fact that people who score high on these so-called tests of creativity also tend to make unconventional career choices or to possess an unusually well-developed sense of humor.

But just as knowledge of word meanings and ability to solve numerical problems hardly summarize the multiplicity of man's intellectual capabilities, neither does fluency in generating a number of distinct ideas or unusual responses capture anything but the barest bones of creative expression. The correlates of these sorts of performances are interesting, to be sure, but other tasks could readily be designed that would reveal abilities equally well described as "creative" yet associated with a quite different set of personal attributes. The problem, in other words, is not to design tests of *some* relevance to creative response; there are already many such tests, and in the execution of empirical studies selection among them is frequently arbitrary. Rather, the problem is to analyze the qualities of creative response in a way that would reveal the range of possible assessment techniques and their relevance, on conceptual grounds, to each other. Unfortunately, the intriguing results obtained with tests of fluency and originality have diverted our attention temporarily from the critical task of considering other criteria, in addition to the production of unusual responses, that are essential to creative behavior.

The exercise of cognitive powers often elicits evaluation. People are continually being informed that they have done well or poorly on intellectual tasks, and the variety of forms these judgments may take is almost as great as the variety of behaviors being judged. These evaluative comments can all be crudely classified, however, into two overlapping categories. On the one hand are judgments having to do with the "correctness" or "rightness" of a person's response. These evaluations deal with the degree to which certain objective and logical criteria have been satisfied. These criteria of correctness tend to be categorical: they usually admit only one answer, or a relatively restricted set of solutions, and regard all other responses as incorrect or in error. On the other hand are judgments having to do with the worth or "goodness" of a person's response. These evaluations deal with the degree to which certain subjective and psychological criteria have been satisfied. The criteria of goodness tend to be continuous: they admit a wide range of responses that vary in their degree of acceptability. Despite the overlap between these classes of evaluation, the two are nonetheless distinguishable, and the distinction between them has important implications for the conceptual separation of intelligent and creative responses.

In the simplest terms, the adjectives *correct* and *good* apply differentially to *intelligent* and *creative* performances. Intelligent responses are correct; they satisfy objective criteria; they operate within the constraints of logic and reality and thus may be considered right or wrong, true or false. Creative responses, in contrast, are "good"; they satisfy subjective criteria. Although they may not necessarily be limited by the demands of logic and reality, they are subject, as we shall point out, to a variety of judgmental standards. But always, as we assess a response's creativeness or "goodness," we are aware of the humanness required to make the judgment. As Santayana (1896) puts it,

> For the existence of good in any form it is not merely consciousness but emotional consciousness that is needed. Observation will not do, appreciation is required. (P. 16.)

And only man, not machine, is capable of appreciation.

The distinction made here between the correct and the good is contained, at least implicitly, in many other discussions of the creative process. Guilford (1957), for one, is particularly aware of it when he says,

> There are different bases or criteria by which a product is judged. One is its logical consistency with known facts. Another is its less-than-logical consistency with other experiences. (P. 116.)

Guilford goes on to imply that logical criteria are applied primarily to scientific products whereas artistic products are evaluated by less-than-logical standards. In the present distinction no such separation between the evaluation of scientific and artistic products is implied. A piano solo may be as incorrect as the solution to a mathematical equation. A scientific theory may be as good as a great novel. The poet's attempt to write a Spencerian sonnet may be both incorrect and poor, as may the engineer's design for a bridge.

In many of the tests currently proposed to assess creative ability, the failure to differentiate between correct responses and good responses leads to unnecessary confounding. Take as an instance the Remote Association Test developed by Mednick (1962). A typical item from this test presents three words, such as *rat, blue,* and *cottage,* and requires the subject to supply a fourth word as a kind of associational link between them. For the example given, the answer is *cheese.* The designer of the test argues that this answer reflects a degree of creativity because it is "remote" and because it is "useful," at least in the sense of meeting specified requirements. We would suggest that the answer reflects an aspect of intelligence because it is correct. To illustrate his point further, Mednick maintains that the answer 7,363,474 to the question, "How much is 12 and 12?" is original but not creative because it is not useful. What seems more important, however, is not that the answer lacks usefulness, but that in the absence of a formal system to justify it, it is wrong. As we use the term, there are no creative answers to the question, "How much is 12 and 12?" The constraints of reality implied in the question only allow for correct or incorrect responses.

Mednick introduces the concept of usefulness because he realizes, as do most researchers in this field (and as you learned in detail in Chapter 6), that the criterion of unusualness or originality is not enough. This quality, as Guilford has shown, takes us beyond the confines of correctness in evaluating cognitive performance, but it is, at best, a first step in trying to understand the good.

CREATIVE RESPONSES AND APPRECIATIVE REACTIONS

Frequency and Fit

No matter what other positive qualities a response might possess, we generally insist that it at least be novel before we are willing to call it creative. Indeed, the conjoining of novelty and creativeness is so deeply ingrained in our thinking that the terms are sometimes treated as synonymous. As a result, novelty is often used as the most common and sometimes the only measure of creativeness.

A two-step operation is required to apply the criterion of unusualness: first, a comparison of the product in question with other products of the same class, and second, a counting of those comparisons yielding similar or identical products. Further, in order to be consistent in the use of these relative frequencies, some standard must be set by which to determine how few is few.

The collection of objects with which the judged object is compared also requires definition. Typically the judgment of unusualness is not made in terms of *all* other objects of a general class, such as all paintings in existence, but in terms of a very small subgroup. When we say, for example, that a child's painting contains an unusual representation of three-dimensional space, our standard of comparison includes only other paintings by children. We probably would not make the same judgment if adult work were the standard. When we consider the possible norms against which the unusualness of a particular object might be judged, it becomes apparent that the relative rareness of the object depends on what it is compared with. With a shift in frame of reference, the same product could be unique in one population and common in another. Clearly, the choice of an appropriate base line or norm group against which to judge a creative work is of utmost importance in applying the standard of unusualness. In short, the infrequency of a response is relative to *norms*, which thus serve as a judgmental standard for evaluating unusualness.

Although the judgment of uniqueness or infrequency is a logical first step in evaluating the creativeness of a product, if we proceeded no further, the total set of products nominated as creative would make a strange collection. It would include, among other things, products that are simply bizarre or odd. Somehow the mere oddities must be weeded out. This task requires the application of a second criterion, also familiar to you from Chapter 6—*appropriateness*.

To be appropriate a product must fit its context. It must make sense in light of the demands of the situation and the desires of the producer. Further, in the case of complex products, the internal elements of a work must also blend together. Thus, internal and external criteria of appropriateness may be distinguished. Indeed, two separate critical stances arise from the relative emphasis on internal or external views of appropriateness.

The chief job of the appropriateness criterion, as it is used here, is to help eliminate from the set of unusual products those that are simply absurd. As a criterion of creativeness, it is used conjointly with unusualness rather than independently. At fairly low levels of creative production—as, for example, in paper-and-pencil tests of divergent thinking—the criterion of appropriateness is not too difficult to apply. When a person is asked, for instance, to think of different uses for a common object such as a paper clip, the response, "Eat it," is obviously inappropriate. When a person is asked to write captions for cartoons and responds by giving the names of colors, again there is little question about the inappropriateness of his reaction. Note, however, that both of these responses would probably be unusual, if not unique, in a statistical sense. In cases where the product has to meet some "reality tests" the application of the appropriateness criterion is not too difficult.

As products become more complex, however, and more responsive to the desires of the producer than to the demands of the situation, the determination of appropriateness also becomes more complex. There are times, of course, when the judgment is still fairly easy to make. It does not require much aesthetic training to judge that the meter of a poem beginning, "Death is here/ Death is there/ Death is lurking everywhere" is inappropriate to its theme. Yet at higher levels of creation the entanglement of sense and nonsense can become so involved that the judgment of appropriateness requires a detailed examination by a highly trained person. Even then there is always the chance that the creator, who is often more aware of the demands that gave rise to his product than the critic is, will disagree with the judgment. As Bruner (1957) has pointed out, "It takes a tuned organism, working with a certain kind of set, to recognize the appropriateness of an idea."

As the term is used in judging creative products, appropriateness deals with much more than the logical fit of the product with its context or of the product's elements with each other (although this kind of fit would be the dominant question in many other applications of the criterion). At times a product violates conventional logic but somehow manages to hang together and to have a logic of its own. Illustrations of this phenomenon abound in modern literature and art.

Thus, although the judgmental standard for evaluating appropriateness is the *context* of the response, this context must be interpreted psychologically as well as logically and should include the producer's intentions as well as the demands of the situation.

Finally, appropriateness is a continuous, not a discrete, quality. It exists in various degrees rather than completely or not at all. In its lower forms, we recognize the appropriateness of a product that is merely "adequate," that bears a clear relation to the environment or to the internal motivations of its producer. In its higher forms, we marvel at the way in which the product reflects not only the massive forces that went into its making, but the more subtle influences as well. At low levels of appropriateness we speak of a product as being "about right," given its sources, the avowed purpose of its maker, and the like. At higher levels we speak of a product as being "*just* right." Indeed, at the very highest level of appropriateness we may experience almost a sense of recognition when we come upon the product. Things are so right they look almost familiar. One critic described such products as having "the handprint of necessity upon them instead of the quickly tarnished sheen of the merely novel, the fetchingly precious, the different" (Dickey, 1963, p. 4). When he comes upon these "handprints of necessity," the viewer may sometimes feel as if his expectations have been fulfilled, whereas what has really happened is that the product has made him aware of what his expectations should have been. Again quoting Bruner (1957), "What makes something obvious is that at last we understand it."

The Transcendence of Constraints

Although unusualness and appropriateness may be necessary criteria for limiting the class of potentially creative products, are they sufficient for making required distinctions in quality and level within the class? Among the products considered both unusual and appropriate some are surely at a higher level of creative excellence than others. One property present in some products but absent, or less obvious, in others is the power to transform the constraints of reality. Some objects combine elements in ways that defy tradition and yield a new perspective. They literally force us to see reality in a new way. These products involve a *transformation* of material or ideas to overcome conventional constraints. The question of how much transformation power a product has can serve, then, as a third criterion of creativeness. Just as the unusualness of a product is judged relative to norms and its appropriateness relative to the context, the transformation power of a product would be judged relative to the strength and nature of the *constraints* that were transcended.

Transformation is more difficult to define than unusualness and appropriateness are. At first glance it might seem to be nothing more than an extreme case of unusualness. But it is unusualness with a difference. It is a type of unusualness that attacks conventional ways of thinking about things or of viewing objects. In its most dramatic forms a transformation involves a radical shift in approach to a subject—the kind of shift, for example, caused by the introduction of the heliocentric theory or Freud's earliest propositions. The conception that man and his earth were not the center of the universe but rather played a peripheral role in a much larger natural order stimulated not only a reformulation of the nature of the cosmos but a reappraisal of man's special position within the biological order and led eventually to a recognition of an evolutionary link between the human and the animal. Similarly, the notion that man was subject to thoughts and impulses beyond his awareness led to a new conception of human motivation—man was no longer a rational being in complete control of his actions—and to new standards of individual and social responsibility.

The difference between a merely unusual product and a transformation may be approached in another way. Things are often unusual in the purely quantitative sense—in the sense of being the most or the least, the largest or the smallest of a preexisting class of objects. (The objects and events described in the *Guinness Book of World Records* offer fine examples of this sort of unusualness.) Products that are unusual in this "record-breaking" sense do not usually qualify as transformations. Transformations are not merely improvements, however unusual, on preexistent forms. Rather, they involve the creation of new forms.

The distinction between transformation and unusualness requires that a further distinction be made between an object that represents a transformation and one that is merely new. If transformation demanded only a new combination of elements, almost any unique collection of things, however derived, would qualify. Mechanical techniques for supplying these fortuitous combinations could be devised, as in the story of the popular writer who obtained the plots of his novels by spinning a set of wheels on which were written adjectives, nouns, verbs, and the like. Generally, however, these new combinations do not qualify as transformations because they are low in heuristic power. They terminate rather than generate thought. They are the occasion for surprise and laughter, but not for reflection and wonder.

The possibility just alluded to—that the presence of a transformation may be determined in part by its effect on the viewer—raises the interesting question of whether the other two response properties, unusualness and appropriateness, might also have distinguishable effects upon the observer. Are there, in short, types of aesthetic responses that somehow parallel the criteria of creativeness? In order to pursue this intriguing possibility we will put aside, for a while, the search for more criteria and focus on how the criteria we have already discussed might strike the viewer. The development thus far is summarized in Table 7.1, which lists the three properties of creative products or responses and the judgmental standards associated with each.

Table 7.1

Response Properties	Judgmental Standards
Unusual	Norms
Appropriate	Context
Transformed	Constraints

The Impact of the Product

Confrontation with an unusual object or event characteristically evokes *surprise* in the viewer. The unusual is attention getting, it "catches our eye," its unexpectedness may shock or amaze us. By definition we cannot be prepared for it, except in a very general way. The impact of first exposure creates surprise and requires a period of adaptation during which the unusual object or event is assimilated into the viewer's experience.

Reaction to the unusual is maximum immediately upon exposure and diminishes rapidly thereafter. Though surprise may occur more than once in response to the same object, the second and subsequent exposures never quite produce the impact of the first. Objects and events whose value is derived almost solely from their unusualness—such as freaks in sideshows or *New Yorker* cartoons—rarely warrant continued viewing.

In this connection it is well to point out that improbability is itself not a sufficient condition for the occurrence of surprise. Most of the events we experience daily are improbable in the sense that they are composed of unusual combinations of elements that are rarely repeated exactly. George Miller points out that a mediocre bridge hand is just as rare, in a statistical sense, as a perfect hand. But the latter surprises us while the former does not (Bruner, 1962). In order for surprise to occur, there must be improbability, to be sure, but improbability that violates the viewer's expectations.

The quality of appropriateness calls forth in the viewer a reaction, which we will call *satisfaction*, that is akin to the general condition of comfort. This feeling of satisfaction would seem to have two major sources. First, there is the recognition that the demands of the creator, the material, and the milieu have been responded to and that the response is not only right, but *just* right. There is a recognition of inevitableness about the product, given the context in which it is embedded. Second, there is the recognition that the product not only is "right" but is complete or sufficient. The first source of satisfaction focuses on the qualitative aspects of appropriateness, on how *well* the demands are met; the second source of satisfaction focuses on what might be considered the quantitative aspects of appropriateness, on how *completely* the demands are met. The satisfied viewer's answer to the first criterion is "just right"; his answer to the second is "enough."

Bruner (1962) describes something close to the meaning intended here in his discussion of what he considers the prime property of the creative act—effective surprise. He states,

> What is curious about effective surprise is that it need not be rare or infrequent or bizarre and is often none of these things. Effective surprises . . . seem rather to have the quality of obviousness to them when they occur, producing a shock of recognition, following which there is no longer astonishment. (P. 3.)

Products embodying a transformation are likely to be *stimulating* to the viewer. The primary value of such products resides in their power to alter the viewer's usual way of perceiving or thinking about his world. Whereas confrontation with the unusual requires the viewer to assimilate the product, to make it part of his world, confrontation with a transformation requires that he revise his world. The new element is not only the product itself but the change in environment the product has caused. Metaphorically, a transformation is something like a stone dropped in water. To a person standing on shore the object of interest is not the stone, which quickly disappears from sight, but the waves it produces. A transforming object invites the viewer to move out, intellectually, in new directions; it stimulates him to consider its consequences.

In review, the first three criteria of creativeness—unusualness, appropriateness, and transformation—may possibly be the source of three types of aesthetic response, which may be summarized by the key words: surprise, satisfaction, and stimulation. The possibility that different types of aesthetic response might be isolated gives rise to two important questions that can only be posed here. First, can the aesthetic responses themselves indicate the presence of the qualities that give rise to them? Can we, for example, take the reaction of surprise to be sufficient evidence for the existence of unusualness? Clearly, the answer to this question has extremely important implications for the assessment of creativity. The second question is whether the aesthetic responses are unique to the viewer of the creative product or whether they also appear in the creator himself. Obviously the creator judges his own product, yet his judgment need not and clearly does not always agree with the verdict of an "external" judge. Before questions such as these can be examined, however, it is necessary to return to the criteria of creativeness and to ask what else needs to be added to the three that have already been suggested.

The Coalescence of Meaning

The properties of unusualness, appropriateness, and transformation in varying combinations characterize a large proportion of the things we are willing to call creative. These dimensions are applicable to products stemming from very divergent sources, from the scientist and philosopher as well as from the craftsman and artist. Yet there is another important quality that does not seem to be covered by these criteria. This quality, which appears in some of the most highly creative products, serves as our fourth criterion: *condensation.*

As was mentioned previously, novelty wears out quickly. The history of fad and fashion is, in essence, an elaborate documentation of the short life and relativity of unusualness. In striking contrast, however, to the ephemeral quality of the novel object is the endurance of the greatest creative achievements of man. These we continually seek to reexamine and reexperience. Although criteria of appropriateness and transformation may partially explain this endurance, something more seems to be involved.

Products that warrant close and repeated examination do not divulge their total meaning on first viewing. These products offer something new each time we experience them, whether they are great works of art or highly developed scientific theories. They have about them an intensity and a concentration of meaning requiring continued contemplation.

Because confusion and disorder also compel the viewer's attention (as he tries to make sense out of what he sees), it is necessary to distinguish between condensation and chaotic complexity. The chief difference would seem to involve the unity and coherence of meaning derived from condensation as compared with the unrelated meanings derived from disorder. An assortment of debris gathered in a junk yard and the ordered arrangement of the same material by an artist serves to illustrate the distinction being made here. Any meaning derived from the random assortment of junk is fortuitous and is obtained either from a chance association between the elements or from irrelevant associations that the material might stimulate in the viewer. By contrast, the ordered arrangement, if it is worthy of artistic notice, contains more meaning than can be understood at first glance. The color and shape of the objects, their texture, their spatial location, and their original function all combine to enhance their aesthetic appeal.

In the highest forms of creative condensation the polar concepts of simplicity and complexity are unified. What appears simple at first glance turns out on closer inspection to possess only *apparent* simplicity. Conversely, that which at first appears complex is found to embody a hidden simplicity that binds together the many complex elements. Some of the more successful poems of Robert Frost and some of the paintings of Klee and Miró illustrate well the use of the simple to represent the complex. The reverse situation, in which initial complexity cloaks a hidden simplicity, occurs frequently in musical works, where repeated listening is often required before the major themes and their variations become apparent.

The condensation achieved by a creative product summarizes essences, and the summary may be expanded and interpreted in a multiplicity of ways—intellectually or affectively, in terms of image or idea. It may be interpreted differently by different viewers or by the same viewer on different occasions. This multiplicity of interpretation and the extensiveness of the expansions generated by the condensation are an indication of its summary power, and an appraisal of *summary power* provides an important judgmental standard for the evaluation of creative condensation.

Parenthetically, it might be noted that the response criteria of transformation and condensation are closely related to the two main mechanisms of the dream in psychoanalytic theory (Freud, 1900). Thus, the present formulation includes elements that, from a psychoanalytic point of view, illustrate the role of primary process or prelogical thinking in creative activity (Pine, 1959; Tauber and Green, 1959).

Before leaving this discussion of condensation, we need to mention two additional points. The first deals with the increased ambiguity and complexity of the criteria of creativeness as we go from unusualness to condensation, and the second deals with their developmental interdependence. At this point the meaning of unusualness appears to be more clearly demarcated than the meaning of condensation, and this is partly because condensation is a more complex concept than unusualness. Indeed, each of the four criteria, in the order presented here, seems to be more complex than the one before it. As it is used here, the term *complex* could be partially defined as "obscure and complicated," but we wish to stress a more derivative connotation, namely "difficult to judge." We recognize that difficulty of judgment is a consequence of complexity rather than its meaning, but such a distinction is unimportant in the present context. The important point is that it is more difficult to make judgments of condensation and transformation than of unusualness and appropriateness; there are more differences in viewpoint, and it is more difficult to reach agreement even within schools of thought. This implies that judges have to know more, or do more, or take more time when judging transformation and condensation than the other two criteria. In this judgmental sense, condensation and transformation are more complex than unusualness and appropriateness.

In addition to this progression in complexity, the four criteria of creativeness are also ordered with respect to developmental interdependence. Each of the four criteria, from unusualness to condensation, is applied in turn conjointly with the previous ones, so that in this sense each is dependent on the ones that precede it. This sequential requirement is only partial, however, in the interdependence of transformation and condensation. The transformations of a creative product must be appropriate and unusual; the condensation must also be appropriate and unusual, but it may not always represent a transformation. If we accept unusualness and appropriateness as necessary properties of a creative product, then the hierarchical ordering of transformation and condensation provides an additional basis, along with degrees of variation within each of the response dimensions, for distinguishing levels of creative attainment within the class of creative products.

Having added a fourth response property, condensation, we return to a consideration of aesthetic responses to examine the possible effect of this new criterion upon the viewer. So far our hypothetical viewer has been surprised by unusualness, satisfied by appropriateness, and stimulated by the transforming qualities of creative products. The question now is how will he react when he confronts a product of high condensation, one that suggests many levels of meaning. The definition of the criterion itself almost describes the viewer's response. A condensed product is an object worthy of pondering; it should be examined slowly, carefully, and repeatedly. In a word, the viewer is called upon to *savor* a condensation. The surprise, the satisfaction, and the stimulation that characterize his response to other aspects of creativeness are present as well in the response to a condensation, but there is an important difference. In the reaction to a condensation these other responses are enduring and intensified. Surprise occurs not only on the first encounter, but also on subsequent ones as new and unusual aspects of the product are discovered; satisfaction deepens with repeated exposure as the appropriateness of each element in the product is more fully revealed; stimulation is enriched as each new reaction to the product builds on those that have preceded it. It is this continued freshness of the product and of the viewer's response to it that makes it an object worthy of savoring.

Sometimes, of course, a viewer returns to a creative product not to experience a new expansion of the condensed essence, but to savor an old familiar satisfaction, to return to the scene of past joys. But this type of savoring is likely to be quite transient, since the initial delight would tend to pale with simple repetition and the appreciation of new expansions and nuances in the meantime would make it difficult to recapture the old experience with its original innocence.

With the addition of condensation to the list of response properties and of savoring to the list of aesthetic reactions, we complete our discussion of creative products and appreciative responses (see Table 7.2 for an outline of the development thus far). One further point needs to be made explicit, however: Just as response properties are relative to judgmental standards, so are aesthetic responses. The degree and character of surprise depends on the norms of expectation in much the same manner as unusualness does. Similarly, satisfaction is relative to the context, stimulation to the nature and strength of the constraints, and savoring to summary power.

It is also likely that a detailed examination of the aesthetic responses described here would reveal that each contains both a cognitive and an affective component. Confrontation with a creative product requires understanding as well as feeling. Customarily, understanding and feeling go hand in hand although, as one student of aesthetics points out (Thomas, 1965), it is possible to understand without feeling and to feel without understanding.

PERSONAL QUALITIES AND COGNITIVE STYLES

Among psychologists, creativity has frequently been thought of as a single dimension or at least a unified cluster of traits, resembling—and to some extent overlapping with—general intellectual ability. Some researchers, particularly factor analysts such as Guilford, have isolated a set of cognitive factors related to different aspects of intellectual produc-

Table 7.2

Response Properties	Judgmental Standards	Aesthetic Responses
Unusualness	Norms	Surprise
Appropriateness	Context	Satisfaction
Transformation	Constraints	Stimulation
Condensation	Summary power	Savoring

tion, but the relation of these factors to creative production is less well delineated. Other investigators have argued that creative behavior depends as much on personality as on cognitive power, and they have accrued evidence to show that the highly creative person is more impulsive, makes more use of fantasy, and is more tolerant of ambiguity than is his less creative peer.

It is commonly recognized that creative expression of the highest quality tends to come from people who limit their efforts to a single mode of expression. The great scientist is generally not also a great poet, the great painter is not also a great dancer, and even the great composer is not also a great conductor. Moreover, in the eye of the public, personality characteristics tend to be associated with a *medium* of expression rather than with a level of expression or any other feature of creative production. Thus, in terms of personality, the outstanding poet seems more like the incompetent poet than like the outstanding scientist, who, in turn, seems more like his less competent colleagues than like the superb composer. Both the professional and the public views, therefore, acknowledge that the maker of creative products is different from his fellow man, but there is little agreement on the form this difference takes. Is it chiefly cognitive or does it involve personality components as well? Is the difference linked to a mode of expression entailing, as it were, a way of life, or is it more closely related to stylistic qualities of the products themselves? Each view of the creative process implies a position about the nature of the creator, which in turn helps to determine the types of variables emphasized in the assessment of creativity.

Within the present context there is a set of personal qualities that may be considered to match, so to speak, the response properties used as criteria of creativeness. The present view is not meant to imply that traits should be used as labels in characterizing people. The appropriateness of that practice depends on such matters as the dominance of the trait in question, its distribution in the population, and so on. Rather, we wish to suggest a relation between personal qualities and properties of the creative response.

The question of whether particular personal qualities are necessary for the production is still another matter. Do particular personal qualities "cause" the appearance of the creative act? Might an infrequent or appropriate response occur by chance, or must it always occur as the result of a particular human condition? The view taken here does not prejudge the answer to this causal question, although it does imply that the consistent production of creative responses cannot occur by chance and that the "cause" of such a phenomenon entails psychological as well as social and environmental influences.

In the present view the person who consistently produces infrequent or unusual responses is thought of as being highly *original*. The relativity of the judgment of unusualness also affects the judgment of personal originality. Persons whose responses look quite unusual when judged against one standard and who would, therefore, be thought of as original, might lose the halo of originality when the judgmental norms are changed. In addition, several personal qualities are predisposing to originality; they increase the likelihood of unusual responses but do not guarantee them. These predisposing characteristics include intellectual abilities and certain cognitive styles, motives, and values. For example, ideational fluency, impulse expression, and cognitive styles of tolerance of unreality, tolerance of inconsistency, and the like appear to predispose the individual toward originality (Barron, 1955, 1963).

The production of an appropriate response would seem to be accomplished most easily by a person who is highly *sensitive* to the demands of his environment and to the subtleties of the material he is working with. His sensitivity may result from a conscious *analysis* of the relations between elements, but it need not. There is some evidence, at least in some fields, that the most sensitive people cannot articulate their awareness with any degree of precision. Their sensitivity is *intuitive*; the person who behaves intuitively is sensitive to cues he cannot identify verbally. Either an analytic attitude or an intuitive predisposition or both in combination could serve as cognitive styles for sensitivity. Thurstone (1924), among others, recognized and discussed the function of intuition in creative performance.

Transformation involves transcending traditional boundaries and limitations. Personal qualities that seem to contribute to the production of transformations are of two sorts, cognitive and noncognitive. Relevant cognitive qualities are those dealing with the stability and fluidity of conceptual systems, intellectual categories, and the like. The production of transformations reflects *flexibility* and calls for qualities not unlike those involved in breaking a mental set. In perceptual terms this type of intellectual fluidity would be reflected in the ability to perceive objects in their own right—independent of their symbolic representation, their stereotyped function, or their relatedness to the immediate needs of the viewer. This kind of perceptual freedom has been given the label "allocentric perception" by Schachtel (1959). At the cognitive and ideological level, this flexibility has been called "openmindedness" by Rokeach (1960).

The noncognitive qualities contributing to the production of a transformation include a playful attitude toward reality and a willingness to expose (even to flaunt) ideas, attitudes, and objects that violate tradition. An attitude of playfulness, a desire to toy with reality, is important because most transformations seem to come as a discovery on the heels of many trials. In that sense, transformations involve an element of "luck," but it is the kind of luck that cannot occur without the predisposing attitudes that lead to experimentation and intellectual play. No single adjective adequately summarizes the personal qualities contributing to the production of transformations. The word closest to describing the cognitive qualities without doing violence to the noncognitive qualities is the adjective: *flexible*.

Just as a condensation often contains a paradoxical union of simplicity and complexity, so does the production of the condensation call for a fusing of contradictory personal qualities. There is first the coalescence of personal and universal concerns, with the unusual result of a loss in self-awareness and a gain in total awareness. Although the product may bear the marks of its maker, his personal needs and interests have been consumed, as it were, by the more abstract relevance of the product itself. Second, there is the intimate interplay, even fusion, of thought and feeling that contributes to a condensation. Even the most "logical" production—such as an elegant mathematical solution to a problem—demands an openness to thoughts and feelings that are only dimly perceived and that may not be easily stated. Third, there is an alternate blending of working styles, a cyclic pattern of patience and passion, of reflection and spontaneity, a continual shifting from total acceptance of one's ideas and actions to a critical rejection of them. In a very useful discussion of the creative process, Erich Fromm (1959) distinguishes between two phases of productive behavior. According to Fromm, the first phase is essentially feminine in quality. It is the birth-giving phase, the moment of conception. Following this, a more masculine phase occurs during which the creator must hone and polish his work to ready it for social judgment. During this second phase irrelevancies and superfluities are eliminated, the uniqueness of the work is more sharply defined, and its content is more effectively expressed. The central theme underlying the production of a condensation involves, then, the unification of things normally thought of as separate—producer and product, personal and universal concerns, cognitive and affective processes, masculine and feminine styles of work.

The complexity of condensations and the personal qualities from which they emerge make it difficult to employ a single adjective to describe the person most apt to produce condensations. Yet, in the interests of symmetry and in order to provide a mnemonic device for summarizing the conceptual scheme presented here, we searched for a word that would come close to capturing the sense of our description. In our opinion, the word that does the most justice to what has been said about the producer of condensations is: *poetic*. Webster's *New World Dictionary* describes a poem, and thus indirectly a poet, as "expressing facts, ideas, or emotions in a style more concentrated, imaginative, and powerful than that of ordinary speech." The adjectives *concentrated, imaginative*, and *powerful* are relevant here and apply of course to many products that would not be commonly thought of as poems. It is this more global implication of *poetic* that we imply when we use the word to characterize people who create effective condensations.

These categories and their relationships are summarized in Table 7.3.

The creative person, his product, and the world's response to it combine to form the drama of human invention. The transaction among these three elements is intimate and our understanding of any one enhances our understanding of the other two. But to examine these elements singly is not sufficient. Social science must work toward a conceptualization that serves to unify the psychological, aesthetic, and social aspects of the creative process. It is not enough, of course, to offer pious hopes for a future ecumenical council whose job it will be to unify divergent views of the process. Before such a grand design is sought, two kinds of preparatory work are necessary. First, we must add greater detail to early attempts at unification, such as

Table 7.3

Predisposing Cognitive Styles	Personal Qualities	Response Properties	Judgmental Standards	Aesthetic Responses
Tolerance of incongruity, of inconsistency	Originality	Unusualness	Norms	Surprise
Analysis and intuition	Sensitivity	Appropriateness	Context	Satisfaction
Openmindedness	Flexibility	Transformation	Constraints	Stimulation
Reflection and spontaneity	Poeticness	Condensation	Summary power	Savoring

the one presented here. The present scheme, at best, is an incomplete outline that must be elaborated more fully if its potential contribution is to be realized. Second, we must initiate empirical studies that will give weight to these efforts at theory and prevent them from deteriorating into mere word games.

In the final analysis, however, it is well to remember that theories of creativity are themselves creative products. As such, they must abide by the same laws as those they are designed to unearth. A realization of this fact should temper our zeal in advocating any single prescription for how best to proceed. The day on which we are certain about how to construct a theory of creativity will also be the day on which we are certain about how to construct a poem.

SUMMARY

One of the most facilitating endowments of man is his capacity for invention, his ability to improve and transform his environment. We are naturally curious about the exceptionally creative person, and for more than a century scientists have investigated various aspects of his history and ability. Studies have been conducted to ascertain the genetic makeup of creative people, the environments that influenced them, their personality and thought processes, their ability to combine previously unrelated concepts, the uniqueness of their associations, and their pathologies as well as their positive traits.

It has become clear that creativity is not the same thing as intelligence. Intelligence tells us something about the "rightness" or "correctness" of a response. Creativity deals with its "goodness," as judged by social and psychological criteria. The matter of stipulating the qualities of goodness is far more difficult than specifying what is right and what wrong, but the task is nevertheless possible. The creative response must, first of all, be *unusual* in terms of predefined norms. It must further be *appropriate to its context.* While the unusual may be merely absurd, and appropriateness alone can lead to banality, these criteria applied together limit the class of potentially creative products.

Two further criteria help us establish the creativeness of a response: first, its *transformation* of material or ideas to overcome the conventional *constraints* of reality; and second, its *condensation of meaning,* which gives the response *summary power,* power that is capable of holding complex and many-faceted concepts in their essence.

A creative product directly affects the viewer, who feels some kind of aesthetic response. The novelty and appropriateness of the product evoke *surprise* and *satisfaction* in the viewer; its transformation and condensation *provoke thought* and yield to the *savoring of content.* These responses, important in themselves, may be useful for determining the very qualities of the creative response.

Clearly, the creative product and the aesthetic response it evokes have a great deal to do with the creative person himself. The personal qualities of the creator, in particular his *cognitive styles,* bear greatly on the creative response. The creative person's *originality* is aided by his *tolerance of incongruity and inconsistency.* His *analytic* and *intuitive* bents increase his *sensitivity* to appropriateness. His *openmindedness* leads to the *flexibility* necessary for the creation of transformations, while his *reflective* and *spontaneous* styles nurture the *poetic* qualities that generate effective condensation.

In sum, a unified view of creativity requires examination of the creative person, his products, and society's appreciation of those products.

GLOSSARY

AESTHETIC RESPONSE—appreciation of and responsiveness to things of beauty.

AFFECTIVE—pertaining to or characterized by feeling, emotion, or mood.

ALLOCENTRIC PERCEPTION—Schachtel's term (1959) for the ability to perceive objects in their own right, independent of their symbolic representation, their stereotyped function, or their relatedness to the immediate needs of the viewer.

ANALYTIC ATTITUDE—a cognitive style that separates things into their component parts.

APPROPRIATENESS, CRITERION OF—ability of a product to fit its context and to make sense in light of the demands of the situation and the desires of the producer; in the case of complex products, the blending together of internal elements as well.

APTITUDE—a capacity for learning; the capacity to acquire proficiency with a given amount of training.

ARTIFICIAL SELECTION—eugenics; selective breeding of the human race.

ASSIMILATE—to take into the mind and to thoroughly comprehend.

BISOCIATIVE—Koestler's (1964) description of the pattern of thought underlying creative synthesis; the recognition of converging associations among previously unrelated dimensions of experience.

BRAINSTORMING SESSIONS—meetings wherein participants blurt out ideas about a particular subject, regardless of their value, as quickly as possible to stimulate themselves and others to produce more ideas (see Chapter 6).

CASE STUDY—a collection of all available evidence—social, psychological, physiological, biographical, environmental, vocational—that promises to help explain a single individual.

CATEGORICAL CRITERIA—criteria admitting only of one answer, or of a relatively restricted set of solutions; all other responses are regarded as incorrect.

COGNITION—that mental process generally called thinking which includes perceiving, recognizing, conceiving, judging, and reasoning.[1]

COGNITIVE STYLE—a consistent and characteristic mode of organizing and regulating thinking.

CONCEPTUAL REORGANIZATION—restructuring of a set of abstract ideas about a phenomenon.

CONSTRAINTS—conventional ways of thinking about or viewing things which must be overcome to obtain "transformation."

CONTINUOUS CRITERIA—in this context, norms that admit a wide range of opinion regarding the acceptability of a product.

CORRECTNESS (OF A RESPONSE)—the degree to which a response satisfies certain objective and logical criteria.

CORRELATE—a thing related to another thing in such a way that a change in one is accompanied by a corresponding change in the other.

CREATIVITY—the process by which ideas are born and new human products created.

CRITERION—a rule or standard for making a judgment.

DICHOTOMOUSLY DISTRIBUTED (DATA)—data that are divided into two classes on the basis of the presence or absence of a certain characteristic.

DISCRETE—changing by individual, separate steps rather than in an endless flow; the steps on a staircase are discrete; a ramp is continuous.

DIVERGENT THINKING—thought processes that break away from conventional mental sets; for example, those that result in seeing a variety of uses for a particular object.

EFFECTIVE SURPRISE—according to Bruner (1962) the prime property of the creative act, having "the quality of obviousness" yet "producing a shock of recognition, following which there is no longer astonishment."

EMPIRICAL—based on factual investigation; experimental.

ENVIRONMENT—the sum of the external conditions and factors potentially capable of influencing an organism.[1]

FACTOR ANALYSIS—a statistical technique for analyzing scores and correlations between scores from a number of tests.

[1] This definition was taken from H. B. English and Ava C. English, *A Comprehensive Dictionary of Psychological and Psychoanalytical Terms*. New York: David McKay Company, Inc., 1958.

FLEXIBILITY—a personal quality not unlike those involved in breaking a mental set; intellectual fluidity; in perceptual terms, allocentric perception.

FLUENCY—a smooth flowing; a property of verbal communications.

GESTATION PERIOD—literally, a period of development before birth; in this context, the development of an idea.

HELIOCENTRIC THEORY—the concept that the sun, and not man or the earth, is the center of the universe.

HEURISTIC—leading to discovery; especially of an argument admittedly imperfect but designed to stimulate further thinking or investigation.[1]

HYPOTHESIS—a tentative explanation of a complex set of data.

IDEATIONAL FLUENCY—the ability to produce ideas easily.

IDIOSYNCRATIC—peculiar to an individual.

IMPROBABILITY—an unusual combination of elements that is rarely repeated exactly.

INTELLIGENCE—the ability to learn; the ability to deal with abstractions and with new situations; the individual's repertoire of problem-solving responses.

INTUITION—a cognitive style characterized by sensitivity to cues one cannot identify verbally.

LONGITUDINAL STUDIES—studies wherein changes in the same person or group of people are examined over an extended period of time.

MENTAL SET—a fixed mental pattern a person follows in organizing environmental stimuli.

METAPHORICAL COMBINATIONS—as used here, connections made between diverse domains of experience by symbols or images.

MNEMONIC DEVICE—a "mental shorthand" which facilitates remembering.

NEUROTIC—of neurosis, a negative abnormality, ill-defined in character, but milder than psychosis.

NORM—a pattern taken to be typical of a large group of things.

NORMATIVE—typical of the behavior of a particular group.

OBJECTIVE CRITERIA—as used here, logical or reality-oriented criteria by which responses can be judged.

[1] This definition was taken from H. B. English and Ava C. English, *A Comprehensive Dictionary of Psychological and Psychoanalytical Terms*. New York: David McKay Company, Inc., 1958.

OPENMINDEDNESS—a cognitive style characterized by perceptual freedom and intellectual fluidity; Rokeach's (1960) term for flexibility.

ORIGINALITY—a personal quality that enables one to produce infrequent or unusual responses.

POETICNESS—a personal quality that, as used here, characterizes people who create effective condensations in a style more concentrated, imaginative, and powerful than that of ordinary speech.

PRELOGICAL THINKING—a mode of thinking that does not follow the standard rules of logic but has a sort of logic of its own; the thinking of children, so-called primitive peoples, and certain psychotics; in psychoanalytic theory, primary process thinking.

PRIMARY PROCESS—prelogical thinking; in psychoanalytic theory, a thought process that seeks immediate satisfaction of an instinctual wish.

PROGRESSIVE EDUCATION MOVEMENT—a reform movement, led by John Dewey and others, which advocated developing an experimental attitude in students, recognizing student individuality, incrementing educational motivation by relating school activities to everyday life, and developing the student's personality.

PROJECTIVE DEVICE—a relatively unstructured test situation in which a person is asked to respond imaginatively to inkblots, clouds, cartoons, vague pictures, play materials, and such; responses are analyzed for personality characteristics.

PSYCHOPATHOLOGY—the systematic study of negative psychological abnormalities.

QUANTITATIVE REASONING—cognitive manipulation of numerical or mathematical material.

REFLECTION—a cognitive style characterized by meditativeness.

REMOTE ASSOCIATION TEST—a test of creativity devised by Mednick (1962) which requires the respondent to provide the associative link between apparently unrelated items.

SATISFACTION—an aesthetic response to the quality of appropriateness; it is akin to the general condition of comfort.

SAVORING—an aesthetic response characterized by slow, careful, and repeated examination of a product; literally, tasting.

SELF-ACTUALIZATION—Maslow's term (1959) for the process of developing one's capacities and talents to the fullest and of understanding and accepting oneself.

SITUATIONAL VARIABLES—variables that are characteristic of a particular situation.

SPONTANEITY—a cognitive style characterized by activity arising without external constraint or stimulus; a predisposing cognitive style for the "poetic" personal quality.

SUBJECTIVE CRITERIA—as used here, psychological (that is, nonobjective and nonlogical) standards by which creative responses can be judged.

SUBLIMATION—a mechanism postulated in psychoanalytic theory by means of which sexual impulses are diverted from sexual aims to new activities having social value.

SUBLIMATION THEORY OF CULTURAL EVOLUTION—Freud's theory that diversion of instinctual energy into creative activities spurs the cultural advancement of civilization.

SUMMARY POWER—the capacity of a creative product to generate a number of interpretations and expansions.

SURPRISE—as used here, an aesthetic response evoked by unusualness.

TOLERANCE OF INCONGRUITY—a cognitive style characterized by the ability to entertain incompatible ideas without anxiety or defensiveness.

TRANSCENDENT FUNCTION—a mechanism postulated by Jung (1946) that governs the interaction of conscious and unconscious processes in the creative act and generally orients the individual toward the realization of potentialities.

TRANSFORMATION—the creation of new forms, of new ways of perceiving things.

UNUSUALNESS—the infrequency of a response relative to norms.

VARIABLE—as used here, a changeable trait or characteristic.

REFERENCES

Barron, F. The disposition toward originality. *Journal of Abnormal and Social Psychology*, 1955, **51**, 478–485.

———. *Creativity and psychological health.* Princeton, N.J.: D. Van Nostrand Company, Inc., 1963.

Bruner, J. S. What social scientists say about having an idea. *Printers' Ink Magazine*, 1957, **260**, 48–52.

———. The conditions of creativity. In H. E. Gruber, G. Terrell, & M. Wertheimer (eds.), *Contemporary approaches to creative thinking.* New York: Atherton Press, 1962.

Dickey, J. In *The New York Times Book Review*, December 22, 1963.

Flavell, J. H. *The developmental psychology of Jean Piaget.* Princeton, N.J.: D. Van Nostrand Company, Inc., 1963.

Freud, S. *The interpretation of dreams.* New York: Basic Books, Inc., 1955. (Original German edition, 1900.)

———. The relation of the poet to daydreaming. In *Collected papers,* Vol. IV. London: Hogarth Press, Ltd., 1948. (Written, 1908.)

———. *Three contributions to the theory of sex.* New York: Nervous and Mental Disease Publishing Company, 1910.

———. *Civilization and its discontents.* New York: Cope & Smith, 1930.

———. *Leonardo da Vinci.* London: Routledge & Kegan Paul Ltd., 1948.

Fromm, E. The creative attitude. In H. H. Anderson (ed.), *Creativity and its cultivation.* New York: Harper & Row Publishers, 1959.

Galton, F. *Hereditary genius.* New York: D. Appleton & Company, Inc., 1870.

Getzels, J. W., and P. W. Jackson. *Creativity and intelligence.* New York: John Wiley & Sons, Inc., 1962.

Golann, S. E. Psychological study of creativity. *Psychological Bulletin,* 1963, **60,** 548–565.

Goldstein, K. *The organism.* New York: American Book Company, 1939.

Guilford, J. P. Creativity. *American Psychologist,* 1950, **5**, 444–454.

———. Creative abilities in the arts. *Psychological Review,* 1957, **64,** 110–118.

———. Three faces of intellect. *American Psychologist,* 1959, **14,** 469–479.

———. Some new looks at the nature of creative processes. In N. Frederiksen and H. Gulliksen (eds.), *Contributions to mathematical psychology.* New York: Holt, Rinehart & Winston, 1964.

Hunt, J. McV. *Intelligence and experience.* New York: The Ronald Press Company, 1961.

Jung, C. G. *Psychological types.* New York: Harcourt, Brace & World, Inc., 1946.

Koestler, A. *The act of creation.* New York: Crowell-Collier and Macmillan, Inc., 1964.

Kris, E. *Psychoanalytic explorations in art.* New York: International Universities Press, 1952.

Kubie, L. S. *Neurotic distortion of the creative process.* Lawrence, Kan.: University of Kansas Press, 1958.

MacKinnon, D. W. The nature and nurture of creative talent. *American Psychologist,* 1962, **17,** 484–495.

———. Creativity and images of the self. In R. W. White (ed.), *The study of lives.* New York: Atherton Press, 1963.

Maltzman, I. On the training of originality. *Psychological Review,* 1960, **67,** 229–242.

Maslow, A. H. Creativity in self-actualizing people. In H. H. Anderson (ed.), *Creativity and its cultivation.* New York: Harper & Row Publisher, 1959.

Mearns, H. *Creative youth.* New York: Doubleday & Company, Inc., 1925.

———. *Creative power.* New York: Doubleday & Company, Inc., 1929.

Mednick, S. A. The associative basis of the creative process. *Psychological Review,* 1962, **69,** 220–232.

Patrick, Catherine. Creative thought in poets. *Archives of Psychology,* 1935, **26,** 1–74.

———. Creative thought in artists. *Journal of Psychology,* 1937, **4,** 35–73.

Pelz, D. C. Relationships between measures of scientific performance and other variables. In C. W. Taylor and F. Barron (eds.), *Scientific creativity: Its recognition and development.* New York: John Wiley & Sons, Inc., 1963.

Piaget, J. *The origins of intelligence in children.* New York: International Universities Press, 1952.

———. *The construction of reality in the child.* New York: Basic Books, Inc., 1954.

Pine, F. Thematic drive content and creativity. *Journal of Personality,* 1959, **27,** 136–151.

Roe, Anne. *The making of a scientist.* New York: Dodd, Mead & Company, Inc., 1952.

———. A psychological study of eminent psychologists and anthropologists, and a comparison with biological and physical scientists. *Psychological Monographs,* 1953, **67,** No. 2.

Rogers, C. R. Toward a theory of creativity. In H. H. Anderson (ed.), *Creativity and its cultivation.* New York: Harper & Row Publishers, 1959.

Rokeach, M. *The open and closed mind.* New York: Basic Books, Inc., 1960.

Santayana, G. *The sense of beauty.* New York: Charles Scribner's Sons, 1896.

Schachtel, E. G. *Metamorphosis.* New York: Basic Books, Inc., 1959.

Stein, M. I. A transactional approach to creativity. In C. W. Taylor and F. Barron (eds.), *Scientific creativity: Its recognition and development.* New York: John Wiley & Sons, Inc., 1963.

Tauber, E. S., and M. R. Green. *Prelogical experience.* New York: Basic Books, Inc., 1959.

Terman, L. M. (ed.). *Genetic studies of genius,* Vol. I: *Mental and physical traits of a thousand gifted children.* Stanford, Calif.: Stanford University Press, 1925.

———. (ed.). *Genetic studies of genius,* Vol. III: *The promise of youth: Follow-up studies of a thousand gifted children* (by Barbara S. Burks, Dortha W. Jensen, and L. M. Terman). Stanford, Calif.: Stanford University Press, 1930.

———. (ed.). *Genetic studies of genius,* Vol. IV: *The gifted child grows up* (by L. M. Terman and Melita H. Oden). Stanford, Calif.: Stanford University Press, 1947.

———. The discovery and encouragement of exceptional talent. *American Psychologist,* 1954, **9,** 221–230.

Thomas, R. M. A rationale for measurement in the visual arts. *Educational and Psychological Measurement,* 1965, **25,** 163–189.

Thurstone, L. L. *The nature of intelligence.* London: Routledge & Kegan Paul, Ltd., 1924.

Torrance, E. P. *Guiding creative talent.* Englewood Cliffs, N.J.: Prentice-Hall, Inc., 1962.

Wallach, M. A., and N. Kogan. *Modes of thinking in young children.* New York: Holt, Rinehart & Winston, 1965.

Wallas, G. *The art of thought.* New York: Harcourt, Brace & World, Inc., 1926.

SUGGESTED READINGS

1. Barron, F. *Creativity and psychological health.* Princeton, N.J.: D. Van Nostrand Company, Inc., 1963. A summary of a decade of research into the "origins of personal vitality and creative free-

dom." Among several topics explored are psychotherapy as an instrument of personal growth and the roles of artistic creation and religious belief in self-renewal.

2. Bruner, J. S. *On knowing: Essays for the left hand.* Cambridge, Mass.: Harvard University Press, 1962. A perceptive series of essays on the functions of intuition, feeling, and spontaneity in the human endeavors of learning, knowing, and creating.
3. Getzels, J. W., and P. W. Jackson. *Creativity and intelligence.* New York: John Wiley & Sons, Inc., 1962. A detailed comparison of two groups of adolescents—one scoring high on tests of intelligence but not equally high on tests of creativity, the other scoring high on tests of creativity but not equally high on tests of intelligence. Findings reveal important differences in values, career aspiration, and family background between the two groups.
4. Golann, S. E. Psychological study of creativity. *Psychological Bulletin,* 1963, **60**, 548–565. A helpful overview of the major empirical studies of the creative process. This article is especially useful in guiding the reader to some of the unresolved issues in the field.
5. Guilford, J. P. Three faces of intellect. *American Psychologist,* 1959, **14**, 469–479. A concise and clearly written exposition of Guilford's factor analytic model of the intellect. This model and the tests derived from it have had a great influence on the empirical definition of creative abilities.
6. Hunt, J. McV. *Intelligence and experience.* New York: The Ronald Press Company, 1961. A study of the extent to which environmental influences shape intellectual performance. The author pays particular attention to the effect of early experience upon subsequent development.
7. Koestler, A. *The act of creation.* New York: Crowell-Collier and Macmillan, Inc., 1964. A brilliant and sweeping treatise on the creative process by a well-known creative writer. In developing his theory of the "bisociative" nature of creative acts, Koestler draws on an exceptionally wide range of human knowledge, extending from the physical sciences to the humanities. Although the book tends to overlook recent psychological research, it is nonetheless thought provoking and a delight to read.
8. Kubie, L. S. *Neurotic distortion of the creative process.* Lawrence, Kan.: University of Kansas Press, 1958. An argument by a psychoanalyst against both popular and scientific views linking creative behavior and psychological disturbances. The author argues instead that creativity is the ultimate expression of psychological health.
9. Miller, G. *Psychology: The science of mental life.* New York: Harper & Row Publishers, 1962. A treatment of the work of several famous psychologists that clearly reveals the historical mainstream of psychological research and links the past to the present. Of particular interest to the readers of this chapter are the sections of the book dealing with Galton, Freud, and Binet.
10. Schachtel, E. G. *Metamorphosis.* New York: Basic Books, Inc., 1959. A decription of the development in some people, from infancy forward, of perceptual defenses that reduce their awareness of the world around them and prevent them from viewing objects and people independently of their usefulness to the viewer. This type of distortion, which is termed "autocentric perception," is contrasted with "allocentric perception," a mode of seeing that is prominent in many creative endeavors.
11. Stein, M. J., and Shirley J. Heinze. *Creativity and the individual.* New York: The Free Press of Glencoe, 1960. A book with an annotated bibliography of the major psychological literature on creativity covering both empirical and theoretical work up to the late nineteen fifties. Each book or article is summarized and the summaries are organized around a useful topical outline.
12. Terman, L. M. (ed.). *Genetic studies of genius,* Vol. IV: *The gifted child grows up* (by L. M. Terman and Melita H. Oden). Stanford, Calif.: Stanford University Press, 1947. A study of a group of gifted children in California that began in the early nineteen twenties and extended into the midfifties.

It is being continued, since Terman's death, by a group of his former colleagues. This work did much to dispel misconceptions concerning precocious intellectual development. In large measure, educational interest in gifted children derives both its impetus and its direction from this well-known longitudinal study.

13. Torrance, E. P. *Guiding creative talent.* Englewood Cliffs, N.J.: Prentice-Hall, Inc., 1962. A book written chiefly for teachers and parents who are interested in fostering the development of creative abilities in children. It contains many examples of creative behavior in children and offers helpful pedagogical advice.
14. Wallach, M. A., and N. Kogan. *Modes of thinking in young children.* New York: Holt, Rinehart & Winston, 1965. A research monograph that investigates the cognitive and personality correlates of a dimension of associational originality that is independent of conventional intelligence tests.

8

Character

DAVID ROSENHAN

PERRY LONDON

Character is a word almost everyone thinks he understands and almost no one tries to define. It is commonly used in several different "jargons," moreover, and though its many different usages share an important core of common meaning, the disparity among them makes the concept, "character," appear more ambiguous than it is. There are three senses in which the term is most often used; one denotes distinctiveness, uniqueness, or peculiarity and is essentially a descriptive term; the second denotes mental and moral attributes of a kind which make it an essentially evaluative word; and the third—more technical—refers to the stability of important personality traits over time.

THE MEANINGS OF CHARACTER

In its purely descriptive sense, *character* refers to a person's *characteristics,* that is, to "the attributes or features that make up and distinguish the individual" (Webster). It is precisely this idea that is conveyed by the vernacular expression, "He's a character!" While such a statement can connote hostile or derogatory meaning, it need not mean any more, to quote the dictionary again, than "a person marked by notable or conspicuous traits." Whether the traits are good or bad does not affect the definition as long as they are conspicuous—and the meaning of the term in this case depends on the observer's intention and not on its own denotation.

In its evaluative sense, *character* is defined by Webster as "the complex of mental and ethical traits marking a person, group, or nation." This definition

Mr. Rosenhan's work on this chapter was facilitated in part by Grant No. HD 01762–01 from the National Institute of Child Health and Human Development. Mr. London was supported by Grant No. 1–K3–MH31–209–01 from the National Institute of Mental Health and Grant No. 1912 from the Wenner-Gren Foundation for Anthropological Research "to aid a study of the sources of altruistic social autonomy."

reflects some of the ambiguity of *character* as an evaluative term by making it sound as if "mental and ethical traits" are obviously related to each other. This is not true, but it is true that the evaluative use of the word *character* may denote both the attributes that are peculiar to an individual and the *moral status* the observer attaches to those attributes. To say, in other words, that a person "has a lot of character" is to imply a positive moral judgment.

This term has still a third meaning, which approaches the technical meaning it usually has in personality theory and the study of psychopathology. This is the notion, introduced in Chapter 4, that certain important personality traits are stable over time. This idea is implied to some extent in the other usages described, but the emphasis here is on the *persistence* of attributes, not on how conspicuous or desirable they are. The expression "he lacks character" does not imply so much that a person is wicked as that he is weak willed and undependable in his attitudes or behaviors and that he otherwise fails to satisfy the standards of conduct or achievement generally approved in our society. That the expression also implies a negative evaluation shows how interconnected the several meanings of *character* are.

The meaning psychologists give to *character*, as might be expected, does not refer directly to social approbation or reprobation but is indirectly connected with them. In the study of personality development, character is generally conceived as a group of behavior dispositions or personality traits which develop early in life and become deeply rooted characteristics of the adult person which are evident in many different situations. In this sense, *character* means only the stability and amplitude of personality traits. But it is rarely used this narrowly even by scientists. Studies of character development are concerned very much with aspects of character that have particular implications for "right conduct" and moral disposition. Even more important, perhaps, the psychopathological conditions called *character disorders* (see Chapter 11) are largely two disturbances technically called "psychopathic personality" and "sociopathic personality." The symptoms attributed to these disorders are mostly the kinds of antisocial, aggressive, dishonest, and deceptive behavior that are connected with criminal conduct. The connection is not accidental.

The concepts of *character* and *temperament* have been interwoven since antiquity, when it was believed that gross personality characteristics were expressions of different combinations of the four basic elements—earth, air, fire, and water—in the physical makeup of an individual. This doctrine of temperament, formulated originally by Galen, accounted for sanguine, choleric, phlegmatic, and melancholy dispositions in terms of the various titers of "humoral" substances in the body. These proportions, in turn, depended on the amounts of the four elements contained in an individual's body.

Nobody today accepts this ancient theory of temperament in its original form, but there is still much scientific effort to associate personality characteristics with temperamental attributes. The notion that criminal or socially deviant character is in some sense hereditary was extremely popular towards the end of the nineteenth century, especially as represented in the work of Lombroso (1891) and Krafft-Ebing (1922). In more sophisticated form, it is reflected in the later researches of Kretschmer (1925), Sheldon and Stevens (1942) (see Figure 8.1), and the Gluecks (1950) on delinquency and body type. And it has even been very recently and popularly revived

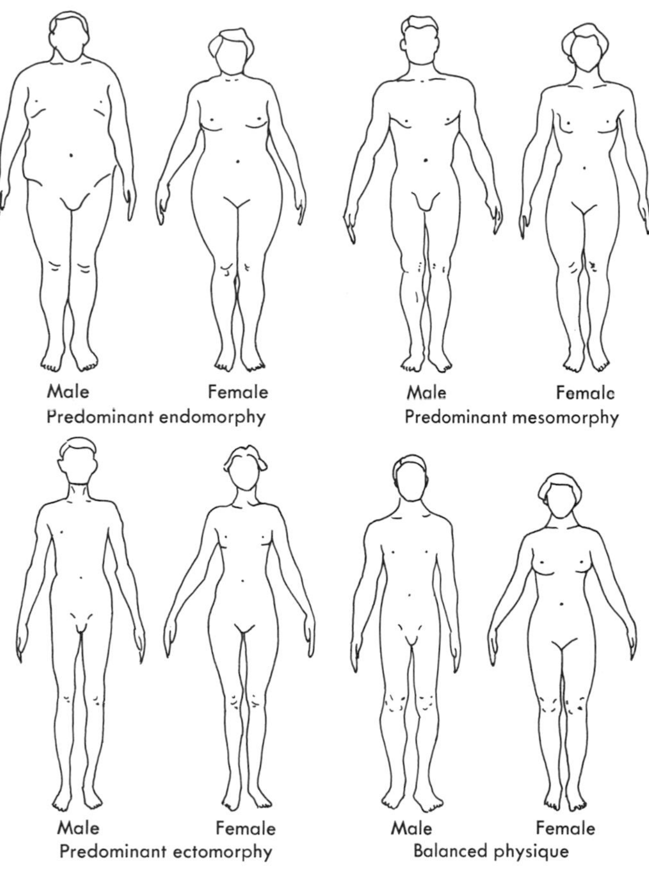

Figure 8.1 Sheldon and Stevens (1942) postulated three body types, or somatotypes: *endomorphy*, prominence of the abdominal region; *mesomorphy*, prominence of muscle; and *ectomorphy*, thinness with prominence of skin and neural tissue. These are here compared with a balanced physique. They also postulated a relationship between temperament and somatotype: *viscerotonia*, or joy in eating, joviality, and relaxation went with endomorphy; *somatotonia*, or joy in competitiveness, energetic movement, and aggressiveness, with mesomorphy; and *cerebrotonia*, or apprehensiveness, restraint, shyness, and hypersensitivity, with ectomorphy. "The Somatotypes" from *Your Heredity and Environment* by Amram Scheinfeld, Copyright © 1965 by Amram Scheinfeld; copyright 1939, 1950 by Amram Scheinfeld. Published by J. B. Lippincott Company and by Chatto & Windus, Ltd.

in Maxwell Anderson's play about hereditary tendencies to murder, *The Bad Seed*.

Opponents of the biological point of view generally interpret criminality or psychopathy as a learned process. Psychoanalytic thinkers have been particularly interested in expanding the concept of character disorder to include a much wider number of disabilities and personality problems. Even so, the focus of their attention has remained upon the kinds of disorders that have most to do with the moral aspects of individual conduct and interpersonal and social relations. Consequently, it is fair to say that, for most practical purposes, psychological usage of the term *character* refers to both the stability and amplitude of traits and their ethical worth. A particular point is made of this in the *Comprehensive Dictionary of Psychological and Psychoanalytical Terms* (English and English, 1958), which defines *character* as "an integrated system of traits or behavior tendencies that enables one to react, despite obstacles, in a relatively consistent way in relation to mores and moral issues," and then goes on to say, "This is the standard, though wavering, current psychological usage. It is distinguished from *personality* by its emphasis upon (*a*) the volitional aspect, and (*b*) morality."

This chapter will use the definitions of character we have spelled out, but it will focus on positive aspects of character, including what are generally regarded as socially desirable character traits like honesty, courage, altruism, and independence of mind. The chapter will not be concerned with delinquency, crime, and psychopathy which, though important in their own right and illustrative of some aspects of character, are generally regarded as psychopathological and are therefore discussed in Chapter 11.

THE CHARACTERISTICS OF GOOD CHARACTER

As difficult as it may be for most people to give a precise definition of *character*, it is not hard at all to conjure up a mental image of what a person of good character might actually be like. *Character stereotypes* are important parts of the legends of any culture, including our own, and are considered critical devices for fostering good character in the young. The personal attributes which define good character in a society are commonly lumped together in the legendary personalities of cultural heroes and transmitted in stories and songs down the generations. Before you identify this method of character indoctrination too strongly with savage tribes around a campfire, consider the public school tales we learn in this country about George Washington's legendary inability to lie and Honest Abe Lincoln's perseverance in educating himself in spite of the impoverished circumstances of his birth. The novels of Horatio Alger, too, however perishable they are as literature, certainly had a powerful effect on the aspirations of an entire generation of late nineteenth century American boys. More recently we have come from Tom Swift and Tarzan, of only a generation ago, to Superman, Batman, and Captain Marvel, who probably inspired both the writers and the readers of this book, and the still unspecified heroes of the space age. This method of character indoctrination is not yet passé, nor is there any reason to think it ever will be. A culture embodies its ideals of good character in the exaggerated form of heroic personalities, real or fictional, who can dramatically capture the imagination of an audience and, one way or another, be easily identified with.

The components of good character are not difficult to identify if they are considered in gross form and in the most general case. Since *real life* situations are often much more complicated than moral adjurations and prescriptions are likely to indicate, the *legendary* culture-hero is a particularly good source for studying exemplary character, often better than a real hero. Legend permits him to limit his activities to situations where the moral imperatives are clear. A composite of culture heroes might yield the following image of good character: First of all, he would be rather *consistent* in both attitudes and behaviors. Not only would his deportment be socially desirable and praiseworthy, therefore, but it would also be *predictably desirable.* At the same time, he would be conspicuously intelligent, at least intelligent enough so that his predictably good behavior would always occur by *choice*, not by chance. This implies that the good character is *actively* rather than passively good. The Boy Scout Oath explicitly embodies most of these ideals:

> On my honor, I will do my best:
> To do my duty to God and my country, and to obey the Scout Law.
> To help other people at all times.
> To keep myself physically strong, mentally awake, and morally straight.

Students of cultural history may already see an element of bias in our portrayal of good character. The good character described here is already beginning to sound rather specifically American, or at least Anglo-Saxon, or certainly Western. All this is true and will become even more evident as the description proceeds. Though many individual attributes of good character that we name are considered socially desirable everywhere, the fact remains that the entire concept of character is closely tied to the ideals of individual cultures and societies. And if this is true when the attributes of character are described in the most general way, as we have done thus far, it becomes even more true and more salient when we examine specific interpretations of these traits in different cultures. The significance of this *caveat* will be clearer when it is illustrated below. Meanwhile, it is important to recognize that the good character epitomized here is one most familiar to Western readers.

The consistency of the good character's makeup, together with his propensity to be active, implies a certain toughness about him also, such that he could be expected to be persistent in the pursuit of his goals. This means, for one thing, that he has a *strong desire for achievement*, in turn implying that he has highly developed *standards of excellence* for evaluating both his own performance and that of others. Since persistence in the pursuit of some objectives may require opposition to the wishes or judgments of others, the good character manifests a high degree of *personal autonomy* or independence of mind, and he also has courage to face obstacles in his path without retreating. These, in turn, imply that he has high *self-regard*, such that he need not rely too heavily on his surroundings for evaluation of himself.

It goes without saying, then, that the good character is a person of *integrity*. But little has been said thus far of the actual content of his aspirations or actions. People may be honest, courageous, and persistent in pursuit of goals which are themselves completely selfish or even destructive of others. Not so the good character of this conception! The objectives of his activity contain some significant elements of *altruism*, that is, of selflessness in serving the needs of other individuals, of society, or of God. The precise focus of his altruistic activities will vary greatly, depending on his background and beliefs, and the actual activities involved will necessarily depend very much on the circumstances in which he lives. The point, in all cases, is that a significant portion of his behavior is motivated and aimed not just at the satisfaction of his personal desires but at the service of persons or ideals beyond himself, which he perhaps serves even at some risk or detriment to himself.

Altruism is not the only limiting content of good character, however; by implication, there are limits on the extent to which a person of good character will inflict pain or frustration on those who stand in the way of his desires, even though he may have no wish to serve their needs. Thus, he will not ordinarily be brutal or personally violent in his persistence, and he will be loathe to engage people in reprehensible conduct merely for the satisfaction of his own desires. Presumably, the man of character wants to accomplish his own purpose in life in ways that will confer maximum benefits on others and on society and minimum detriment on others, including those who stand in his way. This is not easy.

It might well be objected at this point that we have not only identified the good character as an essentially Western gentleman, but have gone further still and injected some gross if unnamed elements of specifically Protestant, Puritanical morality into him to boot—as if his morals were a critical feature of his psychological makeup. So it is, and so we have. And to understand this usage, one must bear constantly in mind the definition of character as "behavior tendencies that enable one to react . . . in a relatively consistent way *in relation to mores and moral issues*." There is no escaping the discussion of moral contents in any comprehensive description of *character*, as it is defined here.

The description of good character we have rendered thus far does not try to specify the right moral stand on any issue; it does try to outline a condition that is likely to underlie any position a man of good character might take on any moral issue. The idea that such a condition is possible may seem foolish or parochial; certainly it is difficult to spell out in theory and often to apply in practice, suggesting that good character is easier to think about than to measure.

In theory, for example, if you say that honesty is a good trait of character and brutality is a bad one, how do you judge a person who is outspoken in a way that is painful to the listener? It may be honest and brutal at the same time. It might be correct in some cases to say that the person who is outspoken to others about their faults (a common practice among vicious people who capitalize on the apparent correspondence between honesty and hostility in this case) is *insensitive*; this makes sensitiveness to others a good character trait. That would be all right, but in itself it implies no particular action. Suppose a person is aware of the pain his outspokenness will cause and speaks out anyway. Then the judgment of how his behavior reflects on his character depends on both his motivation and his sensitivity to the probable consequences of his act. If his motive is hostile and he is sensitive to the probable effect of his behavior, then the judgment of how the act reflects on his character depends on whether the judge values kindliness or awareness more highly. That valuation has not even been clarified by moral philosophers, and in the absence of consensus among them (as among the rest of us), there does not seem to be any very objective way to weight them. (We shall be concerned with these issues again when we examine Mowrer's integrity therapy in Chapter 15.)

As a practical matter, moreover, the traits associated with good character apply differently to different situations. A college student who is scrupulously honest in taking exams places transcontinental telephone calls to himself to let his parents know, courtesy of Bell Telephone, that he has arrived safely back at school. Another who shows unflinching courage in a civil rights demonstration off campus refuses to take part in a different one which his fraternity brothers oppose. A girl who goes out of her way to help other girls in her class with studies refuses to lend her notes to anybody in a course where she learns that grades will be based on competitive examination. A rigid definition of good character in terms of behavior dispositions which are standard across *all* situations overlooks the great complexity of human beings, who, at their best, are still highly variable. A large literature demonstrates that attributes like honesty vary considerably depending upon circumstances like the importance of the event, the degree of temptation confronting the subject, the likelihood of exposure, and the amount of experience he has had with similar or related situations.

It is not the precise moral content of an act that identifies good character, but the moral disposition with which an individual approaches a variety of life situations and the integrity with which he treats them. If this concept has an empirical meaning, as the authors believe, then good character should be identifiable and measurable, not so much by an individual's ability to *verbalize* his behavioral ideals as by the fact that inspection of most of the life situations he encounters where these ideals are relevant reveals that he usually adheres to them *in behavior*, regardless of the particular code he expresses.

THE DEVELOPMENT OF CHARACTER

Good character obviously does not appear full-blown at birth, baptism, or bar mitzvah. Nor can it be identified by a single event or behavior in a person's life. Character develops slowly from early childhood on, and its identification in an adult reflects a dynamic process which is continuously developing and in flux throughout adulthood. The description of good character in the previous section concerns a kind of ideal type who is the apotheosis of character development. Freud (1905) calls this kind of person a "genital character." Fromm (1947) refers to the same type as having a "productive orientation" toward life. Peck and Havighurst (1960) call this kind of person a "rational-altruistic" character. None of these terms are mutually exclusive, and each is meant to identify essentially the same attributes as the others.

The differences between the terminologies used by different students of character reflect different typologies for classifying character traits and different schemes and theories to explain how character develops. For our purposes, the typologies are less useful than the developmental events which obstensibly produce them, but since they are of some interest in their own right we will describe them briefly, together with some of the most important theories of character development.

There are at least two different types of character typologies: one that focuses on the biological or individual aspects of character development, and another that views character primarily as the individual expression of social or cultural characteristics. The biologically oriented position is best represented by Freud, who also presents the most detailed and comprehensive characterology of modern scholars. The socially oriented position is most familiarly portrayed by the character typologies of Erich Fromm in *Man for Himself* (1947) and of David Riesman *et al.* in *The Lonely Crowd* (1950).

The difference between these positions is one of emphasis rather than of understanding. The biological orientation, which is better known, concentrates on the individual's development and internal dispositions as reflections of maturational stages, but it is fully aware that these developments take on form and meaning only in a cultural context. The social orientation, which is more novel (just as sociology is a more novel discipline than biology), focuses on character development as part of the acculturation process, but recognizes nevertheless the importance of temperamental and other biological events in shaping individual dispositions and differences in character development. More important than whether an orientation focuses on the internal bodily events that influence character or the external social events that contribute to it is the fact that both positions see character as *developmental*, that is as *the result of a process of changes over time.*

From either point of view, such changes are not so much of a piece that prediction of adult character is easy in prospect, or that inference of the sequence of events that produced a given character is simple in retrospect. Both positions would agree that character development is highly subject to formal and informal educational processes, on the one hand, and that it is not limitlessly subject to them on the other. To this extent, neither of them is a naïve theory.

The Biological Characterology of Sigmund Freud

Of all his contributions to the study of human behavior, Freud's description of *the genetic process* was among the most important. Although it has been endlessly revised by his followers and assailed by his detractors in the sixty-odd years since it was first promulgated, it remains an intriguing, if not compelling, scheme for understanding the sequence of personality development from birth to adulthood. The sequence of "critical periods" in Chapter 4 is one variant of the concept of genetic stages.

Freud believed that character patterns result from several *stages of infantile development* through which a child progresses more or less regularly in the first six years of life. These stages depend in turn on the physical maturation of the child's pertinent biological equipment—and since the equipment in question is essentially the same for everyone, the things that happen to it provide the same framework for everyone's personality to develop in. The critical parts that successively capture the child's attention in his first years of development are the *mouth*, the *excretory organs*, and the *genitals*; the tensions, pleasures, and anxieties which variously center around them combine at appropriate times to constitute the *oral, anal, phallic*, and *genital* stages. The child's experiences in relation to the external world, especially in relation to the people in it who are responsible for his rearing, give rise to the character traits which will mark him, sometimes conspicuously but often subtly, in adult life.

It is worth noting that Freud's biology is much different from the kind implied by the ancient theory of temperament. Temperament theory says, in effect, that it is the distribution of chemicals, presumably since birth, that accounts for the phlegmatic, choleric, sanguine, and melancholy temperaments. But Freud is proposing that it is the influence of environmental conditions over the span of development that makes the constitutional characteristics of an individual operative. In this respect, he anticipates the modern disdain for the nature-nurture controversy that wasted so many people's time for so long (see Chapter 2). Regardless of the errors of observation and theory that he makes, Freud is clearly proposing that it is the interaction of changing stimulus conditions on the changing physical apparatus of the child that gives rise to the behavior patterns he learns.

The oral stage occurs during the first year of life. The neonate is completely incapable of taking care of his own needs, and for the most part, his cooperation is not even required in order for his needs to be served. The only exception is the satisfaction of hunger. At birth, the muscles necessary for sucking are already well developed, and it is only a matter of a day or so before he is able to suckle actively at bottle or breast. There is presumably a good deal of satisfaction both in eating and in sucking, and it is not surprising that the infant's growing perceptual and sensory apparatus begins to focus on oral processes before others. If the needs connected with oral processes are generally satisfied, then the processes themselves become pleasurable in a way that pervades every aspect of personality development. These needs include a general feeling of security and trust, of optimism, and of confidence in confronting the world. If they are satisfied only irregularly and poorly, then the events connected with orality pervade personality development in a negative way, and the child tends to become insecure, anxious, distrustful, fearful, and doubtful of his ability to hold his own. In the first case, he will be trusting of others and of himself, and consequently able, over time, to develop independence where he needs it as well as mutual and satisfying interdependent relations with others. In the second, the child may grow up distrustful of others, dependent upon them for support and simultaneously fearful that he will not get it or that it will be withdrawn.

The entire system of developmental stages is pyramidal, in the Freudian view; those which occur earlier are more critical to the total development of the child. The stages overlap, of course, so that one begins before another has really ended, and the patterns of behavior that are learned at each stage remain operative in one or another form throughout life.

The anal stage extends from about the end of the first year of life to the end of the third year. During the first year, the infant has gained a good deal of muscular control, and the anal phase, according to Freudian theory, is largely concerned with the further development and testing of muscular control, particularly inhibitory control of the muscles involved in excretory processes. In this stage, the child is asked, for the first time, to give something to the parent rather than to be the passive recipient of care. For the first time, the child has to assume some active responsibility for himself. Bowel and bladder training is, of course, the most critical aspect of this, but virtually all the ideas of cleanliness, neatness, sharing, and obedience which children must learn are first imposed upon them at this time. It is in the anal stage that children begin to form permanent attitudes towards responsibility, cooperation, goodwill, and conformity, on the basis of their experiences of such events during this time. Most important of all, as a result of their cooperative and compliant behavior, they learn to get approval of those who love them.

If the exigencies of the anal period are successfully weathered, the child develops permanent favorable dispositions towards responsibility, autonomy, care of himself and of things, cooperative relations with others. He also learns to defer gratification of his wishes and gets a sense of being able to plan and to work hard and persistently towards the accomplishment of his long-range goals. If the anal period is too stressful and unhappy, on the other hand, if the demands made are harsh and overwhelming, the dispositions born and confirmed there are ones of self-doubt and shame, of grudging hostility toward responsibilities, of laziness or of an offensively rigorous sense of duty, of unwillingness to cooperate and share with other people, of aloofness from others, of selfishness with possessions, of general aggressiveness, and of an inability to formulate and carry out effective long-range plans (compare with "Critical Period II" in Chapter 4).

The phallic stage begins around the beginning of the fourth year and extends to about age six. During this period, the child's concern with his body shifts once again, this time from the anal zone and excretory functions to the genitals and the immature sexual pleasures associated with them. It is at this time, according to Freud, that characteristic differences in sex roles develop between boys and girls; the boy develops a profound love for his mother (which is the prototype of all his future relations with women) and the girl experiences a parallel development in relation to her father. This is the period of the famous "Oedipus complex," of "castration anxiety," and of "penis envy." But most important for character development, and less polemically from the viewpoint of nonpsychoanalytic students of development, it is during this period that children form the powerful *identifications* with the attitudes and behaviors of their parents that serve throughout life as the basis for the formulation and evaluation of their own attitudes and behaviors. It is in this period, more than in any other, that the actual content of adult behavior standards is transmitted to the next generation. It is no accident, in this connection, that in this period children have rather fully developed capacities for the use of language and in fact, start formal schooling (compare with "Critical Period III" in Chapter 4).

There are several more "psychosexual stages" in the Freudian scheme of personality development, but the three mentioned here are the only critical ones for the development of character. Once the phallic stage is completed, according to Freud, the child experiences a period of relative quiet, during which he remains relatively free of severe conflict until puberty and adolescence. Subsequently, if all goes well, the development of mature physical sexuality and of heterosexual relationships will see the evolution in adulthood of an essentially well-socialized, productive, and well-adjusted individual whom Freud calls the "genital character."

It is difficult to identify the precise character types that correspond to various development levels at which an individual may have been "fixated," not so much because Freud's system is imprecise, though it is that, as because the different typologies that result from each stage are so rich, plentiful, and diverse. Under the circumstances, it is more fruitful to see the dimensions of character that are associated with each stage of development. Freud himself did not elaborate these. This task was left for his students, in recent times those called "ego psychologists," and among these mainly Erik Erikson (1959). These character dimensions and the experiences related to them are shown in Table 8.1. The first column presents the psychosexual stages essentially as Freud saw them, and the second depicts the approximate time periods in which they occur. These are paralleled by experiences that Erikson terms "psychosexual crises," which are essentially character dimensions that may arise at each stage of psychosexual development. Significant people and patterns of relationship, as well as subjective elements that gradually become embedded in the individual's character, are shown as "psychosocial modalities."

Critics of the Freudian typology find it hard to believe that particular parts of the body are as important to character development as Freud seemed to think, especially if what makes them so critical is their capacity to yield pleasure. It is difficult, perhaps impossible, to verify firmly or disprove the salience of the particular stages which Freud specified, though there is no doubt that he and many of his students made excessive claims for some. English and Pearson (1937, 1945), for example, have said that the seven stages of psychosexuality—oral, anal, genital, latency, adolescence, adulthood, and senescence—are biologically predetermined and that they are universal among human beings and among cultures. While such claims are exorbitant, the vitality of Freud's concepts remains. Whether or not "oral character" is a precisely meaningful term, certainly *oral*

Table 8.1
Psychosexual Stages and Their Psychological Ramifications[1]

	Psychosexual Stage	Life Stage	Psychosocial Crisis (or Character Dimension)	Significant Relations	Psychosocial Modalities
I.	Oral-sensory	Infancy	Trust *vs.* mistrust	Mother	To get; to give in return
II.	Anal-muscular	Early childhood	Autonomy *vs.* shame and doubt	Parents	To hold (on); to let (go)
III.	Genital-locomotor	Play age	Initiative *vs.* guilt	Basic family	To make; to play roles
IV.	Latency	School age	Industry *vs.* inferiority	Neighborhood school	To make things; to make them together
V.	Puberty	Adolescence	Identity *vs.* identity diffusion	Peer groups and out-groups; models of leadership	To be oneself (or not to be)
VI.	Genitality	Young adult	Intimacy and solidarity *vs.* isolation	Partners in friendship, sex, competition, cooperation	To lose and find oneself in another
VII.		Adulthood	Generativity *vs.* self-absorption	Divided labor and shared household	To make be; to care for
VIII.		Mature age	Integrity *vs.* despair	"Mankind," "my kind"	To be through having been; to face not being

[1] Adapted from Erikson (1959, pp. 120, 168).

characteristics of behavior pervade our entire culture, and at least two habits connected with them, *alcoholism* and *smoking*, have become major issues of public health. Feeding people is characteristically considered a generous need in our society, and allegations of literal anality are commonly made against people who are grudging of themselves or their goods with others. Nor is it particularly uncommon for little girls of five to propose marriage to their fathers or boys to their mothers; and it is widely recognized that, at about that time of life, children first begin to play at what may be their life roles, sometimes external, like nurses, firemen, and grocery clerks, but more often internal, like heroes and heroines born of tales their mothers have told them and inventions they themselves have spun from the life of the family.

The Characterology of Erich Fromm

Unlike Freud, Fromm takes his typology from culture and society rather than from biological phases of development. He posits that all men in Western society are subject to the same critical environmental condition, which he calls "separation from nature."

> Not being able to stand the separation, he is impelled to seek for relatedness and oneness . . . . It is the paradox of human existence that man must simultaneously seek for closeness and for independence; for oneness with others and at the same time for the preservation of his uniqueness and particularity. (1947, pp. 96–97.)

Although Fromm says that his view of the nature of character is generally the same as Freud's, there is actually little resemblance between them.

> The main difference in the theory of character proposed here from that of Freud is that the fundamental basis of character is not seen in various types of libido organization but in specific kinds of a person's relatedness to the world. In the process of living, man relates himself to the world (1) by acquiring and assimilating things, and (2) by relating himself to people (and himself). The former I shall call the process of assimilation; the latter, that of socialization. Both forms of relatedness are 'open' and not, as with the animal, instinctively determined. (P. 58.)

From this base, Fromm develops a character typology containing two general classes: *nonproductive orientation* and *productive orientation.* For each character type he names, Fromm has one term which describes the individual's general disposition toward the acquisition and assimilation of things and another term which describes his disposition toward people. He describes essentially ideal or pure characters, although he allows that in reality, people are blends and mixtures of these types. There are four nonproductive types: (a) *receptive* (dependent), (b) *exploitative* (taking from others), (c) *hoarding* (withdrawn), and (d) *marketing* (exchanging). The single productive type might be called *working,* and the relations of these people with others are characteristically loving and rational.

Receptive orientation. The person belonging to this type believes that the source of all good things lies outside of himself. He is essentially concerned with being loved, believing that if one is loved, one gets what he needs to be secure. He is dependent, uncritical, and fearful of rebuff, primarily because it may terminate his sources of emotional and material supplies. If he is religious, his God is one who gives but requires little or nothing in return. Receptive people, as might be expected, are often quite loyal, but it is "a particular kind of loyalty, at the bottom of which is the gratitude for the hand that feeds them and the fear of ever losing it" (p. 62). This type of orientation corresponds fairly well to the *orally receptive character* in Freudian theory.

Exploitative orientation. Like the receptive character, the exploitative one also believes that the source of all good lies outside of himself. But the exploitative character does not expect to receive these goods as gifts. He feels that the way to get the things you want is to grab or steal them. "Stolen waters are sweeter" is his motto, and he tends to value particularly things that belong to others.

Hoarding orientation. The hoarder is less concerned with the sources of his goods than with the goods themselves. His security lies not in grasping or receiving from others, but in hoarding what he has. Hoarders

> have surrounded themselves, as it were, by a protective wall, and their main concern is to bring as much as possible into this fortified position and to let as little

> as possible out of it. Their miserliness refers to money and material things as well as to feelings and thoughts . . . . [Clearly] their highest values are order and security; their motto: 'There is nothing new under the sun.' (P. 67.)

Finally, they have a special sense of justice which says, in effect: "Mine is mine and yours is yours."

Marketing orientation. The "marketer" is historically a relatively new species, Fromm believes, spawned in the era of modern capitalism. Under the earlier barter system, which was characterized by more personal relationships between people, the value of an object was determined largely by the use to which it could be put. The barter system, however, was replaced by impersonal modern capitalism, in which the individual purchaser's needs are no longer the primary consideration of producers. Production is directed by essentially abstract considerations of supply and demand. We have moved, Fromm argues, from a system characterized by *use* value to one dominated by *exchange* value.

> The market concept of value, the emphasis on exchange value rather than on use value, has led to a particular concept of value with regard to people and particularly to oneself. The character orientation which is rooted in the experience of oneself as a commodity and of one's value as exchange value I call the marketing orientation. (P. 68.)

For marketing kinds of people, competence, usefulness, and skills are by no means sufficient guarantees of success. What is additionally necessary is "personality," which means an appearance of being whatever seems most desirable at a given time and in a particular occupation.

> Success depends largely on how well a person sells himself on the market, how well he gets his personality across, how nice a 'package' he is. (Pp. 69–70.)

The person with the marketing orientation treats himself as an object, as a commodity whose salability increases with his apparent social desirability. His motto is not, "I am what I do," but rather, "I am as you desire me." And he treats others likewise, as commodities with price tags, rather than as people.

The marketing orientation has no counterpart among Freud's character types, but to Fromm's way of thinking, it is one of the most pervasive orientations in modern society. Knowledge itself, he argues, has become a commodity.

> From grade school to graduate school, the aim of learning is to gather as much information as possible that is mainly useful for the purposes of the market . . . . Not the interest in the subjects taught or in knowledge and insight as such, but the enhanced exchange value knowledge gives is the main incentive for wanting more and better education. (P. 76.)

These four orientations—receptive, exploitative, hoarding, and marketing—exist to a certain degree in everyone. They are facilitated by various aspects of the culture and they also have their positive aspects, as Table 8.2 shows. A predominantly receptive person may also be modest, devoted, sensitive, and idealistic, while someone with an exploitative orientation may also be active, self-confident, and captivating. Nevertheless, they are in the main, nonproductive and psychologically debilitating orientations which, in extreme cases, constitute negative abnormalities.

Productive orientation. There is only one productive orientation, and it is positive for the individual and society. Its assimilative aspect is work. It is not concerned with receiving or hoarding or marketing or exploiting; it is concerned with *doing* or *producing*. In its socialization aspect, it is not destructive, masochistic, sadistic, or indifferent: it is *loving* and *reasoning*. In one sense, nonproduc-

Table 8.2

Characteristics of the Four Nonproductive Orientations[1]

Orientation	Positive Aspect	Negative Aspect
Receptive (accepting)	Accepting	Passive, without initiative
	Responsive	Opinionless, characterless
	Devoted	Submissive
	Modest	Without pride
	Charming	Parasitical
	Adaptable	Unprincipled
	Socially adjusted	Servile, without self-confidence
	Idealistic	Unrealistic
	Sensitive	Cowardly
	Polite	Spineless
	Optimistic	Wishful thinking
	Trusting	Gullible
	Tender	Sentimental
Exploitative (taking)	Active	Exploitative
	Able to take initiative	Aggressive
	Able to make claims	Egocentric
	Proud	Conceited
	Impulsive	Rash
	Self-confident	Arrogant
	Captivating	Seducing
Hoarding (preserving)	Practical	Unimaginative
	Economical	Stingy
	Careful	Suspicious
	Reserved	Cold
	Patient	Lethargic
	Cautious	Anxious
	Steadfast, tenacious	Stubborn
	Imperturbable	Indolent
	Composed under stress	Inert
	Orderly	Pedantic
	Methodical	Obsessional
	Loyal	Possessive
Marketing (exchanging)	Purposeful	Opportunistic
	Able to change	Inconsistent
	Youthful	Childish
	Forward looking	Without a future or a past
	Open minded	Without principle and values
	Social	Unable to be alone
	Experimenting	Aimless
	Undogmatic	Relativistic
	Efficient	Overactive
	Curious	Tactless
	Intelligent	Intellectualistic
	Adaptable	Undiscriminating
	Tolerant	Indifferent
	Witty	Silly
	Generous	Wasteful

[1] From *Man for Himself* by Erich Fromm. Copyright 1947 by Erich Fromm. Reprinted by permission of Holt, Rinehart and Winston, Inc.

tively oriented people can be seen as "integumented," as Allport (1960) puts it. The primary and direct concerns are with their own skins, with how they can gain power or riches or popularity for themselves. The productively oriented person achieves his goals by being concerned with things and people outside of himself. He achieves relatedness through interest in other things and other people.

Freud's concern was to illuminate psychopathology, and so he gave little attention to the mature and productive character (he called it the *genital* character, implying, among other things, that the mature individual's concerns extend to reproductivity and relationship). Fromm is concerned to rectify the imbalance. In *Man for Himself* (1947) and in *The Art of Loving* (1956), he elaborates the nature of productive character and particularly the nature of a loving relationship. Most people, he says, think that loving is easy, not much more difficult than finding the right person. That may be true for *falling* in love. *Standing* in love, however, requires several important capacities, foremost among them *care, responsibility, respect,* and *knowledge.* Love that fails to embody care and responsibility is little more than momentary passion, an ephemeral solution to loneliness. Productive love requires concern, not only for another's physical welfare, "but for the growth and development of all his human powers" (p. 100).

Care and responsibility, however, are not enough. With them alone, love deteriorates into possessiveness and domination. Respect (root: *respicere,* to look at) and knowledge are also required, denoting

> the ability to see a person as he is, to be aware of his individuality and uniqueness. To respect a person is not possible without knowing him; care and responsibility would be blind if they were not guided by the knowledge of the person's individuality. (P. 101.)

Social Character: Tradition-, Inner-, and Other-Directedness

The typology which David Riesman and his collaborators, Reuel Denney and Nathan Glazer, have developed in *The Lonely Crowd: A Study of the Changing American Character* (1950) pays more attention to how character is formed than Fromm's does. Riesman and his co-workers discuss the roles of family, peer groups, and other cultural agents. On the other hand, they focus even more than Fromm does on *society* as the agent of character formation and on changes in society as the cause of change in common character types. In fact, *The Lonely Crowd* specifically speaks of "social character" rather than "character," defining it as "that part of 'character' which is shared among significant social groups and which . . . is the product of the experience of these groups" (p. 18). Riesman proposes three character types, each of which is associated with a particular type of society.

Tradition-directed types. Societies that are relatively stable commonly produce tradition-directed people. As long as they do not expand,

> These societies . . . tend to be stable at least in the sense that their social practices . . . are institutionalized and patterned. . . . Since the type of social order . . . is relatively unchanging, the conformity of the individual tends to be dictated to a very large degree by power relations among the various age and sex groups, the clans, castes, professions and so forth—relations which have endured for centuries and are modified but slightly, if at all, by successive generations. The culture controls behavior minutely, and . . . careful and rigid etiquette governs the fundamentally influential sphere of kin relationships. (Pp. 10–11.)

The range of individual choice in such societies is severely restricted even among privileged castes; in all but trivial matters a matrix of social forms determines behavior. Indeed, because such societies change so very slowly, "social character comes as close as it ever does to looking like the matrix of social forms themselves" (p. 13).

Inner-directed types. A period of rapid population growth is also a period of violent transition in social structure. Once advances in hygiene and medicine permit the society's "growth potential" to increase, the traditions that seemed adequate during its slow-moving, stable phase are no longer useful; such transitional societies are characterized by breakdowns in the very structures that formerly contributed to traditional stability. Social and geographical mobility increases; economic and geographic expansion occurs on a vast scale; personal fortunes are made and lost rapidly.

Tradition directedness, which is oriented towards achieving *behavioral conformity,* now gives way to inner directedness, which is goal oriented. "The source of direction for the individual is 'inner' in the sense that it is implanted early in life by the elders and directed towards generalized but nonetheless inescapably destined goals" (p. 15). An inner-directed society provides the individual with a "psychological gyroscope" which, once it is set by socializing agents, keeps him going in a relatively straight line towards his goal. Clearly, the inculcation of inner directedness requires considerably more time and conscious effort from parents and other agents of society than the teaching of tradition directedness does. The latter is simpler and is reinforced by all members of society since its main concern is to produce the same visible behavioral forms in everyone.

Other-directed types. The other-directed individual emerges when a society passes its period of expansion and experiences incipient population decline. When it has sufficient resources to satisfy the immediate needs of its members, its attention turns away from the cultivation of natural resources and materials towards the cultivation of people. The inner directedness that was once so appropriate and useful for an economics of scarcity is no longer of much use in an abundant society. Capital accumulation is now a corporate rather than an individual function. The individual's role is to locate a comfortable niche for himself in Big Society, Big Business, and Big Government. Under these conditions, skills become less useful than personality, the ability to produce less valuable than the aptitude for being liked.

> What is common to all other-directeds is that their contemporaries are the source of direction for the individual—either those known to him or those with whom he is indirectly acquainted, through friends and through the mass media. This source is of course 'internalized' in the sense that dependence on it for guidance in life is implanted early. The goals towards which the other-directed person strives shift with that guidance: it is only the process of striving itself and the process of paying close attention to the signals from others that remain unaltered through life. (P. 22.)

Riesman's other-directed character is Fromm's marketer; they are identical. Both are relatively new character types in the sense that they develop out of economic and social structures that are relatively recent. The child in the other-directed culture has few responsibilities beyond himself, for adults feel no need to inculcate long-range work goals. Families are small and homes efficient; life in the city, where Riesman locates the main force of other-directedness, requires the child to contribute less than the farm and its rural community do. Parents' attentions are therefore directed away from giving children functions and responsibilities ("use values," in Fromm's view) and toward giving them "a psychological radar set," teaching them to be sensitive to the psychological desires of others and able to fulfill them.

There are controlling emotional experiences that, according to Riesman, operate to keep individuals conforming to the norms of their societies. The tradition-directed person is expected to behave in traditional ways, and when he fails to do so, to feel *shame*. The inner-directed type is often deterred from leaving the course of his own conscience by feelings of *guilt*. Other-directed people, like tradition-directed ones, are chiefly responsive to the requirements of their social groups. But where the norms for the tradition-directed are clear and simple, the radar-like sensitivities of the other-directed are severely taxed by the complex array of incoming signals from other people. Often enough, the signals are contradictory, and sometimes they are masked or confused by overlays of "noise." The other-directed character tends to react to this confusion with *anxiety*, a sense of vague fear that he cannot satisfy the many demands to which he is sensitive.

EMPIRICAL STUDIES OF CHARACTER

We observed earlier that character is easier to think about than to measure, and the discussion to this point has not belied this observation. Major characterological descriptions have always been the work of social analysts and clinical psychiatrists whose impressions and theories are broadly conceived. And while many readers will have found these observations on character intuitively compelling and quite descriptive of people they know, they are still lacking empirical evidence for the traits we have described.

Consider the "good" or moral character of our earlier discussion. We noted that the person of good character might be expected to possess such traits as honesty, altruism, and persistence. To what extent do these traits actually occur together in an individual? Are we justified in summing all of them under the one rubric of good character? The evidence on this issue is not as clear as we would like because no study has attempted to measure *all* of the traits we have enumerated. But on the basis of some studies that have measured a few, there does appear to be some relationship between the various traits of good character (Burton, 1963; Hartshorne and May, 1928–1930). The relationship is small because many factors influence the presence, absence, and degree of activity of characterological traits. But the fact that such a relationship exists permits us to refer to *character* without doing injustice to the word.

Following Kohlberg (1964a), we shall distinguish between three overlapping aspects of good character: moral behavior, moral judgment, and moral feeling. We make this distinction because the determinants and correlates of each aspect of character are not identical and because the relationship between these three aspects has never been shown to be substantial. A person who judges that some act is wrong may nevertheless do it and perhaps have little feeling about it. In this regard, character is no different from other aspects of personality; thought, feeling, and action, though somewhat correlated, are not related in a highly predictable manner.

Moral Behavior

Perhaps the most striking finding to emerge from researches that have considered several kinds of moral behavior is that situational conditions are overwhelmingly influential in determining whether a person will observe or violate rules. Studies of the "temptation to cheat" (Hartshorne and May, 1928–30; Sears *et al.*, 1965) have found only moderate correlations (ranging from 0.00 to 0.45) between one tempting situation and another. Children at least, and probably all of us, are not divisible into two neat groups of cheaters and noncheaters. It appears that most people cheat some of the time, a few cheat most of the time, and few manage to resist nearly all temptation. Over and above one's feelings against cheating, whether one succumbs depends greatly on the risk of detection (Hartshorne and May, 1930; Wallace and Sadalla, 1966) and on the potential gain (Rosenhan *et al.*, 1966). Children who cheat in very risky situations also cheat in less risky ones, which suggests that noncheaters may be guided more by cautiousness than by honesty (Kohlberg, 1964*b*).

The examples set by peer and adult models may contribute to violation of all kinds of norms, just as such examples can contribute to their support (Midlarsky and Bryan, 1967; Milgram, 1965; Rosenhan and White, 1966). It is common for children to engage in antisocial acts such as stealing, not because the stolen object is desirable nor from any ignorance that stealing is bad, but simply to conform to group example. Taken out of the group, they follow their own personal habits of honesty or dishonesty (at least as far as the neighborhood five-and-ten is concerned!).

The Effects of Moral Adjuration

It has commonly been assumed that moral education, either in the home or in social institutions, is a critical determinant of moral behavior. Children who display bad character traits are often said not to have "learned any better." While in some sense this analysis must be true, it is by no means as simple as it appears. Hartshorne and May, for example, found no relationship between behavioral tests of honesty or of concern for others and membership in the Boy Scouts or attendance at Sunday School or character education classes. Merely *telling* a child how he ought to behave may be sufficient for *informing* him about what is right and wrong, but it does not influence his actual behavior.

Moral Example

If direct tuition is of little use in establishing moral behavior, what is? Perhaps the most important single means of learning the behaviors which together constitute good character is to observe them in other people and then to imitate them. This prescription is so much a part of virtually universal folk wisdom that sophisticated people are likely to be suspicious of it, but the evidence nonetheless seems to verify that much of the most important learning of childhood begins as attempts to mimic significant figures in the child's life. Nor is this phenomenon limited to human beings alone. Mowrer's (1950) work on talking birds and Harlow's (1958; 1962) more recent studies of affection in monkeys both suggest that imitation is the basis of much significant behavior.

The precise reason why youngsters imitate their elders is not clear; imitation begins at such an early age that it is impossible to believe the child is using it to achieve some rational purpose or solve some particular problem. It is possible that the most primitive kinds of imitation, such as that found in talking birds or very early in human infants, initially occurs at random and only gradually assumes some satisfying property that causes it to be systematically repeated.

Whatever the origins of imitative behavior may be, however, clearly it rapidly comes to function as the primary means by which most social behavior, including language, is learned. Freud (1932) was the first to observe that imitation or modelling is the basis for learning crucial attitudes in childhood, and he interpreted this behavior as an attempt on the child's part to resolve Oedipal anxiety in relation to the parent of the same sex by *identifying himself with the parent* and modelling his behavior accordingly. Thus the term "identification" came to be attached to the process by which a child patterns his attitudes and behavior after others who are significant in his life. (See Chapter 4 for more recent views of identification.)

In all probability, Freud was mistaken in placing the identification process in the phallic stage of development more than in others, but if anything, his error was to underestimate rather than to overstate the importance of this process in the formation of character. Miller and Dollard (1941) consider modelling the central process that guides the learning of social behavior, and this point of view is dominant in the study of personality today (see Bandura and Walters, 1963).

It is easy to see, therefore, why identification should be the basic mechanism by which positive character traits are formed. This process permits a child to emulate the behavior of his parents at a far earlier age than he is able to understand or rationalize it. Since the behavior involved in positive character traits is considered highly desirable, moreover, his parents and other adults are almost certain to reward it. Thus, patterns of desirable behavior are established, along with favorable attitudes towards them, at such early ages that they become part of the normal cognitive equipment of the child whenever he is old enough to form concepts about them. If a child is consistently rewarded for being truthful, open, cooperative, and so forth, and these are behaviors which he takes on in imitation of his parents to begin with, then these patterns are likely to become a permanent part of his behavior repertory.

Several conditions seem to be, if not prerequisite to the formation of positive identifications, conducive to them. These are:

Repeated exposure. A child does not need to observe a parent do something over and over again in order to imitate the action. But the greater his exposure to such behavior, the more likely imitation of it on appropriate occasions becomes. It is also important that he not be exposed to repeated inconsistencies on the part of the model, as these make it difficult for him to determine just what behavior he ought to imitate. (Mischel and Liebert, 1964, 1966; Rosenhan *et al.*, 1966).

Mutual positive affect. The chances that a parent will provide a suitable object of identification for a child are enhanced considerably if there is mutual positive feeling between them. A child will model himself more consistently after a parent he loves and feels loved by than after a despised parent or one he feels rejected by. Though children sometimes identify strongly with parents they fear and hate in order to relieve their fear, such identifications are likely to be full of conflict and anxiety and thus less stable and effective.

Model saliency. The more salient a model is in the eyes of the child, that is the more appropriate an object of imitation, the more modelling will occur. This says, among other things, that a child will be more likely to model himself after an adult whose behavior is like that of other potential models than after one who is conspicuously different. For this reason, conformist models have a better chance of being effective than nonconformist ones—they induce less conflict.

The value of observing a beloved model for establishing moral behavior can be seen in a recent study of altruistic behavior (Rosenhan, 1966). The altruists involved were Negroes and whites who had committed large amounts of time, energy, and financial resources to the Civil Rights movement. All of them had been active in the movement for at least two years and had left their homes or schools to go to the South and participate in voter registration, education, or community organization. They were not simply occasional Freedom Riders or people with casual pro-Negro and pro-Civil Rights sympathies; they were distinguished from such people by the extent of their involvement and activity in the movement.

While they came from varied backgrounds, ranging from the lowest to the highest social class and from minimal to postgraduate education, they appeared to have one experience in common: *nearly all identified strongly with an altruistic parent.* One of them remarked that "my father carried me on his shoulders in the Sacco-Vanzetti parades." Another said his mother "was warmed by Jesus and felt close to him. . . . She devoted her entire life to Christian education." A third distinctly recalled his father's reaction to the outbreak of the second World War: "It was not long after my father learned about the atrocities (in the German concentration camps) that he enlisted. He was nauseated. He couldn't take it any more." Most of these altruists described parents who were socially active in a positive and constructive way, who were, in this sense, socially deviant (see Chapters 1 and 5), and with whom they strongly identified while they were children. During a good portion of their childhoods, they had seen in their parents consistent models of prosocial behavior. At least one parent had set examples that the children had internalized.

We infer from these data that the presence of consistently altruistic models in one's childhood is a potential determinant of commitment to altruistic behavior in adulthood. Exposure to inconsistent models, however, may be relevant to one's own lack of consistency and diffused commitment where altruistic behavior is concerned.

One cannot be certain, of course, that the inferences we make from such retrospective data are, in fact, accurate, but there is some experimental evidence to support them. Mischel and Liebert (1964) found that children who were instructed to reward themselves for a high standard of achievement and who also observed an adult reward himself similarly, uniformly internalized that standard, that is, refused to take rewards for a lower standard of achievement even when they were playing by themselves with no adult present to guide their behaviors. In contrast, where the adult preached a high standard to the children but practiced a low one, many children adopted the adult's practice and rewarded themselves for a low standard. Indeed, a subsequent study (Rosenhan *et al.*, 1966) found that many of the children who were exposed to a hypocritical model not only adopted a low standard but also engaged in dishonest behavior. They took many more rewards than they had earned, and in several instances, stole the rewards outright.

Graded rehearsal. An opportunity to rehearse, and particularly to rehearse in a *graded* manner, is also important for character development. It is more difficult, for example, to resist a powerful temptation than a minor one. and one would expect people to have greater success in resisting major lures if they already had experience in resisting minor ones. Skinner (1948), in his utopian novel, *Walden Two*, proposes that young children might be given lollipops with the promise that if they did not lick them now, they could eat them later in the day. (Powdered sugar on the pop would reveal any cheating, even a "quick lick.") The children would learn that the best way to avoid this kind of temptation would be to put the candy away and out of sight. Having mastered this kind of temptation, they could be confronted with more difficult blandishments that require a capacity for psychological avoidance and strong tolerance for frustration.

Gradually, by rehearsing each step, "ethical training" could be completed by the age of six.

The Soviet educational system exerts greater control over the individual than is possible in the United States, and this control manifests itself in concern for his moral development. A recent manual for kindergarten teachers (in Russia, kindergarten includes four-, five-, and six-year-olds) suggests some moral behavior in which children can be rehearsed:

> The moral feelings of children express themselves in moral conduct. Respect, love, attachment for family and close friends must be expressed through generally accepted forms of attention and respect: greeting people properly and saying good-bye, saying thank you after meals or after receiving a gift or some assistance, . . . letting older people pass or helping younger ones, . . . offering a guest a seat. . . . The teacher must strive to make these habits of moral behavior so secure that the children will behave on all occasions in life in the way in which they were taught. . . .
>
> Certain things must become traditional in the kindergarten, such as greeting classmates on the occasion of a holiday; children in the four-, five-, and six-year-old groups should write letters to sick schoolmates or teachers (the teacher writes while the children dictate) . . . and do the same for friends on their birthdays. (*A Teacher's Commentary*, pp. 124–125.)

While the advice in the Russian manual deals in some respects with what we would call *courtesy*, which may or may not be implicated in moral conduct (depending on your point of view), it is clear that the Soviets urge extensive rehearsal as one method of inculcating this behavior.

Some experimental evidence for the utility of rehearsal emerged in the study of children's charitableness that was referred to earlier (Rosenhan and White, 1966). Children played a game with an adult in which each time either one obtained a high score, he would win two five-cent gift certificates. Each time the adult won, he donated one of his certificates to a charity. The child was free to imitate the adult or not, as he chose. Children who imitated (that is, rehearsed) later donated to the charity when they played the game alone, under no external pressures to donate. On the other hand, children who merely observed the adult donating, but did not donate in his presence, also did not donate in his absence.

Vicarious arousal. The process of identification is the most important single instrument for the formation of good character, but it is not the only one available, and certainly not the one most used by educational agencies of our society. Another technique in wide use is called "vicarious arousal" in reference to the empathic result of emotionally "putting oneself in the other person's shoes."

Vicarious conditioning probably has a powerful influence because it provides the child with a hypothetical figure to identify with. The difference between modelling and vicarious conditioning is that, in the former case, the actual behavior model was available for the child to observe. In vicarious arousal, on the other hand, a child observes or is told about, for example, the victim of oppression or injustice and, without having any direct model of good conduct, emphasizes with the victim and formulates a plan of his own to prevent such suffering in the future. In order for such empathic experience to occur, it is necessary for a child to have had sufficient positive experiences with others to have developed a capacity to sympathize with the unfortunate. Whether or not it is necessary for him to have suffered in order to become sensitive to the sufferings of others is another story. In all probability, just the opposite is the case. The experience of brutality possibly leads to its acceptance in the world, whereas the experience of love and kindness between people disposes one towards loving, kindly, and sympathetic relations with others.

Positive reinforcement. Whether the acts that identify good character initially occur because a child models himself after a parent or for some other reason, they are most likely to become fixed in the behavior repertory if they are directly and positively reinforced, that is, if some reward or satisfaction accrues to the child as a result of performing them (Thorndike, 1927). Positive reinforcement, as such rewards are called, is probably the most important mechanism in the acquisition of any new behavior. The rewards do not need to be material ones, though for some children at some ages rewards such as candy, money, or toys are powerful indeed. Social rewards are even more important—nods and words of approval, the occasional hug—these appear to be the powerful sustainers of moral behavior (Aronfreed and Reber, 1965; Midlarsky and Bryan, 1967; Peck and Havighurst, 1960).

Such reinforcements may, of course, be applied to virtually any behavior with the expectation that, if sufficient reward accrues, the behavior is likely to be learned. Naturally, this principle applies just as well to antisocial as to prosocial behaviors. If the two are in competition for acceptance in the mind of the child, as for instance if he is torn between participating in a gang or going to school, the one which is most immediately and strongly reinforced is likely to win out. In this simple case, it is often going with the gang; the rewards of schooling, though ultimately greater, are also more distant, and, thus, at any given time, weaker.

Aversive conditioning. Just as the learning of prosocial behaviors desirable in character formation depends on positive reinforcement, learning to avoid antisocial and undesirable character traits may require some negative or punitive training. This is a less clear-cut matter than positive reward. It is plain enough that antisocial behavior will not become part of the permanent repertory if it is not satisfying, but it is not so clear that learning it can be altogether prevented by punishment. Certainly, punishment is one of the most widely accepted training methods in our society, but its efficacy is often in question (Bandura and Walters, 1963). Consider, for example, the child who has been caught hitting his brother and gets spanked by his father. Does the child learn that hitting is bad? Or having observed and experienced his father's punishment, does he learn that hitting is all right—so long as you are an adult or can avoid being caught?

At all events, even if antisocial behavior can be inhibited or prevented by punitive means, prosocial behavior does not automatically take its place. In other words, the fact that a child learns to avoid some undesirable act because he has been punished for it does not mean that he will thereby be more prone to perform in a desirable way. Although moral behavior is concerned with both the avoidance of undesirable habits and the promotion of virtue, the inhibition of antisocial behavior does not in any direct way serve the teaching of prosocial behavior.

Generalization. In order for the teaching of character to be maximally effective, it is necessary, once a child has learned some suitable behavior, that he be able to apply it in relatively new and unfamiliar situations. This ought to occur by the process of *generalization,* in which *the experience gained in one situation is transferred to another one that bears some resemblance to it.* Generalized responses require reinforcement just as originally learned ones do if they are to be maintained. There is little actual research on the generalization of moral behaviors however, and our speculations on the role of generalization remain speculations.

Correlates of moral behavior. In examining the components of good character the reader will have sensed that it is probably not an encapsulated aspect of personality, but is related to and perhaps the beneficiary of other positive personality traits. There is some evidence that moral behavior is positively correlated with such positive abilities as intelligence (Hartshorne and May, 1928; Peck and Havighurst, 1960; Sanford *et al.*, 1943), that those who do not cheat in an experimental task are generally more able to postpone gratification (Mischel, 1963) and to control aggressive fantasies (Sears *et al.*, 1965) than those who do, and finally, that ratings of character traits seem to correlate positively with measures of self-esteem and satisfaction with one's surroundings (Havighurst and Taba, 1949).

Moral Judgment

We pointed out earlier that moral behavior and moral judgment are by no means synonymous so that one ought to hesitate before predicting a man's moral behavior from his moral judgments. This is not to say that moral judgment is a trivial thing. Men live in their minds and thoughts as well as in their acts, and what a man thinks is significant and important in its own right.

At the outset, we need to distinguish moral judgment from moral knowledge. People learn moral rules very early in life, and it is probable that by the age of six we have as much moral information as we are going to have. *Moral information* consists of broad social rules, such as, "Don't hit," "Thou shalt not steal," "Say please and thank you," and we are exposed to this kind of information constantly even before we can walk. One's score on a test of moral information reflects things like intelligence, socio-economic station, desire to make a good social impression, and little else.

In many of life's critical situations, however, moral information alone is of little use, primarily because these situations allow the application of two or more conflicting moral rules. For example, should a man steal in order to feed his family? One ought not steal, of course, but neither should one allow his family to suffer hunger. Should one kill in order to defend one's nation? Or obey a law that violates one's conscience? Even such apparently neutral issues as doing scientific research have strong moral underpinnings when the research may be employed for undemocratic (there's a moral rule) or destructive (there's another) ends. And as we shall see in Chapter 15, even the psychotherapies that have called themselves strictly scientific enterprises have such significant moral aspects that psychotherapists in general have earned the title of secular priests (London, 1964).

Moral judgment means the conclusions people reach where moral rules are conflicting or ambiguous; it also includes the reasons they offer to support their conclusions. These reasons and judgments derive from the kinds of people they are and the way they see the world, things that develop independently of moral character but that nevertheless impinge quite directly upon it. Consider the following example: if your brother tells you in confidence of his misdeed, should you tell your father? A young child's thinking might go as follows: "If I tell my father, my brother will hit me. If I don't tell my father, and he finds out that I know, he will hit me." He might then speculate on the probabilities of being caught and on who hits hardest, and arrive at a decision. The horns of his dilemma are ones that hurt physically. An older child might arrive at the same judgment, but for reasons that have more to do with his sympathy for either party, his notions of loyalty, his aversion to "squealing," or his feelings about authority and obedience. Many of these considerations are not possible for a young child because his experiences have not yet provided him with these concepts. His notions of what the world is like, his history, development, and expectations are limited and primitive, and these limitations are reflected in his moral judgments.

Piaget's Views of the Development of Morality

As we have seen, moral judgment cannot be taught and learned by itself, and it changes as personality and cognitive development proceed. This view has long been supported by the work of the Swiss psychologist, Jean Piaget, whose descriptions of children's developing moral judgments (1932) have received considerable attention recently.

Piaget believes that young children from about three to eight years have cognitive limitations that lead them to confuse moral with physical laws as if they were fixed and immutable. Moreover, young children tend to view their parents as perfect and all knowing and therefore to regard parental pronouncements as unchangeable and right. This orientation to authority, combined with a tendency to confuse thoughts and wishes with external realities, makes children moral absolutists. As they grow older, their perceptions of reality and of the role of authority change. They come gradually to recognize that moral rules are instruments of human values and concerns and that, far from being absolute, they are quite relative. Empathy, sentiment, and reciprocity come to play roles in their judgment. Notions of justice and of right and wrong become dislodged from external authority and housed within the individual.

Kohlberg (1964*a*) lists several aspects of moral judgment that are stated or implied in Piaget's work and that have found support in other research. Analysis of them provides a basis not only for understanding alterations in children's moral judgment, but for a developmental theory of moral judgment as well. These facets are:

Intentionality in judgment. Young children tend to judge right and wrong only in terms of results, while older children take intention into consideration. If breaking a dish is wrong, then nearly all four-year-olds would agree that the boy who breaks five dishes while helping his mother is "wronger" than the boy who broke one while stealing a cookie (MacRae, 1954; Piaget, 1932). Of course, actions are easier than intentions for a young child to comprehend. The notion and importance of intention require greater psychological experience, which the young child lacks.

The possibility of multiple judgments. The young child believes there is only one right answer; the older child can see many points of view. Again, the young child comprehends only simplicities, the older one greater complexity.

Contingency of moral judgment upon punitive consequences. A young child will judge the rightness of a behavior retrospectively, that is, according to the consequences it elicits. If you go to jail, you must have committed a crime; and if you've been spanked, you must have done something wrong. For the older child, the moral rule stands independent of subsequent sanctions.

Somewhat related to this is what Piaget calls "immanent justice," the tendency among young children to view accidental misfortunes following a misdeed as punishments willed by God or by other powerful figures, including natural objects. Older children are better able to distinguish accidental from intended misfortunes (Medinnus, 1959).

Painful punishment versus restitution. Younger children advocate a vigorous *lex talionis* ("an eye for an eye") as punishment for misdeeds. Older children tend to favor milder punishments in general and are often concerned to provide restitution for the victim and to reform the transgressor.

The role of reciprocity. A concern for reciprocity and egalitarian belief plays a crucial role in the development of a sense of justice, according to Piaget. For older children, justice is not merely an abstract canon but is derived from and buttressed by feelings of mutual respect, gratitude, and empathy. They use these feelings in judging the rightness or wrongness of an act. Younger children operate more egocentrically; if they have a sense of reciprocity, it tends to be concerned mainly with retaliation or reward (Durkin, 1959).

While nearly all children in all cultures pass from the lower to the higher stages, they may do so at different rates. Relative maturity on one facet does not predict maturity on the others (Johnson, 1962; MacRae, 1954). Personal experiences and cultural teachings may serve to facilitate or retard the process (Havighurst and Neugarten, 1955), but all children seem to leave the most primitive levels and move upwards. However, this does not mean that the processes are necessarily biological. There may be constitutional factors involved in the degree to which a child can ultimately comprehend a complex world, but the processes of moral development are primarily those of learning.

Basing his work on that of Piaget (1932) as well as that of George H. Mead (1934) and J. M. Baldwin (1906), Kohlberg (1963, 1964*b*) has advanced a developmental theory of moral judgment that encompasses three levels, each of which has two stages. In the first level, the child's moral judgment seems entirely dominated by external events. His orientations are principally towards reward and punishment. Subsequently, he moves to the second stage, where his concerns are reflected in "good" or "right" roles and in fulfilling the expectations of others. Finally, he may arrive at the third stage where moral values are upheld because he comes to share socialized beliefs that involve values, standards, rights, and obligations. These stages are elaborated as follows:

Level I. Value resides in external quasi-physical happenings, in bad acts, or in quasi-physical needs rather than in persons and standards.

Type 1: Obedience and punishment orientation. Egocentric deference to superior power or prestige, or a trouble-avoiding set. Objective responsibility.

Type 2: Naively egoistic orientation. Right action is that instrumentally satisfying the self's needs and occasionally others'. Awareness of relativism of value to each actor's needs and perspective. Naive egalitarianism and orientation to exchange and reciprocity.

Level II. Moral value resides in performing good or right roles, in maintaining the convention order and the expectancies of others

Type 3: Good boy orientation. Orientation to approval and to pleasing and helping others. Conformity to stereotypical images of majority or natural role behavior, and judgment by intentions.

Type 4: Orientation toward maintaining authority and social order, to "doing duty" and to showing respect for authority and maintaining the given social order for its own sake. Regard for earned expectations of others.

Level III. Moral value resides in conformity by the self to shared or sharable standards, rights, or duties.

Type 5: Contractual legalistic orientation. Recognition of an arbitrary element or starting point in rules or expectations for the sake of agreement. Duty defined in terms of contract, general avoidance of violation of the will or rights of others, and majority will and welfare.

Type 6: Conscience or principle orientation. Orientation not only to actually ordained social rules but to principles of choice involving appeal to logical universality and consistency. Orientation to conscience as a directing agent and to mutual respect and trust.

These stages were developed on the basis of extensive interviews with children and adolescents about various situations of moral conflict. Kohlberg (1964*a*) offers evidence that these stages correlate only modestly with IQ, but quite highly with age (0.59), indicating that they are influenced by experience and maturation.

How far a child develops with regard to moral judgment will be determined by his experience with life's conditions, but there is reason to believe that most children pass through the lower stages before arriving at the higher ones (Kohlberg, 1963; Turiel, 1966). The learnings and experiences of earlier stages appear to form necessary substructures for the acquisition of newer and more mature modes of moral judgment.[1]

Note that the three levels described in Kohlberg's developmental scheme correspond quite well to the kinds of judgments we might expect from children simply as a matter of growing up. When they are very young, children are merely *reactive* to their own needs and to the requirements of people around them, and we might expect this kind of responsiveness to be reflected in their own judgments. Subsequently they become concerned with maintaining good relationships and with *anticipating* the behavior adults might require of them.

In this second level we see a sort of undifferentiated, global identification: the authority or rewardingness of an adult is taken in "whole hog," as it were. The third level embodies not only the experience of identification, but a considerable amount of intelligent elaboration. Using his earlier experience and identifications as a base, the morally mature person can now develop his own beliefs, which may differ markedly from his parents' or even his society's.

Moral Judgment and Moral Behavior

While we may not expect to find powerful relationships between moral judgment and behavior because so many diverse variables appear to impinge on both, we should be quite surprised if no relationships existed at all. In fact, Kohlberg (1963, 1965) presents a number of findings to support the view that the development of moral judgment is related to moral conduct. For example, girls (but not boys), who cheated while playing a game in which large rewards were given for high scores, were rated lower on the moral development scale than those who did not cheat (Grinder, 1964; Rebelsky *et al.*, 1963). In a study by Brown and others (cited by Kohlberg, 1965), undergraduates who cheated on a test where a small financial reward was promised for a high score tended to make *conventional* (Level II) rather than *principled* (Level III) moral judgments. Note that this finding says nothing about feelings toward cheating. Indeed, attitudes towards cheating were somewhat negatively related to actual cheating; those who felt that cheating was bad tended

[1] The idea of *invariant* developmental stages will trouble those of you who are inclined to believe that these are simply matters of teaching and learning and that the contents of each stage ought to be acquirable regardless of whether one has mastered the previous ones. But while, in fact, there is some evidence that moral absolutists in Piaget's scheme can be trained to become moral relativists (Bandura and McDonald, 1963), the general weight of the evidence tends to support the invariant developmental stage position.

to cheat more rather than less. Moreover, attitudes towards cheating appeared unrelated to maturity of moral judgment.

> Our principled subjects, then, were not principled in the sense of strong verbal endorsement of a cultural role against cheating. Rather they were principled in the sense of being able to base conventional rules upon underlying moral reasons such as the importance of trust, contract, social agreement and equality of reward for equal effort and ability. (Kohlberg, 1965, p. 8.)

If the judgments people make range from the expedient to the principled, then those that hold principled convictions ought to be less willing to change or violate them under pressure than those whose judgments are based on expediency. In an experiment, children who had responded one way to moral conflict stories were pressed by the interviewer to agree that the opposite choice was correct. Those whose judgments were principled resisted pressure much more than those whose judgments were not (Kohlberg, 1965). Similar findings emerged from a study where undergraduates were asked to administer increasingly powerful shocks to a "victim" in an experiment that alleged to study the effects of punishment on memory. The delivery of such powerful punishment clearly violated the moral beliefs of the subjects. Nevertheless, nearly 70 percent of them delivered a seemingly lethal dose simply because the experimenter, who was a legitimate authority, asked them to (Milgram, 1963). (Fortunately, the victim, a collaborator of the experimenter, was not really wired into the apparatus.) Some weeks later, many of the subjects in this experiment were interviewed to determine their level of moral judgment. All but one of them who showed some principled judgment had wanted to quit the experiment, and in fact, 75 percent of those who refused to give the "lethal" shock showed Level III moral convictions. In contrast, less than half of the subjects whose judgments were conventional had been inclined to quit, and of those who did, only 13 percent were in the Level III group (Kohlberg, 1965).

Moral Feeling

There has been some dispute regarding the feelings that sustain or correlate with moral character. One popular view identifies moral character with morality, morality with conscience, and conscience with the Freudian superego. Another view equates moral character with will, personal strength, intelligence, and positive feelings towards others. These traits are considered ego rather than superego functions (Redl and Wineman, 1952; Hartmann, 1960).

The superego view holds that man is constantly beset by asocial and antisocial impulses, starting even before any incestuous desires for his mother and extending throughout life. Primitive, powerful, and unreasoning, these impulses continuously press for expression and need constantly to be contained. The locus of impulse suppression and repression is the superego. Itself harsh, punitive, and unreasoning, the superego is the source of critical self-observation, of self-punishment and censure, and of internal demands for repentance and reparation. Violations of the superego's mandates provoke intense negative affects—guilt, anxiety, shame, and depression—that serve both to prevent misdeeds and to punish when they occur. Man, in this conception, is essentially sinful, self-serving, and impulsive. Were it not for a well-internalized superego, there could be no moral character.

The ego-strength position sees moral character as something positive rather than negative, predicated on experiences of love, reciprocity, and regard for others rather than on guilt and anxiety. The moral character of this conception is relatively at ease with himself and society, gaining much from society and willing to give, with pleasure and occasionally with pain, to it. Indeed, from one point of view (Piaget, 1932), it is precisely the pleasant reciprocities that occur among children which give rise to their sense of justice and fairness.

These two views may be less conflicting than addressed to somewhat different aspects of character. The superego conception is concerned, first and foremost, with *avoidance*—of sin, vice, oftentimes pleasure. Resistance of temptation, honesty, impulse control, particularly of sex and aggression, and the like—these appear to be the primary concern of the superego. The ego conception is addressed primarily to the pursuit of virtue—kindness, altruism, fairness, responsibility, and concern for excellence, among others. The presence of virtue, however, does not automatically guarantee the absence of vice, and contrariwise, the avoidance of sin does not by itself engender virtue. Both ego and superego strength may be requisites to moral character. Both guilt and love have needed places.

Guilt

Most of us have experienced the feeling of guilt following, or in anticipation of, some real or imagined transgression. Its contents are anxiety and self-condemnation often accompanied by shame, revulsion, and remorse, all in various titers and mixtures. For some, it is a fortunately rare experience; many feel it often, and for most of us, it is quite painful.

What function does guilt serve? Is it, as Freud argued, a self-punitive response designed to punish the transgressor as he might have been punished by his parents? Or is it rather an anxiety-reducing response, designed to ward off external punishment?

Recent evidence on responses to transgression appears to support the view that guilt functions, in part, to reduce anxiety. In several experiments, Aronfreed (1963, 1964) has demonstrated that children learn self-critical responses (guilty responses) when they are associated with the termination of punishment, that is, with anxiety reduction. When these responses are associated with the onset of punishment (anxiety induction), however, little learning takes place.

Certain aspects of guilt responses may be acquired because they mitigate the consequences of punishment. Hill (1960) has suggested that confession will be learned when parents reduce the impending punishment, and Levine (Kohlberg, 1963) has shown that, when mothers reward confession in this way, children confess more. Analyses by Aronfreed have shown that the tendency to make restitution can also be acquired in this manner. Other studies suggest that when children confess, it is often in expectation that the parent will forgive them (Sears *et al.*, 1965; Wright *et al.*, 1961).

Given the present state of evidence, however, it would be erroneous to conclude that guilt serves *only* to reduce anxiety. It is possible for a person to violate an important standard, then to experience guilt, and subsequently to alter his behavior so as not to violate his standards again. Certainly the "real guilt" that Mowrer (1961) speaks of when he analyzes neurotic behavior (see Chapter 15) is much more than an anxiety reducer. And several studies have shown that self-blame and self-criticism (both aspects of guilt) on projective tests is positively related to resistance to temptation (Allinsmith, 1960) and nondelinquency (Adorno *et al.*, 1950; Bandura and Walters, 1959; McCord and McCord, 1956). If guilt served *only* to reduce anxiety, these relationships would make no sense. Indeed, one could yield to temptation or be delinquent and reduce the subsequent anxiety by feeling guilty about it. As Aronfreed (1964) and Kohlberg (1963) point out, whether guilt serves more to reduce anxiety or to induce conformity to moral norms may depend upon the way in which it was learned and upon the evaluative responses associated with it.

Love

The positive affects that encourage and accompany good character have not been much studied. Apart from data indicating that positive relationships facilitate identification, which, in turn, is related to moral character, little is known empirically about the role of positive affects.

This is not to say that positive affects have not been of theoretical concern. We observed earlier that Fromm (1947, 1956) defined one aspect of productive character as the capacity for love and its associated traits of care, responsibility, respect, and knowledge. Tomkins (1965) writes of the constructive role of positive as well as negative affect for the altruistic commitments of several pre-Civil War abolitionists.

The modern writer who has been most concerned with character and love is Pitirim Sorokin, an eminent social philosopher and prolific author. His primary interests in this area have been altruism and altruistic love and ways of stimulating these. He writes of altruism from a sociological vantage point as a "meaningful interaction—or relationship—between two or more persons where the aspirations and aims of one person are shared and helped in their realization by other persons" (1954*a*, p. 13). From a psychological point of view, the altruistic relationship is one in which the "Ego or I" of the loving individual tends to merge with and identify itself with the loved "Thee" (p. 10). He speaks of the role of love in terms that appear to have empirical meaning but are not yet amenable to careful examination: "Love is the experience that annuls our individual loneliness," "Love beautifies our life," the "Love experience is marked . . . by a 'feeling' of fearlessness and power" (p. 11). He suggests some twenty-six ways of stimulating altruistic love, among them private and public prayer, exposure to the love of others, meditation, psychodrama and psychoanalysis, rearrangement of group affiliations, and individual creative activity.

Needless to say, the role and usefulness of Sorokin's techniques and theories remain to be tested. His many writings (see Sorokin, 1948, 1950, 1954*a*, 1954*b*) in this area serve at present to direct our concern to the potential role of positive affects in character, but not yet to confirm their importance.

THE AGENTS OF CHARACTER BUILDING

Just as only a limited number of mechanisms operate in the formation of character, only a limited number of agents, individual and institutional, are entrusted with the child's character training. Critical among these, in descending order of importance, are: the family, the community, and the general society.

The Family

Without any doubt, the primary family is the most important agent of character formation in our culture, and within the family, the parents are ordinarily the most important members (see Figure 8.2). The formation of character within the family depends mostly on the process of identification of the child with either or both parents. It is difficult to say with any certainty which parent is likely to exert the greatest influence on the character of the child. Freud's theory would make it seem that the parent of the opposite

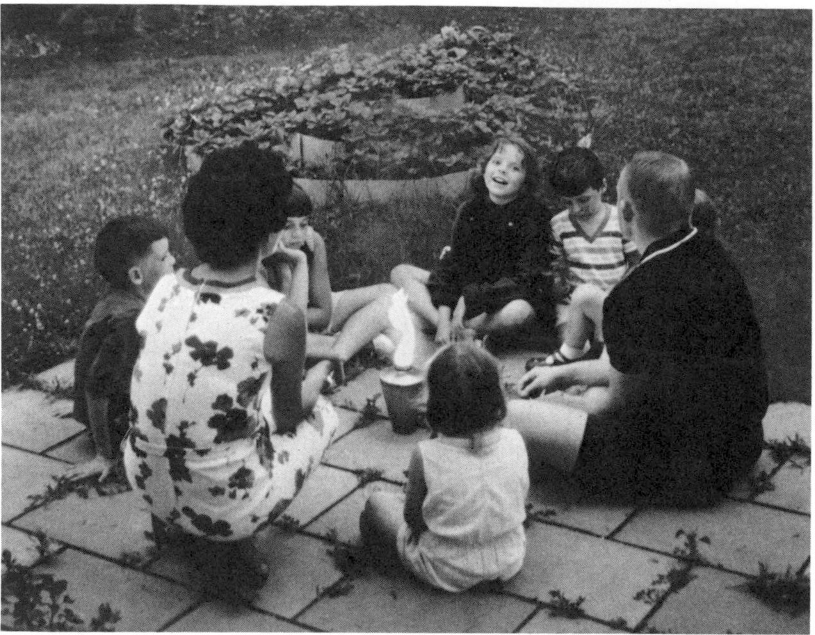

Figure 8.2 **The family is an agent of character building. Photo © Ken Heyman.**

sex is less likely to be critical than the parent of the same sex, since he views identification with the parent as a largely defensive tactic the child uses to alleviate the anxiety caused by his sexual interest in the parent of the opposite sex. Fromm (1956), on the other hand, suggests that the parents differ less in the *amount* of their influence than in the *quality* or *type* of characteristics they influence. In his view, mothers are responsible for the transmission of "feminine" or "maternal" characteristics, for the gentle virtues of love, kindliness, and a positive emotional investment in other people. Fathers are more responsible for transmitting "masculine" characteristics of rationality, concern for justice and righteousness, and presumably the traits of courage and tenacity, which are commonly associated with masculine virtues. Peck and Havighurst (1960) do not assume any theoretical position with respect to relative parental influences on character, but their empirical studies do seem to show that maternal influences are stronger than paternal ones:

> In most families the mother has had a more profound, direct influence on the child's character and personality than has the father. This does not seem to be a case of Philip Wylie's 'Momism,' deliberately fostered by maternal intent. In part, this may be a rather universal effect of the literal absence of the father from home much of the time. As much or more, perhaps, it is due to the cultural assignment of child rearing more and more exclusively to the mother. There appears to be no generally deleterious effects of this matriarchal pattern on the development of character, per se. (P. 180.)

Community Influences

The three main community agencies for character building are (1) the school, (2) the church, and (3) peer-group organizations such as Boy and Girl Scouts, 4-H clubs, and the like (see Figures 8.3 to 8.5). There is not a great deal to say about all of them except that, despite

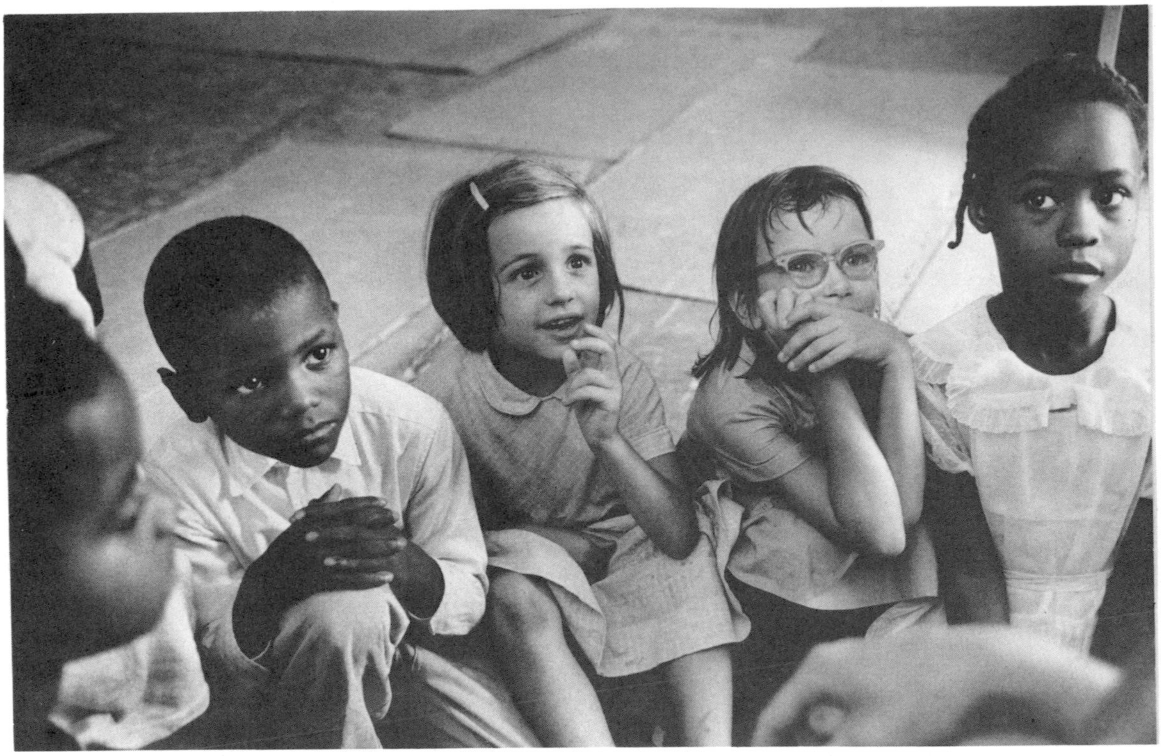

Figure 8.3 School is another agent of character building. Photo © Syd Greenberg, DPI.

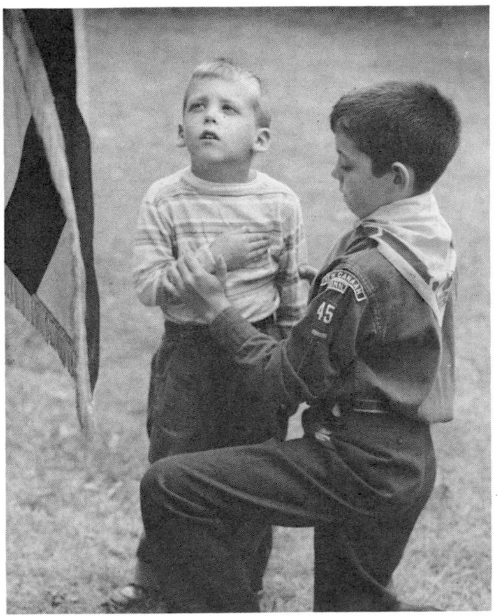

Figure 8.4 The Boy Scouts can be another agent of character building. Photo © Syd Greenberg, DPI.

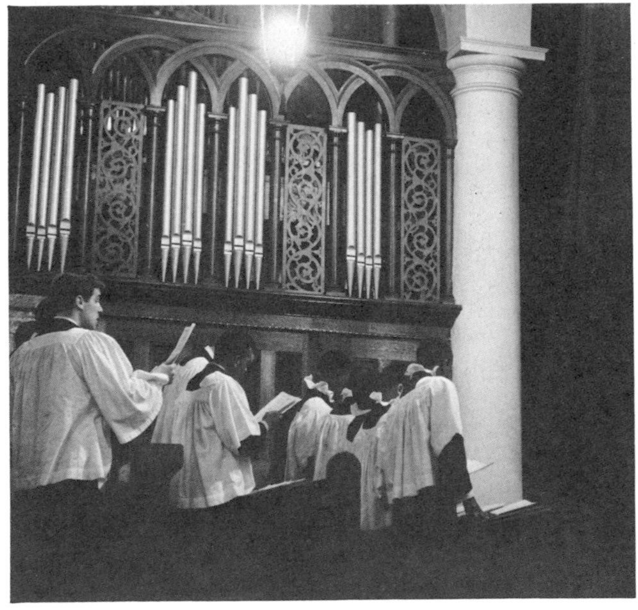

Figure 8.5 Church can be an agent of character building. Photo © Lida Moser, DPI.

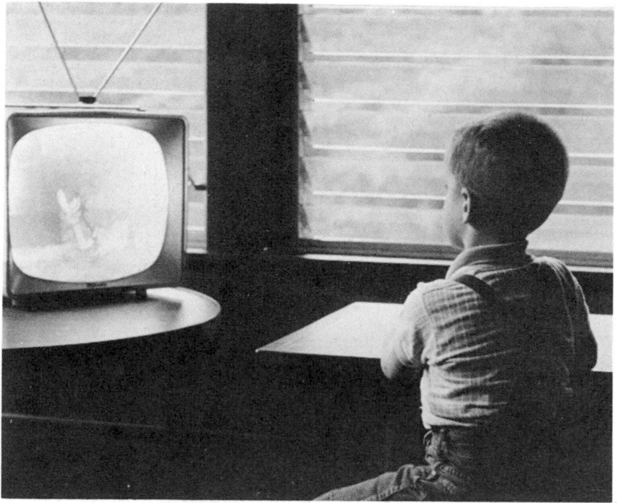

Figure 8.6 Some television programs help to build character. Photo © Burton Berinsky, DPI.

their very explicit intent to influence the formation of good character, they appear to be, as we observed earlier, relatively ineffective. To whatever extent they are effective, the reason is likely to lie less in their organizational structure or intent to teach than in the fact that they expose youngsters to the influence of peers and adults from various backgrounds.

The Generalized Society

The norms for good character of society at large are represented for the most part by mass communication media (see Figure 8.6). As indicated earlier, a reasonable composite of these norms is probably best obtained by observing the heroes of movies, television, comic books, and popular children's tales. Whether this composite merely reflects the culture, or whether it also forms and shapes it, is not entirely clear. Unquestionably it *can* do both, for there is considerable evidence, summarized in Bandura and Walters (1963), that children can acquire novel learnings on the basis of their observation of, and identification with, cartoon or film characters. How long this learning "lasts" and the degree to which it can survive in competition with other, more immediate learnings that press in different directions is yet an unanswered question. But to the extent that such vicarious learning proves robust and enduring, it will be useful to employ it in the service of character formation. Comic books might take to depicting prosocial themes, and television programs for both children and adults might offer altruistic and rational heroes with a view to shaping good character.

Much of this, however, is speculation, and its value remains to be examined in psychological research. For the moment, it is clear that *there is no substitute for parental influence in the process of character education.* The responsibility that devolves upon parents in this case is very grave, and it cannot yet be relinquished to surrogate agencies.

SUMMARY

Character can be expressed in three different ways: in behavior, in judgment, and in affect or feeling. Although there is a positive relationship among these three aspects of character, the relationships reported are not strong enough to convince us that we are dealing with a single dimension. It may be useful, therefore, to specify which aspect of character we are referring to when we discuss the antecedent variables and correlates of good character.

Nearly all theories emphasize the importance of early childhood experiences for the development of character (although they differ about *which* early experiences generate particular character traits). Perhaps the most essential condition in childhood for the development of moral behavior is the presence of a positive model (usually a parent) with whom a child can identify and imitate. Freud was the first theorist to realize fully the significance of the process of identification in the development of character. Beyond Freud, experimental studies have enabled us to list a number of conditions which seem to make identification with a positive model more likely. Among the most important are: frequency of exposure, mutual positive affect, and model saliency. Other mechanisms, such as positive reinforcement and rehearsal, have also been found to encourage behaviors associated with good character.

Developmental stages play a dominant role in character formation. Freud and Erikson have proposed that the child passes through a series of overlapping stages each of which is critical for the emergence of certain character traits. These theorists have also specified environmental events that occur during these stages and determine whether or not particular character traits develop.

Developmental stages are also important in the theories formulated by Piaget and Kohlberg concerning the development of moral judgment. These authors stipulate characteristics of moral judgment, ranging from the hedonistic to the humanistic, that one should find at each developmental stage. Empirical studies appear to have verified both the existence and the sequence of stages these authors describe.

GLOSSARY

Altruism—selflessness; concern for others.

Anal characteristics—behaviors and motivational dispositions that psychoanalytic theory associates with events which occurred during the anal period; these behaviors are said to include stinginess, stubbornness, and meticulous cleanliness.

Anal stage—in Freudian theory, the second of the biologically predetermined psychosexual stages that are crucial for the formation of personality; the anal stage occurs during the second and third years of life and is characterized by the child's preoccupation with his eliminative organs and their products (see Chapter 10).

Anxiety—an unpleasant feeling state usually characterized by increased motility of the gastrointestinal tract, increased heart rate, palmar sweating, shivering, flushing, and muscular contractions (see Chapters 4 and 10).

Assimilation—Fromm's term for the orientation towards acquiring and using things.

Aversive conditioning—learning to avoid or inhibit a behavior on the basis of negative or punitive training.

Biological characterology, Freud's—Freud's description of the genetic process; his scheme for understanding the sequence of personality development from birth to adulthood.

Body type, somatotype—a scheme, devised by Kretchmer and Sheldon, for classification of persons according to their anatomical characteristics; the scheme assumes that certain psychological characteristics are associated with each pattern (English and English, 1958).

Castration anxiety—in the male, the fear of losing one's genitals; in the female, the fantasy of once having had a penis, but of having lost it (English and English, 1958).

Character—descriptively, attributes that make up or distinguish an individual; evaluatively, the complex of mental and ethical traits marking a person, group, or nation; technically, personality traits that are stable over time, commonly such traits as have implications for moral behavior (see Chapters 4 and 11).

Character disorder—a chronic condition, often considered psychopathological, whose only symptoms tend to be socially unacceptable conduct (see Chapter 11).

Critical periods—time periods during which certain events have maximal influence on behavior and development (see Chapter 4).

Developmental stages—periods in an individual's life, each of which is characterized by a specific cluster of traits.

DOCTRINE OF TEMPERAMENT, GALEN'S—the belief that personality characteristics express different combinations of the four basic elements in the physical makeup of an individual: earth, air, fire, and water.

EGO FUNCTIONS—those aspects of personality concerned with relations between the self and external reality (see Chapter 10).

EGO PSYCHOLOGY—a psychoanalytic revision and amplification of Freudian psychology concerned primarily with the ways in which the organism deals with reality.

EGO STRENGTH—a person's relative ability to deal with reality with minimal conflict and anxiety.

EGOCENTRISM, EGOCENTRICITY—behavior that is dominated by one's own needs and which reflects relative insensitivity to the needs of others.

EMPATHY—the capacity for sharing another's feelings or ideas.

EXPLOITATIVE ORIENTATION—one of Fromm's four nonproductive character types; based on the belief that the source of all good lies outside the self and the way to achieve desired ends is to exploit others.

FRUSTRATION—the blocking of, or interference with, an ongoing goal-directed activity (English and English, 1958).

GENERALIZATION—the transfer of learnings acquired in one context to another one that bears some resemblance to it.

GENITAL CHARACTER—Freud's (1905) term for an ideal personality type, the apotheosis of character development; an essentially well-socialized, productive, and well-adjusted individual.

GENITAL STAGE—in Freudian theory, the final biologically determined psychosexual stage in the development of personality; characterized by psychological maturity and the ability to love and to work.

GRADED REHEARSAL—rehearsal of behaviors that gradually increase in difficulty; "shaping."

GUILT—realization that one has violated internalized ethical, moral, or religious principles, together with a regretful feeling of lessened personal worth on that account (see Chapter 4 for a variant of this usage).

HOARDING ORIENTATION—one of Fromm's four nonproductive orientations, consisting of the tendency of the individual to hoard his feelings, thoughts, and belongings because his security resides in "owning" things.

IDENTIFICATION—the process by which a person comes to believe he is like another in some respects, experiences the other's successes and failures as his own, and consciously or unconsciously models his own behavior after him (see Chapters 4 and 10).

IMMANENT JUSTICE—Piaget's term to describe the tendency among young children to view the accidental misfortunes that may follow a misdeed as punishment willed by God or other powerful figures.

INNER-DIRECTED CHARACTER TYPE—one of Riesman's three character types; a person whose values are implanted early in life by his elders and whose adult judgments are based on these internalized ideas.

INTEGRITY—adherence to a code of moral values; moral consistency; honesty and truthfulness.

INTEGUMENTED (PEOPLE)—Allport's (1960) term for people whose concerns are primarily with themselves.

INTERNALIZATION—the process of adopting as one's own the ideas, practices, standards, or values of another person or of society.

LATENCY STAGE, LATENCY—in Freudian theory, the fourth of the biologically predetermined psychosexual stages that are critical for the development of personality; this stage is reached after successful resolutions of the conflicts in the oral, anal, and phallic stages; it lasts generally from ages four or five through twelve. During this stage, sexual impulses are supposedly sublimated (see Chapter 10).

LEX TALIONIS—the law of retaliation; "an eye for an eye."

MARKETING ORIENTATION—one of Fromm's four nonproductive character orientations; it is the tendency of an individual to view himself as an object or commodity whose value lies primarily in its salability.

MODELLING—the process of demonstrating behavior that can be imitated.

NEONATE—newborn infant.

NOISE—in this chapter, the emanation from others of contradictory, masked, or confused signals.

OEDIPUS COMPLEX—in Freudian theory, the repressed desire of a person to possess sexually the parent of the opposite sex; Freud believed it was universal (see Chapter 10).

Oral characteristics—as used in this chapter, aspects of behavior concerned with the mouth; more generally, behavior and personality characteristics that are designed to elicit help from others.

Oral stage—in Freudian theory, the first of the biologically predetermined psychosexual stages that are crucial for the formation of personality; it extends from birth through the first year of life and is characterized by concern with ingestion and with the region of the mouth (see Chapter 10).

Other-directed character type—one of Riesman's three character types; a person for whom others, mainly contemporaries, provide the primary source of direction; he pays close attention to others for cues that might guide him.

Penis envy—in psychoanalytic theory, the female's repressed wish to possess a penis.

Personal autonomy—relative independence of mind; self-regulation; being relatively free from institutional control.

Phallic stage—in Freudian theory, the third of the biologically predetermined psychosexual stages that are crucial for the formation of personality; this stage occurs from ages three to five and is characterized by general concern with the genital organs (see Chapter 10).

Positive reinforcement—that which is rewarding and increases the likelihood that a behavior will be repeated.

Principled moral judgment—judgment in which conformity to conventional standards, rights, or duties is based on such principles as trust, contract, and social agreement.

Productive character orientation—one of the two general character types in Fromm's typology, in which the individual's relation to the world is through his interest in things and in other people; unlike the nonproductive character, the productive one is more concerned with producing rather than with acquiring and consuming.

Productive love—Fromm's term for love that goes beyond concern for physical welfare to "the growth and development of all his human powers"; a loving relationship that is engaged in by those with productive character orientations.

Psychopathic personality—a personality disorder manifested by the chronic inability to delay gratification or to accept conventional norms of behavior.

Psychosexual stages—in Freudian developmental psychology, the five successive biologically-determined stages of development: oral, anal, phallic, latency, and genital (see Chapter 10).

Psychosocial modalities—in Eriksen's developmental scheme, the significant people, patterns of relationship, and subjective elements that gradually become embedded in the individual's character.

Receptive orientation—one of Fromm's four nonproductive character types; a person who believes that the source of all good lies outside himself and is concerned with getting others to provide what he requires.

Senescence—old age.

Social character typology, Riesman's—focused on society as the main agent of character formation, this typology postulates three character types: tradition-directed, inner-directed, and other-directed.

Socialization—generally, the processes by which a child comes to internalize the values, beliefs, and morals of his society; Fromm uses the term to characterize man's relations to others and himself (see Chapter 4).

Sociopathic personality—a personality disorder manifested by failure to have internalized the social or moral norms of a society.

Superego—in Freudian theory, one of the three major dynamic systems of personality representing the learned and internalized moral demands of parents and society (see Chapter 10).

Surrogate—substitute.

Tradition-directed character type—one of Riesman's three character types; a person whose behavior is determined by the stable social forms which have been institutionalized and patterned by the society.

Trait—a personality tendency or disposition.

Typology—any system for the classification of types.

Vicarious arousal—emotion arousal which results from "putting onself in the other person's shoes."

Vicarious conditioning—the process of learning a response by observing others, without practice.

REFERENCES

Adorno, T. W., E. Frenkel-Brunswik, D. J. Levinson, and R. N. Sanford. *The authoritarian personality*. New York: Harper & Row Publishers, 1950.

Allinsmith, W. The learning of moral standards. In D. R. Miller and G. W. Swanson (eds.), *Inner conflict and defense*. New York: Holt, Rinehart & Winston, 1960, pp. 141–176.

Allport, G. W. The open system in personality theory. *Journal of Abnormal and Social Psychology*, 1960, **61**, 301–310.

Aronfreed, J. The effect of experimental socialization paradigms on two moral responses to transgression. *Journal of Abnormal and Social Psychology*, 1963, **66**, 437–448.

———. The origin of self-criticism. *Psychological Review*, 1964, **71**, 193–218.

———, and A. Reber. Internalized behavioral suppression and the timing of social punishment. *Journal of Personality and Social Psychology*, 1965, **1**, 3–16.

Baldwin, J. M. *Social and ethical interpretations in mental development*. New York: Crowell-Collier and Macmillan, Inc., 1906.

Bandura, A., and F. J. McDonald. Influence of social reinforcement and the behavior of models in shaping children's moral judgments. *Journal of Abnormal and Social Psychology*, 1963, **67**, 274–281.

——— and R. H. Walters. *Adolescent aggression*. New York: The Ronald Press Company, 1959.

——— and ———. *Social learning and personality development*. New York: Holt, Rinehart & Winston, 1963.

Burton, R. V. The generality of honesty reconsidered. *Psychological Review*, 1963, **70**, 481–500.

Durkin, D. Children's concepts of justice: A comparison with the Piaget data. *Child Development*, 1959, **30**, 59–67.

English, H. B., and Ava C. English. *A comprehensive dictionary of psychological and psychoanalytical terms*. New York: David McKay Company, Inc., 1958.

English, O. S., and G. H. J. Pearson. *Common neuroses of children and adults*. New York: W. W. Norton & Company, Inc., 1937.

——— and ———. *Emotional problems of living*. New York: W. W. Norton & Company, Inc., 1945.

Erikson, E. H. *Identity and the life cycle*. New York: International Universities Press, 1959.

Freud, S. Three essays on sexuality. In *Standard edition of the complete psychological works*. London: Hogarth Press, Ltd., 1953. First German edition, 1905.

———. *New introductory lectures in psychoanalysis*. New York: W. W. Norton & Company, Inc., 1932.

Fromm, E. *Man for himself: An inquiry into the psychology of ethics*. New York: Holt, Rinehart & Winston, 1947.

———. *The art of loving*. New York: Harper & Row Publishers, 1956.

Glueck, S., and E. Glueck. *Unraveling juvenile delinquency*. Cambridge, Mass.: Harvard University Press, 1950.

Grinder, R. Relations between behavioral and cognitive dimensions of conscience in middle childhood. *Child Development*, 1964, **35**, 881–891.

Harlow, H. F. The nature of love. *American Psychologist*, 1958, **13**, 673–685.

———. The heterosexual affectional system in monkeys. *American Psychologist*, 1962, **17**, 1–9.

Hartmann, H. *Psychoanalysis and moral values*. New York: International Universities Press, 1960.

Hartshorne, H., and M. A. May. *Studies in the nature of character*: Vol. I. *Studies in deceit*; Vol. II. *Studies in self-control*; Vol. III. *Studies in the organization of character*. New York: Crowell-Collier and Macmillan, Inc., 1928–1930.

Havighurst, R. J., and Bernice L. Neugarten. *American Indian and white children*. Chicago: University of Chicago Press, 1955.

——— and H. Taba. *Adolescent character and personality*. New York: John Wiley & Son, Inc., 1949.

Hill, W. F. Learning theory and the acquisition of values. *Psychological Review*, 1960, **67**, 317–331.

Johnson, R. A study of children's moral judgments. *Child Development*, 1962, **33**, 327–354.

Kohlberg, L. Moral development and identification. In H. Stevenson (ed.), *Child psychology: The 62nd yearbook of the National Society for the Study of Education*. Chicago: University of Chicago Press, 1963.

———. Development of moral character and moral ideology. In M. Hoffman and

Lois Hoffman (eds.), *Review of child development research*: Vol. I. New York: Russell Sage Foundation, 1964*a*.

———. The development of children's orientations toward a moral order: II. Social experience, social conduct, and the development of moral thought. *Vita Humana*, 1964*b*.

———. Relationships between the development of moral judgment and moral conduct. Paper presented at the meetings of the Society for Research in Child Development, Minneapolis, Minnesota, March, 1965.

Krafft-Ebing, R. *Psychopathia sexualis*. New York: Physicians and Surgeons Book Company, 1922.

Kretschmer, E. *Physique and character*. New York: Harcourt, Brace & World, Inc., 1925.

Lombroso, C. *Men of genius*. New York: Walter R. Scott, Inc., 1891.

London, P. *The modes and morals of psychotherapy*. New York: Holt, Rinehart & Winston, 1964.

McCord, W., and J. McCord. *Psychopathy and delinquency*. New York: Grune & Stratton, Inc., 1956.

MacRae, R., Jr. A test of Piaget's theories of moral development. *Journal of Abnormal and Social Psychology*, 1954, **49**, 14–18.

Mead, G. H. *Mind, self, and society*. Chicago: University of Chicago Press, 1934.

Medinnus, G. R. Imminent justice in children: A review of the literature and additional data. *Journal of Genetic Psychology*, 1959, **90**, 253–262.

Midlarsky, Elizabeth, and J. Bryan. The development of charity in children. *Journal of Personality and Social Psychology*, 1967, **5**, 408–415.

Milgram, S. Behavioral study of obedience. *Journal of Abnormal and Social Psychology*, 1963, **67**, 371–378.

———. Some conditions of obedience and disobedience to authority. *Human Relations*, 1965, **18**, 57–75.

Miller, N. E., and J. Dollard. *Social learning and imitation*. New Haven: Yale University Press, 1941.

Mischel, W. Delay of gratification and deviant behavior. Paper presented at the meetings of the Society for Research in Child Development, Berkeley, Calif., April 1963.

——— and R. M. Liebert. Effects of discrepancies between observed and imposed reward criteria on their acquisition and transmission. *Journal of Personality and Social Psychology*, 1966, **3**, 45–53.

——— and ———. The role of power in the adoption of self-reward patterns. *Journal of Personality and Social Psychology*, 1966.

Mowrer, O. H. *Learning theory and personality dynamics*. New York: The Ronald Press Company, 1950.

———. *The crisis in psychiatry and religion*. Princeton, N.J.: D. Van Nostrand Company, Inc., 1961.

Peck, R. F., and R. J. Havighurst. *The psychology of character development*. New York: John Wiley & Sons, Inc., 1960.

Piaget, J. *The moral judgment of the child*. New York: The Free Press of Glencoe, 1948. Originally published 1932.

Rebelsky, F. G., W. Allinsmith, and R. Grinder. Resistance to temptation and sex difference in children's use of fantasy confession. *Child Development*, 1963, **34**, 955–962.

Redl, F., and D. Wineman. *Controls from within*. New York: The Free Press of Glencoe, 1952.

Riesman, D., R. Denney, and N. Glazer. *The lonely crowd: A study of the changing American character*. New Haven, Conn.: Yale University Press, 1950.

Rosenhan, D. The origins of altruistic social autonomy. Research Bulletin. Princeton, N.J.: Educational Testing Service, 1966.

———, F. Frederick and Anne Burrowes. Preaching and practicing: The consequences of consistencies and discrepancies in imposed and observed standards. Research Bulletin. Princeton, N.J.: Educational Testing Service, 1966.

——— and G. M. White. Observation and rehearsal as determinants of prosocial behavior. Research Bulletin. Princeton, N.J.: Educational Testing Service, 1966.

Sanford, N., M. Adkins, E. Cobb, and B. Miller. Physique, personality and scholarship. *Monograph of the Society for Research in Child Development*, 1943, **8**, 1–705. (Summarized in R. G. Barker, J. S. Kounin, and H. F. Wright (eds.), *Child behavior and development*. New York: McGraw-Hill, Inc., 1943, pp. 567–589.)

Sears, R. R., Lucy Rau, and R. Alpert. *Identification and child rearing*. Stanford, Calif.: Stanford University Press, 1965.

Sheldon, W. H., and S. S. Stevens. *The varieties of temperament.* New York: Harper & Row Publishers, 1942.

Skinner, B. F. *Walden two.* New York: Crowell-Collier and Macmillan, Inc., 1948.

Sorokin, P. *Reconstruction of humanity.* Boston: The Beacon Press, 1948.

———. *Altruistic love.* Boston: The Beacon Press, 1950.

———. *The ways and power of love.* Boston: The Beacon Press, 1954*a*.

———. *Forms and techniques of altruistic and spiritual growth.* Boston: The Beacon Press, 1954*b*.

Thorndike, E. L. The law of effect. *American Journal of Psychology,* 1927, **29,** 212–222.

Tomkins, S. S. The psychology of commitment. Part I. The constructive role of violence and suffering for the individual and for his society. In S. S. Tomkins and C. E. Izard (eds.), *Affect cognition and personality.* New York: Springer Publishing Co., Inc., 1965.

Turiel, E. An experimental test of the sequentiality of developmental stages in the child's moral judgments. *Journal of Personality and Social Psychology,* 1966, **3,** 611–618.

Wallace, J., and E. Sadalla. Behavioral consequences of transgression: I. The effects of social recognition. *Journal of Experimental Research in Personality,* 1966, **1,** 187–194.

Wright, J., J. Hill, and R. Alpert. The development and expression of conscience in fantasy by school children. Paper presented at the meetings of the Society for Research in Child Development, Pennsylvania State University, 1961.

SUGGESTED READINGS

1. Berkowitz, L. *The development of motives and values in the child.* New York: Basic Books, Inc., 1964. A summary and integration of findings on the development of morality and achievement motivation.
2. Hartshorne, H., and M. A. May. *Studies in the nature of character:* Vol. I. Studies *in deceit;* Vol. II. *Studies in self-control;* Vol. III, *Studies in the organization of character.* New York: Crowell-Collier and Macmillan, Inc., 1928–1930. The data from a classic study of moral behavior. The evidence indicates that morality is situationally based; that there is little relationship between behavior in one context and behavior in another.
3. Kohlberg, L. Moral development and identification. In H. Stevenson (ed.), *Child psychology. The 62nd Yearbook of the National Society for the Study of Education.* Chicago: University of Chicago Press, 1963. An analysis of various theories of morality and its development, with particular attention to the evidence that bears upon them. Kohlberg presents in detail his own view of moral development and the relevant research that supports it.
4. Milgram, S. Some conditions of obedience and disobedience to authority. *Human Relation,* 1965, **18,** 57–75. A description of a series of experiments dealing with the extent to which people will obey a command by a legitimate authority to inflict punishment on an innocent third party.
5. Peck, R. F., and R. J. Havighurst. *The psychology of character development.* New York: John Wiley & Sons, Inc., 1960. A study of moral behavior and moral reputation that accepts developmental stages that are similar to, but not identical with, those presented by Kohlberg and Piaget.
6. Piaget, J. *The moral judgment of the child.* New York: The Free Press of Glencoe, 1948. A description of the development of moral judgment, its transformations with age, and its relations to other aspects of cognition.
7. Riesman, D., R. Denney, and N. Glazer. *The lonely crowd: A study of the changing American character.* New Haven, Conn.: Yale University Press, 1950. A classic description of other-, inner-, and tradition-directedness, their origins, functions in, and contributions to society.
8. Skinner, B. F. *Walden two.* New York: Crowell-Collier and Macmillan, Inc., 1948. Skinner's views on how the ideal community might be achieved and the kinds of psychological training that are necessary for membership in it. While many have described ideal communities, Skinner provides examples of the potential application of his principles to child rearing and education.

9. Tomkins, S. S. The psychology of commitment. In S. S. Tomkins and C. E. Izard (eds.), *Affect, cognition and personality.* New York: Springer Publishing Co., Inc., 1965, pp. 148–197. Two essays examining (1) the motivations and character structure of several famous abolitionists and (2) people's reactions to the death of President Kennedy. The findings from both studies are related to Tomkins' theory of affect and personality.

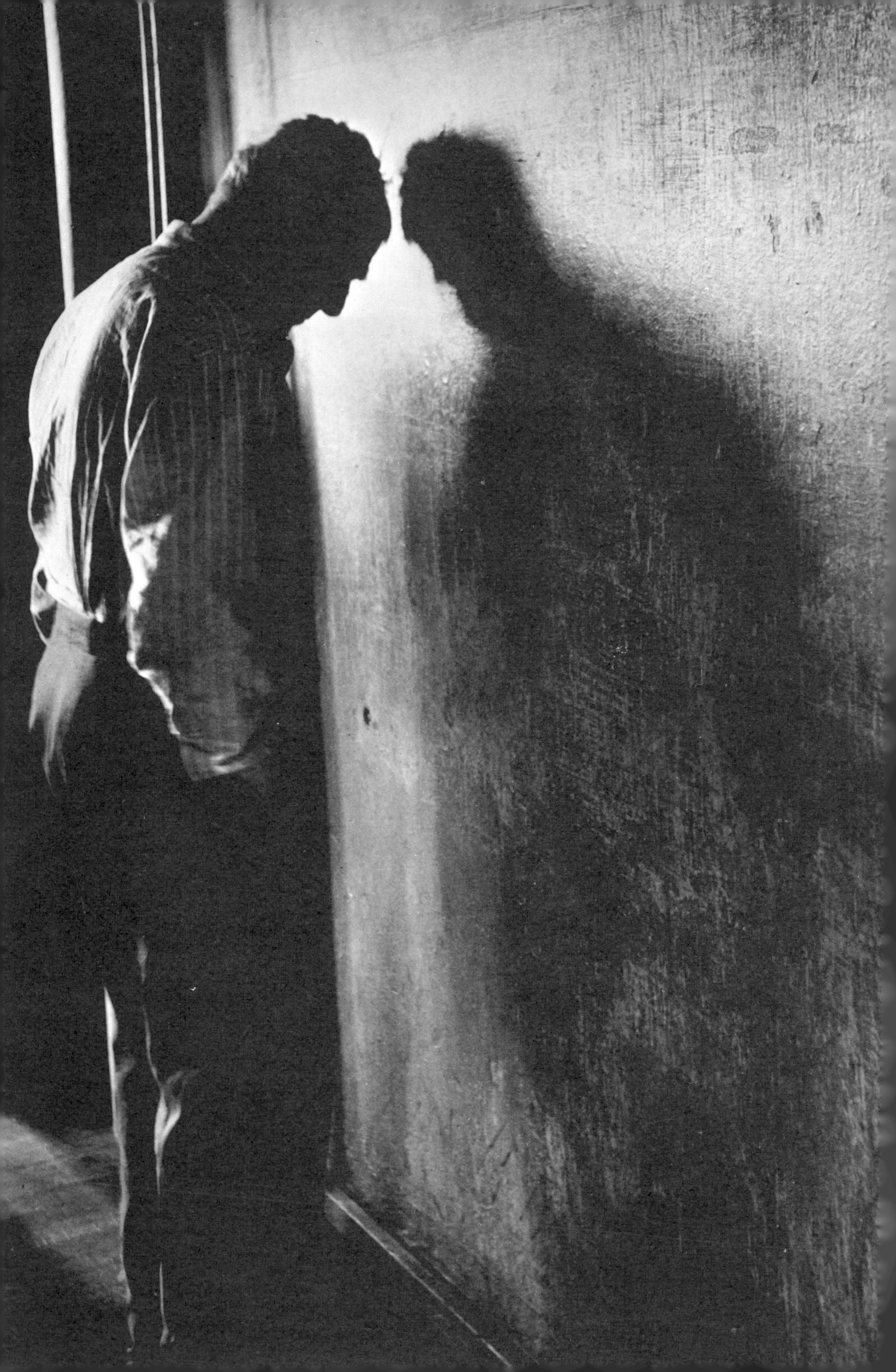

SECTION III

Negative Abnormalities

Depressive stupor. Photo © Jerry Cooke.

9

A Social Learning Interpretation of Psychological Dysfunctions

ALBERT BANDURA

The earliest conceptions of psychopathology viewed it as the manifestations of evil spirits and demons that entered the victim's body and affected his behavior adversely. Treatment efforts, therefore, were directed toward exorcising the demonic spirits by performing various magical and religious rituals or by brutal physical assaults upon the bearer of the pernicious spirits, such as cutting a hole in his skull. Hippocrates supplanted these ideas by relabeling deviant behavior *disease* rather than *demonic* manifestations. Wholesome diets, hydrotherapy, bloodletting, and other forms of physical intervention—some benign, others less humane—gradually and increasingly were used as treatments (see Figure 9.1). This history you have already surveyed in Chapter 1.

Although psychological methods gradually replaced physical procedures for changing deviant behavior patterns, medical notions of health and disease have long continued to dominate theories of psychopathology. They regard behavioral deviations as derivatives or symptoms of an underlying disease process. People who show atypical behavior are therefore called "patients" and are said to suffer from a "mental illness," which generally is treated in a hospital or medical clinic.

Most contemporary theorists and practitioners have adopted this disease model, but they regard the underlying pathology as psychological rather than neurophysiological in nature, that is, lacking physical properties that would permit direct observation and verification. In these thories the underlying disorder functions somewhat like toxic substances that produce symptomatic reactions; the inner disturbing agents are a host of unconscious psychodynamic forces and psychic complexes—ego-alien impulses; infantile images; Oedipal, castration, and inferiority complexes; ancestral unconscious and primordial images; latent instinctual tendencies; counterinstinctual energies; wills and counterwills—somewhat akin to

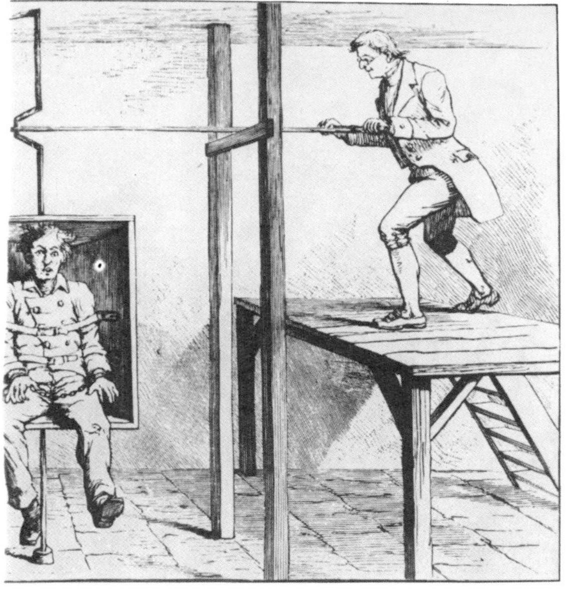

Figure 9.1 Gyrating chair, used by Benjamin Rush to increase the blood supply to the head. From *The History of Psychiatry* by Alexander and Selesnick (Harper & Row, 1966).

the hidden demonic spirits of ancient times. These prevailing theories of psychopathology thus employ essentially an amalgam of the medical and demonological models, which have in common the belief that deviant behavior patterns are external manifestations of underlying pernicious agents.

BEHAVIOR DEVIATIONS: DISEASE SYMPTOMS OR LEARNED REACTIONS?

Although the disease-demonic model has strongly influenced theories of human behavior and psychotherapeutic practice, remarkably little attention has been devoted to the definition of "symptom." Categorizing a pattern of behavior as symptomatic of emotional disorder actually involves a complex set of criteria, most of which are quite arbitrary and subjective. Whether or not an act is considered normal or a symptom of disorder depends upon whether certain social judges, or the person himself, disapprove of it. As we have seen in Chapter 5, the labeling of "symptoms" primarily involves the evaluative responses that a given behavior evokes from others rather than qualities of the behavior itself, so the same response pattern may be viewed as pathological or as normal behavior by persons whose norms and standards differ. Aggressiveness in children, for example, may be rewarded and regarded as a sign of masculinity and healthy social development by parents, while the same behavior is generally viewed by educational, legal, and other agents of society as a symptom of personality disorder (Bandura, 1960; Bandura and Walters, 1959). Similarly, persons who label themselves emotionally disturbed are often judged by others to be functioning at a normal level (Terwilliger and Fiedler, 1958).

Certain properties of a behavior often invite labeling it a symptom of emotional disorder. Responses of *high magnitude*, for instance, generally have unpleasant consequences to others and are therefore more likely to be considered pathological than responses of low to moderate intensities are. A youngster who is continually wrestling and pushing other children may be viewed as exhibiting youthful exuberance; but if his physical aggression becomes more forceful and noxious, he will in all probability be regarded as emotionally disturbed. Although intense emotional responses may be reliably categorized, disagreements are apt to arise in labeling behavior of lesser intensity, and the line of demarcation between normality and abnormality varies with the judge's tolerance.

The *appropriateness* of cognitive or social responses to particular stimuli is also often used in identifying symptomatic disordered behavior, just as it is a basis for judging genius (see Chapter 6). Appropriateness or correctness is generally determined by the degree of divergence from, or conformity to, some social norm of behavior in specific situations. Deviations from norms that do not inconvenience or interfere with the well-being of others are usually tolerated to some degree; deviations that benefit a society, like many technological inventions and intellectual and artistic creations, may be encouraged and given generous material and social rewards. On the other hand, deviance that generates aversive stimulation (unpleasantness) for others elicits strong societal disapproval, is promptly labeled abnormal, and generally results in coercive pressures on the individual to control or to modify the noxious behavior.

The appropriateness criterion, however, poses problems when its judges subscribe to conflicting norms and disagree on what constitutes suitable social reactions. The conforming majority in our society may think the hippie, who refuses to strive for conventionally valued goals, exhibits maladaptive behavior. From the perspective of the hippie, however, the conforming members display symptoms of a "sick" society. Thus, the same pattern of behavior may be assigned the negative status of a symptom by one social group and be positively evaluated as healthy by another. Similarly, when a society radically alters its behavioral norms, both the presence and the absence of the same behavior may be judged inappropriate and pathological. A citizen, for instance, who commits a brutal homicide will be readily diagnosed as suffering from a serious mental disorder, but a military recruit's inability to kill someone on the battlefield may also be viewed as symptomatic of a "war neurosis." This example further illustrates that symptoms can be created by societal norms rather than by any pathology irate to the behavior itself.

Grossly divergent behavior patterns are most apt to be viewed as pathological by persons who do not share the same normative systems as the performers. If the social learning history of the behavior is known, however, there is no necessity for invoking an underlying disease process to explain the deviance. Litz *et al.* (1958) report a case, for example, in which schizophrenic brothers believed that "disagreement" meant constipation. This clearly inappropriate expression was primarily a result of exposure to a relatively bizarre social learning situation rather than an expression of a "mental illness." Whenever the boys disagreed with their mother, she told them they were constipated and required an enema. The boys were then disrobed and given enemas, a procedure that dramatically conditioned an unusual meaning for the word "disagreement." The cases cited by Litz and his associates (Fleck, 1960; Litz *et al.*, 1957*a*, 1957*b*, 1958) provide ample evidence that delusions, suspiciousness, grandiosity, extreme denial of reality, and other forms of "schizophrenic" behavior are frequently learned through direct reinforcement and transmitted by parental modeling of unusually deviant behavior patterns. The significance of modeling in personality development has been emphasized in Chapter 4.

Behavioral deficits are frequently interpreted as symptoms of emotional disorder, particularly when they produce hardships for others. Intellectually adequate children, for example, who are incontinent, or who exhibit deficiencies in verbal and academic skills, and adults who are unable to meet social, marital, and vocational task requirements, all tend to be labeled emotionally disturbed. Moreover, it is generally assumed that the greater the deficits, the more extensive the underlying psychopathology. The arbitrary nature of the criterion for deficit or competence would become readily apparent if one were to vary the standard of competence in any particular situation. If the criterion were set at a very low level, practically all members of a society would be judged healthy and competent, whereas if exceedingly high standards were adopted, the vast majority would suddenly acquire psychopathology. In the latter case, therapists and diagnosticians would devote much time to locating the source of pathology within the individuals.

The presumed *intent* of an action also helps to determine whether others call it a symptom. If a person engages in disapproved deviant behavior that is successful in attaining commonly desired and valued goals, it is less probable that his acts will be regarded as emotional disease symptoms than if his deviant behavior has no apparent utilitarian value. Delinquents who strike victims on the head to extract their wallets expediently are generally considered semiprofessional thieves who are using income-producing *instrumental aggression* responses. By contrast, delinquents who simply beat up strangers but show no interest in their victims' material possessions are supposedly displaying *emotional aggression* of a disturbed sort. It is evident that in many cases of so-called useless aggression, the behavior *is* highly instrumental; that is, it serves the purpose of gaining the approval and admiration of peers and thus enhances status in the social hierarchy of the reference group. Peer group approval is often more powerful than tangible rewards as an incentive for aggressively deviant behavior.

The importance of social rewards in maintaining aggression is clearly revealed in a recent study. Yablonsky (1962) found that the dominant source of reward in many delinquent gangs has shifted from utilitarian antisocial activities to destructive assaults on persons and property executed in a "cool" and apparently indifferent manner. The way in which the threat of loss of "rep" may compel a person to engage in a homicidal assault is illustrated in the following excerpt from an interview with one of the boys selected for study.

> Momentarily I started to thinking about it inside; I have my mind made up I'm not going to be in no gang. Then I go on inside. Something comes up, then here come all my friends coming to me. Like I said before, I'm intelligent and so forth. They be coming to me—then they talk to me about what they gonna do. Like, "Man, we'll go out there and kill this cat." I say, "Yeah." They kept on talking. I said, "Man, I just gotta go with." Myself, I don't want to go, but when they start talking about what they gonna do, I say, "So, he isn't gonna take over my rep. I ain't gonna let him be known more than me." And I go ahead. (P. vii.)

External reinforcement possibilities rather than an internal emotional disease appear to be the major determinants of the behavior of another youth involved in a gang killing.

> If I would of got the knife, I would have stabbed him. That would have gave me more of a build-up. People would have respected me for what I've done and things like that. They would say, "There goes a cold killer." (P. 8.)

It should be noted that prosocial approval-seeking behavior such as athletic achievements or musical accomplishments is seldom labeled emotionally determined, nonutilitarian pathological behavior. Yet certain subgroups have learned to value and reward "stomping" more highly than violin virtuosity.

The dichotomy between instrumental and emotional aggression, therefore, appears to reflect primarily differences in reinforcement conditions and the types of rewards sought, not basic differences in the purposiveness of the behavior itself. Since some members of a society are likely to undergo very atypical learning contingencies, events which are ordinarily neutral or unpleasant for others may become strongly conditioned positive rewards for them. Because the puzzling behavior of these individuals may appear to have little or no instrumental value, it tends incorrectly to be explained by reference to internal psychopathological processes.

Certain *properties of the person*—age, sex, socioeconomic, and ethnic background—also enter into the social judgment of deviant behavior. For example, behavior considered normal at one age level may be regarded as a symptom of personality disturbance at a later period, as in the case of enuresis. It is appropriate, in this connection, to repeat Mowrer's query: "And when does persisting behavior of this kind suddenly cease to be normal and become a symptom?" (1950, p. 474).

The differential cultural tolerance for acting like the opposite sex illustrates the role of sex-of-subject in the assignment of symptomatic status to deviant behavior patterns. The adoption of female apparel by males is supposed to indicate a serious psychological disorder requiring prompt legal and psychiatric attention. On the other hand, females may adopt masculine garb, hair styles, and a wide range of characteristically masculine response patterns without being labeled mentally disturbed. Since, as you saw in Chapter 4, masculine behavior occupies a higher prestige and power position and is more often rewarded in our society than feminine behavior, the acquisition and maintenance of masculine tendencies by females is more readily understandable and, therefore, less likely to be interpreted as a disease process.

It is apparent from the foregoing discussion that the categorization of behavior as symptomatic of an underlying pathology depends upon the judges' normative systems; the social context in which the behavior occurs; its intention, frequency, and intensity; the age, sex, and social background of the person; and many other factors. It is true, of course, that questions of value and social judgment also arise in the diagnosis of physical disorders. But the symptom-disease model is meaningful there because internal organic pathologies do in fact exist and can be directly verified independently of their peripheral correlates (symptoms). Brain tumors and dysfunctions involving respiratory, circulatory, or digestive organs are not hypothetical events. By contrast, psychological pathologies merely represent hypothetical abstractions from behavioral phenomena. So-called symptomatic behavior can be more adequately explained in terms of social learning and value theory than by medical analogizing.

Hypothetical Internal Determinants of Behavior

The questions raised concerning the utility and validity of the concept, "symptom," apply equally well to the psychopathology presumably underlying and causing the troublesome symptom.

As a consequence of focusing attention on hypothetical internal forces, a large number of fanciful psychodynamic theories of psychopathology have emerged. The developmental history of a behavior disorder is rarely known, and attempts to reconstruct it from interview material are of doubtful validity. In fact, the content of such reconstructions is highly influenced by the interviewer's suggestive probing and selective reinforcement of content that accords with his own theories. Heine (1953), for example, has shown that patients interviewed by client-centered, Adlerian, and psychoanalytic therapists tended to account for their behavior in terms of the explanations favored by their interviewers. Thus, a psychoanalytically oriented interviewer is likely to find considerable evidence for an Oedipal complex at the root of things, a Rogerian will find an inappropriate self-concept, and an Adlerian will see feelings of inferiority with compensatory power strivings. Disciples of a "school" are equally unlikely, by the same token, to find evidence for the inner mechanisms emphasized by their rivals.

The persistence of the disease-demonology model and the need for invoking psychodynamic explanatory agents appear to be largely due to lack of knowledge of the genesis of functional behavior deviations. When the actual social learning history of maladaptive behavior is known, the basic principles of learning provide a completely adequate interpretation of many psychopathological phenomena, and explanations in terms of symptoms with underlying disorders become superfluous (Bandura, 1967).

SOCIAL LEARNING TAXONOMY OF PSYCHOLOGICAL DYSFUNCTIONS

Traditional psychodiagnostic labels of nomenclature either describe individuals in terms of motives that hypothetically determine behavior, like passive-dependent, aggressive, and competitive-exploitative, or else order subjects on some form of developmental continuum like oral, anal, phallic, and so on (see Chapters 4 and 8). Still other systems characterize persons in terms of the form and presumed severity of "mental illnesses" like character disorders, neuroses, and psychoses. Finally, some approaches are based on empirically derived homogeneous clusters of behaviors (see "Factor Analysis," Chapter 4). While these different schemes vary somewhat in emphasis, they share in the implicit assumption that social behavior can be mostly understood in terms of *subject variables,* that is, characteristics of the *persons* involved rather than of the *stimulus situations.*

In view of the demonstrated importance of stimulus control over behavior, a social learning taxonomy (classification) of psychopathology must attend to the interaction between behavioral predispositions (subject variables), on the one hand, and stimulus events, on the other. This type of analysis (Staats and Staats, 1963) can help both to explain the acquisition and maintenance of deviant response patterns and to guide therapeutic practices.

Although the specific behavioral problems of individuals may take many forms, their diverse manifestations can be reduced to several distinct patterns, each reflecting a particular type of social learning history and requiring different learning procedures for successful modification. The taxonomic schema presented below, however, is not intended to be exhaustive, nor are its classes without a certain degree of overlap. The categorization of any given case is further complicated by the fact that persons are typically exposed to diverse constellations of social learning experiences, which give rise to varying combinations of deviant behavior.

Behavioral Deficits

Some persons who are called maladjusted simply lack the requisite skills for coping effectively with the social, academic, and vocational demands of their environment. Because of their behavioral deficits, not only may such individuals receive insufficient rewards to sustain what skills they already have, but they are also periodically subjected to negative reinforcement in the form of physical punishment, rejection, ridicule, and loss of income and of other types of social and material rewards. This demoralized condition is frequently reflected in low levels of responsiveness, apathetic, weak performances, or generalized behavioral impoverishment in extreme forms as exhibited by autistic children, (Ferster, 1961; Ferster and De Myer, 1961), chronic psychotics (Ayllon and Michael, 1959; Lindsley, 1960), and institutionalized persons (Freud and Burlingham, 1944; Gewirtz, 1961; Goldfarb, 1943; Yarrow, 1961).

Stable complex patterns of behavior are in part socially transmitted through observation of competent models, and they are then further developed and maintained by *intermittent positive reinforcement* (rewards administered only occasionally, not every time the behavior is performed). Consequently, inadequate modeling and insufficient or poorly managed reinforcements are likely to produce behavioral deficits. Under somewhat better environmental circumstances, deficiencies may be confined to only a few kinds of performance. *Gross* deficits, however, typically result from a reciprocal interaction between a mild behavioral deficit and a social environment that cannot provide much positive reinforcement.

Individuals suffering only from sensorimotor handicaps may likewise manifest performance deficiencies whose unhappy consequences eventually cause them to extinguish or suppress already existing skills (Meyerson *et al.*, 1962).

The mere absence of a specific performance in itself does not necessarily indicate a *learning deficit*. An individual may have developed patterns of behavior appropriate to particular situations but suppressed or inhibited his responses after aversive conditioning. While the observed outcome is still a *performance deficit*, it must be distinguished from one produced by a learning deficiency, particularly when devising treatment programs. The conditions under which inhibitory responses and deficits are acquired and maintained will be discussed later in this chapter.

Defective Stimulus Control of Behavior

People may possess adequate repertoires of responses that could be reinforced by the environment, but still behave inappropriately and therefore go unreinforced or even punished because they fail to respond *discriminately* to important stimuli. Thus, for example, a churchgoer who bursts into operatic arias in the middle of a sermon is apt to receive an extended "rest cure" in a psychiatric facility rather than appreciative bouquets.

During the initial phase of social development most stimuli, except inherently noxious ones, exert little or no influence on behavior. However, specific performances can be readily brought under *discriminative stimulus control* if they are associated with consequences that differ with the presence or absence of particular stimuli. This process is most clearly illustrated in laboratory studies in which response to one stimulus, such as a green light, is regularly correlated with reinforcement, while responses to a second stimulus, such as a red light, are consistently unrewarded. Once the discrimination is learned, the organism responds only to the green light. Thus, by introducing discriminable stimuli that signify the contingencies of reinforcement, that is what will or will not be rewarded, a considerable degree of control has been achieved over the organism's behavior.

In more complex real-life situations, diverse response patterns are each associated with separate schedules and contingencies of reinforcement which, in turn, are correlated with different discriminative stimuli. Effective social functioning requires highly discriminative responsiveness, often to subtle changes in environmental stimulation. Some classes of deviant behavior primarily involve defective stimulus control, due either to faulty social training or to a breakdown of previously established discriminative behavior. This type of disorder and its modification have been studied in the laboratory by Ferster and De Myer (1961), who tried to increase the extremely narrow range of behavior characteristic of autistic children under laboratory conditions.

By performing a very simple response, such as pressing a key, children could obtain coins that served as *general reinforcers*; that is, they could be used to operate a variety of reinforcing devices including a pinball machine, a color wheel, a television set, a phonograph, an electric train, a picture viewer, an electric organ, a candy-vending machine with a separate light and coin slot in each column, and a trinket-vending machine. The responses of the autistic children were studied in relation to gradual changes in schedules (rates) of reinforcement and in relation to simple visual cues showing when the relevant responses would be reinforced.

The development of stimulus control was investigated by making the reinforcing devices operative only when a light was turned on: coins deposited when the light was off not only produced no reinforcers but even extended the machine's inoperative period.

During the early sessions, an autistic boy continued to deposit coins in the devices whether the light was on or not, thus giving no evidence of adapting even with the aid of an easily discriminable stimulus showing the conditions of reinforcement. After repeated exposure to the different reinforcement contingencies, a small degree of stimulus control began to emerge, but it was fully established only after many experimental sessions. However, when similar lights were used as discrimination cues in a more complex task, the previously developed stimulus control broke down completely, resulting in weakened performances and inappropriate responses accompanied by strong emotional reactions. Optimal learning conditions had to be instituted in order to restore and extend gradually the child's limited repertoire.

In marked contrast to the boy described above, a second autistic child, who was somewhat more advanced verbally and socially to begin with, adapted her behavior rapidly to the changing conditions of reinforcement signaled by the lights. Several control subjects, who exhibited no serious behavioral disorders, likewise responded quickly and appropriately to the experimental conditions.

Students of psychopathology are unlikely to be interested in coin-depositing responses *per se* unless they happen to live near Nevada; nevertheless, results of the foregoing laboratory study of the stimulus control process have several important implications. First, the study demonstrates the degree to which certain individuals may remain completely out of touch with the conditions of reinforcement, even in a relatively simple environment with a high potential for positive reinforcement and distinct and reliable discrimination stimuli to facilitate adaptive behavior.

Second, repeated nonreinforcement of inappropriate responses may further impair existing stimulus control and also give rise to a host of deviant emotional responses. The latter findings are in accord with the results of a discrimination experiment on animals reported by Pavlov (1927) many years ago. In his study, a dog was repeatedly rewarded with food following the appearance of a circle, but was not rewarded on being shown other stimuli. After a conditioned response had been well established, the animal was shown successive ellipses which gradually approximated the shape of a circle. He remained undisturbed as long as the circle and the ellipse could be easily differentiated. However, when the differences between the figures were reduced to the point where he could no longer discriminate between them, the animal suddenly exhibited profound behavioral disturbances: the formerly quiet dog thrashed about violently, ripped the apparatus, and barked incessantly when removed from the experimental room. Subsequent tests revealed that his ability to make even simple discriminations was now destroyed and could be reinstated only through a lengthy reconditioning process. Moreover, reexposure to the difficult discrimination again produced the disturbed behavior.

Conventional theories of psychopathology generally assume that most forms of deviant behavior develop in aversive or traumatic conditions. Although this may be true in many cases, it is evident from the findings discussed above that grossly deviant responses can also be generated in an essentially benign and potentially rewarding environment, given defective discrimination functions.

The results reported by Ferster and De Myer on autistic children also reveal the limitations of traditional psychiatric typologies. Although the children who were studied differed markedly in the speed with which they adapted their behavior to the changing environmental conditions, both were nevertheless diagnosed as "autistic."

The psychiatric nosological system is difficult to justify in view of its limited reliability (Ash, 1949; Hunt *et al.*, 1953; Schmidt and Fonda, 1956) and the great behavioral differences among people in the same diagnostic classes.

Because of the importance of symbolic communication in social interactions, most human discriminative behavior is governed by verbal cues. Consequently, persons whose behavior is under defective verbal control will often make inappropriate responses which may have considerable negative consequences. As part of a research program to develop procedures for the modification of psychotic behavior, Ayllon and his associates (Ayllon, 1960; Ayllon and Haughton, 1962; Ayllon and Michael, 1959) provide numerous examples of behavior which is very poorly controlled by relevant verbal stimuli. In one study, a group of schizophrenics with long-standing severe eating problems were totally unresponsive to meal announcements or to persuasive appeals. Prior to the treatment program, these people had been escorted by ward personnel to the dining room, spoonfed, tube-fed, and subjected to electroshock "therapy" and other forms of infantilizing and punitive treatment.

The research staff assumed that the nurses' coaxing, persuading, and feeding was an inadvertent form of positive reinforcement that somehow maintained the eating problems. If so, the same behavior would also tend to reduce the controlling properties of relevant verbal stimuli. All social rewards for ignoring the announcement of mealtime and for refusals to eat were therefore withdrawn; following meal call, the dining room remained open for thirty minutes and any patient who failed to appear during that time simply missed his meal. Under this new contingency, the patients quickly responded to the meal call within the time allotted. Several weeks later, access to the dining room was gradually reduced following meal call until eventually the patients responded in a socially appropriate manner.

It is interesting to note that delusional statements to the effect that the food was poisoned, or that God instructed the patients to refuse to eat, disappeared as soon as the patients began to feed themselves (Ayllon and Michael, 1959). These findings suggest that in some cases delusional responses may be a result rather than a cause of deviant behavior. By adopting a sick role, supported by delusional justifications, the patient may be more successful in compelling the attention and care of busy ward personnel who would otherwise respond in an intolerant and punitive manner. Indeed, the nurses frequently supported and rewarded highly infantile behavior on the assumption that the patients could not be mature and realistic because they were "mentally ill."

The classification and interpretation of objects or events in a given culture is precisely governed by the culture's language and conceptual system. Another form of defective verbal control therefore is evident in cases where inappropriate labels are attached to objects and events. The earlier example of the sibling schizophrenics who believed that *disagreement* meant "constipation" illustrates this type of cognitive dysfunction. Similarly, the verbal labels of a person who insists that a bird has built a nest in his left molar are completely inappropriate to the actual physical environment.

Allusion has already been made to some of the social learning conditions that can give rise to defective stimulus regulation of behavior. Sufficient exposure to different reinforcement conditions correlated with different stimuli is obviously necessary for the establishment and maintenance of discriminative stimulus control. Even though different consequences are regularly correlated with particular stimuli, the desired control still may not be achieved because of the existence of faulty conditions. Thus, as revealed in the Ayllon studies, if failure to respond to a meal call produces positive social reinforcement and prompt response results in loss of attention, the relevant verbal stimuli (the announcements) attain discriminative value but do not acquire the right controlling properties. Similarly, much of the verbal behavior of parents has relatively little influence on their children's social responses. Requests, orders, and directives are continuously issued but generally go unheeded as long as noncompliance is either overlooked or positively reinforced by increased parental attention. The parents' mounting anger usually serves as the cue that further noncompliance will be negatively reinforced. Under these conditions, only verbal behavior of high intensity (yelling) acquires reliable controlling properties.

Previously established repertoires can be reduced or even eliminated completely by high emotional arousal, as revealed in the experiments reported by Ferster and by Pavlov. Additional corroborative evidence for this relationship is provided by Rosenbaum (1953), who found that, under threat of strong painful stimulation, people discriminated more poorly than under mild aversive conditions. A subsequent experiment (Rosenbaum, 1956) further demonstrated that the loss in discrimination from the threat of strong noxious stimulation is greatest among persons who are predisposed to emotional arousal.

Some evidence is also provided by Rodnick and Garmezy (1957) that the loss of discriminative accuracy among grossly deviant people may partly result from the fact that, for this group, negative social reinforcers have powerful emotion-arousing properties. Whereas the *generalization gradients* (graphs of discrimination performance) for "normal" and schizophrenic subjects were similar under conditions of reward, the schizophrenics exhibited discriminative deficits under direct censure (Garmezy, 1952), and even in response to pictures showing different degrees of maternal criticism (Dunn, 1954).

Stimulus control may likewise break

down under extreme conditions of deprivation or when there are marked changes in the social environment and in corresponding conditions of reinforcement (Ferster, 1963). This fact may partly account for the common observation that persons admitted to a psychiatric hospital who initially exhibit highly deviant and disorganized behavior often subside and appear comparatively normal in a short period without any active therapeutic interventions. Removal from a stressful or otherwise unfavorable environment may produce such dramatic changes. The initial disorientation seen at hospital admission may be temporarily enhanced, on the other hand, by the fact that most of the discriminative stimuli which guide the individual's behavior in everyday life are absent, most of his previously rewarded behaviors are no longer appropriate to, or permitted in, the hospital setting, and new performances associated with different and unusual reinforcement contingencies are suddenly required. Even persons who are well equipped to adapt to rapid stimulus changes would experience some feelings of strangeness and disorganization if suddenly confronted with these conditions.

Inappropriate Stimulus Control of Behavior

The preceding section examined behavioral disorders which result from the failure of important discriminable stimuli to acquire the controlling properties essential for adaptive functioning. Another important class of deviant behavior reflects a converse problem arising from the fact that *formerly innocuous and inappropriate stimuli have acquired the capacity to elicit highly intense emotional reactions.* This category includes chronic muscular tensions, intolerable anxiety reactions, and other forms of overactivity of the autonomic nervous system. Such disorders are reflected in a wide variety of somatic complaints such as insomnia, chronic fatigue, gastrointestinal disorders, and respiratory and cardiovascular disturbances of a functional nature. These are discussed in detail in Chapter 13. Most obsessive-compulsive reactions, behavioral inhibitions, phobic and other avoidant response patterns, which occupy much of Chapter 10, are similarly governed by conditioned emotional reactions, particularly while they are being learned. These types of disorder are brought under the control of previously innocuous stimuli through a process of *aversive classical conditioning.* This means that if a formerly ineffective conditioned stimulus (CS) occurs in conjunction with another stimulus which is capable of eliciting unpleasant autonomic responses, the former stimulus itself gradually acquires the power to evoke the same aversive emotional response patterns.

Laboratory studies of *asthma* illustrate how psychosomatic reactions such as asthmatic attacks can be conditioned in the laboratory. Noelpp and Noelpp-Eschenhager (1951, 1952), for example, demonstrated that after repeated pairing of induced asthmatic attacks with an auditory stimulus, many of the animals in the study exhibited symptoms of bronchial asthma to the auditory stimulus alone. Similar conditioned stimulus control of human asthmatic attacks is demonstrated in a carefully controlled experiment by Dekker *et al.* (1957). Two patients suffering from severe bronchial asthma inhaled nebulized allergens to which they were hypersensitive. After repeated inhalations of this allergen extract, which served as the unconditioned stimulus for asthmatic attacks and automatically produced them, inhalation of a neutral solvent, which initially produced no respiratory changes, now elicited attacks of asthma. In later phases of the experiment, inhalations of pure oxygen and even the presentation of the inhaling mouthpiece, both formerly neutral stimuli, had acquired the power to provoke severe asthmatic attacks that were undistinguishable from those induced by the allergen itself.

In the experiment described, asthmatic responses were conditioned to such inappropriate stimuli as the inhalation apparatus simply through contiguous association. It is not surprising, therefore, that the analyses of asthmatic behavior made by Dekker and Groen (1956) showed an extremely varied array of highly specific stimuli eliciting attacks in the group of patients studied; these stimuli included the sight of dust, radio speeches by influential politicians, children's choirs, the national anthem, elevators, goldfish, caged birds, the smell of perfume, waterfalls, bicycle races, police vans, and horses, just to mention a few. Once the critical eliciting stimuli had been identified in a particular case, Dekker and Groen were able to induce attacks of asthma in the laboratory simply by presenting the conditioned stimuli themselves or even pictures of them.

It is particularly interesting that the investigators observed that intense emotional arousal by itself failed to produce asthmatic reactions, whereas exposure to specific conditioned stimuli provoked marked respiratory dysfunction. This observation is corroborated by Ottenberg *et al.* (1958) in a study of the conditioning and extinction of asthmatic responses in animals. Asthma-like attacks, which readily occurred in the presence of conditioned stimuli, could not be induced by means of emotion-provoking procedures involving loud noises, painful stimulation, and electric shock. In view of these findings, one would expect that neutralization of such specific eliciting stimuli through desensitization methods (Walton, 1960) would be highly effective in the treatment of asthma, but that reduction of general emotional disturbances might not have much impact on the respiratory disorder.

Although other forms of human psychosomatic disorders have not as yet been subjected to systematic experimental investigation, almost every form of physiological response that an organism is capable of making has been classically conditioned to innocuous stimuli at one time or another. These have included eyelid reflexes, salivary responses, galvanic skin responses, respiratory changes, cardiac responses, electroencephalogram alpha rhythm, gastrointestinal secretions, and vasomotor reactions (Kimble, 1961). External stimuli like signal lights and buzzers have been used most in classical conditioning experiments, but Russian researchers (Bykov, 1957; Razran, 1961) have recently demonstrated *interoceptive* conditioning, in which changes in the activity of internal organs serve as the signal stimulus (CS). Evidently any discriminable stimulus, whether external or internal, can acquire the capacity to elicit autonomic responses.

Many of the attitudes and emotional responses which people have towards specific objects are not direct results of the pairing of affective experiences with the objects themselves. Some people, for example, may fear snakes without having had any direct frightening experiences with reptiles. Similarly, some people are strongly aroused emotionally at the sight or mention of unpopular minority groups or nationalities, even though they may have had no personal contact. These types of reactions are frequently learned by *higher order classical conditioning,* in which a stimulus, once learned, serves as the basis for further conditioning. For example the Staatses (1957, 1958) have shown that the names of different nations, the names of persons, and even nonsense syllables that had been asso-

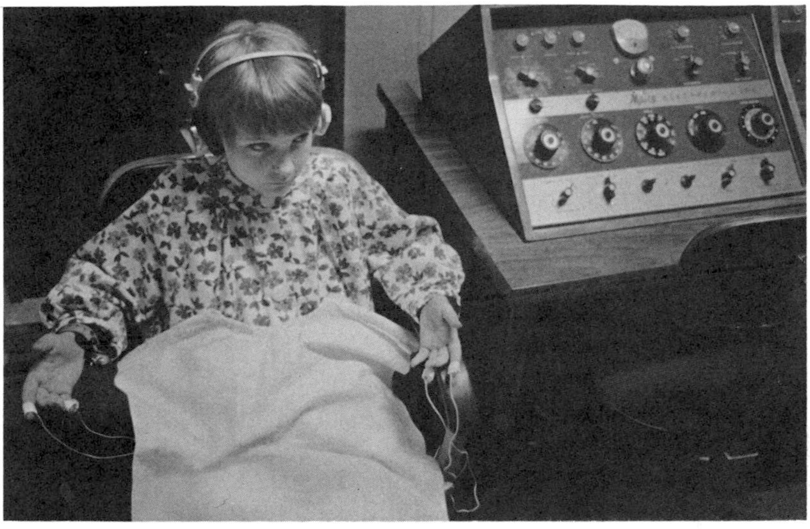

Figure 9.2 Subject with galvanic skin response apparatus. Photo © A. John Geraci.

ciated with words having negative connotations, like "bitter," "ugly," "failure," subsequently tended to be viewed as unpleasant. These same names were rated in the pleasant direction, however, when they had been paired with positively conditioned words such as "pretty," "sweet," and "happy." A study by Das and Nanda (1963) further reveals that higher order conditioned stimuli, once learned, are capable of being generalized to still other situations.

While many emotional response patterns are undoubtedly acquired by direct experience, both first order and higher order conditioning may occur in the case of human learning even without direct stimulation (Berger, 1962) through *vicarious conditioning.*

The process of *vicarious classical conditioning* and the influence of emotional arousal on vicariously acquired responses is shown in a laboratory study by Bandura and Rosenthal (1966). In this experiment, groups of adults observed a single individual who underwent aversive conditioning experiences in which a buzzer sounded at periodic intervals; shortly thereafter he acted as if in pain from an ostensible electric shock. The performer, however, merely feigned pain cues (an arm jerk away from the source of the "shock," wincing) and no shock was actually administered. After repeated pairings of the buzzer (CS) and the performer's pain responses, the observers' conditioned psychogalvanic responses to the buzzer alone were measured in order to test for the acquisition and extinction of emotional responses. (The apparatus used to measure galvanic skin responses is illustrated in Figure 9.2.) Prior to the vicarious conditioning phase of the experiment, the groups of observers had been subjected to different degrees of emotional arousal manipulated both psychologically and physiologically by means of varying doses of epinephrine, a sympathetic stimulant (see Chapter 3).

The results of this experiment provide clear evidence that emotional responses can be transmitted vicariously. Although

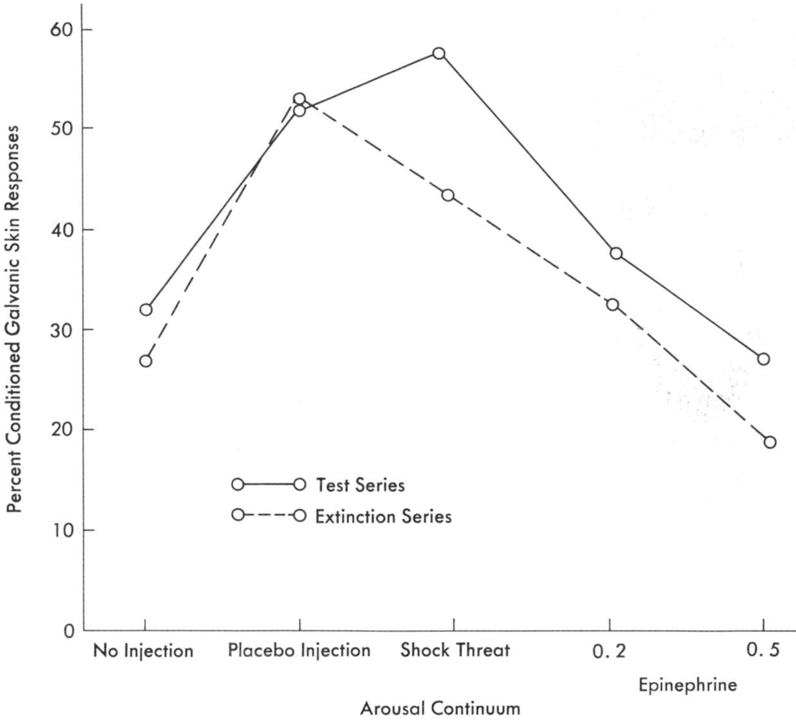

Figure 9.3 Vicarious conditioning and extinction of galvanic skin responses as a function of arousal level. From Bandura and Rosenthal (1966).

the observers had not been subjected directly to the aversive stimulation, they nevertheless endowed the formerly innocuous buzzer with emotion-provoking properties because they had observed another person undergoing painful experiences. In addition, the degree of vicarious conditioning showed a nonlinear graphic relationship to the observer's level of emotional arousal (Figure 9.3). Vicarious responses increased when arousal ranged from low to moderately high, but further increases in arousal were accompanied by progressive decreases in vicariously conditioned responses.

Most stimuli encountered in natural situations are highly complex; that is, they contain a variety of stimulus dimensions, some of which are related and others irrelevant to the existing reinforcement contingencies. If a person happens to attend primarily to the irrelevant dimensions and subsequently generalizes responses on the basis of them, a great deal of inappropriate or maladaptive behavior may occur. Since most reinforcements are of a social nature, the irrelevant cues are most likely to involve some physical or behavioral characteristics of the reinforcing persons. An illustration of this type of inappropriate generalization is provided in the following letter taken from the advice column of a metropolitan newspaper.

Dear Abby:

My friend fixed me up with a blind date and I should have known the minute he showed up in a bow tie that he couldn't be trusted. I fell for him like a rock. He got me to love him on purpose and then lied to me and cheated on me. Every time I go with a man who wears a bow tie, the same thing happens. I think girls should be warned about men who wear them.

Against Bow Ties

Dear Against:

Don't condemn all men who wear bow ties because of your experience. I know many a man behind a bow tie who can be trusted.

In this example, the letter writer had generalized a whole pattern of behavior to bow ties, a stimulus one would not expect to be routinely correlated with negative reinforcement. The journalistic counselor tries to improve the discriminative behavior of her correspondent by emphasizing the *noncontingent relationship* between the sets of stimulus events, that is, the independence of bow ties and masculine trustworthiness.

It is apparent from the foregoing discussion that emotional responses can be brought under the control of relatively complex stimuli. The fact that new stimulus events can become vicariously as well as directly linked to emotional behavior further adds to the complexity of the classical conditioning process. Moreover, once conditioned stimuli have acquired eliciting power, their capacity is transferred or generalized to other sets of physically similar stimuli (Grant and Schiller, 1953; Hovland, 1937; Littman, 1949; Noble, 1950; Watson and Rayner, 1920), to cues related semantically (Diven, 1937; Lacey and Smith, 1954; Razran, 1949), and even to highly dissimilar stimuli that have been regularly associated with them in the person's social learning history (Das and Nanda, 1963). It is therefore not surprising that conditioned emotional responses are often overgeneralized, or generalized on the basis of irrelevant cues, resulting in a chronically unpleasant state of autonomic overactivity.

The discussion so far has been primarily concerned with inappropriate stimulus control of autonomic responses, which are important components of emotional states. After a stimulus has acquired aversive properties, its presentation elicits not only strong autonomic responses, but also efforts to escape and avoid the resultant noxious stimulation. Any response that successfully terminates the aversive state or removes the threatening stimulus will become firmly learned because of the positive reinforcement it receives.

The acquisition of fear-motivated behavior and its extreme persistence even under benign environmental conditions is clearly exemplified in a study by Miller (1948). Rats were given electric shocks in a white compartment of a shuttle box and learned to escape by running through an open door into a black compartment. The once neutral cues of the white compartment rapidly acquired emotion-provoking properties, and the animals continued to run from it long after the shock had been completely discontinued. Escape from the conditioned aversive stimulus (the white compartment) thus reinforced the running. The animals were then placed in the white compartment with the door closed; they could open it by rotating a wheel. Wheel turning was rapidly learned and maintained by the fear reduction that occurred each time they escaped the white chamber. When conditions were changed so that wheel turning no longer released the door, but pressing a bar did, the former response was quickly extinguished and the latter became strongly established. The conditioned aversive stimulus thus sustained a series of avoidance responses, in spite of the fact that there was no longer any basis in reality for emotional reactions once the shock had been completely discontinued. A rodent psychiatrist observing these winded animals dashing through compartments, turning wheels, and pressing bars to avoid a subjectively real, but objectively nonexistent, danger would undoubtedly diagnose a serious psychological disorder in these animals.

The examples of aversive conditioning given so far have all involved independent environmental stimuli like lights, bells, and chambers. Mowrer (1960) has made an important distinction between "place avoidance" and "response inhibition" in terms of where the fearful conditioned stimuli are located. In place avoidance, an individual performs responses designed to escape or avoid an *external* noxious stimulus. If an individual has been repeatedly punished for a particular pattern of behavior, however, the response itself and its cognitive representations gradually acquire the capacity to arouse emotion. Since some of these cues occur early in the response sequence, the very initiation of the act and even thinking about it can come to acquire aversive properties. To avoid this unpleasant experience, individuals learn to suppress the act altogether, and the suppression becomes established through positive reinforcement. Walton and Mather (1963) provide numerous examples in which *obsessive-compulsive* rituals had become conditioned in this way to sexual or aggressive thoughts and behavior.

Response inhibition and the anxiety-eliciting function of response-correlated stimuli described in the previous paragraph tend to be assigned a prominent role in psychodynamic interpretations of neurotic behavior, but it should be recognized that *external* discriminative stimuli, especially social ones, are more typically critical sources of anxiety. Conditioned emotional responses and avoidant acts may, in fact, be elicited by the mere presence of stimuli that signify past traumatic experiences even when the person does not actually engage in the tabooed behavior. The transfer of anxiety-eliciting power to innocuous external stimuli is illustrated in a case reported by Walton and Mather (1963) of a woman who suffered from incapacitating obsessions about being dirty and elaborate hygienic compulsions. The obsessive-compulsive behavior began with her severe guilt and feelings of "dirtiness" because of sex relations in a love affair with a married man. Eventually, a wide range of external stimuli related to urogenital activities and all forms of dirt became aversive to her.

> The main feature was compulsive handwashing which appeared to arise from doubts about contamination of herself by dirt. After every daily activity or whenever she believed she may have touched something which had been handled by another person before her, she would wash her hands four or five times (taking fifteen minutes). Door knobs and taps were particularly anxiety-provoking as they were handled most frequently. Going to the toilet would always be followed by handwashing and additional scrubbing of the nails. Taking a bath and washing her hair would occupy several hours due to continual rewashing of herself, the bath and the washbasin. To avoid contamination, she would ensure that she never brushed against walls or other people's clothing and she always kept her own clothes in a special place untouched by others. Any street or thoroughfare would be examined for patches of dirt. Many such activities, such as turning on taps and opening doors were delegated to her mother. She would in fact never venture outside the house alone lest she were required to handle something and there were no facilities for washing. Sitting on public seats was also difficult for her. (P. 169.)

When broad segments of a person's social behavior have been negatively conditioned for a long time, a wide range of responses eventually gain aversive properties that result either in suppression of the behavior or chronically high states of unpleasant emotional arousal. The passage quoted below (Bateson, 1961), taken from a patient's account of his psychosis, describes vividly an extreme form of self-generated torment. The narrator's scrupulously moralistic upbringing, according to which even most conventional patterns of behavior were considered deviant, sinful, and likely to provoke the wrath of God, elicited dreadful apprehensions about many innocuous acts, such as taking medicine. These, in turn, motivated him to constantly perform exceedingly painful atonement rituals to try to forestall the disastrous consequences he feared.

> In the night I awoke under the most dreadful impressions; I heard a voice addressing me, and I was made to imagine that my disobedience to the faith, in taking the medicine overnight, had not only offended the Lord, but had rendered the work of my salvation extremely difficult, by its effect upon my spirits and humors. I heard that I could only be saved now by being changed into a spiritual body. . . . A spirit came upon me and prepared to guide me in my actions. I was lying on my back, and the spirit seemed to light on my pillow by my right ear, and to command my body. I was placed in a fatiguing attitude, resting on my feet, my knees drawn up and on my head, and made to swing my body from side to side without ceasing. In the meantime, I heard voices without and within me, and sounds as of the clanking of iron, and the breathing of great forge bellows, and the force of flames. I understood that I was only saved by the mercy of Jesus, from seeing, as well as hearing, hell around me; and that if I were not obedient to His spirit, I should inevitably awake in hell before the morning. After some time I had a little rest, and then actuated by the same spirit, I took a like position on the floor, where I remained, until I understood that the work of the Lord was perfected, and that now my salvation was secured; at the same time the guidance of the spirit left me, and I became in doubt what next I was to do. I understood that this provoked the Lord, as if I was affecting ignorance when I knew what I was to do, and, after some hesitation, I heard the command, to "*take your position on the floor again then*," but I had no guidance to do so, and could not resume it. I was told, however, that my salvation depended upon my maintaining that position as well as I could until the morning; and oh! great was my joy when I perceived the first brightness of the dawn, which I could scarcely believe had arrived so early. (Pp. 28–29.)

The above quotation also provides a striking example of how behavior can become completely controlled by fictional contingencies and fantasied consequences powerful enough to override the influence of the reinforcements available from the social environment. Thus, the acceptance of medicine, an act that was later considered a rebellion against the Almighty, generated extremely fearsome hallucinations of torture in hellfire, which would supposedly cease only upon the performance of arduous and bizzare atonements. It is important to bear in mind that fantasied consequences are no less real, or less aversive, to the people who fear them than those associated with external aversive stimuli. Indeed, the intensities of emotion arousal generated by such cognitive activities often exceed those evoked by environmental events. It should also be noted that cognitions can be established, strengthened, and extinguished according to the same principles of reinforcement that govern *overt* responses. The failure of such subjectively experienced threats to come to fruition, as in the case under discussion, undoubtedly serves as the important mechanism maintaining many classes of psychotic behavior.

Given the conjunction of fictional rewards and punishments and a powerful internal reinforcing system, a person's behavior is refractory to environmental control even in the face of powerful external punishments and blatant disproofs of his beliefs.

When I opened the door, I found a stout manservant on the landing, who told me that he was placed there to forbid my going out, by the orders of Dr. P. and my friend; on my remonstrating, he followed me into my room and stood before the door. I insisted on going out; he, on preventing me. I warned him of the danger he incurred in opposing the will of the Holy Spirit, I prayed him to let me pass, or otherwise an evil would befall him, for that I was a prophet of the Lord. He was not a whit shaken by my address, so, after again and again adjuring him, by the desire of the Spirit whose word I heard, I seized one of his arms, desiring to wither it; my words were idle, no effect followed, and I was ashamed and astonished.

Then, thought I, I have been made a fool of! But I did not on that account mistrust the doctrines by which I had been exposed on this error. The doctrines, thought I, are true, but I am mocked at by the Almighty for my disobedience to them, and at the same time, I have the guilt and the grief, of bringing discredit upon the truth, by my obedience to a spirit of mockery, or by my disobedience to the Holy Spirit; for there were not wanting voices to suggest to me, that the reason why the miracle had failed, was that I had not waited for the Spirit to guide my action when the word was spoken and that I had seized the man's arm with the wrong hand.

The voices informed me, that my conduct was owing to a spirit of mockery and blasphemy having possession of me . . . that I must, in the power of the Holy Spirit, *redeem myself*, and rid myself of the spirits of blasphemy and mockery that had taken possession of me.

The way in which I was tempted to do this was by throwing myself on the top of my head backwards, and so resting on the top of my head and on my feet alone, to turn from one side to the other until I had broken my neck. I suppose by this time I was already in a state of feverish delirium, but my good sense and prudence still refused to undertake this strange action. I was then accused of faithlessness and cowardice, of fearing man more than God. . . .

When I undertook this action, I imagined that if I performed it in the power of the Holy Spirit, no harm would result to me, but that if I threw myself round to the right in my own strength, I might break my neck and die, but that I should be raised again immediately to fulfil my mission. I had therefore no design to destroy myself; but, I have often conjectured since, that God in his mercy may have mediated my self-destruction to save me from the horrors he foresaw preparing for me; they were great and intolerable, shocking in themselves, more shocking in my abandonment; I awoke from them as from the grave, to be cut off from all my tenderest ties.

Failing in my attempts, I was directed to expectorate violently, in order to get rid of my two formidable enemies; and then again I was told to drink water, and the Almighty was satisfied; but that I was not satisfied (neither could I be sincerely, for I knew that I had not fulfilled his commands), I was to take up my position again; I did so, my attendant came up with an assistant and they forced me into a straight waistcoat. Even then I again tried to resume the position to which I was again challenged. They then tied my legs to the bed-posts and so secured me. (Pp. 34–35.)

This case material reveals the power of fantasied consequences associated with fictional contingencies. Deviant behavior can also be generated and maintained indefinitely by accidental contingencies involving actual or fictional reinforcements.

Whenever a reinforcing event occurs, any irrelevant behavior already in progress is automatically strengthened. The fortuitous connection in time between an act and its subsequent reinforcement thus increases the likelihood that it will be repeated and again adventitiously reinforced. This type of behavior can eventually come under the control of its reinforcer as precisely and powerfully as if there were, in fact, a causal relation between the two sets of events.

The latter phenomenon was first observed by Skinner (1948) in an experiment in which pigeons received food at regular intervals regardless of what they had been doing during periods between reinforcements. Under these conditions, an amusing variety of nonsensical responses were firmly learned—merely because they happened to occur by chance in close proximity to the reinforcement. The new pigeon habits included hopping from side to side, turning the body counterclockwise, tossing the head upward repeatedly, attenuated pecking movements, turning two or three times between reinforcements, and pendulous movements of the head and body. In one case, a bird hopped from side to side more than ten thousand times before this stereotyped response pattern was extinguished!

The power of adventitious reinforcement in maintaining human deviant behavior is similarly revealed in the operant conditioning experiment of Ferster and De Myer (1961) referred to earlier. One of the autistic children happened to climb over a food reinforcing device just before the machine delivered food. From then on, the child persisted in ritualistic climbing over the tops of the machines between presses of the lever—the only response actually necessary to produce the food. In the absence of knowledge about the accidental contingency responsible for the child's apparently strange behavior, elaborate hypotheses might readily be generated by psychodiagnosticians about the symbolic significance of this peculiar symptom.

The discussion has so far focused on how irrelevant responses become accidentally involved in response chains associated with rewarding consequences, but the phenomenon probably occurs even more often under aversive conditions, as evidenced by the widespread performance of superstitious rituals designed to prevent "bad luck," that is, prospective negative outcomes. In more extreme and socially debilitating forms, such rituals are represented by obsessive-compulsive disorders.

The extreme persistence of behavior learned under aversive conditions is due largely to the self-reinforcing character of avoidance and escape responses. In the first place, successful avoidance provides immediate reinforcement from the dimunition of the aversive stimulation. Second, avoidance tends to be self-perpetuating even when it is no longer realistically justified, as shown by Miller (1948), since prompt or complete avoidance of a formerly noxious situation effectively prevents the organism from reappraising its current status. These types of responses can be rapidly eliminated if the avoidant act can be *prevented* from occurring in the face of the threatening stimuli under new conditions which are either harmless or positive experiences (Bandura, 1967; Eysenck, 1960; Grossberg, 1964; Metzner, 1961; Wolpe, 1958).

In experiments with animals, after avoidance responses have been well established, the noxious stimulation typically is completely discontinued and the animals' behavior has no effect one way or the other on whether it is resumed. On the other hand, in human social interactions, a person's own behavior, especially in anticipation of others' responses, is generally instrumental in provoking counterreactions which may confirm or reinforce his original maladaptive behavior. Our anti—bow tie lady, for example, responds promptly in a hostile, suspicious manner toward men wearing bow ties. In all probability, her behavior evokes hostile and rejecting counterattacks. By contrast, an individual whose anticipatory responses are of a more positive character will undoubtedly encounter greater warmth and friendliness from others. Experimental analysis by Rausch (1964) of sequential interchanges between the antecedent acts of one child and the subsequent acts of another reveals that the proportion of friendly and hostile behavior which children receive from their peers depends largely on their own antecedent behavior. The fact that a person, to a large extent, *constructs his own chains of social reinforcement contingencies through his anticipatory behavior* presents another major obstacle to the elimination of avoidant habits even under favorable conditions (see Chapter 5).

Strong response predispositions not only have social stimulating power, but also influence the perception of interpersonal cues. Most social reactions tend to be somewhat ambiguous, so that a variety of interpretations are possible. This is particularly true of *negative* responses; firm rejection or frank disapproval tends to be inhibited or expressed in indirect and nonverbal forms. Consequently, *nonverbal* cues are typically regarded as more reliable than verbal stimuli; that is, actions come to speak louder than words. Since it is often difficult to know precisely what nonverbal cues mean, one tends to respond to new social events and the behavior of others in accord with prior experiences. There is, in fact, considerable laboratory and clinical evidence (Festinger, 1962; Festinger *et al.*, 1956; Haire and Grunes, 1950; Kelly, 1950; Rokeach, 1964) that people often seize upon very minimal cues as signs of rejection, disapproval, or disinterests; they may go to great lengths to avoid, to deny, or to redefine cues that contradict their beliefs; and they may even do things that provoke from others the necessary confirming experiences to sustain their beliefs. In view of these diverse maintenance mechanisms among humans, it is not surprising that avoidance repertoires are exceedingly resistant to modification without carefully planned relearning experiences.

It is widely assumed that conditioned autonomic reactions, which presumably form the basis of an anxiety drive state, provide the motivation for avoidant behavior and that their reduction reinforces it. Findings from laboratory investigations of avoidance learning in animals whose sympathetic nervous systems have been surgically excised (Wynne and Solomon, 1955) suggest that autonomic feedback plays only a limited role in escape-avoidance behavior and that other physiological systems, particularly the higher brain center, may be more important. In this experiment, feedback functions of the autonomic nervous system were curtailed, and the animals were then trained to avoid an intense shock by jumping over a barrier from one compartment of a shuttlebox to the other. A light served as the main conditioned stimulus. Following avoidance learning, the shock was discontinued in order to see how long it would take to extinguish the jumping response in the presence of the light alone.

A group of unoperated dogs, which served as the comparison group, underwent the same experimental conditions. In addition, two dogs underwent the autonomic blocking procedures and the test for extinction *after* the avoidance response had been well established.

The results disclose that autonomic deprivation had only a partial effect on the learning of avoidance responses and that its effect occurred mainly in the initial phase of learning. Sympathectomized animals took longer than the controls to escape shock, required significantly more trials to learn their first avoidance response, and tended to extinguish more rapidly. However, the speed of extinction in the animals deprived of normal autonomic functioning *after* learning the avoidance did not differ from that of the normal controls. Moreover, no consistent relationship was found between the avoidance-learning pattern and the portion of the autonomic nervous system that was blocked. (A diagram of the autonomic nervous system is shown in Plate 3.)

The fact that all the sympathectomized animals eventually acquired stable avoidance responses suggests that autonomic responsiveness may facilitate the learning of avoidance but does not seem to be a necessary condition for its establishment. The maintenance of already existing avoidance responses is apparently even less dependent upon autonomic feedback. Similarly, the findings of Black (1959) that avoidance responses during extinction persisted long after the related autonomic responses had been extinguished further indicate that avoidant patterns may be maintained without the support of conditioned emotional responses.

It would appear from the studies discussed above that classically conditioned autonomic responses may initially govern the motivation and reinforcement of avoidance behavior. Once instrumental responses are acquired, however, they are probably activated directly by external stimuli and central neural processes rather than by autonomic arousal. Indeed, autonomic responses and accompanying feedback are typically much slower than those of the skeletal response system; consequently, avoidance behavior is typically executed before autonomic reactions could possibly be elicited! This factor alone places serious limitations on autonomic responses as continuing instigators and reinforcers of avoidance repertoires. As has been frequently observed in learning experiments, once an avoidance response pattern has been learned, it becomes highly stereotyped, it is rapidly elicited, and its autonomic and skeletal accompaniments which indicate emotional arousal are markedly diminished or totally absent. In light of these considerations, currently popular theories of psychopathology that consider most deviant behavior motivated by an underlying anxiety drive require revision. A more plausible idea, consistent with recent research findings, would highlight the *direct* eliciting function of conditioned stimuli and their correlates in the central nervous system.

Defective or Inappropriate Incentive Systems

Much, if not most, human behavior is sustained and modified by conditioned positive reinforcers (learned rewards). Neutral stimuli can acquire positive reinforcing properties by classical conditioning, that is, through repeated association with stimuli that already have positive valence.

Some forms of maladaptive behavior are due in large part to the fact that certain potentially harmful or culturally prohibited stimuli have very strong positive reinforcing functions for the individual. These deviations generally take the form of marked attraction to fetishistic or transvestite objects, such as the garments of the opposite sex, to various forms of drugs and intoxicants or to homosexuality. A social learning analysis of several of these disorders will be presented to illustrate the process whereby behavioral repertoires come under the control of unconventional positive reinforcers.

There is considerable cross-cultural evidence (Ford and Beach, 1951) that, in societies where *homosexuality and transvestism* are socially disapproved, masculine and feminine behavioral inversions are relatively rare; by contrast, cross-sex dressing, anal intercourse, oral-genital contacts, and mutual masturbation are regularly practiced by most members of societies in which such behavior is sanctioned. Whereas in our own society inflicting pain on a sexual partner is regarded as a sadistic perversion, in other cultures pain from aggression that normally accompanies coital activities is a powerful sexual reinforcer (Holmberg, 1946; Malinowski, 1929). There is also wide cultural variation in the physical attributes and adornments that become culturally conditioned sexual stimuli. What has been endowed with erotic arousal properties in one society—corpulence, skinniness, upright hemispherical breasts or long pendulous ones, shiny white teeth or black pointed ones, deformed ears, nose, or lips, broad pelvis and wide hips or narrow pelvis and slim hips, light skin color or dark skin color—may be neutral or highly repulsive to members of another social group. The publication of a New Guinea *Playboy* magazine in the United States would unquestionably prove disastrous financially, and conversely, the American version would not be expected to establish sales records among male inhabitants of the South Sea Islands. The cross-cultural data showing the enormous range of preferred sexual reinforcers among human societies provides striking testimony for the influential role of learning variables in the development of sexual responses that may be judged deviant by one or another social group.

Although our society imposes severe restrictions on some forms of behavior that have sexual implications, certain people may, nevertheless, imitate others and experience reinforcements which serve to promote and maintain deviant sexual responses (see Chapter 4). Relevant experimental studies of human sexuality are virtually nonexistent, but a number of observational reports indicate that social learning processes can give culturally inappropriate stimuli and responses very strong sexually reinforcing properties.

Litin *et al.* (1956) describe a case of transvestism in a five-year-old boy, who continually dressed up in his mother's clothes, cosmetics, and jewelry, exhibited almost complete feminine role behavior, and even adopted a girl's name suggested by his mother. Female dressing first appeared following an episode in which the mother, in response to her son's comment that she looked pretty in her new shoes, hugged him and offered him her old shoes. He wore them daily, eliciting considerable maternal approbation. The mother continued to encourage and reward his feminine behavior with affection and approval, while the grandmother and neighbors supplemented the mother's training in transvestism by supplying the boy with generous quantities of old shoes, hats, purses, bridal veils, and other female apparel. When the boy's inverted behavior met with disapproval from other persons, the mother attempted some discrimination training by informing her son, "You must never dress like that in front of company; only in front of the family."

The same authors present the case of a thirteen-year-old boy whose mother actively conditioned voyeuristic behavior toward herself by sleeping with the boy and by being physically and verbally seductive while appearing nude before him. When the boy was six years old, the mother showed him her vagina a number of times, but later discontinued her seductive behavior after the son suggested that they engage in sexual intercourse. The boy's strongly established voyeuristic behavior generalized to the maid and other persons until he was eventually apprehended by the police while peeping from a ladder into a neighborhood bedroom.

Generalization of strongly conditioned homoerotic responses is illustrated in the case of a sixteen-year-old girl whose mother would lie in bed with her, encouraging mutual stroking of the breasts and other erotic play. The mother sought psychiatric advice when she became jealous of her daughter's homosexual attachment to a teacher. Often, homosexual patterns of behavior are fostered in a less blatant fashion. In such instances, the distribution of social power within the family constellation and the pattern of affectional relationships promotes cross-sex modeling; sex-appropriate behavior is unrewarded or punished and, when the parents encourage peer relationships, homosexual associates tend to be selected (Fleck, 1960; Kolb and Johnson, 1955).

A mother's active positive conditioning of deviant sexual behavior is again evident in the case of a seventeen-year-old exhibitionist described by Giffin *et al.* (1954). The mother often showered with her son, engaged him in endless sex discussion, enjoyed exhibiting herself to him, and delighted in looking at the boy's nude body, particularly his "beautiful masculine endowment." A dress fetish was similarly conditioned in a ten-year-old boy by a mother who responded demonstratively whenever the son stroked her dress or complimented women on their attire (Johnson, 1953).

The conditioning of positive sexual reinforcers does not always depend on parental treatment, of course. Oswald (1962), for example, reports a case of a thirty-two-year-old military recruit who was sexually aroused by tying himself up tightly in black shiny rubber. This fetishistic behavior apparently originated in an early experience in which a group of boys seized him, tied a sheet over his head, and masturbated him.

> Since then he had made a practice of tying himself up with rubber groundsheets, a rubber hood and ropes. He came for treatment partly because he feared he might cause his own death, as he had recently had difficulty in releasing himself. (P. 201.)

Except for one occasion when he had sexual intercourse at a brothel equipped with rubber straitjackets, hoods, thongs, and rubber zip suits, masturbation while abundantly attired in rubberized garments was this man's main form of sexual reinforcement. Since heterosexual stimuli had rarely been associated with sexual gratification for him, whereas rubberized stimuli were repeatedly paired with orgasms, it is apparent how the fetishistic stimuli derived and retained their powerful reinforcing function.

The foregoing cases are a small sample of those actually documented. Three social stimulus variables emerge from these reports as important determinants of deviant sexual behavior. First, the degree to which parents themselves model blatant or disguised forms of homosexual, transvestite, fetishistic, or exhibitionistic behavior is often a significant antecedent factor. Second, once the behavior is elicited, whether by direct instigation or modeling, it is endowed with exaggerated sexual significance and strong positive value through repeated association with intense demonstrations of affection, often in the form of physical intimacy. Indeed, in some cases this caused the children to show well-developed patterns of sexual behavior long before the onset of pubescence. The third factor concerns the extent to which parents maintain children's deviant sexual responses over a long period of time through direct and vicarious reinforcement.

Sexual responses of strong positive valence can also become self-reinforcing if their occurrence reduces aversive stimulation. Such diminution of aversive emotional states may involve two somewhat different psychological processes. First, the sexual responses can produce sufficiently intense pleasure to contravene or countercondition feelings of anxiety or frustration. Secondly, sexual behavior also changes the stimulus situation by directing the individual's attention away from the emotion-provoking cues. This shift of attention may itself reduce unpleasant emotions.

Evidence of the emotion-reducing function of deviant sexual responses is seen in a case report published by Cooper (1963). The client characteristically experienced heightened sexual arousal from feeling silken garments. Dressed in women's clothes, he would frequently masturbate to orgasm while straddling a chair. Although initially the transvestite behavior served a sexual function, it later acquired by accident a general anxiety-terminating value. One day while the client was very anxious about a scholastic examination, he discovered that dressing in women's clothes abruptly reduced his emotional upset. Thereafter, a wide range of stressful stimuli elicited transvestite behavior. A number of other authors (Bond and Hutchison, 1960; Conn, 1954) have noted a similar sequence in which mounting tension is abruptly reduced by the execution of deviant sexual acts. These clinical data seem to indicate that very persistent sexual deviance is probably maintained, not only by sexual reinforcers, but also by its aversion-reducing function.

Alcoholism is another prevalent class of behavior disorders. Psychoanalytic theories have generally emphasized the symbolic value of alcohol in gratifying "oral" or "passive-dependent needs," but remarkably little attention has been paid to the *pharmacological* properties of alcohol which, under certain conditions, make it a powerful positive reinforcer.

One set of experiments that has direct bearing on the reinforcing qualities of alcohol concerns its effects on the autonomic nervous system. In these studies subjects' physiological responses are measured before and after ingestion of alcohol. The findings generally show that alcohol in small doses has no consistent effects (Doctor and Perkins, 1961; McDonnell and Carpenter, 1959), but it can result in substantial reduction in emotionality when taken in moderate or large quantities (Carpenter, 1957; Greenberg and Carpenter, 1957).

It is sometimes argued (Chafetz and Demone, 1962) that learning principles cannot adequately explain alcoholism because the long-range social and physical damage from chronic drinking far outweigh its temporary relief value. This argument overlooks the fact that behavior is controlled by its *immediate,* rather than delayed, consequences; and it is precisely for this reason that persons may persistently engage in immediately reinforcing, but eventually self-destructive, behavior.

Further evidence for the emotion-reducing properties of alcohol is provided in experiments with animals designed to study disinhibitory effects and extinction of conditioned avoidance responses. Suggestive findings regarding the conflict-reducing effects of alcohol were reported by Masserman and Yum (1946) in a study of cats that learned to perform complex manipulations to secure food but inhibited these responses after they had been subjected to electric shock at the goal. Administration of small doses of alcohol, however, promptly restored the responses designed to obtain food. In addition, the cats developed a preference for milk cocktails containing 5 percent alcohol to plain milk during the series of shock trials, but reverted to their original preference for nonalcoholic drinks after the aversive conditioning was discontinued and all emotional responses were extinguished.

The results of numerous studies are consistent with the findings that moderate doses of alcohol produce rapid extinction of fear-mediated behavior (Kaplan, 1956; Pawlowski *et al.*, 1961) and reduce the rate of responses designed to postpone the occurrence of aversive stimuli (Hogans *et al.*, 1961; Sidman, 1955). Moreover, the capacity of alcohol to reduce emotional behavior is similar to that of drugs that depress the central nervous system (Korpmann and Hughes, 1959).

A few experiments involving human subjects have also demonstrated the disinhibiting effects of alcohol on verbal expressions of sex and aggression in social drinking situations (Brunn, 1959; Clark and Sensibar, 1955). Among humans, however, the same dose of alcohol may have diverse effects in the types of responses inhibited, in the degree of response inhibition, and on social stimulus conditions which, in part, serve to define and to control appropriate behavior.

Findings from experiments using a forced alcohol regimen, in which the animals' entire fluid intake is restricted to solutions containing various concentrations of alcohol, reveal that alcohol *per se* has no strong inherently reinforcing properties. In these experiments, animals consume small nonintoxicating amounts of alcohol, but they readily revert to other fluids when they become available (Korman and Stephens, 1960; Richter, 1956). The positive reinforcing value of alcohol is substantially enhanced, however, under conditions of aversive stimulation (Casey, 1960; Clark and Polish, 1960; Masserman and Yum, 1946).

The research cited provides ample evidence that excessive alcohol consumption is maintained through positive reinforcement deriving from its depressant and anesthetic properties. The reduction of autonomic and other distressing emotional responses is the significant reinforcing event. Consequently, persons who are repeatedly subjected to aversive stimulation would be more prone to consume anesthetic doses of alcohol than persons who experience less stress, once they have acquired some taste for liquor to begin with.

Prolonged and heavy use of alcoholic beverages produces alterations in the metabolic system which provide the basis for a second maintaining mechanism that is quite independent of the original functional value of alcohol. That is, the withdrawal of alcohol causes very unpleasant physiological reactions including tremulousness, nausea, vomiting, marked weakness, diarrhea, fever, hypertension, excessive perspiration, and insomnia (Isbell *et al.*, 1955). After the person thus becomes dependent on alcohol, he is compelled to consume large quantities of it both to alleviate and to prevent distressing physical reactions. Since the ingestion of intoxicants promptly terminates these "withdrawal symptoms," drinking is automatically and continuously reinforced. At this stage, the major part of the alcoholic's time and resources are devoted to maintaining continuous self-intoxication.

Although reduction of aversiveness and other positive reinforcements which typically accompany social drinking may account adequately for the maintenance of inebriety, an adequate general theory of alcoholism must use additional social learning principles since, obviously, most persons who are subjected to stressful experiences do not become alcoholics. It has been customary to name a varied array of internal determinants such as neurotic personality disturbances and underlying pathologies as the critical conditions which give rise to alcoholism. But the inadequacy of theories of alcoholism which emphasize the role of personality traits and internal dynamics becomes readily evident when we examine the marked cultural and subcultural differences in the incidence of alcoholism. If one accepts the theory that a "neurosis" is instrumental in the development of chronic inebriety, he would be forced to conclude that Jews, Mormons, Moslems, Italians, and members of other cultural groups with similar exceedingly low rates of addictive drinking, are lacking in neurosis, oral deprivations, self-destructive tendencies, latent homosexuality, indulgent mothering, inadequacy feelings, and the other dynamics that supposedly maintain alcoholism. If so, then these pernicious conditions must be highly prevalent among the Irish, who surpass all other ethnic groups in chronic alcoholism (Chafetz and Demone, 1962; McCarthy, 1959; Pittman and Synder, 1962)! Perhaps the most striking evidence that alcoholism primarily represents a learned pattern of behavior rather than a manifestation of some predisposing underlying pathology is provided by the extraordinarily low rates of alcoholism among Jews, who almost certainly experience no less, and in all probability more, psychological stress than members of ethnic groups noted for their inebriety (Glad, 1947; Snyder, 1958). These ethnic and subcultural differences in the use of intoxicants point to the importance of *prealcoholic* social learning of drinking behavior in the development of alcoholism.

The social learning variables take several forms. At the most general level they are reflected in the cultural norms associated with the use of alcoholic beverages. There is considerable evidence, for example, that the consumption of alcohol is significantly influenced by the drinking mores of given social groups. Members of cultures which are highly permissive toward the use of intoxicants, or even consider drinking desirable, display a higher incidence of drunkenness than persons reared in cultures that, for religious or other reasons, demand sobriety. Similarly, within heterogeneous cultures such as our own, the prevalance of chronic intoxication varies with the types of social learning conditions that are associated with class status, religious affiliation, racial and ethnic background, occupation, and area of residence.

Although cultural and subgroup mores obviously play an influential role in determining the extent of excessive drinking, normative injunctions alone do not explain either the relatively low incidence of *addictive drinking* in social groups that sanction alcoholic beverages, or the occurrence of chronic alcoholism in cultures prohibiting or condemning intoxicants.

Cultural and subgroup mores are largely transmitted through the modeling of socializing agents; consequently, one cannot assume that members of a particular social group undergo equivalent learning experiences. Studies of the family background of alcoholics generally reveal an unusually high incidence of familial alcoholism (Fort and Porterfield, 1961; Lemere *et al.*, 1952; Wall, 1936). It might be argued that these data provide support for a genetic interpretation of alcoholism, but in reality the pattern of drinking behavior being modeled and the stimulus conditions that characteristically elicit alcohol consumption are more important than whether or not family members do any drinking. For example, in Italian and Jewish households, dilute alcoholic beverages, particularly wine, are regularly consumed, but in a highly controlled and discriminative fashion. When the use of alcohol is thus restricted primarily to mealtimes and to religious ceremonies and other social and familial practices, its consumption may be brought under sufficient discriminative stimulus control to ensure moderation (Bales, 1946; Glad, 1947; Snyder, 1958). On the other hand, in family situations where alcohol is used extensively for social reasons and as a preferred mode of coping with frustration or stress, a similar type of drinking pattern is likely to be transmitted to the children.

Although drinking is initially most often learned under nonstress conditions, a habitual social drinker will on many occasions experience reduction of distress under alcoholic influence. Once alcohol consumption is thus intermittently reinforced, it will be readily elicited under frustrating or aversive conditions. Therefore, it is not surprising that alcoholism typically results from habituation after prolonged heavy social drinking, especially in families with a history of alcoholism.

The relationship between stress and alcoholism is perhaps strongest among alcoholics who are members of subcultural groups which disapprove of drinking and whose parents have practiced total abstinence. The social learning history of alcoholism under these conditions has never been adequately documented, but there is some evidence to suggest that the drinking pattern in such cases is originally acquired under highly stressful conditions and is then generalized to less acute emotional circumstances (Fort and Porterfield, 1961). Outside the family, moreover, peers who drink may play an influential role in transmitting drinking patterns (Skolnik, 1957).

In this behavioral analysis of alcoholism, aversive stimulation and its prompt reduction through the depressant action of alcoholic beverages are assigned a central role in the development and maintenance of addictive drinking. It should be emphasized, however, that conflict, frustration, and other such stimulus situations may elicit a wide variety of reactions including aggression, dependency, withdrawal, somatization, regression, apathy, autism, inebriation, or constructive action. Persons who exhibit the latter will typically be judged "normal"; in contrast, "neuroses," "deep-seated personality disturbances," and other disease processes are frequently invoked to explain the former patterns of coping. These assumed underlying pathologies represent fictitious causes since the main evidence for their existence is the behavior which they are supposed to explain.

From a social learning point of view, alcoholics are persons who have acquired the habit of alcohol consumption through reinforcement and modeling experiences as a widely generalized dominant response to aversive stimulation. Therapeutic attention would, therefore, be most profitably directed toward reducing the level of aversive stimulation experienced by the client and toward eliminating alcoholic stress reactions, preferably by establishing alternative modes of coping behavior. Given more effective and rewarding response alternatives, the person is less likely to continuously anesthetize himself against aversive or frustrative stimulation.

The discussion so far has concerned the conditions under which certain response patterns are powerfully supported by unfortunate conditioned reinforcers. Another class of behavioral disorders, also reflecting problems of incentive, results from the fact that many of the customary social stimuli which help to establish and maintain human behavior, such as attention, approval, and affection, do not function as positive reinforcers for certain individuals; conversely, negative stimuli such as disapproval, criticism, and censure also fail to serve as negative reinforcers. These types of deficits in incentive systems have been observed most frequently among children usually diagnosed as "autistic" (Ferster, 1961; Ferster and De Myer, 1961; Lovaas *et al.*, 1964; Wolf *et al.*, 1964). For these children, most forms of social approval and censure have either very little effect or unpredictable effects upon behavior. It is often difficult therefore to sustain what reality orientations they have or to develop more complex patterns of social behavior.

The acquisition of incentive value is governed by the frequency with which stimuli are associated with primary reinforcers, the intensity and consistency of affective experiences, the time interval between the originally neutral and the reinforcing stimuli, and numerous other factors. The greatest opportunities for *incentive learning* occur in conjunction with basic caretaking activities, during which parental behavior can have strong reinforcing effects. Since parents of autistic children typically perform these activities in an extremely cold and mechanistic (Eisenberg, 1957), haphazard (Goldfarb, 1961), or restricted (Ferster, 1961) manner, it is not surprising that social stimuli acquire little or no reinforcing value for many of these children. For this reason it is generally necessary to use primary reinforcers like food in the initial stages of treatment programs for autistic and schizophrenic personalities. In fact, the development of conditioned reinforcers constitutes an important initial objective of treatment.

The inadequate development of positive social reinforcers is also frequently seen among antisocial personalities, particularly those for whom dependent and affectionate responses have been negatively conditioned (punished) over a long period of time. As a result, such persons are typically unresponsive or distrusting, hostile, and avoidant to the rewarding positive responses of others (Ackerman, 1944; Aichhorn, 1935; Bandura and Walters, 1959; Thorpe and Smith, 1952).

Evidence that positive social reinforcers may be aversive for persons who strongly inhibit dependency is seen in a study by Cairns (1961). Delinquent boys who exhibited either high or low dependency inhibition participated in an experiment in which correct responses on two tasks were positively reinforced with verbal approval. The boys who were able to express dependency improved on both tasks in response to the experimenter's approval, while the boys high in dependency inhibition showed decrements on both tasks under continued positive reinforcement. In a related experiment with college students, Cairns and Lewis (1962) similarly found that students high in dependency evaluated verbal reinforcing stimuli more favorably and proved more responsive than students low in dependency.

Under conditions of harsh treatment, which appear to characterize the family backgrounds of people anxious about dependency, the very presence of others and their attention gradually become negatively reinforcing. If occasional approval and positive attention are superimposed on a schedule of high negative reinforcement, then these positive social stimuli become unreliable cues which may even assume aversive potency. McDavid and Schroder (1957) indeed found that delinquent boys were less able to discriminate between social approval and disapproval than were boys in an equivalent group of nondelinquents. In view of the fact that conditioned social reinforcers play an important, if not indispensable, role in the social learning process, it is difficult to treat persons for whom social stimuli have only weak or negative reinforcing value.

A final class of incentive problems is reflected in circumstances where the individual has an adequate incentive system but his environment is lacking in reinforcers. This condition usually results in generalized apathy and inattention.

Aversive Behavioral Repertoires

In the introductory section of this chapter, reference has been made to the fact that behavior that generates aversive consequences to others is frequently labeled a symptomatic manifestation of a personality disorder. Consequently, children who are very aggressive, annoying in attention getting, and clinging in dependency, and adolescents or adults who engage in antisocial activities and other forms of socially disruptive behavior comprise a sizeable proportion of the cases regularly referred to treatment agencies. Since most aversion-producing responses are characteristically labeled

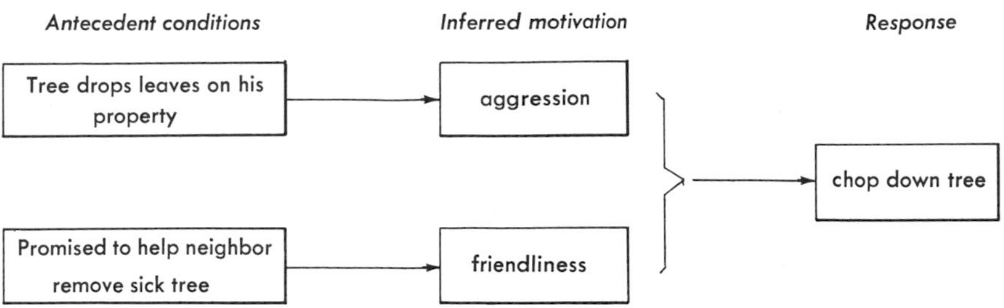

Figure 9.4 Process of inferring motivation.

"aggressive," the social learning conditions under which aggressive responses are acquired and maintained (Bandura and Walters, 1963) will be reviewed briefly.

Much of the theorizing, research, and psychotherapeutic practice relating to aggression has been strongly influenced by Freud's early theory, according to which this form of behavior represents a "primordial reaction" to the thwarting of pleasure-seeking or pain-avoiding responses (Freud, 1920, 1925). Although Freud's later notion of aggression as a manifestation of a "death instinct" (1922) was less widely accepted, the view has persisted that aggression is a natural and inevitable result of frustration.

In later learning theory translations of this *frustration-aggression hypothesis* (Dollard *et al.*, 1939; Miller, 1941), aggression was regarded as a natural, though not inevitable, consequence of frustration, since nonaggressive responses to frustration could also be learned. Nevertheless, aggression was still considered the dominant innate response to frustration, and substitute nonaggressive responses were thought to occur only if aggressive reactions had previously been extinguished or punished. In this formulation, the problems of how aggressive responses are originally acquired and how social learning variables other than frustration influence their establishment, social transmission, and maintenance were largely ignored.

In categorizing social classes of responses, issues of value and fact are generally confounded. Aggression, for example, is typically defined as behavior intended to injure or destroy. The main difficulty with such a definition is that intention is not a measurable property of behavior. Let us suppose that an individual is observed vigorously chopping down a neighbor's tree. By the foregoing definition, it is impossible to tell from the behavior alone whether or not the determined axman is displaying aggression. If one is informed that he has graciously consented to assist his neighbor in removing an infected tree, the chopping would not be labeled aggressive. If, on the other hand, the tree has been dropping leaves and dead branches into his driveway which he is continually forced to clean up, and he is chopping the tree down without the neighbor's consent, his behavior would be considered highly aggressive. The above example illustrates how a complex set of criteria including the form and intensity of responses, their presumed antecedents, and a host of other judgmental factors determine whether or not a given response will be categorized as aggressive (Figure 9.4).

Both children and adults characteristically display wide individual differences in response to stressful or frustrating stimulus conditions. Aggression, dependency, withdrawal, apathy, regression, sexual behavior, somatization, and constructive task-oriented behavior are all common modes of stress responses.

These variations in response patterns are thought by some writers to be primarily determined by constitutional or temperamental factors. More often, however, they are regarded as products of trial-and-error instrumental learning. Some evidence that observed differences in choice and patterning of frustration reactions are partly interpretable in terms of differential reinforcement histories will be presented later. It should be noted in passing that the selective learning interpretation of how persons learn to cope with frustration explains the occurrence of *changes* in existing frustration response hierarchies, but it does not account for the *origin* of different responses to frustration.

Learned patterns of response to stress, frustration, and other forms of emotional arousal frequently originate from the observation of adult and peer models who provide the developing child with ample opportunities to observe their frustration reactions in different stimulus situations. On the basis of such repeated exposure, the child is likely to acquire a hierarchy of frustration responses corresponding to the behavioral examples of his social models. Consequently, when he encounters stressful stimuli he is more likely to respond *imitatively* than in a *random* fashion. Only after a person has learned aggression as a dominant response to emotional arousal will he be likely to show aggressive reactions to frustration.

The influential role of modeling in the social transmission of aggression is demonstrated in a series of laboratory investigations of *vicarious learning* conducted by Bandura and his associates (Bandura, 1962*a*, 1965*a*). In one set of studies (Bandura *et al.*, 1961, 1963*a*), different groups of children observed adult models, presented either live, on film, or as cartoon characters, exhibiting novel aggressive patterns of behavior toward a large Bobo doll. Another group of children viewed the same live model behaving in a nonaggressive, inhibited manner, and subjects in a control group were not exposed to the models. All children were then mildly frustrated, and measures were obtained of the amount of imitative and nonimitative aggression they showed in a new setting where there was no model.

Results of these experiments reveal that exposure to the behavior of models may have several rather different behavioral effects that are reflected in the observers' subsequent behavior. First, a subject may acquire new responses as a function of observing the behavior of another person. Thus, children who had observed the aggressive models displayed a great number of precisely imitative novel aggressive responses, whereas such responses rarely occurred in either the nonaggressive-model group or the control group. Illustrations of the way in which children reproduced the model's behavior with remarkable fidelity are provided in Figure 9.5. The top frames show the female model performing four novel aggressive responses, and the lower frames depict a boy and a girl reproducing her behavior. A related experiment recently conducted by Hicks (1965) further demonstrates that peer and adult models may be equally effective transmitters of aggressive behavior patterns.

Exposure to the behavior of others may also strengthen or weaken *inhibitory* responses in the observer. In the present experiment, for example, children who had witnessed the aggressive models, either live or in pictures, subsequently displayed approximately twice as much aggression as subjects in the control group, or as those who had observed inhibited models (Figure 9.6). Furthermore, the data indicate that exposure to nonaggressive models decreases the probability of aggressive reactions to frustra-

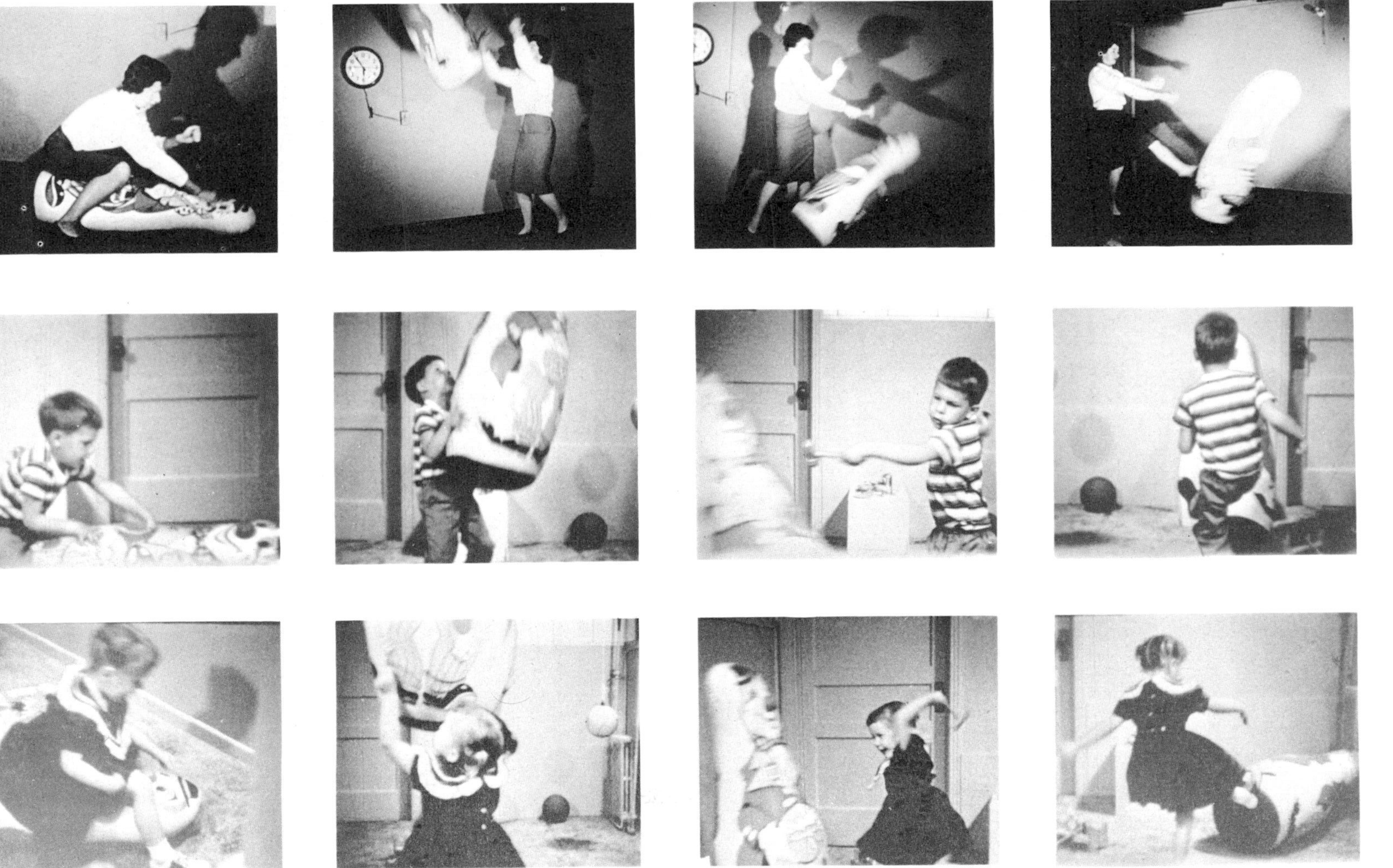

Figure 9.5 Photographs of children reproducing the aggressive behavior that had been exhibited by a female model. From Bandura *et al.* (1963*a*).

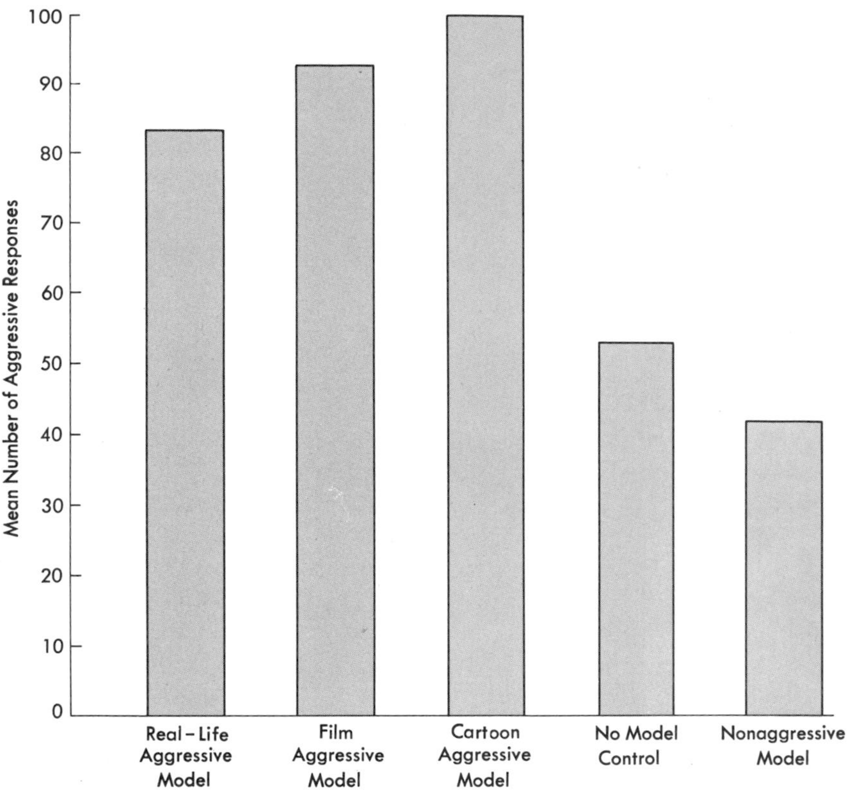

Figure 9.6 Mean amount of postfrustration aggression displayed by control children and by those who had been exposed to aggressive and inhibited models. Reprinted with permission from "The role of imitation in personality development" by Albert Bandura, *Young Children*, Vol. 18, No. 3 (April 1963), p. 209. Copyrighted by the National Association for the Education of Young Children.

tion; children in the nonaggressive condition showed significantly less aggression than subjects in the control group (Figure 9.9). Disinhibitory effects in adolescent and adult subjects of exposure to aggressive models have been reported by Berkowitz and Rawlings (1963), by Hartmann (1964), and by Walters and Llewellyn Thomas (1963).

It is apparent that people do not imitate every model they come in contact with, nor do they imitate every element of behavior exhibited even by models who function as primary sources of social behavior. The occurrence of matching responses is influenced by the types of consequences that have been characteristically associated with the model's behavior. These rewarding or punishing consequences may either follow the model's responses immediately or be inferred from symbols, attributes, and skills possessed by the model that tend to be regularly correlated with differential reinforcements. This has been discussed in some detail in Chapter 4.

The manner in which immediate response consequences to the model enhance or inhibit the imitation of aggression is demonstrated in experiments (Bandura, 1965*b*; Bandura *et al.*, 1963*b*) in which children observed an adult model whose aggressive behavior resulted in either rewarding or highly punishing outcomes. Subjects who witnessed the aggressive model gain rewards preferred to emulate the successful aggressor and showed more imitative behavior, even though they disapproved of his actions, than did children whose aggressive model was punished. The latter group both failed to reproduce his behavior and rejected him as a model for emulation. The effects of witnessing rewarded villainly thus outweighed the acquired value systems of the observers. What happens to a socially deviant model who violates rules and prohibitions determines in a similar manner the extent to which his transgressions will be imitated (Blake, 1958; Walters *et al.*, 1963).

The above laboratory findings are corroborated by anthropological field studies (Bateson, 1936; Whiting and Child, 1953; Eaton and Weil, 1955) which reveal the importance of models in the cultural transmission of both aggressive and nonaggressive reactions to frustration. The role of modeling in the genesis of antisocial aggression is also apparent in naturalistic studies of delinquent subcultures (Cohen, 1955; Yablonsky, 1962; Whyte, 1937) and of the influence of parental modeling on children's behavior (Bandura, 1960; Bandura and Walters, 1959; McCord and McCord, 1958.)

The effects of positive reinforcement on the development and maintenance of aggressive behavior have been demonstrated in numerous laboratory experiments. Patterson *et al.* (1961), for example, found that children who had been verbally reinforced for hitting an inflated doll did more hitting than subjects who had not received training in aggression. The importance of *schedules of reinforcement,* which is abundantly documented in research on nonsocial responses (Ferster and Skinner, 1957), is likewise revealed in a study by Cowan and Walters (1963), who showed that *continuously* reinforced aggressive responses extinguish more rapidly than *intermittently* reinforced ones.

Evidence exists that intermittently reinforced aggressive responses not only are more persistent than steadily reinforced ones but also tend to be generalized to new interpersonal situations. In an experiment by Walters and Brown (1963), boys who were rewarded with marbles every *sixth time* they punched an automated Bobo doll subsequently showed more aggression in two-person competition than did children who had previously been reinforced following *every* hitting response. This study also demonstrates how aggressive responses established in a noninterpersonal context may be employed on future occasions to overcome interpersonal frustrations. Lovaas (1961) also reports that aggressive responses, if positively reinforced, increase in frequency and are generalized from one class of aggressive behavior to another.

In everyday social situations, aggression is not only often rewarded intermittently, but also in a highly discriminative manner. Evidence of direct discrimination training of aggression through differential reinforcement is clearly revealed in a study by Bandura and Walters (1959) of the child-training practices of parents of aggressive and nonaggressive adolescent boys. Parents of the aggressive boys consistently and severely punished any aggression directed toward themselves, but actively encouraged and rewarded their sons' aggressive behavior toward peers and adults outside the home. The excerpt below, taken from an interview with the father of an antisocially aggressive boy, illustrates the pattern of differential reinforcement:

I (interviewer): How much of this sort of thing (verbal aggression) have you allowed?

F (father): I don't allow him to get moody with me because he knows he wouldn't get away with it. They're too smart. They know what they can do and what they can't do.

I: Have you ever encouraged Earl to use his fists to defend himself?

F: Yes, if necessary, I told him many times that if someone wanted to fight with him and started the old idea of the chip on the shoulder, "Don't hit the chip, hit his jaw, and get it over with."

I: Has he ever come to you and complained that another fellow was giving him a rough time?

F: Yes.

I: What did you advise him to do about it?

F: I told him to hit him.

I: If Earl got into a fight with one of the neighbor's boys, how would you handle it?

F: That would depend who was at fault. If my boy was at fault, he'd be wrong and I'd do my best to show that. But if he was in the right I wouldn't want to chastise him.

I: How far would you let it go?

F: I'd let it go until one won. See who was the best man. (Pp. 101, 115.)

A similar discriminative pattern of parental reinforcement of aggression, and discriminative aggressive responses by the children, was disclosed in a comparative study of the social learning histories of very aggressive and behaviorally inhibited preadolescent boys (Bandura, 1960).

It has been well established in both modeling and direct reinforcement studies that aggressive responses are readily acquired under nonfrustrating conditions. The experimental data, furthermore, indicate that frustration may facilitate aggression but is not a necessary condition for it; that is, frustration generally produces a temporary increase in emotional arousal and thus leads to more vigorous responding. The nature of the responses that are elicited and intensified, however, depends to a large extent on the discriminative stimuli present in the situation and the previously acquired dominant responses to emotional arousal.

An experimental study by Davitz (1952) illustrates the inadequacy of the frustration-aggression hypothesis and also the importance of direct training in the development of aggressive modes of behavior. Groups of children were initially observed in a free play situation designed to provide measures of cooperative and aggressive behavior. Half the groups then participated in training sessions in which they were praised for displaying competitive and aggressive responses; by contrast, the remaining groups of children were positively reinforced for constructive and cooperative behavior. Subsequently, all the children were shown a movie during which they were given candy bars. Frustration was induced by terminating the movie just as it approached its climax and at the same time taking away the candy. Immediately following the frustrating experience, the groups of children were again observed in the free play situation. Subjects who had been trained to behave aggressively in the competitive games responded more aggressively to frustration than the groups trained in constructive action. Moreover, children who had been reinforced for cooperativeness responded more constructively following frustration than did the children who had been trained in aggression. These findings are entirely consistent with the view that frustration conditions simply serve as arousal stimuli that will elicit, according to the character of the discriminative stimuli present, the response patterns currently dominant in the subject's behavioral repertoire.

Additional evidence that learning largely determines the nature of responses to frustration is provided in studies by Otis and McCandless (1955), who observed more dominant-aggressive reactions to frustration in children with a strong "need for power" than in children with a prevailing "need for love-affection," and by Block and Martin (1955), who found that undercontrolled children gave predominantly aggressive responses when thwarted, whereas overcontrolled children exhibited constructive behavior. Moreover, the finding (Bandura, 1960) that very aggressive boys experienced no more, and perhaps less, frustration of dependency behavior than withdrawn boys suggests that the two groups of children acquired contrasting patterns of response to frustration as a result of different learning histories and not because of differences in the amount of frustration each group experienced.

Unlike the "frustration-aggression hypothesis," which assumes an initial invariant relationship between thwarting and aggressive behavior, social learning theory (Bandura and Walters, 1963) suggests that one can readily produce a highly aggressive person by merely exposing him to successful aggressive models and intermittently rewarding aggressive responses, even though frustration may be kept at a very low level. Indeed, it is clearly apparent that extreme forms of aggression are increasingly the products of social reinforcement (Yablonsky, 1962). In these instances, the primary functional value of aggression, particularly if performed in a daring and "cool" manner, is to enhance one's peer group status and to win the admiration of in-group members, rather than to achieve material gain or reduce frustration. Similar reinforcement contingencies are frequently noted in other forms of antisocial response patterns.

> "Doing it [breaking into a store] is knowing that the fuzz [police] is coming. I mean any cat can reach in for a bunch of bananas if the Girl Scouts is watching, but the thing is, will you do it when you know the po-leese is just around the corner and coming.
>
> It's like you got to make the scene or the chicks will put you down as nuthin'. I mean you got to go. Ya dig?" (Gavzer, 1964, p. 5.)

Essentially the same set of social learning principles discussed above accounts for the development and maintenance of other classes of undesirable behavior that may not necessarily be categorized as aggressive. The differential reinforcement of responses that are persistent or intense appears to be the factor most often responsible for the unusual resiliency of aversive behavior. Examples from parent-child interactions will serve to illustrate this process.

In many families, children's prosocial responses, and even their mildly deviant behaviors, are likely to go unnoticed or unrewarded. On the other hand, more persistent and intense responses annoy the parents, who are then forced to terminate the troublesome behavior by attending to the child (Bandura, 1962*b*). Numerous vivid illustrations of how children's aversive behavior can come to control their parents' reinforcing reactions is provided in Levy's classic study (1943) of childhood overdependency.

> Patient (4 years, 9 months) rules the household by his screaming and imperative voice. Mother will always comply with his demands rather than hear him scream. . . . The patient is disobedient, hyperactive, impudent to the parents; calls them names, kicks and scratches when not given his way. (Pp. 361–363.)
>
> Mother states that he (10-year-old) was spoiled by herself and maternal grandmother, and later she gave in to his demands for the sake of peace. . . . Whenever refused, he always commands obedience by screaming. . . . After screaming no longer availed, he used the methods of nagging, monotonously repeating his demands. (Pp. 163, 373–374.)

The types of reinforcement situations described above readily generate aversive behavior, which in turn creates the very conditions likely to perpetuate it. Thus, while nature's programming ensured that people's distress would not go unheeded for long, it also provided the basis for the establishment of socially disturbing response patterns.

Aversive Self-Reinforcing Systems

In the taxonomic system presented thus far, we have highlighted the influential role of external reinforcing stimuli in psychopathology. Although the controlling power of such *externally dispensed reinforcers* cannot be minimized, *self-administered reinforcers* may frequently outweigh their influence in governing social behavior, particularly that of older children and adults.

Until recently, self-reinforcing behavior has been virtually ignored in psychological theorizing and experimentation, perhaps because of the common preoccupation with animal learning. Unlike human subjects, who continually engage in self-evaluative and self-reinforcing behavior, rats or chimpanzees are disinclined to pat themselves on the back for commendable performances, or to berate themselves for getting lost in cul-de-sacs. By contrast, people typically make self-reinforcement contingent on their performing in ways they have come to value as an index of personal merit. They often set themselves relatively explicit criteria of achievement; failure to meet them is considered undeserving of reward and may elicit self-denial or even self-punishment. Conversely, individuals tend to reward themselves generously when they attain or exceed their self-imposed standards. Self-administered positive and negative stimuli may thus serve both as powerful incentives for learning and as effective reinforcers in maintaining behavior in humans.

Many people who think themselves maladjusted and seek the help of psychotherapists have relatively competent behavior repertoires under adequate control and are not encumbered by debilitating, externally stimulated inhibitory or avoidant repertoires. Despite their social competence and favorable reinforcement conditions, these people nevertheless experience a great deal of self-generated feelings of misery and self-imposed deprivations. These feelings often stem from excessively high standards of self-reinforcement, standards often supported by unfavorable comparisons with historical or contemporary models noted for their extraordinary achievements. This process characteristically gives rise to depressive reactions, feelings of worthlessness and lack of purpose, and a lessened disposition to perform because of the unfavorable ratio of work to self-reinforcement. In its more extreme forms, this problem is reflected in behaviors designed to escape through alcoholism, grandiose ideation, reluctance to engage in activities that may reflect on one's self-evaluation, and other modes of escape or avoidant behavior.

Self-rewarding responses are partly learned through reinforcements administered initially by external agents. In this learning process, the agent adopts a criterion of what constitutes a worthy performance and consistently rewards the subject for matching or exceeding the criterion level, disregarding or punishing performances that fall short of it. When subsequently the subject is given full control over the administration of reinforcers, he is likely to use the rewards in a similarly contingent manner, with his performance levels serving as the main discriminative stimuli.

The part played by reinforcement patterns and observational learning in the acquisition and maintenance of self-evaluative and self-reinforcing behavior is clearly revealed in recent laboratory studies. Evidence for the direct learning of self-reinforcing responses is provided in a series of experiments by Kanfer and Marston. In one study of

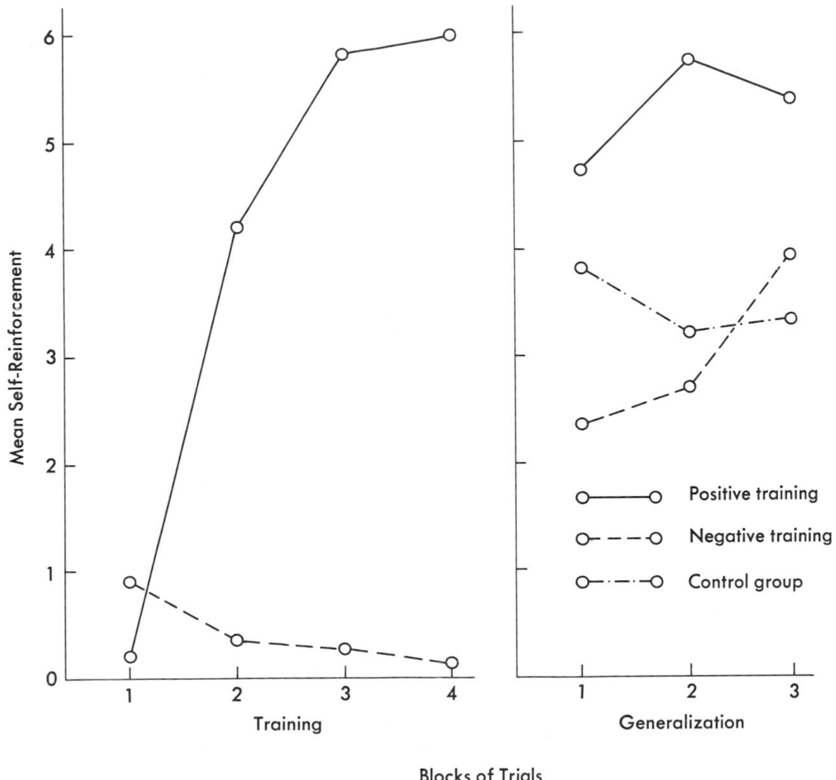

Figure 9.7 Mean self-reinforcing responses in the experimental groups during training and in all groups on the generalization task. Reprinted with permission of author and publisher from F. H. Kanfer and A. P. Marston, "The conditioning of self-reinforcing responses: An analogue to self-confidence training. *Psychological Reports*, 1963, Vol. 13, pp. 63–70.

the relative effects of miserly and indulgent training on the role of self-reinforcement (Kanfer and Marston, 1963*a*), adult subjects performed a subliminal perception task in which there was no apparent correct response nor external feedback about response accuracy. Whenever subjects in one group felt confident that their response on a given trial was correct, the experimenter rewarded them generously with tokens accompanied by approving comments and an indulgent attitude toward self-reward. By contrast, for the remaining subjects the experimenter parted grudgingly with tokens and cautioned subjects against requesting tokens for undeserving performances. A control group of subjects simply reported their guesses and received no reinforcement. Immediately after the training phase, generalization to self-reinforcing responses was tested on a verbal discrimination task for which there were, in fact, genuinely correct answers. In the latter session the subjects initially were rewarded only for accurate responses but later were given complete control over the reinforcers and instructed to reward themselves whenever they thought their responses were correct.

As shown in Figure 9.7, the subjects' rate of self-reinforcement was markedly influenced by the training procedures.

Indeed, in the final block of training trials, subjects in the positive and negative conditions exhibited 58 percent and 0.2 percent self-reinforcements, respectively. Of even greater interest, however, is the finding that, although the groups of subjects achieved the same number of correct responses on the subsequent verbal task, those who had received the positive indulgent training rewarded themselves more than the negatively trained group did.

Various other learning variables have been examined as determinants of positive self-reinforcement. In general, the findings reveal that the frequency of self-reinforcement closely corresponds to the rate of correct responses and decreases with the stringency of the performance standards imposed (Kanfer *et al.*, 1962; Kanfer and Marston, 1963*b*).

The self-evaluation process is often complicated by the fact that many stimulus situations are relatively ambiguous, and consequently it is difficult to determine what constitutes an adequate performance. Considering also that self-administration of positive reinforcers following marginal or undeserving performances is likely to generate negative self-reactions, it is perhaps understandable that subjects engage in less self-rewarding behavior on ambiguous than on structured tasks, but are more inclined to reward themselves when their responses correspond to those of another person in the same situation (Marston, 1964).

Although the studies cited above demonstrate the important role of direct reinforcement in the establishment and regulation of self-rewarding tendencies, it is doubtful that people receive much direct training in self-reinforcement, partly because performances in most situations cannot be evaluated meaningfully independent of the accomplishments of others. A college student, for instance, completes an examination and receives a grade of 70 points. Will he engage in self-rewarding or self-punitive behavior? Without evaluating this performance against the accomplishments of others relative to his self-imposed standards, he would have no basis for either positive or negative self-reactions. If the average performance of the student group is 70, and our subject's aspirations are to achieve no more than most, then he will engage in positive self-reinforcement. If, on the other hand, the subject's adopted standards are relatively high, a score of 70 will be thought undeserving of self-reward and may elicit self-punitive responses. A person's self-evaluations may thus depend upon the degree to which he matches the behavior and standards of models whom he has chosen for comparison.

Some evidence for the influential role of modeling variables in the transmission of self-reinforcement patterns is furnished by an experiment (Bandura and Kupers, 1964) that proceeded in the following manner. Children participated in a bowling game with an adult or a peer model; the scores, which could range from 5 to 30 points, were under the control of the experimenter. At the outset of the game, both the children and their models were given complete control of a plentiful supply of candy, from which they could help themselves as they wished. In one condition of the experiment, the model adopted a *high criterion for self-reinforcement*; on trials in which he obtained or exceeded a score of 20, he rewarded himself with candy and made self-approving statements, but on trials in which he scored less, he refrained from taking any candy and berated himself. In a second condition, the model displayed a similar pattern of self-reward and self-disapproval, but adopted the relatively *low self-reinforcement criterion* of 10 points. There were some minor variations in the amount of self-reinforcement: models helped themselves to one candy when they scored at, or slightly above, criterion, and to two candies when they performed well above the minimum. A control group of children had no exposure to the models.

After completing his trials, the model departed, the experimenter generously refurbished the candy supply, and the child played a series of games in which he received scores ranging from 5 to 30 points according to a prearranged program. In this series, the child was observed to see when he rewarded himself with candy and made imitative positive or negative self-evaluative statements.

Whereas children in the control group administered rewards to themselves more or less independently of performance level, subjects in the experimental conditions made self-reinforcement contingent upon achievements that matched the criteria used by their respective models. Thus, children who had been presented with low-criterion models were highly self-indulgent and self-approving for comparatively low achievements. By contrast, children in the high-criterion condition displayed considerable self-denial and self-derogation following identical accomplishments. The children not only adopted their model's self-rewarding patterns of behavior, but even matched the minor variations in magnitude of self-reinforcement exhibited by the models.

A comparison of the results obtained with adult and with peer models revealed that children were more influenced by adults than by the standard-setting behavior and self-reinforcing responses of peers. Figures 9.8 and 9.9 present graphically the distribution of self-reinforcements as a function of level of performance for each of the three groups of children.

Although in this experiment the children acquired positive and negative self-reinforcing responses without the mediation of direct external reinforcement, the evaluative properties of performances generally are probably the result of past differential reinforcements. Through the repeated pairing of performance deficits with unpleasant consequences, and successful performance with rewards, differential achievement levels *per se* eventually acquire positive or negative valence. It should be remembered, however, that such performance-produced cues have evaluative significance only in relation to some standard of reference. Once the values of different accomplishments are well-established, adequate or inadequate matches are likely to elicit similar self-reinforcing responses regardless of what specific performances are being compared. At this stage the whole process becomes relatively independent of external reinforcement and of the specifics of the original training situations, but it remains dependent upon evaluative cognitions. As shown in the above experiment, children will adopt the particular criteria for self-reinforcement exhibited by a reference model, will evaluate their own performances relative to that standard, and will then serve as their own reinforcing agents.

The criteria for positive reinforcement imposed by a model in relation to his own behavior have been shown by Marston (1964) to affect not only the self-reinforcing behavior of adults, but also the subsequent rate at which they will reinforce another person performing the same task.

People do not always adopt the high standards of achievement and patterns of self-reinforcement that may be displayed by parental and other salient models, despite intensive and continued exposure. A model who displays distinguished achievement may be regarded as inappropriate for self-evaluation by others who, consequently, impose lower criteria

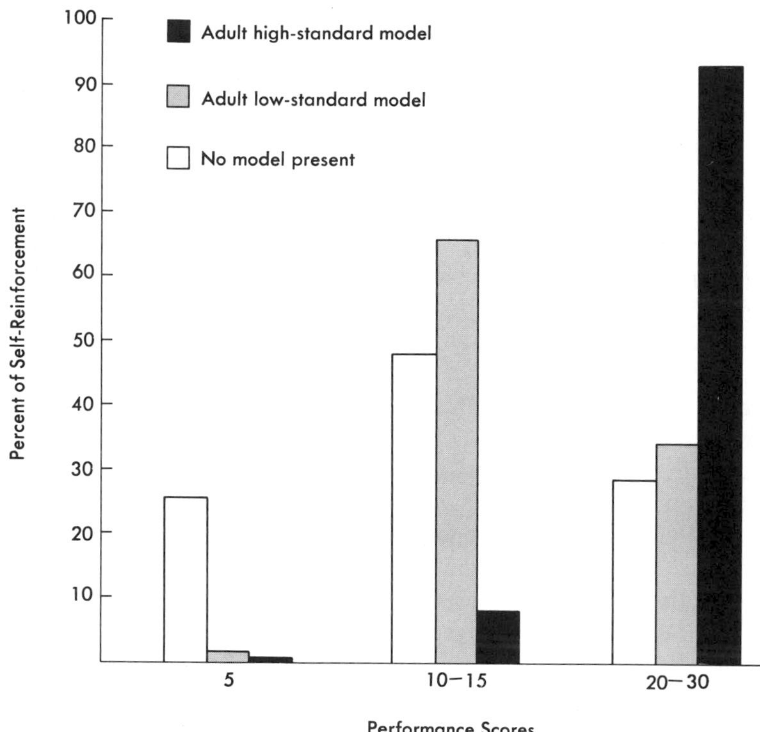

Figure 9.8 Regulation of self-reinforcement as a function of performance level by children in the control group and by those exposed to adult models adopting high and low criteria for self-reinforcement. From Bandura and Kupers (1964).

for self-reward on their own accomplishments. Similarly, persons who have met with repeated failure would not only be inclined to reject models who perform at high levels but, to the extent that they regard themselves as undeserving, would also tend to deny themselves available positive reinforcers.

The interactive effects of prior reinforcement and divergent modeling cues on the incidence of self-reinforcing behavior and self-imposed criteria are demonstrated in an experiment by Bandura and Whalen (1966). Children readily adopted the self-reinforcement patterns displayed by an inferior or an equally competent adult model, but rejected the high-self reinforcement standards of a model who performed at a superior level. Moreover, children who had undergone a series of failure experiences rewarded themselves more sparingly than those who had met with success, particularly when exposed to models exhibiting moderate to high achievements.

Further evidence for the influence of direct training and social models on the development of patterns of self-reinforcement comes from a study by Mischel and Liebert (1964) in which externally imposed and modeled reinforcement criteria were varied simultaneously. In one condition of the experiment, the model prescribed a stringent criterion for the subject but adopted a lenient standard for himself; for a second group of children, the adult imposed a stringent criterion on himself but advocated a lenient standard for the children; and for a third group, both the modeled and imposed criteria

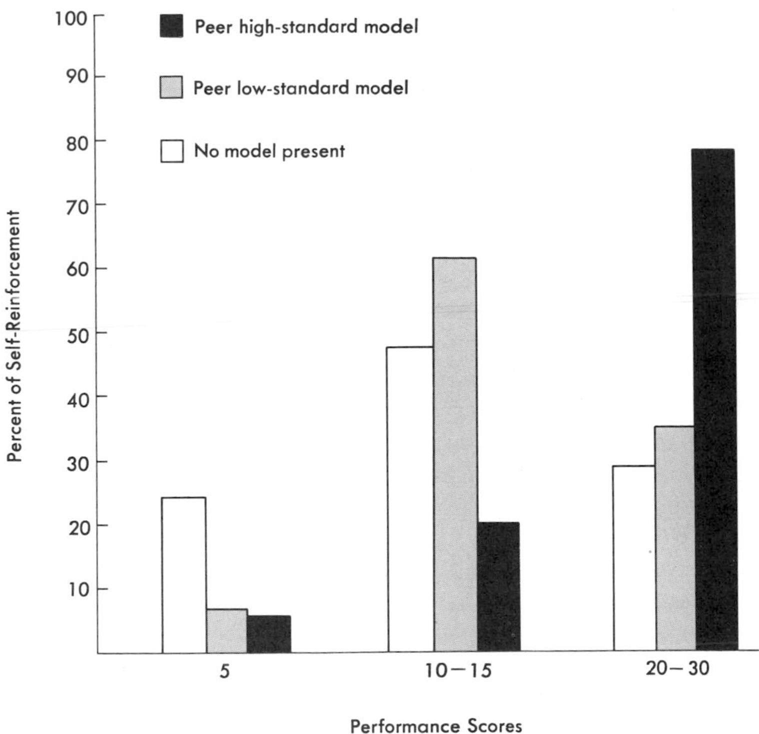

Figure 9.9 Regulation of self-reinforcement as a function of level of performance by children in the control group and by those exposed to peer models adopting high and low criteria for self-reinforcement. From Bandura and Kupers (1964).

were consistently high. After the exposure session, subjects performed the self-reinforcement task in the absence of the model and also served as trainers for another child.

As expected, the lowest incidence of self-rewarding responses was noted among children for whom high standards for self-reinforcement were both modeled and imposed. However, children subjected to equally high standards adopted more lenient criteria if their models had rewarded themselves for low-level performances. The highest rate of self-reinforcing responses was exhibited by children who were themselves treated leniently but had observed the model rewarding himself stringently. On the basis of these findings, we would expect that, under social learning conditions where imposed and modeled standards are consistently low, persons would reward themselves generously for minimal achievements. The data furthermore revealed that subjects imposed on other children the same self-reward contingencies they had adopted toward their own behavior. These findings, which are in accord with those reported by Marston (1964), demonstrate how specific patterns of self-reinforcing behavior can be transmitted by specific models.

The overall laboratory results are also consistent with field studies demonstrating that, in cultures where austerity is the dominant social norm, not only are positive self-reinforcements sparingly administered, but because of the emphasis on personal responsibility for high standards of conduct, self-denying, self-punitive, and depressive reactions occur with high frequency (Eaton and Weil, 1955).

Multidimensional Analyses of Deviant Behavior

In the preceding sections, several distinct classes of psychological dysfunctions and their corresponding social learning antecedents were discussed at length. While the main purpose was to outline a taxonomic schema that would encompass the range of phenomena ordinarily subsumed under the term "psychopathology," it is important to bear in mind that social learning conditions typically combine in a variety of ways to produce different constellations of deviant behavior in different individuals. Thus, a given person's learning history may have produced deficient behavioral repertoires, avoidant response patterns under inappropriate stimulus control, and a powerful aversive self-reinforcement system. On the other hand, another person may exhibit a quite different cluster of deviant behavior as a function of a different set of social learning experiences. For this reason, a multidimensional characterization of behavior disorders will have greater predictive and therapeutic utility than a typological approach.

In a dimensional system, each person is assessed in terms of a series of variables that appear to be important for the establishment and maintenance of social response patterns. The material reported in previous sections of this chapter outlines a set of such variables that are considered functionally important from a social learning viewpoint. Given a set of objective assessment procedures based on each of the constituent factors, one can accurately delineate many patterns of deviant behavior that result from diverse, and often unique, configurations of learning experiences.

This type of multidimensional approach has several distinct advantages. First, it successfully differentiates between individuals who are assigned to a single diagnostic category according to a typological system. Second, it avoids the contradiction into which a typology leads when the majority of cases *do not* fall into clearly defined categories. Since the type of behavioral analysis presented in this chapter focuses on covariations between antecedent stimulus events and behavioral variables that are relevant to the study of social development, its findings can be readily integrated into general psychological theory (Bandura and Walters, 1959). Moreover, in contrast to many psychodynamic formulations, social learning theory does not assume that all disorders are manifestations of a single constellation of developmental experiences (for example, Oedipal complexes, power strivings, inadequate self-concepts, existential anxieties). It does, however, account for the diversity of deviant behavior in terms of an integrated set of social learning principles rather than on the basis of principles eclectically borrowed from widely divergent notions of human behavior. Finally, unlike most existing typologies, which have few specific implications for psychotherapy, the particular deviations comprising the social learning taxonomy require differential procedures for their successful modification (Bandura, 1967).

SUMMARY

In this chapter we have outlined a social learning taxonomy of behavioral phenomena generally subsumed under the term "psychopathology" and discussed the basic principles governing the acquisition and maintenance of response patterns that are labeled deviant either by the individual himself or by society. This theoretical conceptualization differs in several important respects from traditional psychodynamic formulations of deviant behavior.

Psychodynamic theories characteristically lead one to seek determinants of human behavior in terms of hypothetical internal agents, which tend to be regarded as relatively autonomous and, consequently, the first link in causal sequences. The latter formulations employ essentially an amalgam of the medical and demonological models, which have in common the belief that deviant behavior represents external symptomatic manifestations of an underlying pathology.

In contrast, social learning approaches treat mediating events as intervening links, which are lawfully related to manipulable stimulus variables and to response sequences. Moreover, deviant behavior is viewed not as a manifestation of emotional "disease," but as a learned response pattern that often can be directly modified by manipulating the stimulus variables of which both the mediating and terminal behavior are a function. Once the maladaptive behavior is altered, it is unnecessary to modify or to remove any underlying pathology. Indeed, considering the arbitrary and relativistic nature of the social judgment and definition of deviance, the main value of the normal-abnormal dichotomy is in guiding the sociolegal actions of societal agents concerned with the maintenance of an efficiently functioning society. This dichotomy, however, has little theoretical significance since there is no evidence that the behaviors so dichotomized are either qualitatively different or under the control of fundamentally different variables.

In view of the fact that many of the conditions maintaining deviant behavior reside in the environmental contingencies to which the individual is exposed, any taxonomy derived from social learning theory necessarily highlights the reciprocal relationship between stimulus events and behavioral variables. On the basis of the taxonomic schema presented in the present chapter, the specific diverse forms of deviant behavior are reduced to six relatively distinct patterns reflecting (1) deficient repertoires, (2) defective stimulus control of behavior, (3) inappropriate stimulus control of behavior, (4) defective or inappropriate incentive systems, (5) aversive repertoires, and (6) aversive self-reinforcing systems. Since social learning conditions generally combine in diverse and often unique ways to produce multiform configurations of deviant behavior, a multidimensional approach, in which a given person is assessed in terms of each of the above variables, is likely to have greatest value for the prediction and modification of response patterns that are judged to be deviant.

GLOSSARY

ADLERIAN THERAPY—a method of therapy prescribed by Alfred Adler that concentrates on a person's feelings of inferiority.

AGGRESSION—hostile, destructive behavior.

ANTHROPOLOGICAL FIELD STUDIES—social-psychological studies of different cultures as they naturally exist.

AROUSAL—the emotional and cognitive state of excitation and readiness (see Chapter 3).

AUTONOMIC—pertaining to the autonomic nervous system.

CASTRATION COMPLEX, CASTRATION ANXIETY—in the male, the repressed or unacknowledged fear of losing one's genitals; in the female, the fantasy of once having had a penis, but of having lost it.[1]

[1] This definition is taken from H. B. English and Ava C. English, *A Comprehensive Dictionary of Psychological and Psychoanalytical Terms.* New York: David McKay Company, Inc., 1958.

CHARACTER DISORDER—a chronic condition, often considered psychopathological, whose only symptoms tend to be socially unacceptable conduct (see Chapter 11).

CLIENT-CENTERED THERAPY (ROGERIAN)—a form of psychotherapy that is especially nondirective and "nonjudgmental" (see Chapter 15).

COMPULSION—an irrational, repetitive act.

CONDITIONED RESPONSE—a reponse which is not ordinarily elicited by an unconditioned stimulus, but which, because of learning, can now be evoked.

CONDITIONED STIMULUS—an originally irrelevant stimulus that, having been paired with an unconditioned stimulus, becomes capable of evoking the same response as the unconditioned stimulus.

CONDITIONING—the learning of a particular response to specific stimuli which either elicit or reward it.

CONTROL SUBJECTS, CONTROL GROUP—persons who are not exposed to the crucial experimental manipulation but are exposed to as many as possible of the other conditions in an experiment, in order to insure that the obtained effects are not the result of unnoticed considerations.

CORRELATE—either of two things that are related to, or vary with, each other.

COUNTERCONDITIONING—the procedure of conditioning a second response which conflicts with an already conditioned stimulus.

COUNTERINSTINCTUAL ENERGIES—psychic energies used to combat and suppress instinctual urges.

COVARIANCE—the tendency of two variables to change together.

CUE—an event that acts as a signal for some type of behavior.

DELUSION—a belief held in the face of evidence normally sufficient to destroy the belief (see Chapter 11).

DEPENDENCY—extensive reliance upon others for satisfaction of physical and psychological needs (see Chapters 3 and 4).

DISCRIMINATION—the process of detecting or responding to differences in objects or events.

DISINHIBITION—the release of previously suppressed behavior.

DRIVE STATE—a hypothetical state of activity of an organism, or of some of its organs and tissues, that is a necessary condition before a given stimulus will elicit a given class of behaviors.[1]

ELECTROENCEPHALOGRAM ALPHA RHYTHM—the wave form of the EEG (electroencephalogram) from the adult cortex; the EEG records patterns of electrical waves generated in the cortex.

EGO-ALIEN IMPULSES—in psychoanalytic theory, impulses that are "distasteful" to, and rejected by, the self.

ELECTROSHOCK THERAPY—a treatment technique consisting of the application of an electric current to the front part of the patient's head (see Chapter 15).

ENURESIS—bed-wetting.

EXTINCTION—progressive reduction of a conditioned response by withholding of the rewards or reinforcements which usually follow the response.

FRUSTRATION—anything that interferes with goal-directed behavior (see Chapter 3).

GALVANIC SKIN RESPONSE—electrical reactions of the skin, detected by a galvanometer.

GENERALIZATION—the transfer of conditioned responses to stimuli that are similar to those involved in the original conditioning.

GENERALIZATION GRADIENT—the rate of change in the ability of a response to be generalized.

GUILT—the subjective feelings that result from doing something that is forbidden, or from the failure to perform some obligatory act; some writers, particularly psychoanalysts, feel that the *impulse* to deviate from an internalized standard may also give rise to guilt (see Chapters 4, 10, 11, and 15).

HALLUCINATION—a false sensory perception which has a compelling sense of reality.

INFERIORITY COMPLEX—repressed fear and resentment of being inferior, leading to a variety of negative behaviors.

INHIBIT—suppress.

INSTRUMENTAL BEHAVIOR—behavior that effects an alteration in the environment.

INTERMITTENT REINFORCEMENT SCHEDULE—a technique for conditioning a response in which nonrewarding stimuli and rewarding stimuli are irregularly dispensed during the conditioning period; this results in slower conditioning, but also in a slower extinction rate.

LEARNING CONTINGENCIES—variables (like behaviors and rewards) of the learning situation.

MODELING—the process of demonstrating behaviors that are capable of eliciting imitation (see Chapter 8).

MORES—customs.

MOTORIC BEHAVIOR—observable physical movements.

MULTIDIMENSIONAL ANALYSIS (of deviant behavior)—a system whereby a person is assessed in terms of a number of variables that appear to be important for the establishment and maintenance of social response patterns.

NEUROSIS—a negative abnormality, ill-defined in character, but milder than psychosis (see Chapter 10).

NORMS—rules, standards.

OBSESSIVE-COMPULSIVE BEHAVIOR—behavior characterized by intense, irrational, and involuntary repetition of thoughts (obsessions) or actions (compulsions) (see Chapter 10).

OEDIPAL COMPLEX—in Freudian theory, the repressed desire to possess sexually the parent of the opposite sex; Freud believed that it was universal (see Chapter 10).

OVERGENERALIZATION—a nondiscriminative response to *any* stimulus which may occur after that response has been successfully paired with some particular stimulus.

PHOBIC—having excessive or exaggerated fear of some (objectively) relatively harmless object.

PLACE AVOIDANCE—Mowrer's term (1960) for responses designed to avoid or escape an external noxious stimulus; to be distinguished from response inhibition.

PROPRIOCEPTIVE CUES—cues that are sensitive to body position or movement.

PROSOCIAL BEHAVIOR—behavior that is in accordance with society's norms.

PSYCHIC—mental.

PSYCHODYNAMIC—relating to the theories of human behavior, often derived from the work of Freud, that stress motives and drives as determinants of behavior.

PSYCHOGALVANIC—pertaining to electrical responses of the skin to psychological stimuli.

PSYCHOPATHOLOGY—negative psychological abnormalities.

PSYCHOSIS—an ill-defined term, generally meaning any severe negative psychological abnormality (see Chapter 11).

PSYCHOSOMATIC—pertaining to physical symptoms resulting from psychological stress or conflict (see Chapter 13).

PUBESCENCE—the early stage of puberty.

REFERENCE GROUP—the group to whose standards an individual refers in judging his own behavior.

REFLEX—a very simple act in which there is no element of choice or premeditation and no variability save in intensity or time.[1]

REGRESSION—a return to immature modes of behavior, often caused by stress or frustration (see Chapter 10).

REINFORCEMENT—that which strengthens a response.

RELIABLE—consistent, dependable.

RESPONSE HIERARCHY—the ordering of a class of behaviors according to the probability that they will be elicited in a certain situation.

RESPONSE INHIBITION—as used in this chapter, Mowrer's term (1960) for suppression of a response on the basis of internal cues even though the stimuli that would normally elicit it are present; to be distinguished from place avoidance.

RESPONSE-REINFORCEMENT CONTINGENCY—a variable relationship between a response and reinforcement of it.

RITUAL—a well-established pattern of religious or social activity.

SCHEDULE OF REINFORCEMENT—a schedule prescribing when the subject is to be reinforced or rewarded, either in terms of time (that is, how long between reinforcements) or of the order of responses (that is, which of a series of correct responses will be reinforced).

SCHIZOPHRENIA—a group of psychotic reactions characterized by fundamental disturbances in reality relationship and by marked affectual, intellectual, and behavioral disturbances[1] (see Chapter 11).

SENSORIMOTOR—of any act whose nature is primarily dependent on the combined or integrated functioning of sense organs and motor mechanisms.[1]

SKELETAL RESPONSE SYSTEM—specifically, the sensory, neural, muscular, and glandular structures that are coordinated to produce responses in the skeleton of an organism; generally, the motor response system.

SOMATIC—referring to bodily reactions and responses.

SOMATIZATION—the conversion of anxiety into physical symptoms.

SUBJECT VARIABLES—characteristics of an individual.

SYMPATHETIC NERVOUS SYSTEM—the part of the autonomic nervous system that helps regulate the functions of the heart, lungs, blood vessels, and various internal organs.

SYMPATHETIC STIMULANT—a stimulant that

acts on the sympathetic nervous system; for example, adrenaline.

TRANSVESTITE—one who dresses as a member of the opposite sex.

TRAUMATIC—pertaining to any experience that inflicts serious psychological or physical damage upon the organism.

UNCONDITIONED RESPONSE—a response that "naturally" (that is, with minimal learning) follows a stimulus; for Pavlov's dogs, salivation was an unconditioned response to meat powder.

UNCONDITIONED STIMULUS—a stimulus that "naturally" (that is, either innately or with little training) evokes a particular response; for Pavlov's dogs meat powder was an unconditioned stimulus to salivation.

VALENCE—the degree of attractiveness or repulsion an individual, activity, or object possesses.

VASOMOTOR—pertaining to the expansion and contraction of blood vessels.

VOYEURISM—the practice of secretly observing others and thereby obtaining sexual gratification; peeping.

REFERENCES

Ackerman, N. W. Psychotherapy and giving love. *Psychiatry*, 1944, **7**, 129–137.

Aichhorn, A. *Wayward youth.* New York: The Viking Press, Inc., 1935.

Ash, P. The reliability of psychiatric diagnosis. *Journal of Abnormal and Social Psychology*, 1949, **44**, 272–276.

Ayllon, T. Some behavioral problems associated with eating in chronic schizophrenic patients. Paper read at the American Psychological Association, Chicago, September, 1960.

——— and E. Haughton. Control of the behavior of schizophrenic patients by food. *Journal of the Experimental Analysis of Behavior*, 1962, **5**, 343–352.

——— and Michael, J. The psychiatric nurse as a behavioral engineer. *Journal of the Experimental Analysis of Behavior*, 1959, **2**, 323–334.

Bales, R. F. Cultural differences in rates of alcoholism. *Quarterly Journal of Studies on Alcohol*, 1946, **6**, 480–499.

Bandura, A. Relationship of family patterns to child behavior disorders. Progress Report, Stanford University, Project No. M–1734, United States Public Health Service, 1960.

———. Social learning through imitation. In M. R. Jones (ed.), *Nebraska symposium on motivation: 1962.* Lincoln, Neb.: University of Nebraska Press, 1962*a*, pp. 211–269.

———. Punishment revisited. *Journal of Consulting Psychology*, 1962*b*, **26**, 298–301.

———. Behavioral modification through modeling procedures. In L. Krasner and L. P. Ullmann (eds.), *Research in behavior modification.* New York: Holt, Rinehart & Winston, 1965*a*.

———. Influence of models' reinforcement contingencies on the acquisition of imitative responses. *Journal of Personality and Social Psychology*, 1965*b*, **1**, 589–595.

———. *Principles of behavioral modification.* Unpublished manuscript, Stanford University, 1967.

——— and Carol J. Kupers. Transmission of patterns of self-reinforcement through modeling. *Journal of Abnormal and Social Psychology*, 1964, **69**, 1–9.

——— and T. L. Rosenthal. Vicarious classical conditioning as a function of emotional arousal. *Journal of Personality and Social Psychology*, 1966, **3**, 54–62.

———, Dorothea Ross, and Sheila A. Ross. Transmission of aggression through imitation of aggressive models. *Journal of Abnormal and Social Psychology*, 1961, **63**, 575–582.

———, ———, and ———. Imitation of film-mediated aggressive models. *Journal of Abnormal and Social Psychology*, 1963*a*, **66**, 3–11.

———, ———, and ———. Vicarious reinforcement and imitative learning. *Journal of Abnormal and Social Psychology*, 1963*b*, **67**, 601–607.

——— and R. H. Walters. Adolescent aggression. New York: The Ronald Press Company, 1959.

——— and ———. *Social learning and personality development.* New York: Holt, Rinehart & Winston, 1963.

——— and Carol K. Whalen. The influence of prior reinforcement and divergent modeling cues on patterns of self-reward. *Journal of Personality and Social Psychology*, 1966, **3**, 373–382.

Bateson, G. *The Naven.* Stanford, Calif.: Stanford University Press, 1936.

———. (ed.). *Perceval's narrative: A pa-*

tient's account of his psychosis. Stanford, Calif.: Stanford University Press, 1961.
Berger, S. M. Conditioning through vicarious instigation. *Psychological Review*, 1962, **69**, 450–466.
Berkowitz, L., and Edna Rawlings. Effects of film violence on inhibitions against subsequent aggression. *Journal of Abnormal and Social Psychology*, 1963, **66**, 405–412.
Black, A. H. Heart rate changes during avoidance learning in dogs. *Canadian Journal of Psychology*, 1959, **13**, 229–242.
Blake, R. R. The other person in the situation. In R. Tagiuri and L. Petrullo (eds.), *Person perception and interpersonal behavior*. Stanford, Calif.: Stanford University Press, 1958, pp. 229–242.
Block, Jeanne, and B. Martin. Predicting the behavior of children under frustration. *Journal of Abnormal and Social Psychology*, 1955, **51**, 281–285.
Bond, I. K., and H. C. Hutchison. Application of reciprocal inhibition therapy to exhibitionism. *Canadian Medical Association Journal*, 1960, **83**, 23–25.
Bruun, K. Significance of role and norms in the small group for individual behavioural changes while drinking. *Quarterly Journal of Studies on Alcohol*, 1959, **20**, 53–64.
Bykov, K. M. *The cerebral cortex and the internal organs* (translated and edited by W. H. Gantt). New York: Chemical Publishing Co., Inc., 1957.
Cairns, R. B. The influence of dependency inhibition on the effectiveness of social reinforcers. *Journal of Personality*, 1961, **29**, 466–488.
Cairns, R. B., and M. Lewis. Dependency and the reinforcement value of a verbal stimulus. *Journal of Consulting, Psychology*, 1962, **26**, 1–8.
Carpenter, J. A. Effects of alcoholic beverages on skin conductance: an exploratory study. *Quarterly Journal of Studies on Alcohol*, 1957, **18**, 1–18.
Casey, A. The effect of stress on the consumption of alcohol and reserpine. *Quarterly Journal of Studies on Alcohol*, 1960, **21**, 208–216.
Chafetz, M. E., and H. W. Demone. *Alcoholism and society*. New York: Oxford University Press, Inc., 1962.
Clark, R., and E. Polish. Avoidance conditioning and alcohol consumption in rhesus monkeys. *Science*, 1960, **132**, 223.
Clark, R. A., and Minda R. Sensibar. The relationship between symbolic and manifest projections of sexuality with some incidental correlates. *Journal of Abnormal and Social Psychology*, 1955, **50**, 327–334.
Cohen, A. K. *Delinquent boys: The culture of the gang*. New York: The Free Press of Glencoe, 1955.
Conn, J. H. Hypno-synthesis v. hypnotherapy of the sex offender. *International Journal of Clinical and Experimental Hypnosis*, 1954, **2**, 13–26.
Cooper, A. J. A case of fetishism and impotence treated by behaviour therapy. *British Journal of Psychiatry*, 1963, **109**, 649–652.
Cowan, P. A., and R. H. Walters. Studies of reinforcement of aggression: I. Effects of scheduling. *Child Development*, 1963, **34**, 543–551.
Das, J. P., and P. C. Nanda. Mediated transfer of attitudes. *Journal of Abnormal and Social Psychology*, 1963, **66**, 12–16.
Davitz, J. R. The effects of previous training on postfrustration behavior. *Journal of Abnormal and Social Psychology*, 1952, **47**, 309–315.
Dekker, E., and J. Groen. Reproducible psychogenic attacks of asthma: A laboratory study. *Journal of Psychosomatic Research*, 1956, **1**, 58–67.
———, H. E. Pelser, and J. Groen. Conditioning as a cause of asthmatic attacks. *Journal of Psychosomatic Research*, 1957, **2**, 97–108.
Diven, K. Certain determinants in the conditioning of anxiety. *Journal of Psychology*, 1937, **3**, 291–308.
Doctor, R. F., and R. B. Perkins. The effects of ethyl alcohol on autonomic and muscular responses in humans. I. Dosage of 0.5 milliliter per kilogram. *Quarterly Journal of Studies on Alcohol*, 1961, **22**, 374–386.
Dollard, J., L. W. Doob, N. E. Miller, O. H. Mowrer, and R. R. Sears. *Frustration and aggression*. New Haven, Conn.: Yale University Press, 1939.
Dunn, W. L., Jr. Visual discrimination of schizophrenic subjects as a function of stimulus meaning. *Journal of Personality*, 1954, **23**, 48–64.
Eaton, J. W., and R. J. Weil. *Culture and mental disorders*. New York: The Free Press of Glencoe, 1955.
Eisenberg, L. The fathers of autistic chil-

dren. *American Journal of Orthopsychiatry*, 1957, **27**, 715–724.

Eysenck, H. J. *Behaviour therapy and the neuroses*. New York: Pergamon Press, Inc., 1960.

Ferster, C. B. Positive reinforcement and behavioral deficits of autistic children. *Child Development*, 1961, **32**, 437–456.

———. Essentials of a science of behavior. In J. I. Nurnberger, C. B. Ferster, and J. P. Brady (eds.), *An introduction to the science of human behavior*. New York: Appleton-Century-Crofts, 1963, pp. 197–345.

Ferster, C. B., and M. K. De Myer. The development of performances in autistic children in an automatically controlled environment. *Journal of Chronic Diseases*, 1961, **13**, 312–345.

——— and B. F. Skinner. *Schedules of reinforcement*. New York: Appleton-Century-Crofts, 1957.

Festinger, L. *A theory of cognitive dissonance*. Stanford, Calif.: Stanford University Press, 1962.

———, H. W. Riecken, and S. Schacter. *When prophecy fails*. Minneapolis: University of Minnesota Press, 1956.

Fleck, S. Family dynamics and origin of schizophrenia. *Psychosomatic Medicine*, 1960, **22**, 333–344.

Ford, C. S., and F. A. Beach. *Patterns of sexual behavior*. New York: Harper & Row Publishers, 1951.

Fort, Twila, and A. L. Porterfield. Some backgrounds and types of alcoholics among women. *Journal of Health and Human Behavior*, 1961, **2**, 283–292.

Freud, Anna, and Dorothy T. Burlingham. *Infants without families*. New York. International Universities Press, 1944.

Freud, S. *A general introduction to psychoanalysis*. New York: Liveright Publishing Corp., 1920.

———. *Beyond the pleasure principle*. New York: Liveright Publishing Corp., 1922.

———. Mourning and melancholia. In E. Jones (ed.), *Collected papers*, Vol. IV. London: Hogarth Press, Ltd., 1925, pp. 152–170.

Garmezy, N. Stimulus differentiation by schizophrenic and normal subjects under conditions of reward and punishment. *Journal of Personality*, 1952, **21**, 253–276.

Gavzer, B. Defiance of young negroes shows rejection of authority. *Palo Alto Times*, July 27, 1964, p. 5.

Gewirtz, J. L. A learning analysis of the effects of normal stimulation, privation, and deprivation on the acquisition of social motivation and attachment. In B. M. Foss (ed.), *Determinants of infant behavior*. New York: John Wiley & Sons, Inc., 1961, pp. 213–283.

Giffen, Mary E., Adelaide M. Johnson, and E. M. Litin. Antisocial acting out: 2. Specific factors determining antisocial acting out. *American Journal of Orthopsychiatry*, 1954, **24**, 668–684.

Glad, D. D. Attitudes and experiences of American-Jewish and American-Irish male youth as related to differences in adult rates of inebriety. *Quarterly Journal of Studies on Alcohol*, 1947, **8**, 406–472.

Goldfarb, W. Infant rearing and problem behavior. *American Journal of Orthopsychiatry*, 1943, **13**, 249–265.

———. *Childhood schizophrenia*. Cambridge, Mass.: Harvard University Press, 1961.

Grant, D. A., and J. J. Schiller. Generalization of the conditioned galvanic skin response to visual stimuli. *Journal of Experimental Psychology*, 1953, **46**, 309–313.

Greenberg, L. A., and J. A. Carpenter. The effect of alcoholic beverages on skin conductance and emotional tension. I. Wine, whiskey and alcohol. *Quarterly Journal of Studies on Alcohol*, 1957, **18**, 190–204.

Grossberg, J. M. Behavior therapy: A review. *Psychological Bulletin*, 1964, **62**, 73–88.

Haire, M., and W. F. Grunes. Perceptual defenses: Processes protecting an organized perception of another personality. *Human Relations*, 1950, **3**, 403–412.

Harris, Florence R., M. K. Johnson, C. S. Kelley, and M. M. Wolf. Effects of positive social reinforcement on regressed crawling of a nursery school child. *Journal of Educational Psychology*, 1964, **55**, 35.

Hart, Betty H., K. Eileen Allen, Joan S. Buell, Florence R. Harris, and M. M. Wolf. Effects of social reinforcement on operant crying. *Journal of Experimental Child Psychology*, 1964, **1**, 145–153.

Hartmann, D. The influence of symbolically modeled instrumental aggression and pain cues on the disinhibition of aggressive behavior. Unpublished doctoral dissertation, Stanford University, 1964.

Heine, R. W. A comparison of patients' reports on psychotherapeutic experience with psychoanalytic, nondirective and Adlerian therapists. *American Journal of Psychotherapy*, 1953, **7**, 16–23.

Hicks, D. J. Imitation and retention of film-mediated aggressive peer and adult models. *Journal of Personality and Social Psychology*, 1965, **2**, 97–100.

Hogans, A. F., O. M. Moreno, and D. A. Brodie. Effects of ethyl alcohol on EEG and avoidance behavior of chronic electrode monkeys. *American Journal of Physiology*, 1961, **201**, 434–436.

Holmberg, A. R. The Siriono. Unpublished doctoral dissertation, Yale University Press, 1946.

Hovland, C. I. The generalization of conditioned responses. I. The sensory generalization of conditioned responses with varying frequencies of tone. *Journal of General Psychology*, 1937, **17**, 125–148.

Hunt, W. A., C. L. Wittson, and Edna B. Hunt. A theoretical and practical analysis of the diagnostic process. In P. H. Hoch and J. Zubin (eds.), *Current problems in psychiatric diagnosis*. New York: Grune & Stratton, Inc., 1953, pp. 53–65.

Isbell, H., H. F. Fraser, A. Wikler, R. E. Belleville, and Anna J. Eisenman. An experimental study of the etiology of "rum fits" and delirium tremens. *Quarterly Journal of Studies on Alcohol*, 1955, **16**, 1–33.

Johnson, Adelaide M. Factors in the etiology of fixations and symptom choice. *Psychoanalytic Quarterly*, 1953, **22**, 475–496.

Kanfer, F. H., Marcia M. Bradley, and A. R. Marston. Self-reinforcement as a function of degree of learning. *Psychological Reports*, 1962, **10**, 885–886.

——— and A. R. Marston. The conditioning of self-reinforcing responses: An analogue to self-confidence training. *Psychological Reports*, 1963*a*, **13**, 63–70.

——— and ———. Determinants of self-reinforcement in human learning. *Journal of Experimental Psychology*, 1963*b*, **66**, 245–254.

Kaplan, Helen S. The effects of alcohol on fear extinction. *Dissertation Abstracts*, 1956, **16**, 571–572.

Kelley, H. H. The warm-cold variable in first impressions of persons. *Journal of Personality*, 1950, **18**, 431–439.

Kimble, G. A. *Hilgard and Marquis' conditioning and learning*. New York: Appleton-Century-Crofts, 1961.

Kolb, L. C., and Adelaide M. Johnson. Etiology of overt homosexuality and the need for therapeutic modification. *Psychoanalytic Quarterly*, 1955, **24**, 506–515.

Korman, M., and H. D. Stephens. Effects of training on the alcohol consummatory response in rats. *Psychological Reports*, 1960, **6**, 327–331.

Korpmann, E., and F. W. Hughes. Potentiating effect of alcohol on tranquilizers and other central depressants. *A. M. A. Archives of General Psychiatry*, 1959, **1**, 7–11.

Lacey, J. I., and R. L. Smith. Conditioning and generalization of unconscious anxiety. *Science*, 1954, **120**, 1045–1052.

Lemere, F., W. L. Voegtlin, W. R. Broz, P. O'Hollaren, and W. E. Tupper. The conditioned reflex treatment of chronic alcoholism: VIII. A review of six years' experience with this treatment of 1526 patients. *Journal of the American Medical Association*, 1952, **120**, 269–270.

Levy, D. M. *Maternal overprotection*. New York: Columbia University Press, 1943.

Lidz, T., Alice R. Cornelison, S. Fleck, and Dorothy Terry. The intrafamilial environment of the schizophrenic patient: II. Marital schism and marital skew. *American Journal of Psychiatry*, 1957*a*, **114**, 241–248.

———, ———, ———, and ———. The intrafamilial environment of the schizophrenic patient: I. The father. *Psychiatry*, 1957*b*, **20**, 329–342.

———, ———, ———, and ———. Intrafamilial environment of the schizophrenic patient: VI. The transmission of irrationality. *A. M. A. Archives of Neurology and Psychiatry*, 1958, **79**, 305–316.

Lindsley, O. R. Characteristics of the behavior of chronic psychotics as revealed by free-operant conditioning methods. *Diseases of the Nervous System*, 1960, **21**, 66–78.

Litin, E. M., Mary E. Giffin, and Adelaide M. Johnson. Parental influences in unusual sexual behavior in children. *Psychoanalytic Quarterly*, 1956, **25**, 37–55.

Littman, R. A. Conditioned generalization of the galvanic skin reaction to tones. *Journal of Experimental Psychology*, 1949, **39**, 868–882.

Lovaas, O. I. Interaction between verbal and nonverbal behavior. *Child Development*, 1961, **32**, 329–336.

———, G. Freitag, M. I. Kinder, B. D.

Rubinstein, B. Schaeffer, and J. P. Simmons. Experimental studies in childhood schizophrenia: II. Establishment of social reinforcers. Unpublished manuscript, University of California at Los Angeles, 1964.

McCarthy, R. (ed.). *Drinking and intoxication.* New York: The Free Press of Glencoe, 1959.

McCord, W., and Joan McCord. The effects of parental role models on criminality. *Journal of Social Issues,* 1958, **14,** 66–74.

McDavid, J., and H. M. Schroder. The interpretation of approval and disapproval of delinquent and non-delinquent adolescents. *Journal of Personality,* 1957, **25,** 539–549.

McDonnell, G. J., and J. A. Carpenter. Anxiety, skin conductance and alcohol. A study of the relation between anxiety and skin conductance and the effects of alcohol on the conductance of subjects in groups. *Quarterly Journal of Studies on Alcohol,* 1959, **20,** 38–52.

Malinowski, B. *The sexual life of savages in north-western Melanesia.* New York: Harcourt, Brace & World, Inc., 1929.

Marston, A. R. Variables affecting incidence of self-reinforcement. *Psychological Reports,* 1964, **14,** 879–884.

Masserman, J. H., and K. S. Yum. An analysis of the influence of alcohol on experimental neurosis in cats. *Psychosomatic Medicine,* 1946, **8,** 36–52.

Metzner, R. Learning theory and the therapy of neurosis. *British Journal of Psychology,* 1961, Mongraph Suppl. No. 33.

Meyerson, L., J. L. Michael, O. H. Mowrer, C. E. Osgood, and A. W. Staats. Learning, behavior and rehabilitation. In L. Loftquist (ed.), *Psychological research in rehabilitation.* Washington, D.C.: American Psychological Association, 1962, pp. 68–111.

Miller, N. E. The frustration-aggression hypothesis. *Psychological Review,* 1941, **48,** 337–342.

———. Studies of fear as an acquirable drive: 1. Fear as motivation and fear-reduction as reinforcement in the learning of new responses. *Journal of Experimental Psychology,* 1948, **38,** 89–101.

Mischel, W., and R. M. Liebert. Effects of discrepancies between observed and imposed reward criteria on their acquisition and transmission. *Journal of Personality and Social Psychology,* 1966, **3,** 45–53.

Mowrer, O. H. *Learning theory and personality dynamics.* New York: The Ronald Press Company, 1950.

———. *Learning theory and behavior.* New York: John Wiley & Sons, Inc., 1960.

Noble, C. E. Conditioned generalization of the galvanic skin response to a subvocal stimulus. *Journal of Experimental Psychology,* 1950, **40,** 15–25.

Noelpp, B., and I. Noelpp-Eschenhagen. Das experimentelle asthma bronchiale des meerschweinschens: II. Mitterlung die rolle bedingter reflexes in des pathogenese des asthma bronchiale. *International Archives of Allergy,* 1951, **2,** 321–329.

——— and ———. Das experimentelle asthma bronchiale des meerschweinschens: III. Studen zur bedentung bedingter reflexe, bahnungsbereitschaft und haftfahigkut unter stress. *International Archives of Allergy,* 1952, **3,** 108–135.

Oswald, I. Induction of illusory and hallucinatory voices with consideration of behaviour therapy. *Journal of Mental Science,* 1962, **108,** 196–212.

Otis, Nancy B., and B. McCandless. Responses to repeated frustrations of young children differentiated according to need area. *Journal of Abnormal and Social Psychology,* 1955, **50,** 349–353.

Ottenberg, P., M. Stein, J. Lewis, and C. Hamilton. Learned asthma in the guinea pig. *Psychosomatic Medicine,* 1958, **10,** 395–400.

Patterson, G. R., M. Ludwig, and Beverly Sonoda. Reinforcement of aggression in children. Unpublished manuscript, University of Oregon, Eugene, Ore., 1961.

Pavlov, I. P. *Conditioned reflexes* (translated by G. V. Anrep). New York: Oxford University Press, Inc., 1927.

Pawlowski, A. A., V. H. Denenberg, and M. X. Zarrow. Prolonged alcohol consumption in the rat. 2. Acquisition and extinction of an escape response. *Quarterly Journal of Studies in Alcohol,* 1961, **22,** 232–240.

Pittman, D. J., and C. R. Snyder (eds.), *Society, culture, and drinking patterns.* New York: John Wiley & Sons, Inc., 1962.

Rausch, H. L. Interaction sequences. *Journal of Abnormal and Social Psychology,* 1964.

Razran, G. Stimulus generalization of conditioned responses. *Psychological Bulletin,* 1949, **46,** 337–365.

———. The observable unconscious and the inferable conscious in current soviet psychophysiology. *Psychological Review,* 1961, **68,** 81–147.

Richter, C. P. Production and control of alcoholic craving in rats. In *Neuropharmacology: Transactions of the third conference.* New York: Josiah Macy, Jr. Foundation, 1956, pp. 39–146.

Rodnick, E. H., and N. Garmezy. An experimental approach to the study of motivation in schizophrenia. In M. R. Jones (ed.), *Nebraska symposium on motivation: 1957.* Lincoln, Neb.: University of Nebraska Press, 1957, pp. 109–184.

Rokeach, M. *The three Christs of Ypsilanti.* New York: Alfred A. Knopf, Inc., 1964.

Rosenbaum, G. Stimulus generalization as a function of level of experimentally induced anxiety. *Journal of Experimental Psychology,* 1953, **45,** 35–43.

———. Stimulus generalization as a function of clinical anxiety. *Journal of Abnormal and Social Psychology,* 1956, **53,** 281–285.

Schmidt, H. O., and C. P. Fonda. The reliability of psychiatric diagnosis: A new look. *Journal of Abnormal and Social Psychology,* 1956, **52,** 262–267.

Sidman, M. Technique for assessing the effects of drugs on timing behavior. *Science,* 1955, **122,** 925.

Skinner, B. F. "Superstition" in the pigeon. *Journal of Experimental Psychology,* 1948, **38,** 168–172.

Skolnik, J. H. The stumbling block. A sociological study of the relationship between selected religious norms and drinking behaviour. Unpublished doctoral dissertation, Yale University, New Haven, Conn., 1957.

Snyder, C. R. *Alcohol and the Jews: A cultural study of drinking and sobriety.* New York: The Free Press of Glencoe, 1958.

Staats, Carolyn K., and A. W. Staats. Meaning established by classical conditioning. *Journal of Experimental Psychology,* 1957, **54,** 74–80.

——— and ———. Attitudes established by classical conditioning. *Journal of Abnormal and Social Psychology,* 1958, **57,** 37–40.

——— and ———. *Complex human behavior.* New York: Holt, Rinehart and Winston, 1963.

Terwilliger, J. S., and F. E. Fiedler. An investigation of determinants inducing individuals to seek personal counseling. *Journal of Consulting Psychology,* 1958, **22,** 288.

Thorpe, J. J., and B. Smith. Operational sequence in group therapy with young offenders. *International Journal of Group Psychotherapy,* 1952, **2,** 24–33.

Wall, J. A study of alcoholism in men. *American Journal of Psychiatry,* 1936, **92,** 1389–1401.

Walters, R. H., and M. Brown. Studies of reinforcement of aggression: III. Transfer of responses to an interpersonal situation. *Child Development,* 1963, **34,** 563–571.

———, Marion Leat and L. Mezei. Inhibition and disinhibition of responses through empathetic learning. *Canadian Journal of Psychology,* 1963, **17,** 235–243.

——— and E. Llewellyn Thomas. Enhancement of punitive behavior by visual and audiovisual displays. *Canadian Journal of Psychology,* 1963, **17,** 244–255.

Walton, D. The application of learning theory to the treatment of a case of bronchial asthma. In H. J. Eysenck (ed), *Behaviour therapy and the neuroses.* New York: Pergamon Press, Inc., 1960, pp. 188–189.

——— and M. D. Mather. The application of learning principles to the treatment of obsessive-compulsive states in the acute and chronic phases of illness. *Behavior Research and Therapy,* 1963, **1,** 163–174.

Watson, J. B., and Rosalie Rayner. Conditioned emotional reactions. *Journal of Experimental Psychology,* 1920, **3,** 1–14.

Whiting, J. W. M., and I. L. Child. *Child training and personality.* New Haven, Conn.: Yale University Press, 1953.

Whyte, W. F. *Street-corner society.* Chicago: University of Chicago Press, 1937.

Wolf, M., T. Risley, and H. Mees. Application of operant conditioning procedures to the behaviour problems of an autistic child. *Behavior Research and Therapy,* 1964, **1,** 305–312.

Wolpe, J. *Psychotherapy by reciprocal inhibition.* Stanford, Calif.: Stanford University Press, 1958.

Wynne, L. C., and R. L. Solomon. Traumatic avoidance learning: Acquisition and extinction in dogs deprived of normal peripheral autonomic function. *Genetic*

Psychology Monographs, 1955, **52,** 241–284.

Yablonsky, L. *The violent gang.* New York: Crowell-Collier and Macmillan, Inc., 1962.

Yarrow, L. J. Maternal deprivation: Toward an empirical and conceptual reevaluation. *Psychological Bulletin,* 1961, **58,** 459–490.

SUGGESTED READINGS

1. Bandura, A. Vicarious processes: A case of no-trial learning. In L. Berkowitz (ed.), *Advances in experimental social psychology,* Vol. 2, New York: Academic Press, Inc., 1965, pp. 1–55. An explication of the theory and research on observational learning.
2. Bandura, A., and R. H. Walters. *Social learning and personality development.* New York: Holt, Rinehart & Winston, 1964. An amplification of many of the principles described in this chapter and an application of them to the understanding of personality development.
3. Freud, S. A *general introduction to psychoanalysis.* New York: Liveright Publishing Corp., 1920. A presentation of some of Freud's views on the origins and dynamics of negative abnormalities, views that differ greatly from those presented here.
4. Mowrer, O. H. *Learning theory and personality dynamics.* New York: The Ronald Press Company, 1950. An examination of derivations from both learning theory and psychoanalytic theory for their relevance to personality.

10

Neurotic Behavior

L. DOUGLAS DE NIKE

NORMAN TIBER

The task of classifying abnormal behavior patterns has proved to be extremely difficult. Early investigators had hoped to develop a classification system based on etiology, or cause, which would carry clear implications for treatment. Unfortunately, the cause of many common behavior disorders remains a matter of controversy; these conditions have often been described without being explained. This is true for the group of reactions known as the *psychoneuroses* or *neuroses*, which are characterized by anxiety and depression, and various maladaptive techniques people use to escape such feelings.

In this chapter, we shall review the different categories of neurosis. This is not always easy since the differences between them are not always clear. A single behavior may appear in several categories, and in many cases patients exhibit a variety of behaviors which makes it difficult to reliably "place" them in any specific category (Zigler and Phillips, 1961).

In reading these descriptions, the reader will become aware of certain similarities between his own behavior and that described as neurotic. This is to be expected since neurotic reactions are extreme forms of the feelings and behavior that are common to all people. In attempting to meet our own complex needs, each of us develops special ways of avoiding frustration, conflict, guilt, and anxiety. The neurotic is less successful than most people in this respect. He is persistently dissatisfied and ineffectual in his attempts to find satisfaction in important life situations. He remains in contact with reality and rarely requires hospitalization, but he is chronically plagued by his symptoms. He is not crazy, but he is often very unhappy.

NEUROTIC BEHAVIOR PATTERNS

Anxiety States

Anxiety states are characterized by chronic, unfocused, or "free-floating" fear, which varies in its intensity. Their victim appears tense in both posture and facial expression and may report physical discomfort. He seems "jumpy," with hair-trigger reflexes, as if ready to react to some unknown danger. He is afraid of everything and nothing all at once.

For some people in anxiety states, this background of chronic distress is periodically punctuated by attacks of stark terror. One patient described such an acute anxiety attack as follows:

> I feel anxious and fearful much of the time. I keep expecting something to happen but I don't know what. It's not the same all the time. Sometimes I only feel bad. Then, suddenly, for no reason, it happens. My heart begins to pound so fast that I feel it's going to pop out. My hands get icy, and I get a cold sweat all over my body. My forehead feels like it is covered with sharp needles. I feel like I won't be able to breathe, and I begin panting and choking. Everything gets black. I feel like I am going to faint or die. It's terrible, so terrible! I can go along for a while without too much difficulty, and then suddenly, without any warning, it happens.

In most cases, an acute anxiety attack lasts only a little while, and the patient then returns to his usual state of anxious anticipation.

Protracted neurotic anxiety states are not very common, but almost everyone has experienced mild versions of them. Any time you find yourself bothered by a nagging mental discomfort whose origins are hard to explain and which seem to have no definite object, you are undergoing a greater or lesser anxiety attack. College students seem to have them mostly when they are not mentally occupied and commonly shake themselves free of anxiety by some kind of distracting activity.

Phobic Reactions

Phobic reactions are specialized anxiety states in which the patient experiences intense fear when confronted with a *particular* object or situation. Unlike "free-floating" or general anxiety, the source of fear is specific and can be identified. The patient, along with most other people, sees it as unreasonable, however, and cannot account for his overwhelming fear. He is dominated by the need to avoid the fearsome object, and his daily life is regulated so as to minimize contact with it.

Almost any object or situation may become a phobic stimulus. Some people show phobic avoidance of animals, others of heights, and still others of open spaces, vehicles, household objects, dirt, and schools. In extreme cases, people have become incapacitated by the difficult detours and abstinence necessary to avoid phobic stimulus situations. One such patient described the following experience:

> I was riding in my husband's car and I suddenly became terrified. I felt as if I would die. I made him turn around and take me home. I ran into the house and suddenly felt safe. I could not understand what had happened. I had never been afraid of cars. The next day it happened again and it kept getting worse. Finally, just being on the street and seeing a car would bring on a terrible feeling. Now I just stay at home.

Phobias are among the most common of all psychological disorders. Almost everybody has some irrational fears which are extreme enough to be classified this way. But the phobias of everyday life are not commonly considered neurotic because they do not ordinarily interfere with important activities. Many people are phobic about snakes, for example, and will even panic at the sight of a garter snake, which they know is harmless or, for that matter, at the sight of a snake pickled in formaldehyde. We do not ordinarily regard this kind of phobia as pathological, however, since modern Americans have no need to maintain good relationships with snakes in order to get on with their affairs. A phobia about being outdoors, on the other hand, or about water (Shaffer and Shoben, 1956) interferes with the routines of life too much to be taken so lightly and is therefore the subject of considerable attention in the study of neuroses.

Phobias are among the oldest known neurotic conditions, and they have long been identified in medical terminology by Greek and Latin names. *Altophobia* or *acrophobia* is fear of heights, *agoraphobia* is fear of open places, *claustrophobia,* fear of confinement, and so forth, for as many fears as there are Greek and Latin words to name them. These terms add nothing to our understanding of the conditions, but they are useful for impressing friends, colleagues, and patients.

Obsessive-Compulsive Reactions

These disorders are characterized by the intense, irrational repetition of thoughts (obsessions) or acts (compulsions). The patient frequently is tormented by recurrent thoughts of illness, impulses to commit crimes or other antisocial acts, and sexual ideas that evoke anxiety and guilt. In addition to such obsessive ruminations, he may carry out a variety of compulsive acts.

The compulsive neurotic develops rituals by which he attempts to avoid intense anxiety. He may count compulsively, recite some ritual formula, touch certain objects in a ritual fashion, or dress, eat, or sleep in some precisely defined manner. The variety of obsessive-compulsive symptoms is practically unlimited; almost any idea or act may be incorporated into the neurotic pattern. In severe cases, almost all aspects of daily life become seriously affected and the individual feels trapped by his own thoughts and actions. This was verbalized by one patient as follows:

> I have reached the point where I don't care anymore. For the past year, I have become so worried about getting ill. I keep thinking about what will happen to my wife and children, and how much I will suffer. It's become so bad that I worry about what I'm touching, how I'm dressing, and what I'm eating. If a plate looks a little greasy, I have to wash it over and over again. I'm so afraid of germs, I wash my hands till they are red and sore. I'm terrified that they have germs on them. I just feel chained and I don't know how to get out.

Obsessive-compulsive neuroses are rarely seen in their most virulent forms, but mild versions of them are common enough to be considered part of what Freud called "the psychopathology of everyday life" (Freud, 1938). Most of us are familiar with the common compulsive rituals of childhood, like not stepping on the cracks of the sidewalk, or touching every telephone pole as one walks along. In adulthood, such overt practices tend to give way to the more subtle rituals of obsessional thinking. In mildest and commonest form, these include things like tunes that keep repeating themselves over and over in one's head, or license plate numbers that we casually glanced at on the street, or stray nursery rhymes, or the punch lines of jokes. As with phobias or anxiety states, these trivial obsessions and compulsions have no pathological significance until and unless they begin to interfere with the important routines of our lives. Washing one's hands several times a day probably protects one from disease, but washing them several dozen times a day will create an ailment where none existed before. Getting out of bed before falling asleep to check whether the door is locked probably helps ensure a restful night—the first time it is done—but if it is repeated fifty times, it prevents sleep altogether and is then the symptom of a neurosis.

Hysterical Reactions

Early modern studies of neurotic reactions focused on rather dramatic cases of hysteria. The symptoms of this disorder, which is probably the earliest known psychological disability (see Chapter 1), are a variety of physical symptoms called *conversion reactions* and disturbances of memory called *dissociative reactions*. Symptoms usually appear rapidly in response to emotional stress.

Conversion reactions take the form of physical ailments like pains in different parts of the body, paralysis of limbs, blindness, deafness, or muteness, or even malfunctions of internal organs like the kidneys or genitals. The variety of symptoms is extensive and frequently mimics the patient's view of some physical disorder rather than the true symptoms of organic illness. In an interesting demonstration, students were asked to act out some bodily injury. The sham symptoms they produced were characteristic of hysterical reactions (Henderson and Batchelor, 1962). However, hysteria must be distinguished from *malingering*, that is from the deliberate simulation of illness, since in hysteria the individual believes himself to be physically afflicted.

Any of the senses may be involved in a conversion reaction producing either a heightening or a loss of sensitivity to certain stimuli. Visual disturbances, for example, may involve total or partial blindness, or excessive sensitivity to light. The same variability is found in disturbances of hearing, smelling, tasting, and touching. The latter frequently takes the form of "glove" or "stocking" anesthesia, that is, loss of sensation in the hands or feet only, while most of the body is generally unaffected.

The anesthesias frequently accompany another major group of conversion reactions which result in motor symptoms. The patient suddenly becomes unable to perform voluntary movements of his head, hands, feet, or entire body; or he may become completely unable to speak or to speak above a whisper. In addition to total or partial paralysis, hysterical motor disturbances also appear as disordered movements ranging from slight tremors and tics to severe fits which resemble epileptic seizures.

Finally, conversion reactions may produce a variety of visceral symptoms. Some mild ones are hiccups, air swallowing, regurgitation, constipation, and extremes in appetite. More severe hysterias of internal organs can include sexual impotence, incontinence, menstrual problems, and, on rare occasions, false pregnancy, complete with morning sickness and swelling belly, but with no vital ingredients.

A number of factors allow conversion reactions to be distinguished from organic disorders. First, no organic malfunction can be identified to account for the patient's symptoms. Second, conversion reactions often leave their victim with some voluntary control of a kind that makes his behavior inconsistent with that of an individual who has a truly organic disorder. Thus, in hysterical blindness, the pupillary (eyeblink) reflex usually remains intact; also, the patient rarely bumps into obstacles placed in his path. Third, hysterical patients frequently appear unconcerned about their illness, demonstrating what Charcot called *la belle indifference*, the beautiful indifference. Lastly, hysterical symptoms often can be temporarily induced or removed by hypnotic suggestion.

The following description reflects the development of a hysterical reaction:

> I was uncomfortable living at home with my family so I left. Things went along fairly well, even though I had some difficulty in getting a good job. I finally became the secretary to the vice-president of a leading company. Everyone was so nice and I really loved my work. As time went on, my employer became interested in me and we became quite friendly. I really thought he would marry me. I know he loves me. One night we were out and discussing marriage. I acciden-

> tally bumped my leg. It hurt a little while and there was a bruise mark. The next morning I found that I could not move my leg at all. I didn't think the bump was that bad. I called George and he brought me here to the hospital. I haven't been able to move it since. There's no pain, but it just won't move.

No organic basis for the paralysis could be identified.

Dissociative reactions are characterized by disturbances in memory which result in a loss of awareness of personal identity. There are four main patterns of dissociation: *amnesia, somnambulism, fugue states,* and *multiple personality.*

In *amnesia,* the individual loses all memory for a particular period in his life. This occurs suddenly and may last for a few days or for many years. It is as if part of the patient's life had been cut away. Traumatic experiences frequently stimulate these reactions, and events before or after traumatic experiences may be forgotten. In severe cases, the individual loses all sense of personal identity. He does not know his name, address, or occupation and fails to recognize his family and friends.

Somnambulism, or sleepwalking, is a common occurrence during childhood that may reappear periodically throughout life. In its simplest form, the person arises from his bed and engages in some activity. Frequently, this is nothing more than walking, but occasionally it involves more complicated activities. These reactions usually are of short duration and terminate in return to bed. The next morning the individual may vaguely recall some of the events which occurred.

In *fugue* states, the person suddenly leaves his usual environment and loses all sense of identity. As in amnesia, the patient cannot recall the events which occurred during the fugue period. Usually, the reaction is limited to a few hours or days. The person suddenly finds himself in a strange place and cannot account for the events which brought him there. In extreme cases, however, the fugue state may last for months or years. The individual may take up residence in a new community and develop a completely new life. This will continue until he is found or suddenly recalls the prefugue period and regains his original identity.

Lastly, we come to the *multiple personality* reactions, which are extremely rare. The patient presents two or more alternating "personalities" which characterize his behavior at different times. These are usually quite distinct, like Dr. Jekyll and Mr. Hyde. These "personalities" appear to operate independently of each other, although one "personality" may be aware of the others.

The following experience described by a soldier reflects the development of a dissociative reaction:

> We were all running up the hill. The next thing I know I'm back at the soup kitchen drinking coffee. When the O.D. asked me what company I was with, I just told him. He then asked me why I hadn't moved out and I didn't know what he was talking about. I don't know what happened. I just don't remember anything. I wish someone would help me.

Under hypnosis, the soldier recalled leaving the battle and returning to the safety of camp.

Extreme hysterical reactions are every bit as rare as extreme obsessive-compulsive disorders. Although the reasons for it are not entirely clear, there is no doubt that the incidence of hysterical neuroses has declined very drastically in the United States over the past fifty years or so. This may be related to the great increases in general education that have occurred during this period. Hysteria seems to be an especially common disorder among relatively poorly educated and socially naïve people. Perhaps because of its apparent similarity to malingering, perhaps for other reasons, it seems to have become socially stigmatized to the point where sophisticated people simply cannot afford to be branded as "hysterical" in the technical sense.

Despite its decline as an extreme condition, there are two forms in which mild hysteria is still quite common. One of these occurs among children, and the other takes the form of mild symptoms among otherwise mentally healthy adults.

It is quite common for children who are afraid of a new or difficult situation to try to escape it by feigning illness. Outright malingering, however, is too closely associated with lying in the minds of most children for them to be able to do it with aplomb; what they may do, therefore, is to actually become sick in the sense that they convince themselves that their protestations of aches and pains are real. Since concerned parents are likely to give the child the benefit of the doubt in such situations and therefore permit him to miss school or whatever, he is reinforced positively for a variety of aches, pains, and discomforts which may become patterned for him in the future when he finds himself about to face stressful situations.

Such childhood experiences probably do not give rise to full blown hysterical neuroses in adulthood, but they probably do support the subclinical symptoms which many adults develop in response to psychological threats. Headaches, sore throats, spells of weakness, and other minor troublesome symptoms which do not incapacitate people very seriously may still free them of the anxiety aroused by some distressing life situation. The headaches that kept a fifth grade girl from having to deliver a school report she had not prepared may save her in college from a date she does not desire. Such symptoms are first cousins to hysteria.

Neurotic Depressive Reactions ("Reactive Depression")

Neurotic depressions occur in response to some severe personal loss, such as the death of a loved one, losing a job, failure to be admitted to college, or financial reversal. Almost everyone feels depressed at one time or another, but "reactive depressions" differ from ordinary depressions in both their intensity and duration. The individual feels listless, lonely, and helpless to cope with his problems. He may have difficulty sleeping and eating and weeps at the slightest provocation. Some depressed people contemplate suicide as the only solution for their misfortunes, and some actually do kill themselves. The reaction frequently produces fatigue, an apathetic attitude towards life, and paradoxically, a great concern about one's general health.

One man who had recently been fired from his job commented about his situation as follows:

> I don't know what I'm going to do. I know I can never get another good job again. No one will want me. I feel like my life is over. I just cannot begin again. I sit up all night knowing that I've failed and I don't know what to do about it. I wish I were dead.

Having briefly reviewed the neurotic reaction patterns, we shall now turn our attention to the two major theoretical systems which try to explain the origin and treatment of neurosis.

PSYCHODYNAMIC AND LEARNING ACCOUNTS OF PSYCHOLOGICAL DISORDER

Most current explanations of maladaptive behavior may be grouped under one of two main theoretical headings: *psychodynamic* theories stemming from Freudian psychoanalysis and its derivatives, and *learning* theories developed largely from experimental psychology. The term *psychodynamic* refers broadly to theories which stress internal motives or drives as determinants of behavior (English and English, 1958); *learning* approaches are relatively more concerned with behavior as a function of external stimulation. As will be evident from the discussion which follows, there is some commonality between these two sets of formulations, and much diversity within each set. However, the fairly distinct cleavages between psychodynamic and learning approaches are presently matters of central concern for the mental health professions. As we have seen to some extent in Chapter 5 and 9, the two approaches imply different schemes of classifying and treating mental disorders. This section describes the main features of both systems.

Freudian Psychodynamics

Sigmund Freud (1856–1939) developed a monumental set of hypotheses concerning human motivation, development, and psychopathology. Although his formulations have undergone substantial revision by others (Munroe, 1955), they remain the wellspring of the psychodynamic approach. Freud derived his doctrines chiefly from the practice of psychoanalysis, a therapy which he invented, developed, and viewed as a method for the scientific study of personality. In psychoanalysis the analysand (patient) typically lies on a couch and attempts to say whatever comes into his mind; that is, he tries to give *free associations* without omissions or distortions. These, along with dreams and reports of experiences, are explored and interpreted to him by the analyst as he understands and assimilates them. The course of psychoanalysis typically consists of from one to six hour-long sessions per week during a period of two years or longer. Freud conceived of psychoanalysis as a way of providing the analysand with intellectual and emotional insight or self-understanding. Since he observed that the attainment of such insight was sometimes accompanied by the remission or cure of neurotic symptoms, psychoanalysis soon evolved into a distinct form of psychotherapy which attracted wide attention.

The Freudian View of Personality

Freud and later writers in his tradition held that human personality is governed by the interaction of three major dynamic systems: (1) the *id*, which consists of unconscious inborn sexual and aggressive instincts; (2) the *superego*, representing the learned and internalized moral demands of parents and society, also largely unconscious; and (3) the *ego*, which develops as a control system to provide for the orderly satisfaction of the strong conflicting demands emanating from the id, the superego, and external reality. The id is characterized by the amoral pursuit of immediate instinctual gratification, that is, pleasure; the superego by unrelenting demands for moral perfection; and the ego by the demands of external reality (see Figure 10.1). Despite the ego's orientation to reality, Freud considered it basically subservient to the unconscious dictates of the other two. Thus, man's orientation to reality—his goal striving—is fundamentally organized around the pursuit of pleasure and the avoidance of guilt and anxiety. The transition from id dominance to ego functioning in the course of development, in Jones's words (1955, p. 314), "betokens not an abrogating of the pleasure principle, but the providing of a more secure basis for it." The ego's most basic means of controlling id impulses is through *repression*, whereby unacceptable sexual and aggressive desires are "pushed into the unconscious." Freud saw psychoanalysis as a means of bringing unconscious material to consciousness. By

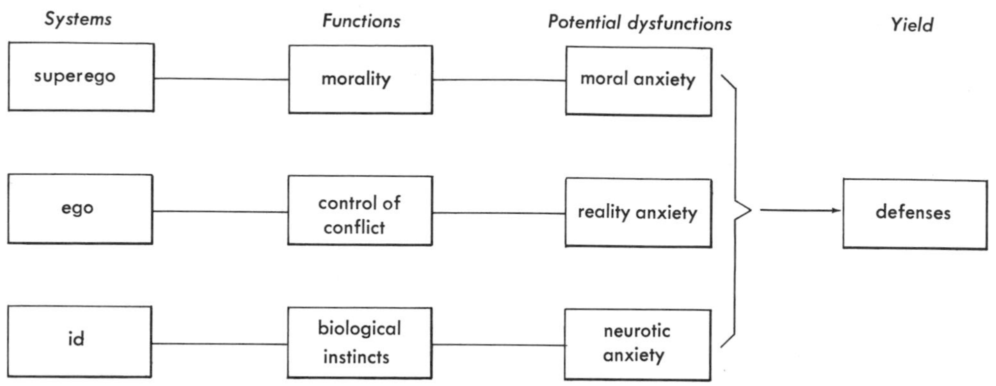

Figure 10.1 Diagram of the Freudian conception of personality.

enabling the patient to accept this material and its emotional significance, analysis could give him control over it and end its covert domination of his personality. In Freud's phrase, "Where id was, there shall ego be." Behind this phrase there was, for Freud, a profound, and central faith in the ultimate power and importance of man's *rational faculties* to control his behavior. Even though it is typically walled in by defenses and preoccupied with scheduling ordinary life activities, the ego, as Freud saw it, is potentially capable of steering a full and integrated existence. If there is a single central tenet of Freudian therapy, it is that complete consciousness brings about adaptive behavior change.

In Freudian developmental psychology, the first five years of life are considered crucially important for the formation of personality. In this interval, the young child develops through biologically predetermined "psychosexual stages." These successive stages are characterized by a concentration of interest and instinctual energy, called *libido*, on particular parts of the body. The first, or *oral* stage, goes from birth through the first year of life; at this time, the infant is concerned with its mouth and the incorporation of food by sucking and biting. The *anal* stage, during the second and third years of life, is reflected in the child's preoccupation with his eliminative organs and their products. The *phallic* stage is typified by concern with the genital organs; it lasts from about ages three to five. During this stage, the child goes through the conflicts of the *Oedipus complex*, involving sexual attraction toward the parent of opposite sex, hostility toward the parent of the same sex, and anxiety over the dangerous consequences of expressing these impulses.

Through traumatic experiences of one kind or another, personality growth may be *fixated* at one of these early psychosexual stages, or regression back to an earlier stage may occur. For example, a child whose needs for sucking have been frustrated in the early oral stage might remain psychologically dependent on oral things as an adult, drawing psychological "nourishment" from other people or from oral food substitutes such as alcohol and tobacco. Coercive toilet training in the anal stage is presumed to result in obsessive-compulsive neatness in later life or, through rebellion, in resentful messiness. Failure to resolve the Oedipal crisis is thought to result in the inability to assume a mature sex role and in ambivalence toward authority figures. Successful resolution of these early conflicts enables the child to pass on to the *latency* stage, lasting from around age six until adolescence. After adolescence, the normal adult has achieved the *genital* or mature psychosexual stage, which Freud summed up as the abilities "to love and to work."

The Mechanisms of Ego Defense

It was mentioned above that Freud conceived the ego as a relatively weak, compromising system whose task is to integrate the chaotic pleasure-seeking impulses of the id and the stern perfection-demanding injunctions of the superego with reality. The ego may be threatened in its operations by potential loss of self-esteem, by depressive feelings, and by anxiety stemming from three sources: *neurotic anxiety,* that is, fear that id impulses will get out of control and erupt into unacceptable behavior; *moral anxiety,* or guilt feelings from the superego about culturally disapproved behavior; and *reality anxiety,* or fear of dangers in the external world. The ego is aided in dealing with these various threats by diverse *mechanisms of defense.* Defense mechanisms ordinarily operate unconsciously. They neutralize the potentially upsetting impact of threatening events or ideas by distorting reality in small but significant ways. While some other Freudian doctrines have been extensively revised or largely discarded with time, the concept of ego defense, formally spelled out by Freud's daughter, Anna, in *The Ego and the Mechanisms of Defense* (1937), enjoys wide acceptance today.

As Freudian psychology has become more widely known, the idea that defenses and "defensiveness" are generally bad, weak, and neurotic has spread in popular culture. However, psychoanalytic theory has always recognized the potentially large positive value which particular defenses have for personality stability and productivity. In the discussion below, bear in mind that defensive modes of adjustment are universal in human personality, and that whether a particular defense is helpful or harmful for a given individual really depends on the life circumstances in which it appears and the purposes it serves. The material may call to mind illustrations from your own life and the behavior of friends and relatives; this should by no means carry the implication that you or they are in need of psychological help.

No really complete schematization of defenses is possible because different authors vary in the number and definition of defenses they recognize. To provide a general orientation, we shall begin with *repression,* which Freud considered the root of all other defenses. We shall next discuss defense mechanisms which primarily affect *thinking,* and then defenses primarily affecting *overt behavior.* Within each of these categories mechanisms are grouped according to whether they are primarily *personal, interpersonal,* or *general.* This schema only approximates the scope of particular defenses because some reactions, such as phobias and obsessive-compulsive symptoms, have both thinking *and* behavioral components, and indeed all defenses have some properties in each sphere.

Another limit on the usefulness of our scheme is the likelihood that the utility of any given classification of neurotic symptoms declines with time. Changing social conditions seem to change symptomatology. For example, the hysterias seem more prevalent among individuals and groups relatively unsophisticated in psychology and have retreated in incidence since the Victorian era, in which Freud began his work. There has been a relative upswing in the occurrence of what has been termed "existential symptoms"—in which the patient is distressed at the lack of meaning in life and social relationships but is without serious symptoms of anxiety, depression, or other specific complaints. Also, perhaps partially because of the permissive aura of psychoanalytic theory and practice, there has been a relative upswing in—and need to reformulate—the "character disorders," which have shown their presence in alarming current levels of crime, divorce, and alcoholism and other addictive symptoms. A listing of the major mechanisms of defense follows. (Italicized terms other than the initial words in each paragraph are discussed elsewhere in this section.)

Repression: the basic defense. Repression is the selective deep forgetting, or "pushing into the unconscious," of painful, embarrassing, or anxiety-provoking experiences. The concept of repression plays a key role in Freud's analysis of neurotics. The need for psychoanalytic treatment to "make the unconscious conscious" arises because traumatic experiences and unacceptable impulses have been repressed. The release of repressed memories is clearly illustrated in the treatment of combat neuroses. Hypnosis or certain drugs may render repressed memories of combat once more available to consciousness; their recall is often accompanied by dramatic explosions of feelings. Freud held that such recall, accompanied by full emotional awareness, which he termed "abreaction" or "catharsis," is prerequisite to successful treatment. Repression may be very specific and circumscribed, as in the case of a person who is only amnesic for the few hours in which traumatic events took place. However, in Freud's view, unconscious conflict over repressed sexual and aggressive impulses gives rise to anxiety, and the ego attempts to guard against this anxiety by invoking a host of other defense mechanisms. For Freud, repression was the basic defense, and all other such mechanisms were seen as secondary outgrowths of repression. That is, all other neurotic defenses are seen as defenses against the eruption of previously repressed material into consciousness or behavior. Presumably if an individual were aware of and comfortable with all of his formerly repressed memories and drives, he would have no need of neurotic defenses and would hence be healthy. But defenses are not seen as totally pathological. The stresses and anxieties of reality, let alone of the id and the superego, are sometimes so pressing that the afflicted individual needs mental defenses to make life bearable when he cannot change it. Thus, the defense mechanisms have potentially adaptive roles if they are not used to excess.

Defensive thinking: personal thinking. *Rationalization* is the invention of plausible but fictitious reasons for one's own more or less irrational, immoral, or inept behaviors or attitudes. A familiar instance of it is the "sour grapes" phenomenon of devaluing unattainable goals; also, the reciprocal attitude of making a virtue of necessity is a form of rationalization. It may be noted in passing that both of these are special cases of *dissonance reduction* (Brehm and Cohen, 1962; Festinger, 1957), a process whereby a person's attitudes and future actions are made consistent with his past actions and commitments. The accommodation of belief to behavior was noted by Saint Paul, who in exhorting early Christians to contribute to the church said, "Where your treasure is, there will your heart be also."

Isolation is the process whereby inconsistent beliefs or values are kept from clashing with each other in a person's thinking. For instance, a person who claims adherence to Christian ideals of human brotherhood may practice racial discrimination; or one who claims that extremist doctrines are too silly to attract a significant following may advocate suppression of these doctrines. Such inconsistencies are kept isolated from each other in the person's mind. When they are pointed out, usually one or another *rationalization* is invoked to justify the disparity (Westie, 1965).

Narcissistic defenses are characterized by a seemingly unshakeable habit of excusing one's own faults and "blowing one's own horn," often accompanied by impulsive and irresponsible behavior. Narcissistic defenses frequently accompany manic activity. They sometimes cloak underlying feelings of inferiority and inadequacy or protect the individual from guilt feelings after he has acted irresponsibly. Some degree of narcissistic self-infatuation is probably useful in getting work out of oneself and one's subordinates. The belief that one's work is very important justifies putting great effort into it; thus, the frequent association of high achievement with very high self-esteem.

Identification is a process in which a person believes himself to be like another in some respects, experiences the other's successes and defeats as his own, and consciously or unconsciously models his own behavior after him. Freud held that the child normally resolves his Oedipal conflicts by repressing his desire for the parent of the opposite sex and identifying with the parent of the same sex, thus participating vicariously and unconsciously in the adult sexual role. The fact that there is emotional involvement with the other person distinguishes identification from mere imitation; many children and some adults are dejected when their baseball heroes lose and elated when they win. The process of identification has been discussed in detail in Chapter 4.

Introjection involves adoption of the beliefs or attitudes of powerful others after an initial period of resistance or hostility to them. Introjection is thus a special case of identification, enabling one to escape from conflicts with the powerful others in question. Prisoners in Nazi concentration camps sometimes displayed the same brutality, and even the same mannerisms, as their guards toward other prisoners. The brutal acts might be explained as an instance of displacement, but the imitation of mannerisms would seem more explainable through the concept of introjection.

Defensive thinking: interpersonal thinking. *Displacement* is the transfer of feelings or actions from their original source to an object which arouses less anxiety. For example, excessive concern about the mouth may indicate underlying concern about the genital organs (Menninger, 1947). "Scapegoating" is a kind of displacement in which some other person or group is unjustly blamed for one's own failings. Displacement is also seen when anger originally aroused by a parent, authority figure, or stronger person is "taken out" on a weaker person, an animal, or a helpless object. The displacement of aggression is known to occur among animals as well as people. Miller (1948) trained two rats to attack each other in order to turn off an electric shock in their cage. When one of the rats was removed, the remaining animal attacked a rubber doll that was put in the cage.

Projection is the attribution of one's own unacceptable traits to other people or groups. For example, a person with unconscious homosexual impulses might see others as making subtle homosexual advances towards him. Sometimes the term *projection* is used to denote the scapegoating process: by projecting his own hostility onto certain others and accusing them of being hostile, a disturbed person may "justify" his aggressive impulses against them; such a process seems frequently to occur in racial or religious prejudice and in the international tensions that precede wars. Although it is not usually considered a defense, *idealization* is worth mentioning in the same context as projection. Idealization is the attribution of desirable traits to another person or group; it is the opposite of projection, which is concerned with the unacceptable. Idealization has its defensive function in masking from the individual those faults in others which might make him anxious. The person who is so idealized often unwittingly cooperates in maintaining his admirer's impression; sometimes he exploits it.

Paranoid defenses involve unwarranted feelings of personal importance or the false belief that others are hostile. Paranoid symptoms severe enough to produce gross distortions of reality are given the technical name *delusions*. One speaks of "delusions of grandeur" and "delusions of persecution." Persecutory ideas may result from *projecting* one's own hostility onto others; the idea that one is important then helps to rationalize why others may be "out to get" him. Freud hypothesized a connection between paranoid ideation and latent (unconscious) homosexuality: to control his repressed homosexual impulses, the patient may come to believe that he is hated by others of the same sex, thus building a protective wall of mutual hostility.

Defensive thinking: general thinking. *Denial* is refusal to accept the truth of a negative evaluation of oneself or of something one values. For example, a girl might indirectly reveal mixed feelings about her boyfriend, but when a friend calls it to her attention, profess unalloyed and undying devotion to him. Presumably she makes a defense against recognizing her ambivalence because it would occasion guilt or anxiety that the relationship might be further strained.

Emotional insulation is the process whereby a person reduces his degree of emotional involvement in situations that might provoke anxiety, anger, or disappointment. This mechanism is visible in the behavior of adolescents who strive to maintain a "cool" or "sophisticated" pose no matter what the situation. A great many social roles require a high degree of emotional insulation for their proper performance. Thus a characteristic problem of sophisticated modern man seems to be a tendency to retain such detachment when genuine effect and intimacy are called for, as with friends and family.

Intellectualization, a form of emotional insulation, refers to a number of "intellectual" ways of defending against threatening feelings. A person may describe an anxiety-provoking event in abstract generalities that make it "distant" or treat it as a general human problem without admitting its very personal reference. Intellectualization also refers to compensation for deficiencies through intellectual achievement and to the process of crowding anxiety-laden thoughts from consciousness by ruminating on unrelated matters. Thus, prisoners in concentration camps may engage in heated debates on matters having no bearing on their current plight; unrecognized thinkers may console themselves by constructing theoretical schemes of great scope. One notable characteristic of intellectualizers is their excessively involved use of words. This is, as one might expect, a defense frequently employed by intellectuals. Perhaps the circumlocutious quality of intellectualized speech is due partly to the fact that direct self-expression is associated with anxiety and partly to the individual's feeling that he can best master this anxiety by conceptualizing his problems within a complicated, and therefore distracting, abstract theory. When the user of very elevated language is motivated less by anxiety than by desire to impress others, this style may more properly be called pedantry.

Phobias operate as defenses, according to psychodynamic theory, by permitting the individual to displace onto a specific set of feared objects, such as snakes, elevators, or crowds, fears originally aroused by some repressed sexual or aggressive stimulus. While some phobic symptoms are symbolic expressions of repressed feelings, there is much evidence that most phobias are acquired directly through conditioning.

Fantasy may act as a defense by permitting the harmless indirect release of tensions arising from the unfulfilled goals of real life. Fantasies of fame, riches, sexuality, and unpunished aggression are very common among normal people, and they are facilitated by movies, books, and other media. Fantasy is used creatively by a person who turns his dreams into concrete achievement. However, fantasies blend into the pathological process of *delusion* and *withdrawal* if the individual comes to believe them on insufficient evidence or if he unduly substitutes them for actual accomplishment.

Delusion consists of a manifestly false belief which resists all argument or evidence. A *delusional system* is a set of interlocking false beliefs. Delusions tend to make the believer feel more important, to rationalize his failures, to provide a justification for hostility towards others, or to otherwise explain events. Some beliefs of extremist political and religious groups may be considered socially shared delusions. In the severely disturbed, hallucinations (false perceptions, such as "voices" and "visions") may be part of a delusional system.

Defensive action: self-oriented behavior. *Compensation* is the process whereby a person makes up for his deficiencies and inferiority feelings by striving for superiority along certain lines. This mechanism, like many others, may be of substantial positive value if it is not overdone (see Figure 10.2)—in this case, by adoption of overly perfectionistic standards with consequent depression on failure to meet them. An example of compensation might be drawn from Charles Atlas, the "ninety-seven pound weakling," who by body building became a "he-man." Alfred Adler (1870–1930), a disciple of Freud, built his theory of neurosis around the concept of compensation for inferiority through aggressive striving for power. He later held that the best expression of compensation was interest in the common social good (Adler, 1929).

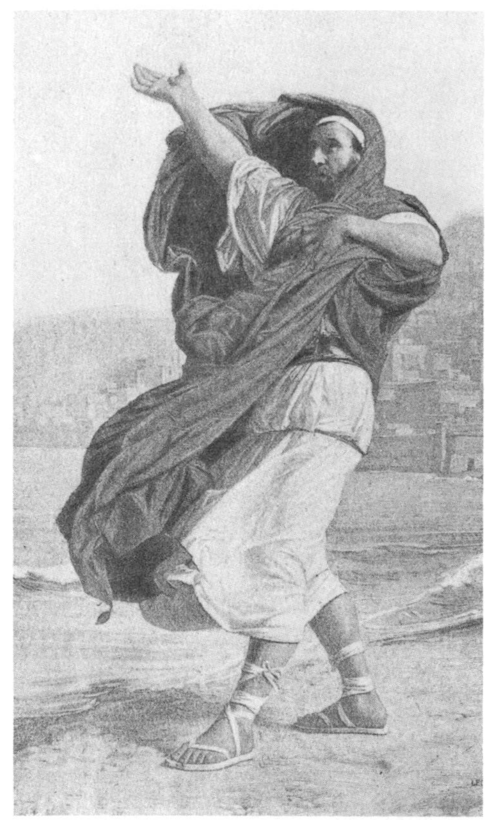

Figure 10.2 Demosthenes (384?–322 B.C.), one of the greatest orators of all times, practiced speaking with pebbles in his mouth so that he would speak extremely clearly as a *compensation*. Photo courtesy of the Granger Collection.

Turning against the self is the acceptance of guilt or blame resulting in feelings of low self-esteem, depression, anxiety, and a search for expiation through *compensation* or *undoing*. In extreme forms, this defense may lead to profound depression, self-punishing behavior, or even suicide. Since depressive states are fostered by many physiological causes, such as endocrine changes and metabolic

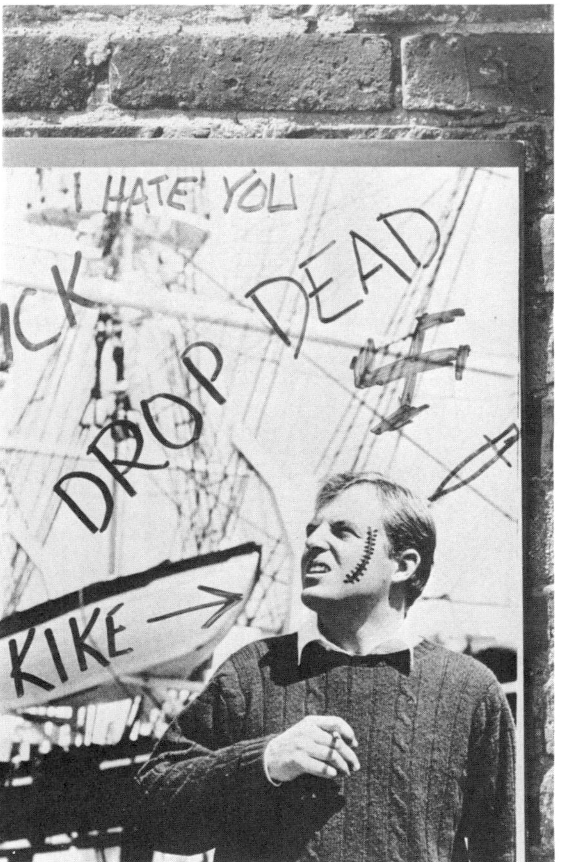

Figure 10.3 Some people *act out* their conflicts by defacing ads and other prominently displayed objects. Photo © WESKEMP.

disorders, as well as psychological ones, turning against the self should be accepted as a pertinent explanation only when guilt has clearly helped precipitate a depressed condition.

Regression is the return to early immature modes of behavior. It may be caused by stress, frustration, or simply environmental reward of such immature behavior. An example of the latter is the practice of some mental hospitals of spoon-feeding psychotic patients who would otherwise feed themselves. Sometimes regression is hard to distinguish from simple imitation of an immature model: the older child may imitate the new baby who gets all the attention by crying and bed-wetting. Regression has the general defensive purpose of evading the challenges and problems of maturity. However, it appears that temporary and voluntary "regression in the service of the ego," as in "immature" party behavior and in sexual intimacies, valuably renews the individual for further mature coping and creativity (Hartmann, 1950).

Somatization includes defenses which involve the formation of symptoms of physical illness. In conversion hysteria, an individual may develop a back pain or other complaint, with the incidental or secondary result that he is able to avoid an unpleasant situation. If there is an underlying sexual maladjustment, for example, such a symptom may "excuse" the patient from the sexual activity he finds unrewarding. Somatization should be distinguished from malingering since the patient genuinely believes himself to be afflicted, although medical examination reveals no clear-cut organic basis for his symptoms. Some somatizers seem to gain considerable indirect satisfaction, called secondary gain, from their complaints, as in hysteria. *Hypochondriasis* is a term designating a fairly stable tendency of some people to complain about vague aches and pains, to constantly seek medical attention, to take all kinds of medication, and to oblige others because of their "illness" to cater to their wishes. *Neurasthenia* consists of fairly constant feelings of weakness and fatigue without apparent organic basis. Some psychotic patients give bizarre somatic complaints along with other delusions, but neither hypochondriasis nor neurasthenia, are typical of psychotics. A rather different form of somatization is involved in cases of ulcers, asthma, and other psychophysiological reactions in which psychological stress brings on identifiable physical pathology; such reactions are discussed in Chapter 12.

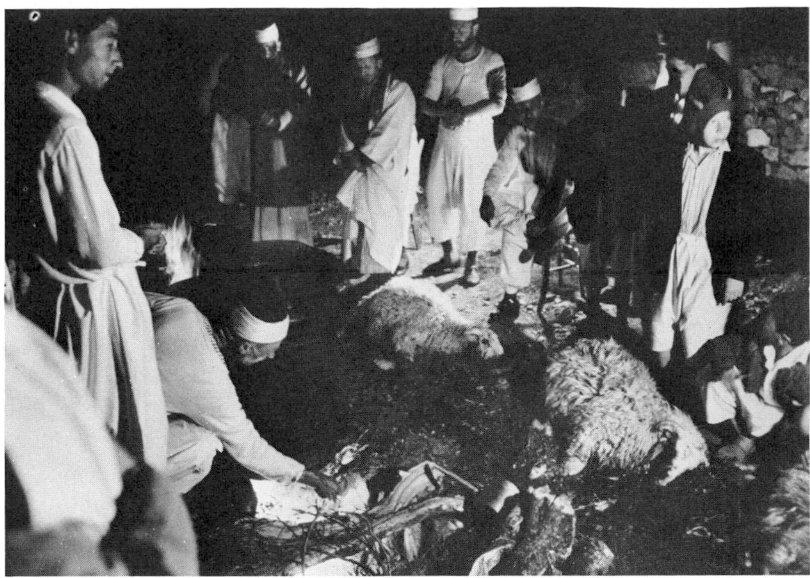

Figure 10.4 The Samaritans, a Jewish sect that survives today in very small numbers in Jordan, practices ritual sacrifice, an example of *undoing*. Photo © Frank Horvat, courtesy of *Life* magazine.

Defensive action: interpersonal behavior. *Acting out* consists of aggressive, sexual, or self-damaging behavior performed as a means of reducing anxiety. This defense mechanism gains its name from the supposition that the individual "acts out" or symbolizes his otherwise unconscious conflicts in overt behavior (see Figure 10.3). The adolescent with hostile feelings toward authority, for example, may deface the statue of a general. Through guilt and the consequent need to be punished, a thief may bungle a crime so that he gets caught. More commonly, acting out may reduce tension by enabling an individual to "blow off steam" or forget his troubles temporarily (in this regard see *manic behavior* below). Acting out is generally viewed negatively by clinicians, but even this defense may sometimes have adaptive features. We know that expressing resentments assertively can sometimes re-balance a chronically irritating situation, for example. It is probably not true, on the other hand, that people need or require aggressive acting out as an "outlet," nor does such behavior lessen the long-term disposition to engage in further aggression (Berkowitz, 1962).

Undoing is the guilt-inspired attempt to atone for or neutralize the damage done by one's misdeeds. For instance, if a child felt that his "bad" thoughts or behaviors were to blame for the death of a parent, he might strive with great fixity of purpose to become a doctor. On the everyday level, we strive to be especially nice to someone we have inadvertently slighted. Freud regarded religious rites for the expiation of sins as examples of undoing (see Figure 10.4). It will be seen that the concept of undoing is akin to *compensation* and *reaction formation.*

Reaction formation is excessive behavior or concern in the opposite direction from one's underlying motives. Children who are jealous of younger brothers or sisters sometimes show an exaggerated preoccupation with ensuring their safety. An alcoholic on the wagon

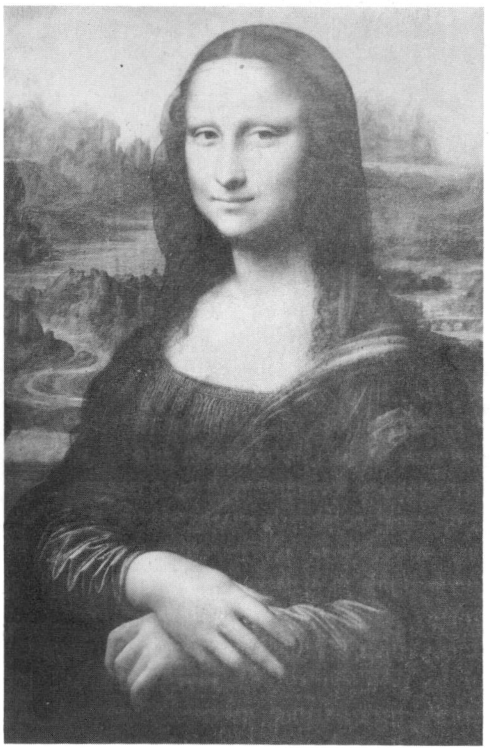

Figure 10.5 The *Mona Lisa* of Leonardo da Vinci shows a smile that is sometimes thought the result of *sublimation*, a form of *substitution*. Photo © Photographie Bulloz.

may go out of his way to denounce drink or to avoid going past the tavern door. In the early stages of love, mild rejections lead readily to such statements as "I hate him." Mothers who covertly reject their children may exert smothering control and protection over them.

Defensive action: general behavior. *Manic behavior* refers to overdriven "busyness" in work or play which blocks out feelings of anxiety, depression, or hostility. The restless energy of manic behavior may be put to constructive or destructive use; it might be said to characterize many successful people, but also many whose energy is expanded in a relatively pointless quest for adventure and pleasure, often at others' expense. Some people block out pervasive fears of sexual inadequacy by repetitive sexual conquests; their pursuit of the opposite sex has the "driven" quality typical of manic behavior.

Substitution is the acceptance of substitute goals in place of those originally sought. Sublimation is a special case of substitution in which the substitute goals have a higher social utility than the original goals (see Figure 10.5). For instance, a nun may sublimate her unfulfilled maternal drives by becoming an excellent teacher or nurse. Sublimation is considered a relatively adaptive defense, but some forms of it may create difficulties. A person who sublimates hostile impulses by becoming a soldier or a surgeon may at times abuse his role under the influence of such unconscious motivation. For Freud, sublimation was the closest man could come to a genuinely altruistic form of motivation; he held that in principle all more "exalted" motives could be reduced to derivatives of sexual or aggressive drives.

Obsessive-compulsive defenses, as we have seen, are actions that have to be repeated many times to keep the sufferer from being overwhelmed by acute anxiety. Freudians usually interpret obsessive-compulsive symptoms as symbolic of underlying conflict or guilt; a symptom such as repetitive hand-washing to "*undo*" the guilt-arousing act or thought of doing some "filthy" thing (see Figure 10.6). In mild form, obsessive-compulsive traits are useful in many occupations; they assure attention to detail, punctuality, and orderliness. Working up to the degree of compulsiveness necessary for many present-day skilled occupations is a source of strain for many people, while the more compulsive person may accept such job demands without complaint.

Withdrawal encompasses a number of response patterns typified by passive failure to accept challenge, narrowing of interests and activities, and retreat into fantasy and solitude. Whether or not a particular manifestation of withdrawing behavior should be considered pathological depends on the context in which it occurs. Retreat from lost causes is only sensible; withdrawal from necessary activities may indicate the presence of depression or of deeper problems. Withdrawal, like regression, serves the defensive function of temporarily enabling a person to avoid the problems of life activities.

Difficulties in Anxiety-Defense Formulations

The psychoanalytic-psychodynamic approach has provided some genuine and unmistakable advances in our understanding of psychological disorder. The concept of defense is one of these. When we try to understand many of the particular actions of neurotic people, it is unquestionable that defense formulations are sometimes extremely useful. But in overall application, the anxiety-defense model of psychological disorder presents substantial difficulties which indicate the need for reformulation of some psychodynamic doctrines.

In the first place, it is not always clear under what defensive heading a particular trait or symptom should be classified. In part this inclarity stems directly from the intrinsic complexity of human behavior and motivation. Failure in school may represent a punitive turning against the self for real or imagined sins, or it may be a by-product of manic preoccupation with extracurricular activities, or it might be an indirect form of acting out, unconsciously intended to make parents feel uncomfortable, or it might stem from depression related to still other causes. A feeling of personal importance may stem from paranoid ideation, from deservedly high self-esteem, or from a manipulative sociopathic makeup. Moreover, as we earlier pointed out, normal

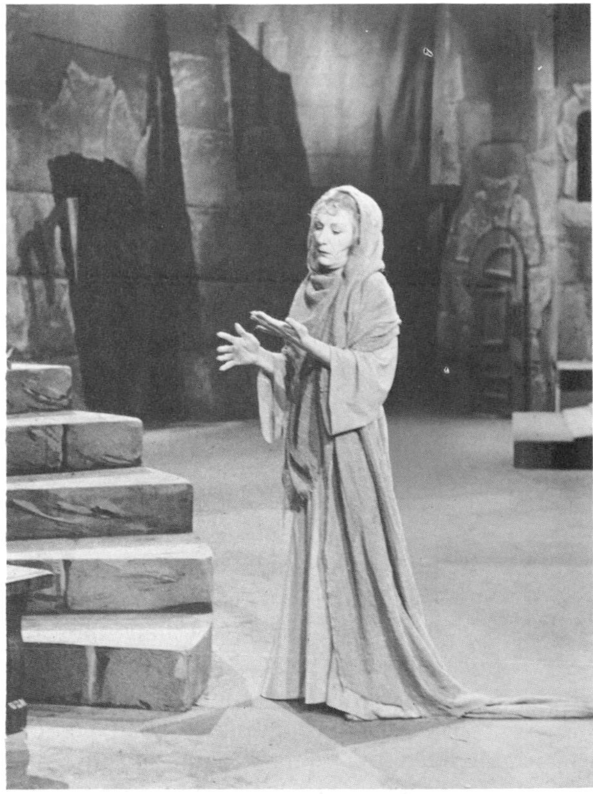

Figure 10.6 Lady Macbeth's hand-washing can be seen as an *obsessive-compulsive reaction.* Photo courtesy of NBC.

people as well as those requiring psychological help make extensive use of various defense mechanisms. Thus, it is not possible to clearly differentiate well-adjusted and poorly adjusted people simply on the basis of the presence or absence of particular defense mechanisms, nor can we plan treatment directly from such information. In fact, most symptoms bear no direct relation to defense mechanisms and most defense mechanisms have no simple relation to diagnosis and treatment. These conclusions are underscored by the consideration that the most seriously disturbed individuals, those with psychotic disorders, are considered in psychodynamic theory to have suffered a *loss* of the more adaptive defenses, such that they are prey to impulsive behavior, deep depression, uncontrolled anxiety, or substantial regression. This last consideration is a major reason why the distinction between "neurotic" and "psychotic" defenses, once sharply made, has tended to break down.

Anxiety-defense formulations have contributed to our understanding of psychopathology by pointing out that sometimes what the patient *is not doing* is more important than what he is doing. For example, a hospitalized patient may busy himself in occupational therapy making clay pots and thereby avoid the interactions with others which are his real problem. However, the activity itself might erroneously suggest that the patient had obsessive concerns with the female genitals, symbolized by the pots, perhaps with anal overtones, since the clay used to make the pots might be viewed as a substitute for feces. Given the numerous possible interpretations offered by psychodynamic theory, it is possible to ascribe a number of defensive or symbolic significances to many kinds of behavior. In part this problem reflects the genuine complexity of human phenomena, but it is evident that the problem remains a central concern for those attempting to make scientific sense of psychodynamic principles.

Given the elaborate range of possible defenses, psychoanalytic and related theory does not offer a comprehensive account of how the patient comes to settle on one or a few particular characteristic ones. Moreover, dynamic theory tends to assume that the organism becomes neurotic mainly in reaction to traumatic, conflicting, or depriving life circumstances. The question of what the sufferer gains by his symptoms—that is, the question of so-called "secondary gain" —is not usually given enough attention as a *main* source of disorder. This point will become clearer in the discussion of operant conditioning and neurotic "games" later in this chapter.

It is incumbent upon the thoroughgoing psychoanalytic theorist to demonstrate sexual, aggressive, or anxiety motives underlying essentially all cases of psychological disorder. This is no small job; often, on the plausible basis that the anxiety, sexuality, or hostility is repressed, psychodynamic theorists assume without evidence that such drives are operating. Such assumptions may give rise to drawn out therapeutic efforts to steer the patient slowly toward the therapist's own ideas about the meaning of the symptoms. When at length the patient verbalizes the same concept, it is sometimes hard to tell whether he has achieved a valid insight or has simply been "trained" to talk in the same way as his therapist.

Since psychoanalytic therapy hinges on the premise that constructive behavior change should follow upon proper intellectual and emotional insight or consciousness of repressed motives and memories, once the patient verbalizes the sources of his symptoms and appropriately "works through" this material, he should become free of symptoms. The fact that insight often does not result in such behavior change raises a critical question about the adequacy of psychoanalytic formulations. Other approaches, which do not posit that consciousness plays a necessary role in mediating new behavior, are not so challenged.

Psychoanalytic and related therapeutic techniques bear only a loose relation to the personality theories which are claimed to underlie them. Moreover, laboratory investigations of psychoanalytic concepts, perhaps partly because of the limitations of their settings, have yielded relatively few unequivocal results which support Freudian personality theory (Adams, 1957; Eriksen, 1962; Sears, 1944).

For all these reasons, the contributions of psychoanalytic and related doctrines to our understanding of psychological disorder has been limited. The next section discusses the characteristics and limitations of the other principal group of clinical psychological formulations, those derived from various theories and principles of learning.

The Learning of Psychological Disorder

An amazing proportion of human behavior is determined by learning. Practically everything we do depends in part on the "teaching" influences which surround us. Studies of other cultures and developing children reveal that our getting hungry at noon, our concepts of colors, our concepts of past and future times, and our ability to see a straight line are all influenced by social experiences; none of these seemingly basic matters is determined by biology alone. By "learning" we refer not simply to instructional learning in educational contexts, but to the broad spectrum of behavior-acquisition principles that govern how the human organism changes in his social context; further discussion of learning in relation to motivation is found in Chapter 3. The principles of human learning include instruction, self-instruction, inference, suggestion, persuasion, imitation, conditioning, generalization, and extinction.

Although the psychodynamic theory of mental disease sprang directly from the genius of Freud, learning accounts of psychological disorder were developed only after the primary principles of learning had been laid down by men who were not themselves clinicians. E. L. Thorndike and I. P. Pavlov are centrally linked with the development of the principles of conditioning, including generalization and extinction, while the psychology of conscious cognitive learning is closely associated with the contributions of William James and E. C. Tolman. Other learning principles, such as suggestion, persuasion, and imitation, are diversely associated with pioneers in the fields of hypnosis, social psychology, and developmental psychology. Since current research and theory have gone far beyond the founding formulations of these men, we will not discuss the history of these developments.

Instruction. A major source of our learning is what we are told about the world by parents, friends, teachers, and others. Although most such instruction is either helpful or harmless, some instructions may have unfortunate consequences, especially if communication is not clear. Many young children have experienced some disturbance because they got the idea, through an unclear explanation, that kissing leads to pregnancy or that defecation is equivalent to miscarriage (Erikson, 1950). In many cases, the child has been too upset to ask for clarification, with the result that others have been unaware of his distress. Well-intentioned parents may unnecessarily inhibit the child by blanket taboos. If the child is instructed that all strangers or all animals are dangerous, he may develop such generalized avoidance tendencies that his life activities become severely restricted. Similarly, if one is exposed repeatedly to racist indoctrination, he is likely to have interpersonal difficulties with members of other racial groups.

Instruction may lead to psychological disturbance by any of several routes. The child who thinks kissing results in pregnancy has learned a *false causal relation.* The child who has been told all animals are dangerous has acquired a *generalized avoidance tendency* with similar results; the same is true of the highly prejudiced individual. On the other hand, a superstitious person who surrounds his life activities with magical rituals might be said to be handicapped by *surplus discriminations*; he makes distinctions where none are necessary, and thus modifies his behavior in special ways which are not called for by the demands of reality. Inept instruction can also lead to *generalized approach tendencies* based on inadequate discrimination; a child who is told that the candy-flavored children's aspirin *is* candy is likely to seek it out in the medicine cabinet. As might be predicted, if the individual fails to learn important discriminations by instruction —such as the difference between moving and stationary automobiles—he may later learn the hard way by conditioning, and perhaps thereby acquire generalized avoidance tendencies.

Self-instruction. People not only learn from what others tell them; they gather a great deal of knowledge on their own. Some of this self-acquired information develops through experimentation or *trial-and-error learning,* as when the child learns to take apart and put together a Chinese puzzle by randomly trying out different possibilities. But much self-instruction involves the incorporation of knowledge from books, magazines, television, and other sources of information. People tend to choose these sources to conform with their preconceptions; they more rapidly forget facts which do not comport with their previous beliefs than those which do (Levine and Murphy, 1943). Thus, in the absence of balanced social contact, a person may select for self-instruction only materials which strengthen his pathological predilections and biases. The evidence is strong, for example, that television, movie, and comic book violence incites violent behavior in some, but not all, children (Bandura and Walters, 1963). Thus, self-instruction may become the vehicle for learned psychological disorder.

As a result of either self-instruction or instruction from without, the individual may rehearse, practice, and act on what he has learned either alone or in social situations. This again is a normal process which will have unfortunate consequences only to the extent that the original learning was incorrect. In many cases, however, rehearsal may become a fairly continuous process of anxious or hostile self-indoctrination: the individual ruminates obsessively on the consequences of some irrational premise such as, "There's nobody you can trust," or again, "It is absolutely necessary that others like me." As is usual in so-called logical thinking, such premises are typically so far buried in the consequences that spring from them that they themselves are never directly examined. Hence the habitual emotional rehearsal of such ideas may become sources of long-standing anxiety and maladjustment (Ellis, 1962).

Inference. If we know that all men are mortal, and that Socrates is a man, we are able to *infer* that Socrates is mortal. If we know that Jones is a Baptist, and that most Baptists believe in heaven and hell, we are able, by the process of inference, to conclude that Jones *probably* believes in heaven and hell. If we overhear a conversation about something that swims and flies and waddles and quacks, we can make a confident inference concerning its identity (it is a swimflying waddlequacker). Inference enables us to generate many correct or probably correct conclusions about matters not explicitly stated or observed. In social relationships, we tend to rely rather heavily on inference, since people are normally not completely candid about themselves and others.

The accuracy of inferences, however, depends crucially on the accuracy of the premises and theories which constitute the working material from which they are drawn. If an individual reasons from erroneous premises and inaccurate theories, he will almost invariably come to false conclusions. The dubious steps by which we ordinarily draw conclusions from our often questionable assumptions are a continuing horror to the logician and the scientist. The variety of fallacious inferences are treated in many books on logic. The problems of unreliable inference are compounded if the person reasoning is strongly motivated to believe certain things or is inclined to accept *post hoc ergo propter hoc* reasoning, that is, the idea that if one event is followed by another, the first event must have caused the second. For example, at the very instant when the 1965 power failure struck the Northeast, a child hit a light pole with a stick. The city plunged suddenly into darkness, and the child ran home crying guiltily because he had not meant to knock out all the lights! If a business recession follows the election of a particular party to power, its political opponents will be quick to blame it for "causing" the recession. A child may believe that his resentful feelings magically caused the injury or death of a family member. If the boss clears his throat with the wrong inflection or inadvertently fails to say "Good morning," several of his employees may experience twinges of anxiety. Such examples illustrate the many ways in which erroneous inferences may foster emotional difficulties.

Suggestion and persuasion. Suggestion is a process of drawing attention to a possible course of action without particular exhortation or coercive pressure. Persuasion implies the same pointing-out process accompanied by a greater degree of emotional appeal or insistence. Suggestions and persuasive appeals are often ignored, but many are not, and these are important sources of learning. To a suitably predisposed individual, advertising may suggest that he is more likely to fail if he is not dressed in the latest style, driving a particular new car, or whatever. To a certain extent, relief from some kinds of physical and emotional symptoms can be effected through suggestion or autosuggestion, with or without the aid of hypnosis. The "power of suggestion" is also illustrated by the *placebo* effect: a chemically inert substance which the patient believes has curative powers will frequently induce symptomatic relief (Nash, 1959). Some initial gains in psychotherapy appear to be due to the powerful indirect "prestige suggestions" emanating from the expert mien of the therapist and the trappings of his office. People differ widely in their susceptibility to suggestion and persuasion of different kinds; some are relatively autonomous and immune. Lowered self-esteem renders most people relatively more suspectible (Krech *et al.*, 1962); thus the practitioners of both brainwashing and psychotherapy seek at times to engender anxiety in people who are too self-confident to want to change.

In brainwashing, several principles of behavior modification are subverted in order to bring about political or ideological indoctrination. Since work achievement is a source of identity, self-esteem, and physical fitness, the new arrival at a prisoner-of-war camp may be told that he need not work. Seduced by this initial "kindness," he is encouraged to be insubordinate to prisoners of higher rank and to inform on fellow POW's. The undermining of self-esteem, organization, and trust among prisoners isolates the individual to a point where he is susceptible to a combination of threats, promises, torture, and small rewards for collaborating with his captors and adopting their views. Suggestions and persuasions in this context have heightened effect because of the physical deprivation and isolation of the prisoner; dissonance reduction enables the prisoner to justify to himself what he has done and to make the enemy's viewpoint more plausible (Meerloo, 1951).

Suggestion and persuasion effects tend to be short lived and are thus in relative disfavor as primary vehicles for psychotherapeutic change. However, some

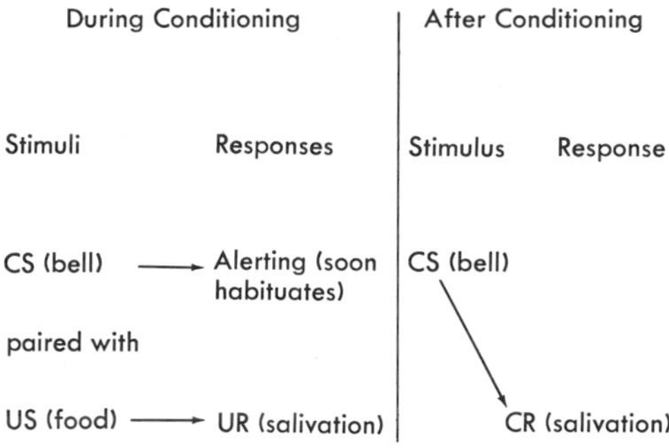

Figure 10.7 The conditioning sequence.

therapeutic techniques (for example, Ellis, 1962), make extensive use of persuasion, and some methods of suggestion involving hypnosis appear to be at least as effective as other forms of psychotherapy for particular disorders and patients (Estabrooks, 1962; Gordon, 1967).

Imitation. Children and adults model their behavior around the visible attributes of people they like or admire. The behavior they imitate may be noble or base, or anywhere in between. Little girls scold and mother their dolls as their mother does them; teenagers emulate the good and bad qualities of movie stars and athletes. Children raised in an environment lacking proper models for law-abiding behavior may be influenced toward crime by older delinquents. Neurotic as well as delinquent behaviors may be learned by imitation. A child may pick up from a parent a habit of hypochondriacal complaining about health or a norm of lying to policemen. Irrespective of the character of the behavior involved, parents become more efficient models for their children by rewarding them and by engaging in rewarding interactions with them. Fuller discussion of imitation and the related process of identification is found in Chapters 4 and 9.

Conditioning. Conditioning refers to the development of a particular type of response as a consequence of specific stimuli which either elicit or reward it. Two major kinds of conditioning are omnipresent in human learning and thus constitute major means of both causation and treatment of psychological disturbance.

In *classical conditioning,* sometimes called "respondent conditioning," an arbitrary stimulus comes to elicit a similar response to that elicited by another stimulus which it preceded. The prime example of classical conditioning is found in Pavlov's technique for developing a conditioned salivary response in the dog. Pavlov knew that blowing meat powder into a dog's mouth would elicit salivation. He found that virtually any signal regularly given just before the meat powder would eventually elicit some salivation. The basic elements of classical conditioning are always (1) an arbitrary stimulus, the *conditioned* or *conditional stimulus* (CS), that is presented shortly before another stimulus, (2) the *unconditioned* or *unconditional stimulus* (US), which is known to produce (3) a given reaction in the animal, the *unconditioned* or *unconditional response* (UR). With repetition, the conditioned stimulus will evoke a response similar to the unconditioned stimulus; that is, it will evoke (4) a *conditioned response* (CR). (See Figure 10.7 and the discussion of conditioning in Chapter 3).

The significance of the classical conditioning process for psychopathology stems from the fact that our emotional reactions are often the victims of accidental and maladaptive classical conditioning. A child who has been bitten by a dog may come to fear all dogs, a manifestly unrealistic and handicapping state of affairs. In this instance, the sight of the nearby dog is the *CS,* the bite and its pain is the *US,* and the resulting CR is fear, leading to withdrawal, at the sight of any dog. Only one conditioning trial may suffice to produce a stable CR, which unfortunately is likely to be *generalized* to other dogs and perhaps even to other animals. If an individual has been treated punitively by his parents while growing up, he may by generalization respond with fear and resentment to other authority figures as well. His fear and resentment may lead him to behave in a hostile or truculent manner and thus to elicit the very punishment he wishes to avoid. Such a maladaptive sequence may become a vicious circle in which both the expectation and the probability of punishment grow with each experience involving authority figures. Thus fear and its ramifications, which follow traumatic classical conditioning, may lead to a great variety of neurotic outcomes (Eysenck, 1960; Wolpe, 1958) and not simply to anxiety or avoidance.

Operant or *instrumental* conditioning consists of the regular presentation of reward, called positive reinforcement, following some specific behavior of the organism. The basic operant conditioning paradigm is illustrated by the laboratory rat in the "Skinner box": the animal learns to repeatedly press a lever which causes food pellets to drop into his dish (Figure 10.8). By contrast with classical conditioning, operant conditioning depends on the animal's making an appropriate response, here pressing the lever. The response involves the skeletal musculature, the so-called voluntary muscles. Although the evidence is still incomplete, operant conditioning in humans seems to occur only when the individual knows or has some idea of what he is being reinforced for (Spielberger and DeNike, 1966).

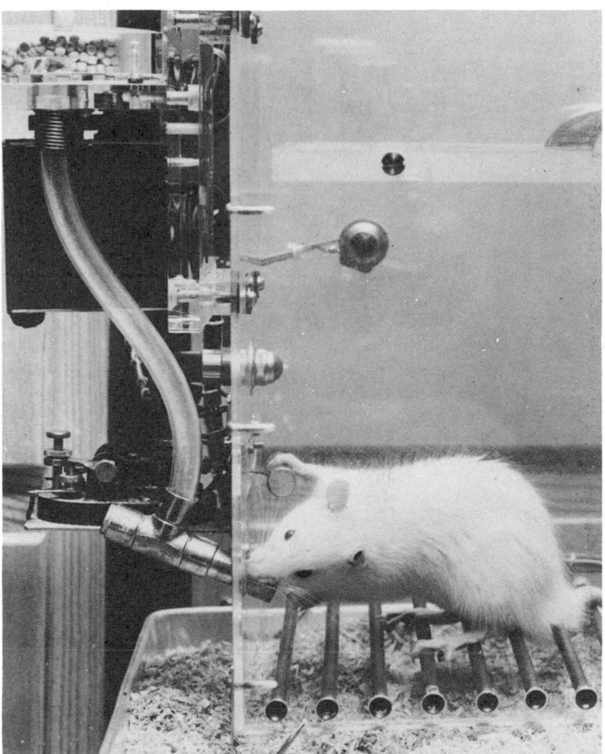

Figure 10.8 The Skinner box apparatus. A trained albino rat presses a lever to obtain food as part of a behavioral research program at the Pfizer Medical Research Laboratories, Groton, Connecticut. Rats such as this one are fed tranquilizers, stimulants, antidepressants, and test compounds and are then tested to compare the actions of the drugs on the rat's behavior. The results of these tests may prove useful in the discovery of new mental drugs and may shed new light on mechanisms of human behavior. Photo courtesy Chas. Pfizer & Co., Inc.

If the young child who brushes his teeth is rewarded by a shiny new penny, the rewarding figure is practicing operant conditioning. Many times, however, maladaptive behavior is established by an unrecognized pattern of operant conditioning. If a child finds that he can more readily maneuver one parent than another, and if parents do not agree on their rules and reinforcement schedules, the child will learn by the difference in rates of obtaining permissions to approach the more manipulable parent and to steer clear of the other. If a tense and depressed person is reinforced by the temporary vanishing of his problems when he imbibes alcohol, the response of drinking will be strengthened. If one spouse is reinforced in making unjust demands by the yielding of the other spouse, the unjust demands will continue

Extinction Paradigm

Time			
1	Stimulus	No Reinforcement →	Response
2	Stimulus	No Reinforcement →	Response
3	Stimulus	No Reinforcement →	Response
4	Stimulus	No Reinforcement →	Response
	Stimulus	No Reinforcement →	Response
	Stimulus	No Reinforcement →	Response
	Stimulus	No Reinforcement →	Response
	Stimulus	No Reinforcement →	Response
	Stimulus	No Reinforcement →	Response
	Stimulus	No Reinforcement →	Response
N	Stimulus	No Reinforcement →	Response

Figure 10.9 Extinction paradigm. Upon repeated presentation of a stimulus without reinforcement the response gradually weakens.

to be made and will probably become more and more arbitrary. One successful theft encourages the next. Maladaptive operant conditioning is better understood in the light of three basic principles noted in laboratory experiments. First, reward for small acts of any kind is likely to increase the probability of larger acts of the same kind; a dictator who has "gotten away with" small-scale injustices will be emboldened to do greater evils, and a timid person who experiences some interpersonal success will be emboldened to strive further to improve his adjustment. This is the so-called *principle of small steps*. Second, immediacy of reward greatly enhances the learning process. An obese person who experiences the immediate satisfaction of the taste of food is not likely to be swayed from his eating pattern by the more remote consequences of being fat; thus overeating may continue indefinitely. Similar observations apply to other habitual or addictive behaviors such as alcoholism, drug addiction, cigarette smoking, and gambling. Thirdly, an operant response seems to become more stable if it is reinforced sporadically instead of regularly, the so-called *partial reinforcement effect*. It is speculated that the uncertainty creates a stronger preference for the operant activity itself through dissonance reduction (Brehm and Cohen, 1962).

Generalization of conditioned responses. It was mentioned earlier that in classical conditioning, the organism may transfer conditioned responses to *CS*'s similar to those involved in the original conditioning. Generalization has either positive or undesirable effects, depending on the context. It is desirable that a dog be conditioned to avoid chasing automobiles, but if his fear is generalized to the mere sight of automobiles so that he cannot be induced to travel in one, problems may be created. In operant conditioning, it is desirable that a child be rewarded for looking things up in books, but it would be unfortunate if this behavior was generalized so that it also took place during exams in school. It is apparent in both instrumental and classical conditioning that we must learn elaborate discriminations or sets of cues which determine the appropriateness of a particular act. The mastery of discriminative cues prevents overgeneralization of learned responses.

Extinction and counterconditioning. Extinction refers to the weakening or elimination of a conditioned response. In classical conditioning, extinction is accomplished by repeatedly presenting the *CS* without the *US*; in time, it no longer elicits a *CR* (Figure 10.9). If a phobic patient who is afraid of elevators (*CS*) can bring himself to take elevator rides (*CR*) of gradually increasing duration, his fear should eventually disappear. In setting up the extinction trials (the elevator rides), the individual might take

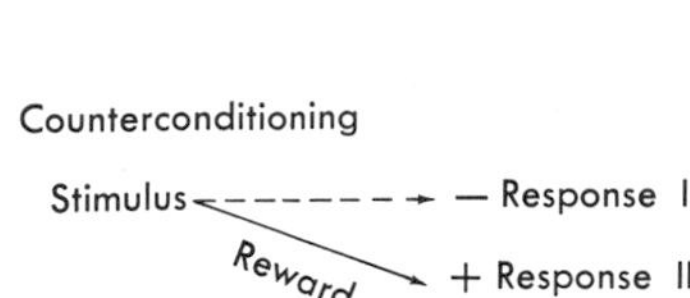

Figure 10.10 Counterconditioning paradigm. A rewarded positive response gradually replaces a negative response.

advantage of the principle of small steps, first by merely looking briefly at an elevator, then later walking by it, then pushing the button but not boarding, and so on up to the response of taking repeated trips in the elevator. The process of overcoming the elevator fear could be speeded up if other people were reassuring or if tranquilizing drugs helped to overcome the person's initial fears. Also, an attempt to condition elevator-related *CS*'s to positively toned *US*'s might be deliberately arranged. For example, the individual could be shown pictures of elevators and elevator-related words, each closely followed by pictures of attractive women or other beautiful scenery. This procedure would illustrate classical *counterconditioning,* or conditioning opposite from the fearful conditions in which the person presumably originally learned to fear elevators (Figure 10.10). Operant counterconditioning might operate by rewarding the individual during or after each elevator ride, or by rewarding a child for staying home and doing his homework to counteract the rewarding effects of playing with his peers down the street. In operant conditioning, extinction consists of simply omitting the rewards. If a child's tantrum behavior is perpetuated by the reinforcement of getting the parents' goat or obtaining concessions from them, then parents can extinguish tantrums by learning to control their tempers while denying concessions.

Analysis of symptoms in learning theories of disorder. Once such factors as brain injury or other physical diseases have been ruled out, learning-oriented interpretation of maladaptive symptoms proceeds to investigate whether the disordered behavior in question was acquired through faulty information, faulty inference, bad models, maladaptive conditioning, or some combination of these or other learning principles. Following such an analysis, treatment focuses on reorganizing the reinforcement patterns in the person's life, providing good models for imitation, correcting faulty instruction or inference, counterconditioning in a desirable direction, and so on. While this might seem to be a fairly straightforward process, "diagnosing" a psychological problem in learning terms *or* psychodynamic terms demands a thorough scrutiny of the patient's symptoms in relation to his environment and general adjustment. Learning-oriented therapists must be ready to reformulate their interpretations of the patient's symptoms, and thus their treatment plans, in the light of new evidence. For example, in the case of a child's refusal to go to school, which is generally termed "school phobia," the causes leading to this symptom may invoice a bully or a punitive teacher at school, a desire to stay with the mother which she may unwittingly reinforce because of loneliness, a fear that something might happen to the mother while the child is away at school, the child's inability to compete successfully in peer group activities, and so on. All these possibilities should be checked. The things disturbed individuals find positively reinforcing are often surprising. Children who get an insufficient amount of positive rewarding attention will find even punishing attention from adults reinforcing. Adult neurotics may find reward in discovering flaws in others, in keeping their spouse or child emotionally disturbed and inadequate, or in creating pain and humiliation in their sexual relations. If such aspects of problem situations are not brought to light, learning-oriented therapy will presumably fail. Eric Berne, in a stimulating book titled *Games People Play* (1964), has called attention to the paradoxical goals neurotics often aim for in their interpersonal relations. There would appear to be no simple means of discovering neurotic aims, however, other than careful assessment both before and during treatment. Often, neurotic maneuvers result from covert fears. The alcoholic's wife may want him to remain alcoholic because she fears that, if he were really adequate, he would reject her. The compulsively active businessman may drive himself to a heart attack because he is terribly afraid of potential ridicule from competitors. If fears of this sort can be identified, appropriate means may be set up for relieving them. While some such specific problems may be diagnosed in a way which is reminiscent of psychodynamic anxiety-defense theories, the following section will serve to point up contrasts between the learning and dynamic approaches.

Comparison of Psychodynamic and Learning Theories

In theory, the best comparison of psychodynamic and learning theories of psychopathology would be a carefully controlled study of treatment outcomes based on each class of methods. However, it is impossible to compare results adequately in any direct and simple way. Eventually it may be possible to determine the relative merits of dynamic and learning theory therapies, but for the present, we must be content to specify certain broadly uniting and differentiating characteristics of the two approaches as they are now articulated.

1. *There is no absolute distinction between "dynamic" and "learning" approaches; both have much subject matter in common.* Psychodynamic and learning accounts both recognize certain biologically based motives and learned derivatives of them. In Freudian theory, these are considered id impulses; in learning theory, they are called drives, and the especially powerful reinforcing properties of sexual and aggressive drives are conceded. Both approaches accept the concept of unconscious motivation and the importance of conflict between motives. Moreover, both approaches recognize the fact that motives may become chained; a person may be motivated to catch a bus to buy some flowers for his wife to make her sexually receptive; thus the basic sexual motive may be transformed into motives with various subgoals. While there is disagreement concerning the number and relative independence of certain motives or needs, learning theory rests on much the same motivational base as psychodynamic theory.

2. *Psychodynamic theory stresses early childhood experiences and psychosexual development; learning theory emphasizes the recent past and the perpetuation of symptoms by current conditions.* Learning theorists are inclined to deny the primary determination of behavior by the first five years of life and are prone to dismiss the notion of biologically determined psychosexual stages. They point out that the same parents who are supposedly responsible for infantile trauma remain with the child for years afterward, and thus may influence his personality development far after such events as weaning and toilet training have been forgotten. Thus correlations between infant care and later personality might have no

direct causal significance, but rather might only indicate that the same parents contributed to both (Orlansky, 1949). Learning theorists look for current fears, reinforcements, and misconceptions as the perpetuators of current symptoms, although they concede that adult symptoms might have been learned in childhood.

3. *Psychodynamic therapies are oriented toward general personality change; learning theory therapies toward specific symptom relief.* Psychodynamic diagnostic formulations frequently imply that the symptoms are only the surface manifestation of psychological disease or retarded development in the total personality. Thus, therapeutic goals are couched in terms of a slow "recovery of health" or a slow growth of psychosexual maturity achieved by the arduous "working through" of much repressed material. Learning-oriented therapists stress the probable independence of the patient's problems from the rest of his personality. In the case of multiple symptoms, they may set up multiple treatment programs, but they do not conceive of themselves as reconstructing the total personality or large parts of it. They tend to deny the efficacy of psychodynamic approaches, saying that such methods often achieve neither symptom relief nor basic personality change; and they tend to treat patients for much briefer periods of time than psychodynamic therapists do. Psychodynamic theorists reply that the symptomatic relief effected by learning therapies is only temporary, or that it will give rise to new "substitute" symptoms since basic conflicts remain unresolved. But while learning techniques sometimes fail to effect permanent changes, there is no clear evidence that the changes induced by extensive psychoanalytic therapy are more permanent; moreover, there appears to be relatively little "symptom substitution" as a result of symptomatic relief in learning therapies (Yates, 1960). Wolpe (1961), in reviewing the permanence of improvement after nonpsychoanalytic therapy for neurotic symptoms, found that 173 of 177 patients who had benefited from treatment maintained their gains through follow-up periods ranging from one to fifteen years. Thus it would appear that both relapse and symptom substitution are rare among neurotic patients who initially profit from nonpsychoanalytic therapy. Even in the treatment of addictive disorders, in which relapse rates commonly range from 20 to 50 percent or even higher, the development of substitute symptoms is quite unusual (Blake, 1965; Rachman, 1965). Moreover, symptom substitution is not encountered to any significant extent in the treatment of habit disorders such as nocturnal enuresis (Jones, 1960; Lovibond, 1963) or writer's cramp (Sylvester and Liversedge, 1960). Frequently positive, rather than substitute negative, personality changes are seen after successful symptomatic treatment (Davidson and Douglas, 1950); apparently freedom from some specific disabilities permits the individual to handle remaining problems more successfully. Hence for a broad range of psychological problems, the notion of symptom substitution has little empirical foundation and may generally be more the exception than the rule.

4. *Psychodynamic theorists emphasize the symbolic aspects of symptoms, while learning theorists tend to see the same behaviors as nonsymbolic.* Especially with respect to phobias, obsessive-compulsive symptoms, hysterias, and delinquent behavior, learning-oriented therapists tend to see the symptoms as directly and specifically learned, whereas psychodynamicists see them as symbolizing deeper disturbances. For example, psychodynami-

cists might view a child's stealing as representing an attempt to steal the love of which he had been deprived. Learning theorists would view the same behavior as an event reinforced by its consequences—the stolen objects themselves, peer group approval, distress to disliked parents—and insufficiently inhibited by the combination of disapproval, good example, reinforcement for impulse control, and so on which normally operates to control such behaviors. While learning-oriented therapists might recognize symbolism in the patient's words and his responses to personality tests, they would not ordinarily attempt to treat the patient by means of symbolic interpretation. Instead, they would concentrate on changing the particular behaviors and subjective distresses which trouble the patient or those around him.

5. *Psychodynamic formulations focus on the appearance of relatively novel behaviors; learning theories on the perpetuation of behaviors as maladaptive habits.* If a hitherto normal person without warning declares himself to be Christ, we tend to invoke psychodynamic processes to explain his act; we hypothesize that some stresses led him to the sudden eruption of delusional defenses. If, on the other hand, we hear of a patient who has gradually relinquished more and more of his duties on the excuse of illness, without organic basis, we tend to think of this as the gradual acquisition of an avoidance response. In general, sudden shifts in behavior tend to evoke psychodynamic explanations; while slow changes make us think of conditioning or extinction. In part, this distinction is the accidental consequence of the fact that learning approaches to clinical phenomena have stemmed mainly from behavioristic models that emphasize gradual acquisition of responses. Cognitive processes have been left to the province of psychodynamics despite their foundations in the psychology of learning. To some extent, the same can be said of imitation and suggestion processes, and of instruction and self-instruction. Thus, learning theory explanations, with some significant exceptions, are largely couched in the language of classical and instrumental conditioning. This one-sided emphasis will probably lessen with time as learning-oriented therapists come to assimilate the psychology of cognition and perception into their position.

One factor which has prolonged the artificial partition of learning and dynamic explanations has been the phenomenon of generalization, coupled with the ancillary concept of response equivalence. If a person solves a problem even remotely similar to other problems he has previously mastered, the gradualist explanation is that certain habits have been transferred from the old to the new problem, without "insight" or cognition. If a child lacks a toy hammer and uses a toy baseball bat instead, it is an open question whether he had a "bright idea" or simply generalized habits learned with one object to another similar one.

If an individual is unable to telephone and sends a telegram instead, this too may be described without reference to thinking processes by the notion of a *class* of responses—in this case, "notification responses"—that have been learned *as a class* in similar reinforcement circumstances. Thus, even responses for which the individual has manifestly never been reinforced, such as murder, suicide, or claims to divinity, may be considered extensions of past-rewarded destructive response repertoires or pretensions to higher status that have been rewarded in the past. For many such phenomena, no precise differentiation between learning and psychodynamic approaches is possible; either could be invoked in explanation.

6. *Psychodynamic and learning explanations differ on the general efficacy of*

insight and on the interpretation of phenomena attributed to insight. Early and extreme formulations of psychoanalytic doctrine appeared to make the attainment of intellectual and emotional self-understanding both necessary and sufficient for therapeutic behavior change. Behavioristic psychology, on the other hand, has tended to deny the primary efficacy and sometimes even the existence of such cognitive insight (Skinner, 1963). More recently, psychodynamic therapies are becoming freer in their use of systematic behavior modification plans, while behavioristically oriented therapists have become more alert to the cognitive aspects of their patients' behavior. We might predict with some optimism an eventual confluence of these currents and an eventual predominance of the view that psychotherapy involves changes in both thinking and behavior, and that either one may, under certain circumstances, elicit changes in the other. Further research should clarify the conditions under which insight leads or fails to lead to constructive behavior change. For the present, some speculations might be made concerning the eventual role of insight within a sophisticated learning theory.

A. Insight may lead to constructive behavioral change by causing the patient to reclassify something from a threatening to a nonthreatening category. When a medical patient is told by an expert diagnostician that the growth on his skin is not cancer, his anxiety subsides. When a man is told by an expert psychologist that his boy's misbehavior is due to anxiety rather than to sheer cussedness, the parent's frustration and counter-hostility may give way to sympathy, enabling him to weather tantrums and to reconstruct a positive relationship with his son. Such phenomena do not necessarily depend upon the truth of the interpretations offered, but rather in large part upon their acceptance—A mere diagnostic "label" sometimes enables a patient to experience a reduction in anxiety because the expert is confidently able to assess the condition. Should a patient in another land be told by a witch doctor that his manic states and hallucinations are manifestations of rare spiritual gifts, he may become stabilized in the role of mystic or soothsayer.

B. Again irrespective of its truth value, insight may function as reward or punishment, as inflater or deflater of self-esteem. Insight achieved partly or wholly through one's own efforts carries with it the intrinsic reward associated with any successful tackling of a problem. If a truculent patient is convincingly told that his behavior problem stems from incestuous impulses toward his mother, this in itself may be shaming or frightening enough that the problem disappears. But a poorly timed or incompetently communicated confrontation with "Oedipal material" may result in anxiety, seriously undermined self-esteem, and depression to an insecure patient. Psychoanalysis may have a relatively built-in potential for generating anxiety and depression in some patients, since the primary motivations to which it typically traces problem behaviors are socially undesirable and primitive. This is not meant as an implication about the truth or falsity of psychoanalytic formulations, but only about their possible effects on some patients. A minister might achieve positive therapeutic results by assuring a depressed patient that his inferiority feelings reflect Christian humility, and that the last shall be first in the kingdom of heaven, whether or not his words are true.

C. Exclusive reliance on insight methods may lead to chronic self-excuse, intellectualization, depressive rumination, and self-consciousness, narcissistic preoccupation with one's own mental state, or chronic dependency on the therapist. Some fairly stereotyped behavior patterns appear to grow out of long-term psychotherapy. One is seen in the person who adopts the psychoanalytic premise that his early childhood is the cause of his present blemishes. He then routinely excuses himself for his lapses, since obviously he can't change his early childhood. Another is seen in the individual who achieves insight at the expense of self-acceptance, and who adopts a coldly intellectual attitude toward himself and others, seemingly involving much emotional insulation. Still another pattern is the agitated defeated reaction of the individual who constantly and self-punishingly analyzes his motives, responses, and failures, who seems to prepare himself for failure through the paralyzing or disrupting self-consciousness involved for him in analyzing past mistakes. A pleasanter form of preoccupation with oneself, but still a limiting one, is seen in people whose therapists' interpretations has been generally rewarding rather than punishing. Their treatment supplies them with endless fascinating material about themselves, which they assume is equally fascinating to others. Any of these patterns of response to therapy may occasion increased dependency on the therapist, and indeed some psychotherapists believe that a highly dependent therapist-patient relationship is prerequisite to improvement. However, in long-term insight therapy, the therapist may unwittingly prolong treatment through interpretations which alternately flatter the patient and arouse anxiety, a partial reinforcement schedule which may perpetuate his coming for therapy.

The Case of Little Hans

Psychodynamic and social learning theories may be illustratively compared with reference to the case of Little Hans, originally reported by Freud in 1909. This case is particularly significant because Freud thought it provided direct evidence of the role of sexual urges in the development of phobic reactions.

Hans's father had contacted Freud because the child suffered from a "nervous disorder," which basically meant that he was terrified at the prospect of being bitten by a horse. In those horse-and-buggy days, this phobia was quite damaging to his everyday functioning. The treatment of Hans was carried out by his father, a physician, who kept Freud informed in written reports and consultations. Freud himself only saw the boy once during the entire treatment. According to Freud, the basis of Hans's phobic reaction was the Oedipus complex. Little Hans was assumed to be experiencing both love and hatred for his father. The hatred, Freud maintained, stemmed from Hans's being

> a little Oedipus who wanted to have his father "out of the way," to get rid of him so that he might be alone with his handsome mother and sleep with her. (P. 253.)

Thus, little Hans is portrayed as being in conflict because of ambivalence: love and hatred directed towards the same person. The situation, however, is even more complex. In addition to being ambivalent, little Hans is also afraid that his father will retaliate against him for having incestuous impulses. This fear is experienced by the child as castration anxiety. Thus, little Hans is portrayed as being in conflict because of his ambivalence towards his father, his incestuous desire for his mother, and his fear of castration. Freud maintains that this conflict was handled by Hans's ego through the repression of his ambivalent and incestual impulses and through the mechanism of displacement. The fear of castration by the father is displaced to its symbolic representation, the fear of being bitten by a horse.

In contrast to Freud, Wolpe and Rachman (1960), who rely on Freud's descriptive material in building their case, explain Hans's phobia in terms of social learning theory. His fear of horses is seen simply as a conditioned anxiety response. The reader should keep in mind that the disagreement between the psychoanalytic and the social learning views is theoretical, not empirical. The behavioral data have not changed, but the selection and interpretation of data have.

Freud indicated that the onset of the phobic reaction could be traced to a bus ride. Hans was with his mother and became very frightened when the horse which pulled the bus fell down and was hurt. Hans is quoted as saying,

> I only got it [the phobia] then. When the horse and the bus fell down, it gave me such a fright, really. That was when I got the nonsense. (P. 146.)

This was confirmed by the boy's father and mother. Freud interprets this incident as merely the precipitating cause of Hans's phobia. He maintained that the real basis lies in the intrapsychic conflict which was evident in little Hans during the Oedipal period.

Wolpe and Rachman, however, maintain that this incident is, in fact, "the cause of the entire disorder" (p. 146). They point out that Hans had previously a number of unpleasant experiences which probably sensitized him to horses. These involved seeing horses beaten, being hurt while playing "horses," and being warned by a friend's father to avoid horses because they might bite him. In other words, a fear response had partially been conditioned, and the incident on the bus represented the final learning trial which established it. Once established by classical conditioning, the phobic response was maintained by operant conditioning: each time Hans successfully avoided a horse, his anxiety was reduced and his avoidance behavior reinforced.

PSYCHOLOGICAL DISTURBANCES AND CONTEMPORARY SOCIETY

Psychology defines itself primarily as the science of the behavior of individual organisms. As such, it is not its concern to focus centrally on the group, ethnic, societal, and cultural influences that affect large numbers of people. Yet precisely because these factors operate so pervasively, it is important that they receive careful consideration. The significance of large-scale social *changes* is doubly important to emphasize to the college student because his life experience may not be sufficiently long or broad to enable him to observe firsthand the depth and rapidity of change in contemporary society. It is only in the perspective of the past, and of other societies, that many of the characteristic aspects of our own way of life become clear. What most pervades our existence may be least contemplated simply *because* it is so omnipresent; it is only when we consider societies in which different generations of a family live together, or in which the entire economy is dependent on the world price of coffee, that we gain a comparative understanding of our own family customs and our own economic systems. In this connection, it has been said, "The fish will be the last to discover the water." The disciplines of anthropology, economics, history, philosophy, political science, sociology, and theology have each made unique and extensive contributions to man's understanding of his condition. This section will treat very briefly some of the principal factors discussed in these fields pertinent to the problem of individual maladjustment and disturbance in modern America. The discussion will center around three interrelated topics: (1) the rapid growth and change in science, technology, and population; (2) heterogeneity and evolution in normative standards; and (3) intergroup and international tensions. To highlight some of these factors, we first present fictional abstracted descriptions of three contemporary Americans differing in *socioeconomic status*:

Hurlburt High. Hurlburt High was born to fashionably placed parents. His great-grandfather had accumulated the family fortune by means his father found it inconvenient to discuss. Hurlburt's father, highly placed in the family firm, devoted much of his time to political and philanthropic activity. At private school and college, Hurlburt associated with friends from similar backgrounds and became a connoisseur in matters of dress and the arts, and also in sex, liquor, and tobacco. His political beliefs were conservative: certainly he could not see turning over the country, for which his ancestors fought the Revolutionary War, to upstart minorities. His attitude toward society was generally one of bemused indifference; he made it a point to take nothing too seriously. He planned for a career in finance, for which his family contacts stood him in good stead. Sometimes he lamented the fact that his middle-class acquaintances in college were too grubbily oriented toward careers, lacked a breadth of knowledge or else spouted it competitively, and were vaguely uncomfortable in his rather bland presence.

Hurlburt made a suitably decorous marriage with a similarly placed girl to whom, as to everything else, he was not overly attached. His wife felt he preferred the company of his old college and prep school chums, some of whom she suspected of being homosexual. She managed to develop her own sphere of life, actively presiding over social events, enjoying travel, and developing an excellent collection of antique silver and crystal. Occasionally she experienced fits of depression and drank heavily, and was discreetly treated by a psychiatrist friend of the family.

Raising a family, Hurlburt found his son developing too great an interest in sports cars and wenching with girls of inferior station. He managed to have various legal scrapes involving his son hushed up, including the traffic death of a little girl. Mr. High's influence was widespread; he was unknown to the inhabitants of the South American country whose dictatorial government was supported by the concern in which he owned considerable stock, but then he was not himself especially aware of the more questionable operations of this company. In his own circle, he was widely respected for his substantial volunteer efforts for charity, and as a valuable man for advice on picking a bank president, an investment portfolio, or a good cigar.

Arthur Average. Arthur Average was the child of industrious middle-class parents who strove to give their children the advantages they themselves had lacked. His mother, constantly concerned over what the neighbors thought, always kept the house and children scrupulously neat. Arthur was toilet trained rather early and was taught by his mother to be very neat in many other ways. Because he saw little of his father, who worked in the city each day, Arthur's early conceptions of what grown-up men did were derived principally from television, comic books, and movies. The family placed considerable emphasis on good grades in school, and Arthur felt considerable tension about them but usually managed to do passing work. He competed with his brothers and sisters for the rewards of praise, intermixed with sometimes humiliating admonitions administered by his parents.

On coming into adolescence, Arthur knew little about girls, but acquired what he thought was adequate knowledge from his buddies. In high school, Arthur discovered that his parents were fairly rigid and did not understand him, also that there were important things to be learned outside the schoolbooks emphasized by his parents and teachers. He questioned family political and religious beliefs, but soon learned the advantages of keeping nonconformist thoughts to himself. In college, Arthur's fraternity friends thought much as he did, and he settled on a career in engineering, forgetting in time his political and religious iconoclasms, which he had espoused mainly for shock value anyway.

Following graduation and marriage, Arthur found that the duties of his job were more preoccupying than he had expected. The workaday worries and family crises seemed somehow to be met; somewhat surprisingly, he found himself thinking and acting much as he recalled his father. He had little time for reading except as it touched on his work; he did not feel deeply religious, but attended church regularly, largely because of his wife's influence. He was active in local businessmen's groups. Arthur's goals centered around the advancement of his career; his work associates, largely through challenging banter, kept the edge on his achievement drive. When he received a promotion, Arthur felt it necessary to sever certain social ties, and every so often the family moved to a better house in a different part of town. Mr. Average felt somewhat uneasy about the ephemeral character of his friendships and at the extent to which his social life was taken up with entertaining people from the office, but he did not really have either the time or the inclination to reflect deeply on such matters. His wife occasionally annoyed him with suggestions that he change certain things to comport with the higher station to which he had ascended. Realizing that he was able to give little of himself to the family because of work pressures, in the domestic sphere he usually acceded gracefully to his wife's judgment. New innovations in engineering at first attracted his keen interest, but as years passed, Arthur felt that new developments were getting away from him. Moreover, he was now principally an administrator rather than an engineer and felt conflicted and strained by human relations problems for which he was not trained. Three times in the course of his career he was promoted to a branch factory in a different city. The children had mixed feelings about these moves, but by now possessed the adaptability and social skills to make new friends readily. Mr. and Mrs. Average saw little of their parents and sometimes felt bad about this. But since the older generation appeared to be getting steadily more stodgy and harder to get along with anyway, they reluctantly concluded it was just as well their visits were infrequent and brief.

Mr. Average developed tension headaches during his strenuous work activities and worried about his blood pressure. He found that a few drinks helped to steady his nerves, but his wife objected to alcohol, so he switched to tranquilizers. Mrs. Average worried about Arthur's tendency to berate and make off-color jokes about minority groups, which was especially noticeable when a younger Negro co-worker received a promotion Arthur had sought.

Mr. Average was beginning to wonder about his declining energies in relation to the increasing financial requirements necessary to see his children through college. He felt that it was difficult to communicate with his children, and Mrs. Average also worried that they were moving with too fast a crowd. One of the sons seemed to be drifting in the direction of bohemianism and radical politics. Mr. Average did not have the reading time necessary to rebut his son's arguments, so he resorted to sloganizing, which impressed the son not at all. At times, the home seemed to Mrs. Average to be principally a refueling station for its members, who would eat, sleep, and watch television without really communicating or sharing each other's lives. Every so often all of the family members wondered about international tensions. Discussions on this topic ended in stereotyped disagreements, coupled with a feeling that nobody could do much on his own to change the situation. Defense contracts accounted for a substantial percentage of Mr. Average's firm's business.

Lonnie Lowe. Lonnie Lowe never knew his real father. The man who lived with his mother said little to Lonnie and was inclined to answer questions with a slap. Lonnie quickly learned not to ask questions and spent most of his childhood on the streets and doorsteps of his slum neighborhood. His first two years of school were a frustrating experience because of a perceptual-motor problem which was unrecognized by the teachers or school authorities; they atttributed his reading disability to a combination of mental retardation and a trouble-making attitude. After the true nature of the problem was diagnosed, his mother was bilked by a quack doctor who promised a miraculous cure. Because the family's income was low, treatment had to be postponed another year.

The things his schoolbooks contained seemed very distant and unreal to Lonnie, and to salvage his hurt feelings when he failed to read satisfactorily, he pulled girls' hair and created commotions to get some attention. As he neared adolescence, he was beaten up by a teenage gang that came from a few blocks away. Lonnie and his friends organized their own gang in self-defense. In a "rumble," Lonnie acquired a scar which made him look tough to boys but which repelled girls. Lonnie found that he could still impress some girls by being tough with them. To supplement the family income, Lonnie dropped out of high school as soon as he could. He was barely passing anyway. Realizing that promotion was unlikely in his job as a gas station attendant, Lonnie joined the army just ahead of the draft. He took poorly to discipline and was discharged "at the convenience of the government" after serving time in the stockade. Returning to civilian life, Lonnie found his lack of education and bad service record an effective bar to employment. In a publicly supported job training program, his perceptual-motor problem reappeared, apparently because of the emotional stress of the situation coupled with his desperate desire to succeed. He moved in with relatives, then lived briefly with a woman whose husband deserted her. When his promises ran out, he was arrested on a charge of narcotics possession. In prison, he learned a lot about techniques of crime and was forced into homosexual activity at the point of a handmade knife. Knowing that he will be unemployable on his release, Lonnie presently contemplates getting into the numbers racket in his home town, whose operations he has been familiar with since early childhood.

These brief and abstracted life pictures may serve to illustrate the general cultural climate in which some kinds of contemporary maladjustments originate. Such longitudinal descriptions may also convey some impression of the progressive and self-reinforcing nature of past experience on the individual. Nothing succeeds like success and nothing fails like failure. Initially disadvantageous circumstances lead, in the absence of intelligent and persistent efforts to the contrary, to increased likelihood of failure, decreased communication, alienation, and hostility. Early mischance is perpetuated in the individual's anxiety that he will again be found inept and rejected. To defend against this anxiety, he may beat others to the punch by rejecting them first. Another general observation which might be drawn from these descriptions is that certain kinds of psychological disorders are more prevalent in certain social strata. The most severe incidence of disorder is found in the lowest socioeconomic stratum (Hollingshead and Redlich, 1958; Riessman *et al.*, 1964). It is one of the great ironies of our time that the poor, who are most in need of mental health services, are "served" chiefly by inadequate educational facilities, hostile police, untrained ministers, and overworked health and welfare workers.

The Rapid Growth of Technology and Population

It has been estimated that 90 percent of all the scientists that ever lived are alive today. The growth of each science facilitates the growth of others, and the net result has been a "knowledge explosion" which at once provides for a rapidly growing population and vastly accelerates the process of technological change. In the previous chapter, Bandura has noted that, as standards of role adequacy change, the number of people defined as inadequate or "mentally ill" does also. The central standards of adequacy in our society are occupational, and automation and other processes of innovation constantly make many work skills obsolete. Hence individuals are displaced in large numbers not merely from jobs but often from their basic identity, neighborhood, and community standing. Those remaining in a given line of work must update their skills continually to "keep current" and maintain a competitive position in the labor market. The displaced suffer simultaneous interruptions in income, prestige, and way of life generally. Automation and technological advance create high-level job opportunities as they destroy low-level positions; however, the burden is chiefly upon the individual to acquire the new skills necessary to take advantage of such opportunities. Thus, the rapid growth of knowledge has made life easier and more varied outside the occupational sphere but harder and more complicated within that sphere. Nor does the housewife escape its effects. She must acquire up-to-date information in order to understand her husband's job and her children's homework. The need to relate to the community and to raise her children according to the best current knowledge makes it incumbent upon the contemporary woman to involve herself in a variety of activities. This picture is complicated by the frequent changes of address and status that a geographically and socially mobile family experiences. Mobility itself is a product of educational, technological, and economic progress, of course, and makes possible the attainment of many desirable goals at the same time that it necessitates many adaptations on the part of individuals.

Population growth, which in America results partly from the economic success of the culture as a whole, brings multiple problems in its train. At the present time, population growth coupled with advanced means of transportation has given rise to super cities or "megalopolises" of tremendous size. While the central portions of the cities strive to maintain their livability in competition with the more habitable suburbs, their tax base is eroded by the flight of wealthier residents to suburbia and the demolition of taxable property for freeways. The cities of necessity become the mecca for poor people, many of whom are not native urbanites, but are displaced from agriculture by technological obsolescence or discrimination; caring for these immigrants further strains urban welfare budgets. Yet it is plain that the core of the nation's mental health problems lies in the lower socioeconomic classes (Harrington, 1963; Hollingshead and Redlich, 1958). Unless adequate means are achieved for providing necessary educational, occupational, and other opportunities for this group, we may expect more rioting in the slum areas of cities, such as that which cost millions of dollars in property damage and thirty-four lives in Los Angeles during the summer of 1965. Beyond the cities, population growth and rapid means of transportation press upon available living space and are rapidly destroying the beautiy of the environment (Caudill, 1963; Dasmann, 1964). They raise the specter of various scarcities and threaten new dimensions of stress which will have still unknown, but definitely untoward, effects on the psychological adjustment of the population.

The Flux in Normative Standards

One of the by-products of the rapid expansion of knowledge is that many of the traditional religious and ethical values which formerly operated to control the behavior of individuals have been called into question. Religion as a source of transcendental values is threatened and finds it difficult to maintain its relevance to the contemporary world. Individuals, seeing the widespread disagreements and shifts in normative standards in modern times, may find it hard to attribute such values to the will of an eternal deity. Moreover, the means by which religious values are transmitted to individuals have become attenuated as geographical mobility makes church affiliations transitory and more social than spiritual. In such a mobile society, people tend to look for values in the standards of their neighbors or peers, rather than in traditional authority. America is a nation of movers. When a family moves, it leaves behind some or all of the friendships and social structure that gave meaning to its existence, helped to control its behavior, and guided it in crisis. Although the family chooses its new residence and church affiliation to perpetuate as much as possible the standards to which it is accustomed, there will undoubtedly be some differences from the past. For children, tending as they do to view moral precepts as absolute rather than relative, conflict is fairly unavoidable.

Two special aspects of normative flux deserve special attention. The first is that in a culture where new occupational specialties are constantly emerging, the things people actually do for a living are less and less visible and comprehensible to outsiders. Thus, resources for intelligent understanding of others are more limited. One cannot engage in very deep communication with a person beset by the problems of being an electron microscopist unless one understands in detail what an electron microscopist does. The increasingly esoteric nature of problems associated with occupational roles, even the occupations of husband and wives, cuts down the amount of rapport possible between people. As a result, the opposite sex appears more opposite than ever, and occasions for misunderstanding between spouses are more frequent. Neighbors are harder to talk to because they have fewer common interests, even if they don't move out before very long. Parents are more readily perceived as ignorant and thus ignorable by their children since the old folks don't understand the new math (Morison, 1967), and ministers appear even farther "out of it" unless they make strenuous efforts to keep current.

Another major aspect in the contemporary flux is the interaction between anonymity, transportation, and deviant behavior. It is hard to misbehave in a criminal or sexual way close to home; it is relatively easier on the other side of town, or in the next town, which can be readily reached by car. Anonymity and the automobile provide a context for deviance and escape. It has been said that the invention of the automobile had more influence on standards of sexual behavior than the invention of contraceptives did. These factors, plus the increased proportion of young people in the total population, have accounted for a substantial part of the alarming rise in the crime rate.

While the increasing number of young people contributes to the magnitude of problems like juvenile delinquency and educational failure, advances in technology and the health sciences have given rise to new challenges at the other end of the age continuum: older persons have difficulty finding employment once they lose a job because all skills obsolesce faster and because taking on employees close to retirement encumbers company retirement funds, which are already widespread. As medical science makes it possible for many more people to live well past the typical retirement age of sixty-five, the existence of older people is long on time but short on meaning. Often involuntarily retired at a certain age, they are cut off from the social contact and feelings of adequacy they got from working. In an earlier time, grandparents had the valuable functions of passing on to the young the lore, history, and technology of the society. But since rapid technical change makes their knowledge in many ways passé, the younger generation frequently bypasses or ignores its elders, eliminating yet another source of meaning in their lives. Through the growth of retirement communities and nursing homes, contemporary society has attempted to pass on some of the problems of the elderly to professionals, with mixed results.

Intergroup and International Tension

Modern transportation has created a "shrinking world" in which one might expect people to develop cosmopolitanism through increased contact with those of differing backgrounds. While this trend may be noted, if one lacks skills for relating with other groups and has been further crippled by learning intolerant attitudes, contact will only increase conflict and a fearful sense of "encroachment" on all sides. Religious and racial differences, which give rise to stereotyped misconceptions, become foci for bigotry. Differences between rich and poor nations are seized upon as excuses for plunder by either side. The artificial separation of peoples, or segregation, is at best a temporary and self-defeating solution, since prejudice and negligence thrive when an outgroup is confined to a ghetto on the other side of town. On both the intergroup and the international level, problems of group hostility have been greatly exacerbated by modern developments in weaponry. In a city where practically anyone over fifteen years of age can procure a gun, make firebombs, and drive a car, suppressed minority groups are capable of wreaking widespread damage. International suspicion coupled with the development of nuclear, biological, and chemical weapons deliverable by missiles has generated an accelerating arms race which will require our most strenuous cooperative efforts to reverse (Fisher, 1964; Gardner, 1966). It is likely that man's involvement in the increased complexities of earning a living has increased his likelihood to think evil about outgroups, at the same time that it has rendered him too busy and too competitively oriented to relate readily to those who differ in nationality, race, or social status.

Sociological Factors and Symptom Formation

Anxiety, Tension, Fatigue, and Irritability

As life grows more complex, is lived at a faster pace, and presents more diverse demands, the individual may react with a constant low-level fear that something, including some lapse of his own, will harm him. It was pointed out earlier that attention to detail was characteristic of obsessive-compulsive personality; conversely, detailed work that demands unswerving attention and high productivity brings on obsessive-compulsive anxiety and tension. Muscle tension has been found to be a primary component of anxiety and a prime contributor to nervous fatigue (Jacobson, 1964). Attempts to lessen anxiety or obtain quick relaxation and escape from tension can be readily inferred from the billions spent annually in the United States on alcoholic beverages, cigarettes, and tranquilizing medications. Additional indices of the widespread tension in contemporary society are found in the continuing demand for psychotherapy and religious-philosophical inspiration. A common focus for anxiety, readily exploited by advertising, is social status. Thus myriad products from automobiles to artichokes are marketed through advertised promises to exalt or maintain social status, job performance, or personal attractiveness.

Tensions consume both energy and patience, so that the productive individual may have little enthusiasm left for his family and for nonoccupational areas of existence. Thus when his children misbehave, he may be suddenly and excessively punitive. Or he may react away from his irritations and be subtly hostile and rejecting under a mask of rather bland and overcontrolled propriety. Again, he may have little stomach for the parental business of rewarding positive behaviors in his children; this makes it likely that they will force his attention through misbehaviors or simply ignore him. In other spheres, the tense individual may seek surcease in escape from the family setting through selfishly pursued hobbies, divorce, or desertion. But even if he simply sleeps a good proportion of his off-duty hours, his family suffers somewhat. His wife may feel that she is obliged to assume inordinate responsibility for raising the children; if she communicates this too insistently to her husband, his avoidance of the domestic situation may become more pronounced. It may be noted in connection with the recent increase in the divorce rate that of some factors which historically contributed to the stability of the family have declined in importance. In the farm setting, the husband needed his wife's domestic labor, which is now largely aided by household appliances and commercial services such as cleaners. Children, an economic advantage as helpers in the farm setting, are economic liabilities in a predominantly urban culture where their education is long and expensive.

Low Self-Esteem and Depression

In the competitive work setting, the individual may constantly feel overchallenged by his associates or superiors. In the elaborately subdivided flow of work, his own contribution to the process may be so small that he takes no pride in his job; and yet his own specialized task may be so necessary to the total operation that it requires constant attention. Necessary concentration on work may distract him from relationships with co-workers, so that he feels socially marginal. If a person has low self-esteem, he is less likely to associate with others for fear of revealing his inferiority; thus substantial lower-class areas of cities are inhabited by families who may know little about their neighbors, and thus may have little sense of community solidarity. The physical settings of some jobs, or their requirements for maintaining status distinctions, may create physical or social barriers to conversation during work hours and afterward. The growth of the "coffee break" to offset these stresses may be of little value to the truck driver on the superhighway, or the men in the control tower at a busy airport. If individuals do not gain through home, friends, church, or community activity the social rewards and purposes lacking in their job settings, they may suffer from lowered productivity, feelings of futility, and the various mental and physical indices of depression. If a person is always rather sad-faced, not enjoying life, others may avoid him. The individual with low self-esteem and many worries may thus drift toward a marginal social position; he feels his own alienation from others but has reduced capacities to counteract it. Pervasive low self-esteem may lead one to be suspicious of, or to devalue, those who are friendly toward him —"He can't be much himself if he likes a jerk like me"—or to punish himself for receiving more than he gives in a relationship.

Neurotic Game-Playing

If a person gets insufficient gratification from healthy goals such as work achievement, family and friends, and fulfilling hobbies, he may orient his life to a greater or lesser degree to neurotic satisfactions. The goals of neurotics are, among other things, to gain satisfactions from feeling superior, to aggress subtly or openly against others, and to control others and themselves by disguised means. Behaviors that are engaged in repetitively for such usually unconscious ends have been termed "games" (Berne, 1964). Even people ostensibly seeking psychological help may play games to justify their neurotic ends. Mental health practitioners must be alert to the game-playing aspects of symptoms. A woman patient may come initially complaining of anxiety and fatigue; however, seeking help may be an indirect means of gaining control over her husband by enlisting the professional's righteous indignation toward the brute she subtly describes.

Existential Symptoms

With increasing frequency in modern times, individuals without very specifiable handicaps or problems request psychological help. Generally from upper-middle and upper socioeconomic levels, such people complain of pointlessness or emptiness in their lives, a feeling that their work and play have become mechanical and uncreative and that they are alienated from meaningful and joyful existence. Often cultured and talented, they search for a positive psychological health over and above mere freedom from specific handicapping symptoms.

There is some question as to whether existential complaints should be considered symptoms at all; this is the question of whether psychological techniques can or should deal with problems of the overall meaning of life. While this question has no definite answer at present, it would appear that with advancing knowledge of the prevention and treatment of particular psychological disorders, increasing attention will be paid to more general and less focused kinds of discontent. In recent years philosophical, humanistic, and existential psychology has sought to establish a new identity and orientation to psychotherapy (Bugental, 1965; Maslow, 1962; May *et al.*, 1958). Existential therapists claim that their methods are broader, less tainted with the mechanistic presuppositions of industrial society, and more attuned to the patient's inner experience than other approaches. Their critics argue that the existentialists have introduced a new antiscientific theory composed of philosophical esotericism and obscurantism and tied to expensive long-term treatment methods which are out of the question for dealing with the central, massive mental health problems of the day.

Existential psychology, with its emphasis on the individual's phenomenological perception of his world, raises another pointed query with which this chapter may well close. This is whether the patient's view of his problems can serve as a basic orienting feature of the therapy, or whether essentially part of the patient's problem is his viewing his problems in unresolvable terms. With regard to existential symptoms, the psychologist of a learning persuasion would probably "translate" the patient's complaints of lack of meaning into such formulations as inadequate reinforcing agents, unconscious avoidance tendencies, and so on. For example, a successful businessman who had "gone stale" might be found to have no acquaintances who were his intellectual peers, who could genuinely stimulate him. Or again, he might have artistic talent, but this might be buried beneath the long unexamined premise that artistic people are irresponsible beatniks or fairies. In either case, the patient might become once again joyful and creative if he were encouraged to reach out to yet untapped sources of reinforcement, to new activities and friends. That very talented people can go for decades without utilizing some of their talents reflects a salient characteristic of American society, to wit, the phenomenon of stereotyped role behavior. Under the ever-present pressures to appear hardheaded, practical, and masculine—or in women, to fulfill some sterile caricature of the role of wife, mother, and hostess—individuals may chronically neglect their spontaneous, speculative, artistic, and truly emotional side. The result is sexual and other kinds of apathy. Thus here as elsewhere we may see the interplay between psychological disorders and the sociocultural milieu in which they originate.

The less disabling psychological problems of American society reflect a rapidly changing sociocultural milieu. While the achievements of the physical sciences are primarily responsible for this state of affairs, all the resources of the social sciences will be needed for its resolution. But more importantly, the individual must bear much of the main burden of improving the psychological health of his family, community, and nation. Neurotic disorder is most emphatically not something which can safely be left to experts. Mental health in fact depends on such a variety of environmental factors that it is, in a very real sense, everybody's responsibility.

SUMMARY

Psychoneurosis, or neurosis, is characterized by feelings of anxiety, depression, or inadequacy and by some disordered techniques of escaping such feelings. While classification is difficult, neuroses may roughly be divided into: (1) anxiety states, (2) phobic reactions, (3) obsessive-compulsive reactions, (4) hysterical reactions, and (5) reactive depression.

Two chief bodies of theory have developed to explain neurotic behavior. The first of these is *psychodynamics*, which emphasizes the role of internal motives or drives; the second is *learning theory,* which focuses on external stimulus conditions. Psychodynamics has evolved and developed from the genius of Freud. In Freud's psychoanalytic theory, three major dynamic systems interact in producing either neurotic conflict or normal growth. Unconscious conflicts centering about social constraint versus sex and aggression are normally reconciled by the conscious *ego.* The ego is aided in its functioning by various *mechanisms of defense,* which neutralize threatening or conflicting stimulation, at greater or lesser costs in overall attunement with reality. The most basic mechanism of defense is repression or motivated forgetting, which since it is incomplete, provides the basis for later conflicts. In Freudian theory, the child in growing toward maturity passes through various *psychosexual stages* in which his interests and behaviors are organized about different bodily organs and aspects of sexuality. Defense mechanisms are more or less "abnormal" in any negative sense only in the light of their context and consequences for a given individual's adjustment. Defenses may be approximately classified on the basis of their relative contributions to thinking and behavior and also in terms of their general, personal, or interpersonal character.

Learning theories of neurosis stem from experimental psychology. The chief forms of learning by which disordered behavior is acquired are instruction, self-instruction, inference, suggestion-persuasion, imitation, and conditioning. "Diagnosis" in learning terms, as in psychodynamic terms, requires an extensive scrutiny of the individual's problems in relation to his environment. Within the framework of learning theory, search is made for faulty information, false inference, malign suggestions, bad models for imitation, and traumatic or otherwise unwholesome conditioning processes.

Psychodynamic and learning approaches have much subject matter in common. They differ, however, in their emphasis on the developmental or genetic factors in neurosis, their interpretation of the significance of symptoms, their view of symbolism, and their capacity to deal with sudden versus gradual abnormal changes in behavior. A perhaps unfortunate focus of debate is the role of insight in therapeutic change. In discussing Freud's case study of an infant's phobia in terms of both psychodynamic and learning theory principles, we reveal our bias toward learning theory.

Neurotic disturbance has a societal matrix in various salient aspects of contemporary American culture, particularly in growth, normative flux, and intergroup tensions. The contributions of sociological and cultural factors to symptom formation can be seen in (1) stress effects, (2) failure effects, (3) neurotic satisfaction systems or "games," and (4) existential symptoms.

GLOSSARY

ABREACTION—see Catharsis.

ACROPHOBIA (ALTOPHOBIA)—fear of heights.

ACTING OUT—a defense mechanism in which aggressive, sexual, or self-damaging behavior is used as a means of reducing anxiety; an adolescent with hostile feelings toward authority may deface the statue of a general.

AGORAPHOBIA—fear of open places.

ALTOPHOBIA—see ACROPHOBIA.

AMBIVALENCE—the tendency to experience simultaneous feelings or attitudes toward the same object.

AMNESIA—loss of memory for a particular period in one's life; amnesia occurs suddenly and may last for a few days or for many years.

AMORAL—irrelevant to moral considerations.

ANAL STAGE—in Freudian theory, the second of the biologically predetermined psychosexual stages that are crucial for the formation of personality; the anal stage occurs during the second and third years of life and is characterized by the child's preoccupation with his eliminative organs and their products.

ANALYSAND—in psychoanalysis, the patient.

ANALYST (PSYCHOANALYST)—a professional practitioner of psychoanalysis.

CASTRATION—removal of the genitals.

CATHARSIS—in psychoanalysis, the release of anxiety by emotionally reliving the events of the past.

CLAUSTROPHOBIA—fear of confinement.

COGNITIVE PROCESSES—mental processes that involve perceiving, recognizing, conceiving, judging, and reasoning; the processes required for being aware and knowing.

COMBAT NEUROSIS—a disorder brought on by the stress and anxiety of combat.

COMPENSATION—a defense mechanism by which a person makes up for experienced deficiencies and inferiority feelings by striving for superiority along certain lines.

COMPULSION—an irrational, repetitive act.

CONVERSION REACTIONS (CONVERSION HYSTERIA)—a form of neurotic behavior which involves both the belief that one is physically ill and the manifestation of symptoms of such illness; the symptoms may consist of paralysis, blindness, deafness, and such; to be distinguished from malingering, which consists primarily of simulation of physical illness without belief that one is ill.

COUNTERCONDITIONING—inhibition or extinction of previously acquired conditioned responses.

DELUSIONAL SYSTEM—a set of interlocking false beliefs which resist all argument or evidence; they tend variously to make the believer feel more important, enable him to rationalize his behavior, provide a target for hostility, or explain events which he finds otherwise inexplicable.

DENIAL—a defense mechanism whereby a person refuses to accept a true, but negative, evaluation of himself or something he values.

DISPLACEMENT—a defense mechanism involving the transfer of feelings or actions from their original source to another object that arouses less anxiety.

DISSOCIATIVE REACTION—an aspect of an hysterical reaction characterized by disturbances in memory which result in a loss of awareness of personal identity; amnesia, somnambulism, fugue states, and multiple personality are dissociative reactions.

DISSONANCE REDUCTION—a process of integrative thought whereby a person's attitudes and future actions are made consistent with his past actions and commitments.

DRIVES—predisposing forces in the individual, both biological and learned, that sensitize him to certain classes of stimuli within the environment.

EGO—a control system which provides for the orderly satisfaction of the conflicting demands emanating from the id, the superego, and external reality; in Freudian theory, one of the three major dynamic systems of personality.

EMOTIONAL INSULATION—a defense mechanism enabling a person to reduce his emotional involvement in situations that might provoke anxiety, anger, or disappointment.

ETIOLOGY—the study of the causes or origins, for example of a disease.

EXISTENTIAL SYMPTOMS—distress about the lack of meaning in life and in social relationships, but without serious symptoms of anxiety, depression, or other specific complaints.

EXTINCTION—the weakening or elimination of a conditioned response either by repeated presentation of the conditioned stimulus without the unconditioned stimulus or by withholding reward.

FANTASY—an imagining of a complex event or object.

FREE ASSOCIATION—in psychotherapy, a sequence of ideas and images verbalized with minimal constraint; saying everything that comes to mind.

FREE-FLOATING ANXIETY—chronic and unfocused fear; fear that is fairly constant but lacks a specific stimulus.

FREUDIAN PSYCHODYNAMICS—explanations of behavior that derive from Freud's theory of personality.

FUGUE STATES—a neurotic syndrome in which a person loses memory and identity and leaves his usual environment; the person suddenly finds himself in a strange place and cannot account for the events that brought him there.

GENERALIZATION—the transfer of conditioned responses to stimuli that are similar to those involved in the original conditioning.

GENITAL STAGE—in Freudian theory, the final, biologically determined psychosexual stage in the development of personality, characterized by psychological maturity and the ability to love and to work (see Chapter 8).

HALLUCINATION—a false sensory perception which has a compelling sense of reality.

HYDROPHOBIA—fear of water.

HYPNOSIS—a complex interpersonal process commonly involving focused attention, relaxation, and heightened receptivity to suggestions made by the hypnotist.

HYPOCHRONDRIASIS—exaggerated concern for one's health, frequently manifested in magnified complaints regarding minor aches and pains.

ID—in Freudian theory, one of the three major dynamic systems of the personality; unconscious inborn sexual and aggressive instincts.

IDENTIFICATION—process by which a person comes to believe he is like another in some respects, experiences the other's successes and defeats as his own, and consciously or unconsciously models his own behavior after him; the presence of emotional involvement distinguishes identification from imitation (see Chapter 4).

INCEST—sexual intercourse between closely related members of a family.

INCONTINENCE—loss of bowel or bladder control.

INTELLECTUALIZATION—a defensive process involving the exclusion of affect (commonly negative affect, but occasionally even positive) from experience, with the result that only the intellectual aspects remain.

INTROJECTION—a defense mechanism involving the adoption of the attitudes or beliefs of powerful others, often after a period of resistance or hostility.

ISOLATION—a defense; in psychoanalytic thinking, the separation of an idea from its affect.

LATENCY STAGE—in Freudian theory, the fourth of the biologically predetermined psychosexual stages that are crucial for the formation of personality; this stage is reached after the successful resolutions of the conflicts in the earlier stages (oral, anal, and phallic) and lasts from age six to adolescence.

LEARNING THEORIES—theories of animal and human behavior derived mainly from laboratory exploration that seek to explain behavior in terms of stimuli and responses.

LIBIDO—in Freudian theory, instinctual energy.

MALINGERING—deliberate simulation of illness, commonly in order to avoid undesired consequences or responsibilities.

MANIC BEHAVIOR—excited and hyperactive behavior which commonly serves to block out anxiety, depression, or hostility.

MORAL ANXIETY—in Freudian theory, anxiety that occurs because of actual or anticipated violations of conscience.

NARCISSISM—self-love; a defense characterized by placing an overly high value on one's self and one's qualities; often results in boastfulness and in tendencies to excuse one's own faults easily.

NEURASTHENIA—a neurotic syndrome involving constant feelings of weakness and fatigue that are without apparent physiological basis.

NEUROTIC ANXIETY—in Freudian theory, the fear that impulses might erupt into unacceptable behavior for which the individual might be punished.

NEUROTIC DEPRESSIVE REACTION (REACTIVE DEPRESSION)—depression that occurs in response to a severe personal loss; differs from normal depression in its greater intensity and duration.

NOCTURNAL ENURESIS—involuntary discharge of urine at night.

OBSESSION—an irrational, repetitive thought.

OBSESSIVE-COMPULSIVE REACTION—a disorder characterized by intense, irrational, and involuntary repetition of thoughts.

OEDIPUS COMPLEX—in Freudian theory, the repressed desire of a person to possess sexually the parent of the opposite sex; Freud believed it was universal.

ORAL STAGE—in Freudian theory, the first of the biologically predetermined psychosexual stages that are crucial for the formation of personality; it extends from birth through the first year of life and is characterized by a concern with ingestion and with the region of the mouth.

PARANOID DEFENSES—unwarranted feelings of personal importance or the false belief that others are hostile.

PHALLIC STAGE—in Freudian theory, the third of the biologically predetermined psychosexual stages that are crucial for the formation of personality; this stage occurs from ages three to five and is characterized by general concern with the genital organs.

PHOBIC REACTIONS—irrational, fearful reactions.

PLEASURE PRINCIPLE—in Freudian theory, the demand that an instinctual need be immediately satisfied, either directly or by fantasy.

PROJECTION—the attribution of one's own traits to other people or groups; the attributed traits are commonly those present in but unacceptable to the self.

PSYCHODYNAMIC THEORIES—theories of human behavior, often based on the work of Freud, that stress motives and drives as determinants of behavior.

PSYCHOPATHOLOGY—the negative psychological abnormalities.

PSYCHOSEXUAL STAGES—in Freudian developmental psychology, the five successive biologically determined stages of development: oral, anal, phallic, latent, and genital.

PSYCHOTHERAPY—the use of any psychological technique in the treatment of mental disorder or maladjustment.

PUPILLARY REFLEX—eye blink.

RATIONALIZATION—a defensive process that involves assigning socially desirable reasons for one's behavior that impartial analysis would not substantiate.

REACTION FORMATION—a defense that involves a behavioral display that is directly opposite to a presumed (unconscious) motive; thus, aggression may be a reaction formation to fear.

REALITY ANXIETY—fear of dangers in the external world.

REGRESSION—the return to early, immature modes of behavior caused by stress or frustration, with the general defensive purpose of evading the challenges and problems of maturity.

REGRESSION IN THE SERVICE OF THE EGO—in psychoanalytic thinking, a temporary return to an earlier mode of perceiving, thinking, or functioning in order to serve the needs of a realistic goal; distinguished from defensive regression by the absence of clear conflict and by its realistic problem-solving character; often associated with creativity (see Chapter 8).

REINFORCEMENT—that which strengthens a response.

REPRESSION—the exclusion of psychological contents (memories, feelings) from awareness, commonly because they provoke anxiety.

SCAPEGOATING—a type of displacement in which some other person or group is unjustly blamed for one's own failings.

SKINNER BOX—a device for studying learning; used primarily with animals.

SOMATIZATION—the formation of symptoms of physical illness as a defense.

SOMNAMBULISM—sleepwalking; a form of dissociative reaction.

SUBLIMATION—a special case of substitution in which the substitute goals have higher social value than the original ones.

SUBSTITUTION—the acceptance of substitute goals in place of those originally sought.

SUPEREGO—in Freudian theory, one of the three major dynamic systems of personality, representing the learned and internalized moral demands of parents and society.

SYMBOLIC INTERPRETATION—in psychoanalysis, a method for interpreting a person's behavior, thoughts, dreams, and so on on the basis of the belief that what one observes is a disguised representation of an unconscious conflict.

TIC—a nervous twitching that cannot be voluntarily controlled.

TURNING AGAINST THE SELF—a defensive action which results in punishing the self (with anxiety, depression, and feelings of low self-esteem) for real or imagined guilt.

UNCONDITIONED RESPONSE—a response that "naturally' (that is, with minimal learning) follows upon presentation of a stimulus; for Pavlov's dogs, salivation was an unconditioned response to meat powder.

UNCONDITIONED STIMULUS—a stimulus that "naturally" (that is, either innately or with little training) evokes a particular response; for Pavlov's dogs meat powder was an unconditioned stimulus to salivation.

UNCONSCIOUS—a loosely defined collective term that characterizes activities and mental functions and contents of which a person is not aware.

WITHDRAWAL—a broad defense that encompasses a number of response patterns, among them passive failure to accept challenge, retreat into solitude and fantasy, and narrowing interests and activities.

REFERENCES

Adams, J. K. Laboratory studies of behavior without awareness. *Psychological Bulletin*, 1957, **54**, 383–405.

Adler, A. *Problem of neurosis*. London: Routledge and Kegan Paul, Ltd., 1929.

Bandura, A., and R. H. Walters. *Social learning and personality development*. New York: Holt, Rinehart & Winston, 1963.

Berkowitz, L. *Aggression: A social psychological analysis*. New York: McGraw-Hill, Inc., 1962.

Berne, E. *Games people play: The psychology of human relationships*. New York: Grove Press, Inc., 1964.

Blake, B. G. The application of behavior therapy to the treatment of alcoholism. *Behaviour Research and Therapy*, 1965, **3**, 75–85.

Brehm, J. W., and A. R. Cohen. *Explorations in cognitive dissonance*. New York: John Wiley & Sons, Inc., 1962.

Bugental, J. F. T. *The search for authenticity*. New York: Holt, Rinehart & Winston, 1965.

Caudill, H. *Night comes to the Cumberlands*. Boston: Little, Brown & Company, 1963.

Dasmann, R. F. *The destruction of California*. New York: Crowell-Collier and Macmillan, Inc., 1965.

Davidson, J. R., and E. Douglas. Nocturnal enuresis: A special approach to treatment. *British Medical Journal*, 1950, **1**, 1345–1350.

Ellis, A. *Reason and emotion in psychotherapy*. New York: Lyle Stuart, 1962.

English, H. B., and A. E. English. *A comprehensive dictionary of psychological and psychoanalytical terms*. New York: David McKay Company, Inc., 1958.

Eriksen, C. W. *Figments, fantasies, and follies: A search for the subconscious mind*. *Journal of Personality*, 1962, **30** (Suppl.), 3–26.

Erikson, E. H. *Childhood and society*. New York: W. W. Norton & Company, Inc., 1950.

Estabrooks, G. H. (ed.). *Hypnosis: Current problems*. New York: Harper & Row Publishers, 1962.

Eysenck, H. *Behaviour therapy and the neuroses*. New York: Pergamon Press, Inc., 1960.

Festinger, L. *A theory of cognitive dissonance*. New York: Harper & Row Publishers, 1957.

Fisher, R. (ed.), *International conflict and behavioral science*. New York: Basic Books, Inc., 1964.

Freud, Anna. *The ego and the mechanism of defense*. London: Hogarth Press, Ltd., 1937.

Freud, S. *Collected papers*, Vol. 3. London: Hogarth Press, Ltd., 1950 (originally published 1909).

———. The psychopathology of everyday life. In *The basic writings of Sigmund Freud*. New York: Random House, Inc., 1938.

Gardner, R. N. (ed.), *Blueprint for peace*. New York: McGraw-Hill, Inc., 1966.

Gordon, J. E. (ed.). *Handbook of clinical and experimental hypnosis*. New York: Crowell-Collier and Macmillan, Inc., 1967.

Harrington, M. *The other America: Poverty in the United States*. New York: Crowell-Collier and Macmillan, Inc., 1963.

Hartmann, H. Comments on the psychoanalytic theory of the ego. In Anna Freud *et al* (eds.), *The psychoanalytic study of the child*, Vol. 5. New York: International Universities Press, 1950, pp. 74–96.

Henderson, D., and I. R. Batchelor. *Textbook of psychiatry*. New York: Oxford University Press, Inc., 1962.

Hollingshead, A., and F. C. Redlich. *Social class and mental disease*. New York: John Wiley & Sons, Inc., 1958.

Jacobson, E. *Anxiety and tension control: A physiologic approach*. Philadelphia: J. B. Lippincott Company, 1964.

Jones, E. *The life and work of Sigmund Freud*, Vol. 2. New York: Basic Books, Inc., 1955.

Jones, H. G. The behavioral treatment of enuresis nocturna. In H. J. Eysenck (ed.), *Behaviour therapy and the neuroses*. New York: Crowell-Collier and Macmillan, Inc., 1960, 377–403.

Krech, D., R. S. Crutchfield, and E. L. Ballachey. *Individual in society*. New York: McGraw-Hill, Inc., 1962.

Levine, J. M., and G. Murphy. The learning and unlearning of controversial material. *Journal of Abnormal and Social Psychology*, 1943, **38**, 507–517.

Lovibond, S. H. The mechanism of conditioning treatment of enuresis. *Behaviour Research and Therapy*, 1963, **1**, 17–21.

Maslow, A. H. *Toward a psychology of*

being. Princeton, N. J.: D. Van Nostrand Company, Inc., 1962.

May, R., E. Angel, and H. F. Ellenberger (eds.). *Existence: A new dimension in psychiatry and psychology*. New York: Basic Books, Inc., 1958.

Meerloo, J. A. M. The crime of menticide. *American Journal of Psychiatry*, 1951, **107**, 594.

Menninger, K. A. *The human mind*, ed. 3. New York: Alfred A. Knopf, Inc., 1947.

Miller, N. E. Studies of fear as an acquirable drive. I. Fear as motivation and fear reduction as reinforcement in the learning of new responses. *Journal of Experimental Psychology*, 1948, **38**, 89–101.

Morison, R. S. Where is biology taking us? *Science*, 1967, **155**, 429–433.

Munroe, Ruth. *Schools of psychoanalytic thought*. New York: Holt, Rinehart & Winston, 1955.

Nash, H. The design and conduct of experiments on the psychological effects of drugs. *Journal of Nervous and Mental Disease*, 1959, **128**, 129–147.

Orlansky, H. Infant care and personality. *Psychological Bulletin*, 1949, **46**, 1–48.

Rachman, S. Aversion therapy: Chemical or electrical? *Behavior Research and Therapy*, 1965, **2**, 289–299.

Riessman, F., J. Cohen, and A. Pearl (eds.), *Mental health of the poor*. New York: The Free Press of Glencoe, 1964.

Sears, R. R. Experimental analyses of psychoanalytic phenomena. In J. McV. Hunt (ed.), *Personality and the behavior disorders*, Vol. I. New York: The Ronald Press Company, 1944, pp. 306–332.

Shaffer, L. F., and E. J. Shoben. *The psychology of adjustment*, Ed. 2. Boston: Houghton Mifflin Company, 1956.

Skinner, B. F. Behaviorism at fifty. *Science*, 1963, **140**, 951–958.

Spielberger, C. D., and L. D. DeNike. Descriptive behaviorism versus cognitive theory in verbal operant conditioning. *Psychological Review*, 1966, **73**, 306–326.

Sylvester, J. D., and L. A. Liversedge. Conditioning and the occupational cramps. In H. J. Eysenck (ed.), *Behavior therapy and the neuroses*. New York: Crowell-Collier and Macmillan, 1960, pp. 334–348.

Westie, R. F. The American dilemma: An empirical test. *American Sociological Review*, 1965, **30**, 527–538.

Wolpe, J. *Psychotherapy by reciprocal inhibition*. Stanford, Calif.: Stanford University Press, 1958.

———. The prognosis in unpsychoanalyzed recovery from neurosis. *American Journal of Psychiatry*, 1961, **118**, 35–39.

——— and S. Rachman. Psychoanalytic "evidence": A critique based on Freud's case of Little Hans. *Journal of Nervous and Mental Disease*, 1960, **131**, 135–148.

Yates, A. Symptoms and symptom substitution. In H. Eysenck (ed.), *Behavior therapy and the neuroses*. New York: Pergamon Press, Inc. 1960.

Zigler, E., and L. Phillips. Psychiatric diagnosis: A critique. *Journal of Abnormal and Social Psychology*, 1961, **63**, 607–618.

SUGGESTED READINGS

1. Berkowitz, L. *Aggression: A social psychological analysis*. New York: McGraw-Hill, Inc., 1962. A summary and analysis of theory and research on aggression.
2. Fenichel, O. *The psychoanalytic theory of neurosis*. New York: W. W. Norton & Company, Inc., 1945. A compressed and comprehensive psychoanalytic view of the origins and dynamics of neurotic behavior.
3. Festinger, L. *A theory of cognitive dissonance*. New York: Harper & Row Publishers, 1957. An important treatise on attitude and cognition which examines the effects of discrepancy between belief and behavior.
4. Freud, S. The psychopathology of everyday life. In *The basic writings of Sigmund Freud*. New York: Random House, Inc., 1938. An examination of such matters as slips of the tongue, superstition, and ordinary forgetfulness for their relevance to psychological processes.
5. Shaffer, L. F., and E. J. Shoben. *The psychology of adjustment*, Ed. 2. Boston: Houghton Mifflin Company, 1956. An introductory text on personality and adjustment.

11

The Major Psychological Disorders

PERRY LONDON

The difference between a major and a minor psychological disturbance is, like beauty, in the eye of the beholder. Some people who suffer from major disorders, such as psychoses, feel pretty good much of the time. And many more whose problems are like those described in the previous chapter often feel miserably unhappy. It is not much easier to distinguish these classes of disorder objectively than it is subjectively (Noyes and Kolb, 1958). In general, conditions like psychosis are more disabling than the neuroses, more likely to result in loss of job, inability to succeed in school, and need for hospitalization. To that extent, such conditions can be treated objectively as major disorders. On the other hand, it is hard to imagine a psychosis more disabling than agoraphobia (fear of going outdoors), a mere neurosis, and the world is full of people who lose jobs, school grades, careers, and love relationships because they suffer from moderate anxiety and respond to it in just the wrong ways in just the wrong situations.

Despite the many logical difficulties that stand in the way of clearly distinguishing major from minor psychological disabilities, there are fairly widespread conventions, at least among professional mental health experts like psychiatrists, for making some such distinctions. By and large, there are four large categories of disability in common parlance in addition to the neuroses: organic disorders, mental retardation, functional psychoses, and "personality" disorders. Organic disorders are commonly subdivided into those involving damage to the brain or central nervous system and *psychosomatic* conditions, the subject of Chapter 13. Mental retardation is covered in Chapter 14.

This chapter focuses chiefly on the functional psychoses, especially *depression* and *schizophrenia*, and briefly on personality disorders, especially psychopathic or deviant behavior patterns and addictive disorders. About half of all cases of major psychological disabilities in American hospitals are diagnosed in one or the other of these two categories (see Chapter 12), and most of the layman's ideas of insanity are likely to derive from behavior that most psychiatrists would diagnose as psychotic.

As must be apparent from previous chapters, virtually all psychiatric conditions have acquired a large mass of technical terminology, some of which is supposed to aid in understanding the conditions and some of which seems intended chiefly to prevent people from understanding them. The latter serves no purpose but to awe the listener (for example, by saying "dysphoric affect" for "bad feeling"), and even much of the legitimate technical language is now valueless to students and doctors who do not understand Greek or Latin. Even the *Psychiatric Dictionary* recognizes that plain English is adequate to most descriptive purposes; it cross-references ponderous blather like *oniomania* "under its popular English equivalent," *buy, impulse to* (Hinsie and Campbell, 1960, p. v). This chapter tries to avoid technical terms which do not serve to improve understanding of the material. Where they are used, however, as they sometimes are because they are so popular professionally that it is necessary to be acquainted with them, an effort is made to provide clear and accurate definitions in unvarnished English.

The purpose of the chapter is to provide a descriptive overview of the major clinical features of psychosis and personality disorders in the light of current knowledge about their development, diagnosis, and characteristic course, as well as to confront the student with some of the peculiarities of custom and logic that make it impossible to comprehend these disorders very thoroughly. Reaching this goal may leave the reader dissatisfied, for the state of knowledge in the field is endlessly dissatisfying. It is impossible to talk authoritatively about the theoretical underpinnings of the major disorders because there are no satisfactory theories of psychosis or of personality disorders. Empirical research on these disorders is probably too voluminous by this time to be read in the lifetime of any one person. But even though much of it is well conceived and well executed, few research findings are simultaneously very reliable and very general. Even classification (taxonomy) and description, the starting points of all sciences and the areas in which by far the most work has been done on the major disorders, are unsatisfactory. Although *dynamic* descriptions are ultimately the most valuable ones for planning treatment, the dynamics of many of these disorders cannot be described because they are obscure or extremely variable. *Genetic* (developmental) descriptions, which are most valuable for predicting the occurrence and course of a disorder, are often equally impossible because origins are so often unclear, patterns variable, and outcomes (prognosis) unpredictable. Symptomatic descriptions, which group disorders together chiefly in terms of their superficial relations to each other, are of necessity the most widely used, both in psychiatric practice and in textbooks (including this one), but they are very unsatisfactory, as we shall see. It is often terribly difficult to be certain whether a particular behavior is symptomatic of any disorder, or which of two or three or fifteen different symptoms of different disorders is the most representative, or whether it makes sense to call a particular behavior a "symptom of disorder" merely because a legal tradition or convention of public morals regards it as undesirable. Yet as Szasz (1957) puts it,

> Such dissimilar concepts are now all subsumed under the heading of "psychiatric diagnosis." . . . In my opinion, this is one of the reasons why the taxonomic system known as "psychiatric nosology" does not work and why attempts to improve it—which have not taken this factor into account—have failed to satisfy anyone but their authors.

Until an enormous increase in knowledge makes a more unified understanding possible, therefore, one can only try to develop a brief catalogue of generalities from the facts that are more or less clearly substantiated at this time and a very critical mental set towards all representations about them which pretend to be either authoritative or complete.

Whether we are talking about the overall subject of mental disorders or about a particular kind of them, there are some common problems of classifying and diagnosing, of describing symptoms accurately, of explaining the course of development and the dynamics of disorder, and of prescribing useful treatments. We shall first discuss these problems in general and then in connection with individual disorders (treatment, however, is not fully discussed until Chapter 15).

CLASSIFYING MENTAL DISORDERS

The study and treatment of mental disorders has always been plagued by the great difficulty of making meaningful diagnoses of them (Hoch and Zubin, 1953). Modern psychiatry is barely more than a hundred years old (the first modern text on the subject appeared in 1845), and its modernity is largely defined by its emphasis on the importance of good diagnosis (Griesinger, 1845). Unfortunately, diagnosis is not a great deal better today than it was sixty years ago. The most important work on psychiatric classification was written by Emil Kraepelin (1856–1926) and published in 1907. Kraepelin's classification scheme made a number of incorrect assumptions about the nature of mental disorders, such as that they were all organic, and about the "course of illness," such as that schizophrenia inevitably gets worse and worse. It was nevertheless very carefully constructed from meticulous observations of thousands of patients, and while it fell short of its precise aims, it represented the best effort to date at a comprehensive diagnostic system. As Zigler and Phillips (1961) put it:

> A brief glance at its history indicates that the original purposes and goals in the construction of this schema went far beyond the desire for a descriptive taxonomy. . . . Kraepelin not only studied the individual while hospitalized, but also the patient's premorbid history and post-hospital course. His hope was to make our understanding of all mental disorders as precise as our knowledge of the course of general paresis. He insisted on the classification of mental disorders according to regularities in symptoms and course of illness, believing this would lead to a clearer discrimination among the different disease entities. He hoped for the subsequent discovery of a specific somatic malfunction responsible for each disease. For Kraepelin then, classification was related to etiology, treatment, and prognosis.

Since Kraepelin's time, psychiatric thinking about the origins (etiology), treatment, and probabilities of recovery or deterioration (prognosis) has advanced considerably from most disorders, but our ability to describe the actual *symptoms* of disorder is not a great deal better than it was then. The American Psychiatric Association made a very serious effort to revise Kraepelin's diagnostic schemes on the basis of its enormous accretion of experience during World War II in selection and treatment of men in military service. The outcome was an official manual of psychiatric diagnosis, *Mental Disorders: Diagnostic and Statistical Manual*, published in 1952. But the basic schemata of this manual, which is still the more or less official basis for classification in American mental hospitals (and textbooks on psychopathology), do not differ very much from those of Kraepelin's original work. It is thus almost certainly correct to refer to the different diagnostic entities used in American psychiatry as "Kraepelinian categories."

There are many different bases for evaluating and criticizing the diagnostic classification system. One of the most important of these under current discussion is the problem of whether a *disease* model is really appropriate for thinking about mental disorders. Chapters 5, 9, and 10 all raise serious objection to the idea that mental illness really is illness in the usual sense, and Chapter 9 presents the alternative view that most functional disorders can be understood best as the results of socially undesirable learning experiences. Whether or not the disease model is a good one, however, the conventional psychiatric diagnoses may still be useful so long as they dependably describe the different disorders well enough to keep them from being confused with each other. This is the problem of *reliability*.

There have been many studies of the reliability of psychiatric diagnoses, and the upshot of them is that the broad categories are fairly dependable and the narrow ones are not. In other words, two psychiatrists are likely to agree readily that a certain person is psychotic rather than neurotic, but they are less likely to agree about what kind of psychosis he has. A more detailed survey of studies of diagnostic reliability is presented in the next chapter, but the matter is neatly summarized by Zigler and Phillips (1961):

> In evaluating the body of studies concerned with the reliability of psychiatric diagnosis, one must conclude that so long as diagnosis is confined to broad diagnostic categories, it is reasonably reliable, but the reliability diminishes as one proceeds from broad, inclusive class categories to narrower, more specific ones. As fine discriminations are called for, accuracy in diagnosis becomes increasingly difficult.

The reliability of diagnosis presents less serious difficulties than does the problem of validity or meaningfulness of diagnosis. This is a special concern of this chapter because we attempt here to describe the more severe functional disorders, and the question is, "What are the criteria of severity?"

It is possible to consider one condition more serious than another because it involves greater *subjective distress*, but that is not a very useful criterion. The common cold is more distressing subjectively than sleeping sickness, but the latter is considered more serious because it is often lethal. The most acceptable criteria for the severity of a disorder involve more than how the victim feels about it. Usually, they include something about the effects of the disorder on the person's behavior.

In the case of mental disorders, one conventional criterion of severity is whether or not the person has to be institutionalized. This is not an altogether good standard of severity, because some neurotics have to be institutionalized and some psychotics do not and also because it would consider ordinary criminals as severely ill as psychopaths. Even so, the criterion is a useful if not self-sufficient one; it seems clear that if a person needs to be removed from everyday activities because of his mental condition, the disorder is serious (Erikson, 1957).

The need for institutionalization presumably arises because the patient is so disabled by his condition that he is unable to take care of himself outside an asylum or might even be dangerous to himself or others. The presumption, which is not always warranted (Szasz, 1961), is usually made that such a person has "lost contact with reality." It is this notion that chiefly distinguishes neurotics from psychotics (English and Pearson, 1963). Neurotics are supposedly overly prone to anxiety and overly inclined to make use of the ego defenses in their efforts to fight it. Their behavior may be unrealistic, but only with respect to a fairly limited set of symptoms or conditions. On the whole, their aberrations are sufficiently few or mild so that they can maintain normal intercourse with society in most respects. Psychotics, on the other hand, appear to be so overwhelmed by whatever stresses precipitate their condition that their general behavior is unusual to the point of being bizarre.

Another way of stating the same distinction is that most of us are able to see more kinship between our own behavior and neurosis than between ourselves and psychotics, which is why we are made much more uncomfortable by reading about the defenses and neurotic adjustments than by reading about the greater but less familiar miseries of psychosis. In fact, the phenomena which characterize the aberrations of sensation, perception, cognition, and motor behavior which we associate with psychosis are really exaggerated forms of experience common in all our lives but sufficiently mild and transient so that we usually pay little or no attention to them.

The purely descriptive difference between neurosis and psychosis suggested here seems to imply that psychosis is more *unconventional* than neurosis and that, for practical purposes, what distinguishes them is that psychiatrists regard psychosis as a more serious trouble. That is true, but it is stated in a misleading way. The case is more accurately put if we say that when psychiatrists observe mental disorder which is so serious that its victim seems to have generally lost contact with reality, they are likely also to observe that he is behaving in a very unconventional way and to recommend that he be hospitalized for his own protection. When the disorder is plainly less disabling, the victim is also probably acting more conventionally, and the diagnosis is much more likely to be neurosis.

All of these distinctions are rudely empirical ones; that is, they do not really refer to any theoretical or qualitative difference between minor and major disorders. Some attempts have been made to draw fine scientific distinctions between them. The best known may be that of Hans Eysenck, who did an elaborate study of the characteristics of mentally disordered people and, using the techniques of factor analysis, claims to have identified both *psychoticism* and *neuroticism* dimensions of personality; according to his report, these factors are entirely unrelated to each other, which would mean that diagnosing a person as neurotic would not preclude observing psychotic components in his behavior, and vice versa (Eysenck, 1960). The more conventional psychiatric view of these diagnostic entities is that they are more or less mutually exclusive, at least to the extent that a neurotic person is not ordinarily in danger of becoming psychotic. The evidence for either position is equivocal (Buss, 1966).

The so-called *personality disorders* occupy a place all by themselves among psychiatric disabilities. They are usually not classed with the neuroses because they do not seem to involve the use of ego defenses or, for that matter, to be particularly tied up with the problems of anxiety and how to avoid it. They are not readily classed with the psychoses, on the other hand, because they do not conspicuously involve a loss of contact with reality or necessarily appear so severe or bizarre that they require hospitalization (or imprisonment). They are regarded as severe disorders, from the point of view of this book, not because they incapacitate the individual (some of them do, some don't) but because they represent serious social problems. Just how serious will become evident in the statistics of the next chapter.

DEVELOPMENT OF SEVERE DISORDERS

Once some useful classification system is devised, it becomes possible to make systematic inquiry into the development of psychological disorders and to see whether some systematic means of treatment is more useful for one kind of problem than another. Treatment methods are dealt with in Chapter 15 and will not be discussed here, but the problem of development deserves some attention at this point.

Knowing how a condition develops has no necessary connection with doing anything to alleviate it, but it does tend to have a significant psychological effect on those responsible for it. In the case of mental disorders, this has proved particularly true. There are two dominant and opposing views among psychiatrists about the development of psychopathology, and each view has given rise to a quite different perspective on treatment. The *organic* view, whose major modern sponsors were men like Greisinger and Kraepelin, attributes virtually all mental disorders to one or another kind of hereditary misfortune, constitutional accident, or physical damage or disease. As we have already seen in Chapters 1 and 2, there is some truth to this position in connection with some disorders. Its eighteenth and nineteenth century proponents, on the other hand, were too prone to assume that custodial managements and physical treatments were the only possible approaches of merit for what were literally *mental* illnesses, and progress in scientific research and treatment were undoubtedly delayed considerably by this view of the problem. (Bockoven, 1956; Joint Commission, 1961).

The *psychological* or *dynamic* view, chiefly sponsored by Charcot and Janet but boosted to acceptance by Freud, views the major disorders as defects in the *functioning* of people who are *organically* quite sound. The psychoanalytic position and its revisionist variations tend to regard the disorders as the outcome of unhappy events in childhood which are expressed when the individual cannot withstand the stresses and strains of his life circumstances (Munroe, 1955). As we have seen in Chapters 4, 9, and 10 in particular, there is a lot of truth to this position also. At its extreme, however, it fails to make use of the treatment aids that are available in drugs and other "physical assault" methods. Research now in progress on control of behavior through electrical stimulation of the brain (Delgado, 1964) holds the promise of powerful methods of physical treatment in the foreseeable future (see Chapter 16).

Whatever the implications for treatment in either orientation towards the major disorders, it is important for the modern psychologist to recognize that both organic and dynamic factors are often critical.

Organic factors. Although their precise status with respect to most psychoses and all personality disorders is questionable, it is clear that *genetic factors* can play an important role in mental disorders (see Chapter 2). Other biological factors can also operate: *noxious chemicals, physical injury,* and *deficiencies of vital substances* ranging from oxygen to vitamins can precipitate serious mental aberrations (Sourkes, 1962). In all probability, so can extreme stress (Selye, 1956).

Stress, injury, and chemical intoxication or deprivation are all *precipitating* factors in mental disorder, which means that they all *produce* disorders in people who otherwise would not have been likely to get them. Genetic factors are more of a *predisposing* kind, which means that they tend to make some people more *prone* to disorders than others, whether or not they actually develop them. *Constitutional* as well as genetic factors may also predispose people to various disorders, although the evidence for this is less clear (Rees, 1961).

The difference between a constitutional and a genetic event is that the former reflects an anatomical or physiological condition which may or may not have some known genetic basis. *Body type* is the constitutional event most widely studied in connection with personality and behavior disorders. Modern work on this subject was begun by Kretschmer (1925), but it is currently most commonly associated with Sheldon (1942). Kretschmer distinguished four main body types, two of which, *asthenic* (lean and bony) and *pyknic* (stocky and rotund), he thought were particularly susceptible to schizophrenia and manic-depressive psychoses, respectively. Sheldon identified three major body types: *endomorphic,* which corresponds to pyknic; *mesomorphic,* which is muscular, like Kretschmer's *athletic* type; and *ectomorphic,* which corresponds to asthenic. Like Kretschmer, but with more sophisticated methodology, Sheldon attempted to relate his body types to personality traits and disorders. He and his collaborators not only discovered, like Kretschmer, that endomorphy was related to affective disorders (depressions) and ectomorphy to schizoid conditions, but also that paranoia was related to mesomorphy (Wittman *et al.,* 1948). In addition, extensive research by Glueck and Glueck (1956) has turned up some evidence that mesomorphy is found significantly more often and ectomorphy less often among juvenile delinquent boys than among others.

Numerous studies have attempted to relate physiological rather than anatomical functions to mental disorders with varying degrees of success. Some of these, such as the Funkenstein test of autonomic reactivity to Mecholyl, have been discussed in Chapter 3. In general, the results of such studies are tenuous, not because there are no anatomical or physiological correlates of the functional disorders, but because they are likely to be so subtle that only a very refined and elaborate technology can discover them. The very reason these disorders were called "functional" in the first place is that their organic correlates were not obvious to anyone. They have not become very evident, for the most part, to date. Critiques of the methodology and conclusions of the anatomical (Humphreys, 1957), biochemical (Kety, 1959*a* and *b*), and genetic (Jackson, 1960) studies of mental disorders have found most of them wanting. This situation is almost certain to change within the next several years as biological knowledge expands, but there have not been any major breakthroughs yet.

Psychological factors. Psychological factors that give rise to personality disorders have been discussed in detail in Chapters 3, 4, 9, and 10. Conflict, frustration, and the learning of inappropriate or socially undesirable response patterns seem to account for most disorders. Childhood experience is particularly important, as we have seen, in that some periods of development are more critical than others for the learning of specific patterns of behavior. As with biological factors, however, precipitating events are easier to identify than predisposing ones, which makes it easier to associate immediate or gross effects of the environment with mental disorders than early or subtle effects. This fact is reflected in detail in the next chapter, which identifies some of the most important social and environmental correlates of the major disorders: war, employment, marital status, residence, and assimilation in the general culture.

THE FUNCTIONAL PSYCHOSES

The official diagnostic manual of the American Psychiatric Association (APA) lists four main types of functional psychoses and eleven subtypes, nine of which are kinds of schizophrenia. In fact, the first of the four main headings, "involutional psychotic reactions," is a fictional category: it really refers to any functional psychosis that sets in around middle age. As Cameron (1963) puts it,

> All that this designation means is that, if one of the psychotic reactions . . . appears for the first time in middle or late middle life, it may be called involutional. At this period of life, a psychosis is most likely to be depressive or paranoid. . . . Although one is warned in the 1952 diagnostic manual not to include psychotic reactions in this category "merely because of their occurrence within this age group," . . . there is no cluster of symptoms that can conceivably be regarded as distinctive. Age remains the only criterion in spite of the manual's warning. (Pp. 628–629.)

So there are really three main kinds of functional psychosis, not four (1) *affective reactions,* which include depressive and manic emotional states, (2) *schizophrenic reactions,* which account for the vast bulk of psychotic disorders, and (3) *paranoid reactions,* which are dramatic and interesting but so rare in actual occurrence that almost no clinical psychiatrist or psychologist has ever seen one.

General Characteristics of Psychosis

For practical purposes, then, there are really two main kinds of psychotic reaction that require separate discussion (paranoia can be tucked under "paranoid schizophrenia"). Even these involve a common core of experiences that mark them as pathological. Landis (1964) tried to identify "the nature of subjective experience commonly called psychopathological" and concluded that these states possess three common qualities:

> (1) a disturbance in thought process, (2) an uncertain emotional feeling state, and (3) some degree of apprehension about one's ability to control voluntarily one's thoughts and actions. (P. 15.)

A more conventional way of identifying psychosis, as we have seen, is in terms of "loss of contact with reality," which means the development of sensory, perceptual, cognitive, or motor peculiarities. Sensory and perceptual aberrations are commonly known in psychiatric terminology as *hallucinations,* and cognitive aberrations are referred to as *delusions.* The difference between them is that a hallucination involves the subjective *experience* of some strange sight, sound, smell, or the like, while a delusion is a strange *idea* about what is going on rather than a direct experiencing of such events. Most aberrations of motor control are connected with organically based disorders, such as brain damage; but a few, like *catatonic stupors* (Figure 11.1), which are rigid or bizarre postures, are found among functionally psychotic people.

The presence of delusions or hallucinations is one index of psychosis, but it is not easy to diagnose a psychosis only on the basis of such peculiarities. The reason for this difficulty is that it is sometimes hard to tell the difference between a psychotic delusion and a creative inspiration. Sometimes, indeed, the one is also the other and, as was implied in Chapter 6, the distinction is only made in retrospect. Suppose Hitler had succeeded and Alexander the Great had failed. The judgments of history would have been reversed as to who was the military genius and who the maniac. At another time or even today in other places, the same criticism could be made of some things we call hallucinations. Even religious Americans, by and large, do not believe in prophecy, and easily conclude that a man who claims to have spoken with God is crazy. In fact, they would probably consider him at least a little warped if he merely claimed to have had a prophetic dream; everybody has dreams, of course, but many people would regard prophetic interpretations as delusions. The point is that our judgments of what is delusory or hallucinatory are based on an implicit consensus among us about what is real or valid. The reason these things are relevant to psychosis is not that they are untrue or invalid in any absolute sense, but that they lack consensual validation; that is, they may reflect an inability on the part of the person who experiences them to share the common consensus of what reality is in our society. This in turn may reflect an inability to get along by satisfying the minimum demands of society for work, personal interactions, and public obedience to laws. The failure to develop a refined system of consensually validated interpretations of reality, as Harry Stack Sullivan (1953) brilliantly defined mature development, predisposes an individual to bizarre mental experience; in lay terms, it means he is crazy. But it is only the social disability that results from his craziness, not the mental experiences themselves, that bring him to public attention and make psychosis the subject of vital public concern.

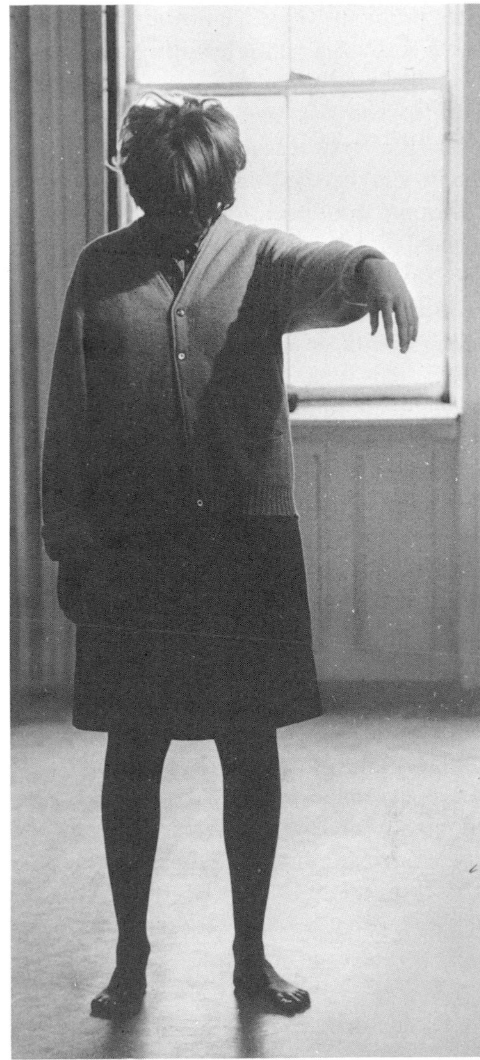

Figure 11.1 Catatonic stupor. Photo © Ed Lattau.

Moreover, the fact of psychosis is much more important than the particular diagnosis (Quay, 1966). Quite aside from the problems of diagnostic reliability, there really is a good deal of symptomatic overlap between conditions, and to some extent, people's symptoms change, so that they may reasonably be put in one diagnostic category at one time and a different one at another time. At all events, and in all cases, it is the presence of the subjective experiences which Landis (1964) has observed, coupled with severe social disability and, more often than not, the presence of delusions or hallucinations, that conspire together rather than singly to identify psychosis.

Just as the categories overlap, there are a number of kinds of breakdowns or severe disorders that do not fit very neatly into any diagnostic category at all, except perhaps the general one of psychosis. *Postpartum psychosis,* for example, sometimes looks like depression, sometimes more like schizophrenia, but its truly distinguishing characteristics are that (1) it is a psychotic condition and (2) as its name implies, it is precipitated by giving birth. Though psychiatrists are always constrained to label disorders as one thing or another, the variety of human miseries still exceeds that of diagnostic categories.

The Affective Psychoses: Depression and Mania

The affective psychoses offer a convenient entry into discussion of specific functional syndromes for two reasons: (1) they easily evoke empathy because they are obvious exaggerations of everyone's experience, and (2) they clearly illustrate the continuity of major and minor disorders.

There are several different ways of classifying affective disorders, none of them very precise. The APA diagnostic manual, in addition to specifying involutional reactions as a separate type, divides *affective reactions* into *manic-depressive* and *psychotic-depressive* subtypes, and also includes a *depressive reaction* subtype under *psychoneurotic disorders.* These classifications are honored by most textbooks on psychopathology, and at least one text devotes an entire chapter to neurotic depressions (Cameron, 1963). In fact, all these disorders share a single critical feature: *their victim undergoes a tremendous change of mood with consequences that are disabling.* In many instances, the resulting condition is so severe that the victim must be adjudged psychotic. In most cases, psychotic or otherwise, the dominant symptoms are those of depression. In some, the main symptom is mania, an excess of excitability, activity, and, superficially, boundless good spirits. And in some cases, depression and mania alternate with each other in a repetitive cycle of misery. This cyclic condition, which had been recognized for hundreds of years, was named *manic-depressive psychosis* by Kraepelin, the great taxonomizer, and it has been popularized as the most common of the affective disorders. In fact, it is not; depression is.

Virtually everything in the affective disorders is experienced with sufficient poignancy by ordinary people to enable them to understand the symptoms of these disorders. Everybody has moods and mood swings; everybody knows what it is like to feel dejected, mournful, lethargic, despondent, guilty, inept, unworthy, and on the verge of illness. The whole array of morbid sentiments, which can be considered as *dejection, self-deprecation, lethargy,* and *bodily ailing,* add up to the experience called depression. The difference between ordinary depressions, such as you and I admit to, and the miserable states labeled neurotic and psychotic depressions, rests entirely on how often they occur, how profound they get, and how long they last. Despite efforts to describe qualitative differences that distinguish neurotic from psychotic depressions, the only real difference between them is their depth. Psychotic depressions are so profound that they are accompanied either by *delusions* or by *motor aberrations*. In neurotic depressions, to put it tritely but correctly, the patient is plainly miserable but not plainly crazy. In both, the experience is enough more profound, frequent, and lasting than among normals that depressives often threaten and commit suicide, even before anyone succeeds in deciding whether they are psychotic or merely neurotic (Shneidman and Farberow, 1959; Farberow and McEvoy, 1966). On very rare occasions, they have committed murder and suicide.

Mania is more deceptive than depression because its symptoms are less likely to be what they seem—expressions of happiness. Even so, they are also easily understood from our everyday experience. All of us (I hope) have had periods of great energy, have felt terribly excited and full of pep for no obvious reason and in connection with no specific event, have been elated in a "nothing-can-stop-me" mood, have felt touched by a lucky star that privately filled us with a sense of confidence and inevitable success, have been full of puns and quips and felt our minds racing at breakneck speed in flashes of brilliance, wit, and delightful disorder, have been certain that nobody around us could keep pace with us mentally or match our repartee or help but be overwhelmed with awe and admiration for our beauty, brilliance, verve, and nerve. It is this combination of *activity* and *grandiosity*, which, run away with itself, constitutes mania. Cameron points out that the diagnostic manual does not have a special category for *neurotic* mania, which is foolish if it is going to have one for neurotic depression. In this case Cameron distinguishes

> between mild and severe manic reactions without calling one neurotic and the other psychotic. . . . Minor, slight manic reactions, usually called *hypomania*, are too much like the mild elations and episodes of self-assertion which a majority of adults at some time experience to make them convincing illustrations of psychopathology. Indeed, some persons appear to remain in a more or less constant mild manic state, and to perform a prodigious amount of work or play because of this. (1963, p. 560.)

On the face of it, manic and depressive conditions are opposites, related only by the fact that they are both disorders of mood. But that is not the case at all, and it is no accident that a single manic-depressive cycle has been considered most representative of the disorder, even though it is statistically the rarest of the affective reactions. In fact, the origins and dynamics of manic and depressive states seem to be almost identical, and the choice of symptoms may depend upon which ego defenses have been most strongly habituated and perhaps upon differences in temperamental energy levels. Both conditions seem to occur in the same kinds of people (the main difference between normals and others for this disorder may be in personality traits that make some people more prone to it than others), both involve the same dangers of violence and suicide, even murder, and both have an extremely high rate of recovery, treated or not. Also, even at their worst, affective psychotics do not seem to be as disturbed as schizophrenics.

Depression

Psychotic depressions occur more often in women than in men, but they happen in large numbers to both sexes (see Chapter 12). Onset is usually gradual but may take place in a matter of a few days, especially after some kind of personal disaster. The course of the condition is likely to be, first, a general loss of enthusiasm and slowing down of activity, accompanied by feelings of despondency and complaints of bodily ailments. The depression becomes more evident as lethargy changes to dejection and feelings of ill health become secondary to expressions of guilt and self-deprecation. Lethargy, technically known as *psychomotor retardation, despondency*, and *guilt* are the chief symptoms of clinical depression. The diagnosis of psychotic depression is not usually made until these symptoms deepen to the point where lethargy becomes stuporous and guilt and dejection become delusional.

Psychiatrists frequently distinguish between *agitated depressions* and *retarded depressions*. In the former, the onset of disorder is not lethargy but tense and anxious excitement and, rather than passive and stuporous misery, more of wailing and wringing of hands and gnashing of teeth. If you picture the mourning at a funeral—how some people are violent in their grief while others are quiet and withdrawn—you will have some idea of the difference in appearance between *agitated* and *retarded* depressions. But the mourning here is for oneself, and it is always colored by a morbid blend of feelings that one deserves this misery on the one hand and is infinitely pitiable on the other. There is no important difference in the underlying dynamics of agitated and retarded depressions; the patterns are quite interchangeable, so that a person who starts with one may shift to the other in due course. It is during more agitated phases, of course, that depressive delusions are most readily reported, and it is probably during them that the greatest risk of suicide occurs. In the extremes of retarded depression, however, inactivity, withdrawal from others, the inability to maintain a conversation, and the general picture of hopeless misery give way to *depressive stupor* (see the figure at the beginning of this section), in which the patient may be so unresponsive that he has to be completely cared for and may look just like a catatonic schizophrenic. In most depressions, extreme loss of appetite and sleeplessness are common. Extreme fatigue, lack of sleep, and hunger, in fact, probably dispose even normal people to mild depression. Students might do well to remember this when they find themselves feeling "down" and to undertake the therapy of a good night's sleep and a good meal.

Delusions are the commonest indices of psychosis among depressed people. Almost all of these are concerned with the patient's guilt and worthlessness, with the implication that his current misery is justly deserved, that he will never recover from it, and that its exposure to other people permanently separates him from them and demonstrates the justice of the secret contempt in which he knows they have always held him.

At an even greater extreme, the delusions may become grandiose and sharp. The patient may describe himself as a monumental failure, sinner, or criminal, who has wrought enormous destruction and deserves excruciating punishment, which in turn may be described in sadistic detail. He may feel that he has been doomed by an immanent destiny, that he is undergoing terrible changes, and that the world around him is being horribly transformed and becoming unreal. These feelings may be largely concentrated on his own body in what are called *somatic delusions*, which may take the form of feeling that he is fatally ill with (undiagnosed) cancer or some painful and multilating disease, and he may experience the fearful events in and around him as ghastly transformations within his body. Since depressed people inevitably become haggard from sleeplessness, poor eating, and often constipation, along with perhaps more subtle changes in physiological functioning, it is easy for such delusions to gain reinforcement.

Hallucinations are less common than delusions in affective psychoses. In other words, the bizarre material produced is more in the nature of bizarre ideas and beliefs than sensory or perceptual aberrations. The depressed psychotic may believe that God intends his destruction, but he is unlikely to have had a vision or heard a ghostly voice bearing such news. In this sense, affective disorders are considered less severe than schizophrenia, where delusions often give way to outright hallucinations.

The origins and dynamics of depression. If there is any single content or idea that characterizes depression, without a doubt it is the idea of *guilt*. Virtually the entire theme of the depressed person's mental life is his own guilt or something that can be traced to a byproduct of his guilt. But depressions are not precipitated by obvious misdeeds, on the whole, but by catastrophic events in a person's life which profoundly threaten (1) his dependency needs, like the need for love from others or economic security, or (2) his self-esteem. The precipitating events in depressions tend to be things like the death of a loved one, rejection in a love relationship, losing one's job or enforced retirement (a common cause among older people), failure to be admitted to college (once a major cause of *seppuku*, or dishonorable suicide in Japan), or, more rarely, appointment to new responsibilities or the receipt of great honors, called *promotion depression*. Why, then, does the subjective misery of depression revolve around guilt and unworthiness? *Is guilt a consequence of depression or a cause of it?*

The predominant view among both dynamically and biologically oriented students of the subject is that guilt is a result of depression or a partial precipitator of it rather than a disposing factor. Concordance studies (see Chapter 2) indicate that there may be some genetic predisposition, advocates of Kretschmer and Sheldon certainly support the notion of a constitutional factor, and there are some changes in brain wave patterns during depressions, though there is no evidence that these changes reflect a predisposition toward depression (Shagass and Schwartz, 1962).

Dynamic theorists are more prone to regard depression as a learned pattern of response to the threat of losing the source of satisfaction of dependency needs. This would be most likely to happen, of course, to people who developed exaggerated dependency needs in childhood, perhaps by being repeatedly threatened with the loss of nurture if they did not comply with parental demands. An effective way to handle this threat and maintain parental love, as we have seen, is to identify with parents and introject their standards of conduct (Chapter 4). For some people, however, this would be very trying. It would result in their developing an overly severe conscience, becoming excessively dependent for self-esteem on other people's approval, thus very conforming, and also nursing a large but hidden bundle of resentment against others for constraining them to be forever "good." In the face of disaster, such people might become dejected at the loss of love and simultaneously feel that they were guilty of causing it and resent that it was happening. Since they are habituated to the use of introjection, the resentment would not be directed against others but against themselves and thus would exaggerate the guilt. Exaggerated expressions of guilt are certainly common among depressed people, who often recall trivial misdemeanors of the past as if they were major crimes.

An important and stimulating alternative explanation of guilt in depressions is presented by O. H. Mowrer (1966), who, in addition to having a distinguished career as a clinical psychologist and an experimental psychologist of learning, himself underwent a severe *promotion depression* some years ago. Mowrer proposes that guilt is a critical predisposing factor in depression, so much so that, whatever the physiological or personality correlates underlying it may be, *people never undergo clinical depressions unless they have a substantial history of misconduct to be guilty about.* The critical disposing dynamic, in his view, is not the threat to one's *dependency* but to his *integrity*. The symptoms of depression occur when a person is so reviled by the totality of his transgressions against his own principles that he is likely to be overwhelmed by any life crisis that forces him to confront his personal inadequacies. The attack of depression is much like a fever, in which the individual struggles with his own infected personality and, through self-torture, expiates his guilt. It has long been known that electric shock has almost (and only) immediate effects in lifting depression (Szalita, 1966). Though painless, this treatment is terrifying, and the reason it works so well in depressions is possibly that it is seen as punitive and therefore expiative.

If a psychotic episode serves as an expiative punishment, then it is easy to understand why depressives, unlike other psychotics, almost invariably recover *with or without* treatment. But Mowrer's theory goes a great deal further than others by offering a self-consistent explanation of why depressions are likely to recur, a perennial problem to students of this condition. If the depression is a response to *real transgressions* of the patient's morality, and the guilt is not just a fanciful introjection of unexpressible hostility towards loved ones, then the feverish syndrome of depression is itself *a fanciful expiation of guilt,* whose results at best can only be temporary because the patient's integrity has not been healed. The depression as such is sheer wasted energy unless it functions to direct its victim towards an active reconstruction of his life. His mental state, in Mowrer's view, depends ultimately on his behavior. The therapy he proposes is one of teaching the patient to be open with others instead of deceptive, that is, teaching integrity, and then helping him to direct his life activities in constructive ways, deliberately expiating his misdeeds wherever he can (1961, 1964). This is an *action* therapy, of course, whose theoretical basis is behavioristic in the sense that it rests more on the psychology of learning than on a psychodynamic theory of personality (see Chapters 9 and 15).

Mowrer's theory is important not only in its effort to understand depressions but because it views depression as a paradigm for *all* functional disorders. It has been widely observed that virtually all neurotics are inordinately prone to *feelings* of guilt, apparently in great disproportion to their *actual* behavior. Freud labeled this phenomenon "moral anxiety," and treated it as a neurotic response to fantasized misbehavior which was never performed and not even always conscious (Freud, 1911). If so, therapy should attempt to free the patient of unrealistic guilt and, in so doing, alleviate his neurosis. Mowrer proposes, on the other hand, that guilt is almost inevitably a realistic rather than a neurotic sentiment, reflecting one or another act the person has performed in violation of his integrity. In that case, therapy should be aimed at exposing the *behavioral* source of guilt and encouraging its expiation. Research derived from this theory has aimed at examining the behavioral history of functionally disordered people rather than only their mental experience and has indeed demonstrated that Mowrer's argument has some real basis in fact (Mowrer, to be published).

Mania

As we have indicated, the origins and underlying dynamics of manic states seem to be identical with those of depression; therefore the differences between them are, in that respect, superficial. Still, the symptoms are so strikingly different that we consider them important enough to observe.

While depressions may appear to differ in kind, manic attacks seem to differ only in degree of severity. Depressions may appear to be either agitated or retarded, but manic states are always agitated. Their diagnostic names reflect the degree of agitation. As we noted, *hypomania* is not clearly a pathological condition at all, but an elated mood which almost everybody undergoes from time to time. *Acute mania* is the label most often applied to severe manic states, and *delirious mania* is the term given to blatantly psychotic episodes of mania. The difference between acute and delirious mania is basically one of *activity rate*: if a person's activity speeds up beyond a certain point during a manic episode, he loses all semblance of self-control in a frenzy of activity which becomes so wildly unintelligible and incoherent that he is virtually delirious. This does not happen very often or last very long for the same reason that *all manic episodes are necessarily acute*: people quickly wear themselves out by the profligate expenditure of energy in all directions which defines a manic attack. When it does occur, nevertheless, delirious mania is quite terrifying to see and is indeed quite dangerous. So it is no wonder that it is the essence (rather accurately) of the stereotype of a "raving maniac."

Because they are so dramatic and noisy, not to say frightening or irritating to others, manic attacks draw people's attention more rapidly than other personality disorders. Friends, relatives, and neighbors all quickly realize that there is something seriously wrong with a person in an acute manic state, and his wild excitement is as likely to cause them to refer him to the police as to a psychiatrist. Manics may, in their excitement, injure or kill themselves or others—more likely themselves. If not forcibly restrained, moreover, acute mania may rapidly produce exhaustion from lack of sleep and sometimes from starvation. A somewhat less acute but more prolonged attack is likely to go unrestrained longer, in which case there is some likelihood that the victim will get involved in zany financial and sexual adventures. He may, for example, commit all of his income and assets to harebrained get-rich-quick schemes, or he may get involved in quick succession with several different sex partners, perhaps even marrying a few simultaneously. Since ambitious, energetic, and outgoing people in our society are normally more likely than others to get involved in unorthodox financial, social, and sexual affairs anyway, it may not be easy in any given case to tell from these events alone whether a person is entering an acute manic episode or just expanding the scope of his normal activities. Manic patients are characteristically more energetic, ambitious, and outgoing than normals even before they become disturbed (Becker, 1960), and the disorder may therefore be even harder to recognize.

As with depression, it is the mood of mania which identifies it, not any change in style of living: its components are great *excitability*, *apparent high spirits*, and a degree of *grandiose self-assertiveness* which seems *oblivious to social constraints*. The mood can be considered psychotic when the grandiosity reaches delusional proportions and the patient starts making fantastic claims of his own achievements, or of his unlimited powers, or of his absolute rights to do anything he wants. These assertions always have the air of childish bragging or of something closer to buffoonery than to any calculated plotting or purposeful fantasy because they are always delivered in a breezy self-inflated manner and, more important, because manics are so easily distracted that they cannot stick to the subject even of their own grandiosity long enough to make anyone take it seriously. The *flight of ideas* from one thing to another which becomes apparent in the endless talking of manic people makes it impossible to mistake their delusions for plans and gives their entire speech a tenor of grandiose chatter.

Even so, there is a kind of monomania in mania such that, however trivial and flighty his discourse might be, the manic individual is frustrated and infuriated by any interruption of it or interference with anything he does. Even small frustrations may incite him to violent anger, during which he may be quite dangerous. Fortunately, he is as easily distracted from anger as from anything else, and such outbursts are always brief.

The psychotic delusions of mania are ultimately less important than the feverous pitch of activity that is unique to this disorder. Manic speech is not merely flighty and rapid; it may become so swift and wild that it is completely incomprehensible. Manic sex behavior may involve endless frantic masturbation or repeated frenzied copulations; one acutely maniacal man was hospitalized as a result of frenzied sex relations with his wife. He would leap out of bed after having relations and mark "the score" on the wall with a large crayon; it exceeded something like fifteen or twenty sex acts a night. Religious frenzies are also common in this condition. Manic patients, sometimes inspired by visions, will preach endlessly to their families, on the streets, or in the hospital, the actual content of their message often degenerating into gibberish. In his excitement, the manic may rip off his clothes, cut or scratch himself without noticing, or break furniture.

The point at which acute mania passes into delirious mania (in those cases where it does at all) is difficult to discern, but the loss of all semblance of control over speech or action seems to be the best rule of thumb for labeling the difference. In manic delirium, the patient may be completely *disoriented,* not knowing or caring where he is or when, oblivious to what is going on around him, insanely wild, alternately shouting, screaming, singing, breaking things, pacing up and down, ripping his clothes apart, urinating on the walls, or throwing or smearing his excreta about the room in wild extravagance. He may rub his genitals until they bleed, will not sleep at all, and either starves or gobbles food like a brute beast. It is for conditions like this that the *strait jacket* and *padded cell* were designed and are sometimes tragically necessary. I have seen cases of manic delirium in which it took six large men to restrain a medium-sized patient whose outburst would surely have brought serious injury to himself or to others.

Acute mania is likely to wear itself out without giving way to delirium, and the clinical picture of grandiose elation is more common to this condition than that of absolute frenzy. But the elation is itself a lie, as is the grandiosity, and the increasingly frantic activity of manics is probably only an increasingly desperate effort to maintain the falsehood of good spirits. Beneath the boisterous cheer lies a profound depression. To some extent, this can be seen in clinical interviews with manics, where it usually becomes quickly evident that their exaggerated statements of good feeling and their swift actions are not accompanied by appropriately happy affects. Their laughter is boisterous but hollow, their movements are rapid but not blithe, and any suggestion of disbelief that they are as happy as they say is likely to arouse fury and insult. As you know, the affective disorders are sometimes cyclic, and in fact, when they are, mania gives way to depression much more often than depression changes to mania, suggesting that depression is more likely to be the underlying condition. Finally, the life situations which precede manic attacks tend to be precisely the same as those preceding depressions.

Ego Defenses in Affective Disorders

Aside from any unknown organic causes that may differ in depression and mania, the choice between them in people who are susceptible to either seems to depend upon the kind of defense mechanisms habitually used. *Denial* and *reaction formation* seem to be more prominent in the response habits of manics than of depressives; life conditions which would otherwise precipitate a depression in them arouse these defenses in particular. To avoid being overwhelmed with guilt at the confrontation of his own inadequacies or loss of love, the manic person denies all such bad feelings and, to reinforce this denial, reacts with apparently opposite feelings and mentally reconstructs the world on the basis of them. Thus his grandiosity: instead of being inadequate, he is superadequate; instead of being unloved and unlovable, he is irresistibly attractive and the darling of others; instead of being doomed and damned, he is God's chosen emissary to save or condemn others. And if he can work intensely enough at creating these impressions, maybe he can convince himself and others that they are true. Thus the manic's frenzy, and his obliviousness to the needs or responses of others. Beneath it all, but not far enough beneath to preserve his sanity, is the blitter gloom of depression.

Schizophrenia

Most hospitalized psychotics are schizophrenic, not just because schizophrenia occurs more commonly than other psychoses but also because recovery from it is slower and more doubtful. Most schizophrenics, on the other hand, are probably never hospitalized at all because they are never formally diagnosed and because they are able to make quietly miserable adjustments to life which keep them from being the objects of adverse public scrutiny. Unlike the affective disorders, the schizophrenias, by and large, are quiet tragedies, whose victims tend more to be withdrawn, isolated, and turned into themselves than to drench the world with their unhappiness (Figure 11.2). In fact, the *secondary symptoms* of schizophrenia, delusions and hallucinations, are more likely to cause hospitalization than the *primary symptoms*, disordered thinking and social and emotional withdrawal, because secondary aspects of these disorders attract most attention. But there are schizophrenics aplenty in brothels and hobo jungles, on the skid row of every major city, in county jails and transient labor centers, and sitting quietly in middle-class homes watching television sixteen hours every day. These are the most pervasive—and puzzling—of the functional psychoses.

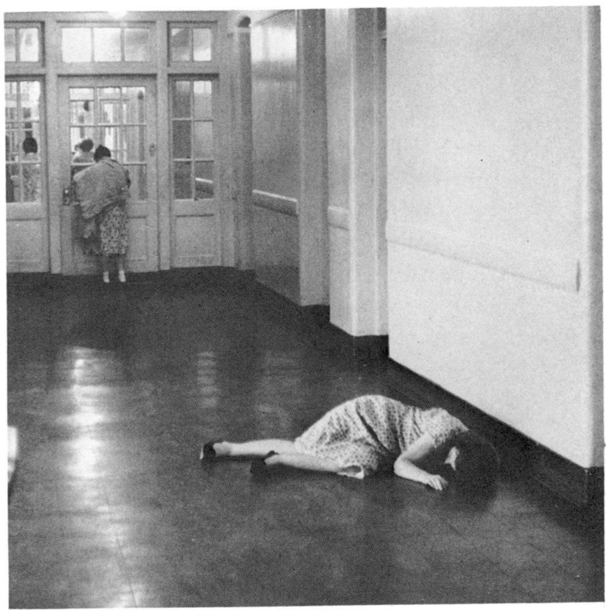

Figure 11.2. Schizophrenic withdrawal. Photo © Ken Heyman.

The nine different subtypes of schizophrenic reactions listed by the APA diagnostic manual generally refer to different typical symptom patterns, but some of them have no such justification. There is, for example, a "childhood type," which simply refers to "schizophrenic reactions occurring before puberty." There is also a "residual type," which simply refers to the persistence of mild symptoms in a person previously severely disturbed. "Schizo-affective type" refers to a combination of affective and schizophrenic psychoses but since symptoms and types of psychoses generally tend to be somewhat interchangeable, this type has no special significance. Finally, there are two "waste basket" subtypes, that is, categories defined by the refusal of their victims to fit into other categories: the "acute undifferentiated type," in which onset is sudden and symptoms may either "disappear or develop into another type," and the "chronic undifferentiated type," in which symptoms are prolonged (that is, the onset of disturbance is slow) and "no single type predominates." This leaves four types of schizophrenia whose symptoms are distinct enough to require separate attention—simple, catatonic, hebephrenic, and paranoid—and we shall look at each of them individually. The others overlap too much with each other and with these four to be considered useful diagnostic categories in their own right—a *child* may undergo an *acute schizo-affective reaction*, but it would not make sense to say that he has three kinds of schizophrenia.

General Symptoms: Primary and Secondary

There seems to be a common core to all the conditions that go by the name of schizophrenia. Kraepelin incorporated them under the single heading, *dementia praecox*, that is, precocious insanity, or insanity of the young. Unfortunately, the common core of *his* observation, that the disorder had an early onset and progressive deterioration, was wrong. It tends to occur, or to be diagnosed at least, mainly between the ages of about fifteen and forty-five, and it does not necessarily result in deterioration at all. One important reason for Kraepelin's observation may be that conditions of hospitalization in his day tended to be so abominable that the very fact of incarceration and humiliating or impersonal treatment tended to make schizophrenic people withdraw even further into their private worlds. This is often true today also; even some of our best mental hospitals contain "snake pits," which almost inevitably contribute to the deepening of psychotic states.

The most definitive work on the subject was written shortly after Kraepelin's text by Eugene Bleuler, a Swiss psychiatrist, whose *Dementia Praecox: Or the Group of Schizophrenias* (1911), both gave the condition its modern name and identified its primary and secondary characteristics. *Schizophrenia* means "split mentality," and it refers to a splitting from the environment or from reality, not to the dissociative hysterical condition technically called "multiple personality" (see Chapter 10). Bleuler recognized that neither early onset nor deterioration were critical features of the disorder, whereas disturbances in thinking were. These could take many different forms, but the upshot of all of them is that the thoughts and feelings the schizophrenic displays are so thoroughly individual that they fail to communicate conventional meanings to other people. The affects he shows seem inappropriate to the demands of the situation. The thoughts he expresses are so strange, illogical, in violation of the conventions of syntax, or full of newly coined words (neologisms) that they may constitute a veritable "word salad." The general impression he conveys is one of emotional distance or withdrawal from the world around him, and the content of his communications is "autistic," that is, so personal in its origins and meanings that it has significance only for himself. Many different names and descriptions have been assigned to the varieties of intellectual disarray that make up schizophrenic speech and that imply a similar disarray of thoughts and feelings: "cognitive slippage" (Meehl, 1962), "paralogical thinking" (Vigotsky, 1934), and "overinclusion" (Cameron, 1947) all describe different aspects of schizophrenic communication that give it an *autistic* character. Autism is perhaps best summarized, however, by saying that it reflects what Freud (1933) called *primary process thinking*, that is, thoughts, images, and the like that are dictated by internal states rather than by the nature of external reality. Realistic thinking, which develops as children learn language, was called *secondary process* by Freud; it is the same consensually validated thinking that Sullivan (1963) described, and the lack of it is the most evident and critical symptom of schizophrenia.

The secondary symptoms which Bleuler identified are mostly of the same kind as the secondary symptoms of affective reactions: delusions and hallucinations. They are secondary both in the sense that they are less important in identifying schizophrenia and also that they are less likely to occur in all cases. All schizophrenics show autistic thought disorders, but not all of them have hallucinations.

Comparison of Schizophrenia and Affective Reactions

The secondary symptoms tend to be much more severe in the schizophrenias than in affective psychoses; they start earlier, take more varied and distressing forms, and last longer. What is more, hallucinations occur even more often than delusions. They are more serious symptoms, you will recall, because the direct experience of fantasied events is even further removed from reality than the belief in them (delusion). Auditory hallucinations are more common than other kinds, probably because they are the easiest to have—all of us have heard someone calling our name when nobody was, have listened to meaningless sounds in the night that seemed full of (ominous) content, or have been certain the telephone was ringing or the doorbell buzzing when it was not. Visual hallucinations are not so easily come by for most people, and even schizophrenics tend to have them, along with taste, smell, and tactile hallucinations, only in more acute phases of the disorder.

Two other kinds of secondary symptoms are seen more in schizophrenics than in other disorders and are suggestive of the greater severity of this condition. These are tremendous anxiety along with apparent inability to derive any pleasure from anything (this is *not* like the frantic but short-lived despondency of depression), called *anhedonia*, and a more rarely seen but weird-seeming inclination to imitate the speech or movements of other people, called respectively *echolalia* and *echopraxia*. These are not ordinarily detailed imitations of complete sentences or complex movements; they are more often partial imitations, delivered faintly or blandly, and suggesting that the behavior of the person imitated has been registered on the brain of the patient without being understood. It is as if a defective robot were faultily copying its mentor.

At their worst, the secondary symptoms of schizophrenia give way to completely *regressive* behavior, and the person has to be cared for altogether. But the regressed schizophrenic who smears his feces on the wall does not do so with the frantic passion of mania, but with the absorption of a child in finger paints or the indifference of a preoccupied artist doodling his fingers in his oils. He may eat them with the same abstracted air. Schizophrenic regression is in no sense a return to childhood, as was once commonly thought by psychiatrists. But this is a more regressed condition than affective regression in that the behavior of the schizophrenic is more primitive; it reflects a lower level of general functioning, less ability to get along in the world, and, to some extent, less hope of recovery. A "maturity index" comparing affective and schizophrenic psychoses would distinguish them on at least four counts: (1) the spontaneous recovery rate is very high for the former, low for the latter; (2) the more common secondary symptoms of affective reactions (delusions) are less regressive than those of schizophrenia (hallucinations); (3) the premorbid needs and capacities of manics and depressives is for intense and warm interpersonal relationships whereas *schizoid* people (people with withdrawn, inward-turned personality traits) have low needs and abilities to form close interpersonal relationships; and (4) guilt is a more mature primary symptom than withdrawal in that it has more potential for contributing to some reconstruction of the person's life.

Another important difference between schizophrenic and affective disorders is in the course of the disorder. Affective disturbances, as we have seen, can be described as "attacks" both because their onset is relatively sudden after some specific precipitating incidents and because they last for a fairly limited time. Although this is sometimes the case with schizophrenic reactions, it is not the characteristic pattern. The onset of disorder tends to be very gradual, more an extension of already well-established patterns of behavior and personality than an explosive extrapolation from them. Cameron, in fact, states that "a slow, indefinite, insidious onset is common in schizophrenia," and that "sudden onset is often more apparent than real" (1963, pp. 603). Schizophrenia tends *not* to originate in an attack, does *not* undergo clear-cut stages, and does *not* necessarily disappear after any given duration, if at all. The clinical personnel responsible for its management and treatment tend to speak of "improvement" rather than "cure" and, when a schizophrenic seems to recover altogether, which is not infrequent, to describe him as "in remission," that is, having merely given up his symptoms: the implication is that his recovery may be an altogether temporary thing. It often is, but the same is true of affective disorders. This common conservative way of discussing recovery from schizophrenia reflects the relatively poor success that has been had in accomplishing permanent cures.

Perhaps the main reason why schizophrenia has a predominantly gradual onset is that its victims tend, to begin with, to be schizoid people whose personality patterns and habits of social and emotional withdrawal and isolation are already of such long-standing familiarity to those around them that it never occurs to anyone that they are "crazy" unless their behavior takes a strong turn for the worse and secondary cognitive symptoms or bizarre acts become evident. Once this happens and the victims come to the attention of mental health experts, it often turns out that they have long since undergone a serious thought disorder which only now is revealed. The population of *ambulatory* schizophrenics, that is, unhospitalized and often undiagnosed, is unknown but must be quite large, perhaps larger than that of schizophrenics who come to hospitals and clinics.

When schizophrenic "breakdown" does occur, it does not run through clear stages. Rosen and Gregory (1965) propose, however, that three fairly distinct stages are typical of chronic schizophrenia. The first is *breakdown,* where the patient experiences anxiety and confusion about strange things happening to him, ranging from bodily ills to hallucinations, whose reality he may still doubt. It is hard to classify subtypes of schizophrenia at this point. Secondly, there is a *setting-in* stage, where the patient comes to accept his symptoms as realities and to systematize them in relation to each other. At this time he is classifiable. And last is a *deteriorating stage,* where his more dramatic cognitive and perceptual symptoms may disappear along with most other signs of agitation and liveliness. In this stage, he tends to be very regressed, sometimes requiring custodial care for routine physical functions, and shows virtually no feeling about anything; technically, this is called *flattened affect.* Again, he cannot be classified very easily and, in most hospitals, is relegated to a "chronic" or "back" ward, where little hope is held out for recovery. Such people are known in the polite language of the trade as *regressed* schizophrenics, and colloquially are called *back-ward* or *burned-out* schizophrenics.

The terminology of mental hospitals is somewhat confusing, however. Most chronic schizophrenics are kept on open or unlocked wards as they can take care of themselves, are not endangering anyone, and are in reasonably good contact with reality most of the time. "Chronicity" properly refers more to the duration of the disorder than to its severity. Locked wards are not necessarily the same as back wards, although back wards are always locked; the former generally have more patients with acute disorders who require intensive management. Usage varies with hospital customs, but the term *open ward* always refers to a place for patients with relatively mild and hopeful cases and *back ward* to the opposite.

Schizophrenic Subtypes

Despite the common core of thought disorder, autism, and withdrawal which unites the schizophrenias, they continue to be divided into subtypes. Moreover, the division is hallowed, on the one hand, by clinical tradition and experience, which does indeed find clusters of symptomatic differences between patients and, on the other hand, by the evidence of systematic research, which also demonstrates rather consistently that subtypes are necessary, though perhaps not the subtypes used in clinical psychiatric practice. For research purposes, in fact, Maher (1966) concludes that "there appears to be little justification for continuing to use the grosser category of schizophrenic versus nonschizophrenic" (pp. 388–389), and it goes without saying that, for clinical purposes, diagnosticians appropriately wish to assign the most defined labels possible. Four of the subtypes of the diagnostic manual contain the major clinical typologies of schizophrenia: *simple, catatonic, hebephrenic,* and *paranoid.*

Simple schizophrenia. Most ambulatory psychotics are probably simple schizophrenics, because these are the least conspicuous kind. They are also the most easily confused with mental retardates because their withdrawn manner is easily taken for stupidity; unless they demonstate some overtly disordered thinking or active delusions or hallucinations, in fact, there is usually no way to distinguish them from retardates. Simple schizophrenics generally do tend to have rather low IQ's, for whatever reason, and to function at a sufficiently high level to be anonymous. The clinical picture usually is one of apathy and simplicity, not of active psychotic symptoms. These people can often get along at unskilled jobs, especially ones that require little interpersonal communication. In addition to hobo jungles, brothels, and the like, they may be found clustered in the downtown areas of large cities, where they may live isolated lives in cheap rooming houses and eke out a living dishwashing, "policing" refuse in parks, and perhaps collecting unemployment checks between jobs. Most people in such life situations are not psychotic, but ambulatory psychotics can often adjust to life outside of institutional settings by restricting themselves to such circumstances and activities. From the point of view of the patient, this is probably a healthier adjustment pattern than that of hospitalization, which is more likely to result in decline than in remission. From the viewpoint of society, it is almost certainly cheaper, since in addition to being relatively self-sufficient economically, simple schizophrenics are not likely to harm themselves or others.

If it were not for the fact that they sometimes develop specific symptoms, there is little chance that simple schizophrenia would be classified as a functional psychosis at all. It would probably be contained under the heading *schizoid personality* and be regarded as a personality or character disorder.

Catatonic and hebephrenic schizophrenia. Describing catatonic and hebephrenic schizophrenia is chiefly a matter of academic interest because these conditions are now rare. A search of first admission records over the past five years at one large mental hospital failed to produce a single case of either kind. How much commoner they were many years ago is hard to say, but it is always important to remember, in discussing the incidence of psychoses, that *hospital conditions often promote insanity* and that brutal and impersonal hospital management was certainly more common years ago than it is now. Thus, many people who were hospitalized with milder symptoms may have developed catatonic or hebephrenic symptoms which better treatment could have prevented. We cannot know.

Hebephrenia is probably even less common that catatonia, and what cases there are are most likely to be seen on the back wards of large mental hospitals. They tend to be quite unmistakable. Hebephrenics appear idiotically happy—they may wear a nearly perpetual grin, giggle or babble from time to time, and have extremely bizarre delusions and hallucinations, generally pleasantly tinged and often of sex or of bodily changes. The condition tends to be deteriorative, so that eventually the patient becomes incontinent and incapable of managing himself, but generally does not give up the bizarre mannerisms that identify the type. Since the relatively high activity level of hebephrenia and the apparent joviality do not look much like those of mania, these conditions are usually easy to distinguish. Nor does the grinning or giggling suggest much affect in these people; it is conspicuously inappropriate and bizarre.

Catatonic symptoms are as dramatic as those of hebephrenia but less ominous. If treated early, catatonics show more frequent recovery than any other schizophrenics, especially if the onset of symptoms was fairly sudden. (Notice that, with all the functional psychoses, there seems to be a favorable correspondence between speed of onset and likelihood of recovery.) The symptoms of catatonic disorder are chiefly motoric, and the condition cannot always be distinguished from agitated or retarded depressions, especially if its victim does not speak, a condition called *mutism. Catatonic stupor* is a condition of immobility and apparent apathy. The patient may show *waxy flexibility*, meaning that his limbs can be moved to strange and unusual positions, which he will then retain like a wax statue. He may require total care. A less stuporous catatonic may be mute and *negative,* refusing to follow any instructions given him, or may show the echolalia or echopraxia mentioned earlier. On very rare occasions, catatonic immobility may suddenly give way to violent hostility, in which the patient can be quite dangerous.

In some cases, at least, catatonic symptoms seem to be psychotic efforts of the patient to defend against expressions of his pent-up hostilities. The reports that recovered patients give of their fantasies and delusions during catatonic stupors seem to bear this out; they often have gloomy anticipations or experiences of misery, death, and universal catastrophe, including thoughts that they are already dead. One patient explained his immobility by saying that he was afraid that if he had moved the world would have come to an end.

The stuporous condition may give way suddenly to *catatonic excitement,* and vice versa. The excited state looks like delirious mania but is more dangerous; the patient may kill himself or others or, what is more likely, may mutilate himself. Like mania, the condition burns itself out through sheer energy expenditure, but patients have been known to die of exhaustion during such fits.

Paranoid schizophrenia. Because paranoid schizophrenia is the occurrence of paranoia in a schizophrenic, we had better talk about paranoia. The diagnostic manual lists *paranoid reactions* as an independent class of functional psychosis, along with *schizophrenic, affective,* and *involutional reactions,* but it is not really clear whether this independent listing is justified. Certainly, the difference between true paranoia and paranoid schizophrenia is subtle enough so that Rosen and Gregory (1965), at least, consider it a matter of degree rather than kind. At all events, paranoid reactions which do not manifest any of the symptoms of schizophrenia are quite rare, and the conditions share far more similarities than differences.

The essence of *paranoia* (which we are not distinguishing here from "true paranoia," "classical paranoia," or "paranoid states") is that the patient suffers from delusions which are organized into a tight logical and perceptual system around which his entire life revolves. Although we commonly think of these as delusions of persecution, that is not always the case; they may be delusions of grandeur, wealth, or power, called *megalomania,* or of sex or jealousy or virtually anything else whose nature places him in a fantasied unique position relative to other people. As his delusions take shape, the paranoid person increasingly comes to perceive everything that happens to him as systematically related to his delusional ideas; that is, he refers all his experiences to his major preoccupation. These *ideas of reference* are then used to reinforce and further elaborate the basic delusion.

In its purest, and rarest, form there is evidently nothing at all wrong with the paranoid person except that he has inflated a *single insane idea* until there is space for nothing else in his consciousness. Paranoid single-mindedness is the technical meaning of *monomania,* and it is the only symptom of this disorder.

Comparison of paranoia and paranoid schizophrenia. Aside from some statistical differences of unknown significance (paranoid reactions seem to occur at older ages than paranoid schizophrenic ones, and more among women than among men), the only sure basis for distinguishing paranoia from paranoid schizophrenia seems to be the generally better functioning which characterizes the former. Paranoids are generally intellectually intact, and their social behavior, except with reference to their delusional systems, is more adept and appropriate than that of paranoid schizophrenics. The prognosis for recovery with any kind of treatment is very poor compared to paranoid schizophrenia (and most other disorders), but this may itself be a function of the paranoid's generally high level of functioning. In other words, general intactness may be so great that it permits effective maintenance of a singular delusion in spite of outside influence or persuasion. By the same token, the paranoid schizophrenic may have a somewhat better prognosis *because* of his thinking disorder, which may keep him from getting his delusions down pat, that is, from systematizing them beyond any possibility of change.

About half of all diagnosed cases of schizophrenia are of the paranoid variety. The average age of onset is higher than for other types of schizophrenia, though the paranoid type may occur from puberty on; and relatively acute onsets, with their corresponding favorable prognoses, are fairly common. Paranoid schizophrenics are considerably more intact than other schizophrenics; their delusional systems are not well organized, compared to those of paranoids, and are both modified by the very conspicuous disturbances of thought process which identify them as schizophrenic and bolstered by hallucinations to a much greater degree than is ever found in paranoid states. Although paranoid schizophrenics are more able and willing than other schizophrenics to communicate, communication is not necessarily easy because their delusional and hallucinatory experiences dominate their consciousness and their disturbed thinking often results in very autistic verbal productions. The condition is not especially deteriorative, but difficulties in understanding the meaning of paranoid schizophrenic ideas are likely to increase with time because the delusional material often becomes less systematic and more fragmentary and autistic, whereas early in the course of the disorder it is more plainly an outgrowth of the patient's impulses and concerns. At all events, this type of schizophrenia is characterized by a relatively good ability to communicate, and almost all of the extensive clinical literature of patient reports and of artistic production during psychotic states is concerned with paranoid schizophrenics.

Research Approaches to Schizophrenic Typologies

The schizophrenic typologies of the diagnostic manual are derivatives of observations first systematized by Kraepelin, who based his taxonomy more or less completely on similarities among symptoms. Typologies may have other bases, of course, as we have seen in the previous two chapters, and recent research suggests that one particularly useful way of classifying schizophrenics is in terms of their prepsychotic history rather than of their symptoms. The most detailed and sophisticated research on the *premorbid social competence* of severely disturbed people has been done by Phillips and Zigler and is described at length in the next chapter. In general, it tends to demonstrate a positive relationship for all kinds of disorders between level of functioning before the onset of disorder and the prognosis for recovery from it.

A similar typology, but one more specific to schizophrenia, makes a distinction between *process* and *reactive* schizophrenia. Process schizophrenia includes cases in which, to begin with, the victim is socially inadequate and the onset of symptoms is gradual. Prognosis is poor in such cases. Reactive schizophrenia happens to people whose social functioning has been good and whose symptoms develop relatively suddenly after some stressful or traumatic experiences. Prognosis here is relatively good (Chapman *et al.*, 1961). Considering the Kraepelinian subtypes, *simple schizophrenics* (and hebephrenics) would generally be *process* types and *paranoid* (and catatonic) cases would more often be *reactive* types.

The Origins and Dynamics of Schizophrenia

By implication, the process-reactive and social competence typologies are attempts to develop taxonomies that get at the dynamics or origins of schizophrenia rather than merely group its superficial manifestations together. The same conflict about origins applies to schizophrenia as to the affective reactions, but it is much more complicated in this case. Cameron (1963) reports that there have been more than *fifteen thousand* professional articles and books written about schizophrenia! As we might expect, therefore, the evidence is prodigious in all directions. There is plenty of reason to think that genetic factors play an important role in at least some kinds of schizophrenic disorders, and while there is no evidence of causality, there are certainly some subtle metabolic and other biochemical and anatomical differences between schizophrenics and others. At the same time, it is even clearer that patterns of interpersonal relationships, especially within families and especially in parent-child relationships, are critical determinants of schizophrenia in many cases, and as we have seen in Chapter 10 and shall see again in Chapter 12, there are many dynamic influences within the culture as a whole that contribute to the development (and prevention) of psychological disorders.

The problem of identifying the origins and unraveling the dynamics of schizophrenia, even more than with other functional disorders, is not that there is a lack of good research but that the subject matter is enormously complicated and confusing. All affective reactions are *reactions*, but simple schizophrenia tends to be more of a *life style* and may not fit neatly into any dynamic formulation of psychosis which presumes that it involves an *escape* or *retreat* from reality. One dynamic interpretation of paranoid schizophrenia, for example, is based on Freud's idea that paranoia is a defense against one's own homosexual impulses (1911), and there is some evidence, albeit equivocal, to support the notion. But since simple schizophrenia lacks any of the clear symptomatology of the paranoid type, there is no basis for applying that kind of dynamic interpretation to it. To find a psychological basis for it, therefore, one must try to explore the more distant background of familial and other interpersonal experiences. Here the problems of reliability and comprehensiveness of information become enormous, just as they do with pedigree and concordance studies that try to identify a genetic basis for schizophrenia. It is quite likely that we are actually dealing with more than one kind of entity under the single heading of schizophrenic reactions, and this helps to confuse things (Buss, 1966; Szasz, 1957). Still more confusion arises from the fact that many adherents of the psychological or the biological view of schizophrenia present their cases with monomaniacal enthusiasm, which may discourage their students from developing a balanced perspective on the problem.

Infantile Autism and Childhood Schizophrenia

The problem of how many different entities are really lumped together as schizophrenia is emphasized particularly by considering *infantile autism*. The diagnostic manual has no such classification; it speaks only of childhood schizophrenia and means by it nothing more than schizophrenic symptoms occurring in children. Kanner (1944), however, observed that there is a rather rare syndrome of childhood psychosis, almost invariably diagnosed as schizophrenia, which really differs quite remarkably from it. He named it "early infantile autism." Rimland (1964) conducted a prodigious survey of all the literature on this phenomenon and concluded not only that infantile autism is drastically different from childhood schizophrenia but that its basis is *entirely* genetic as well! Ferster (1961; personal communication, 1965), however, who has formulated the theory that childhood schizophrenia reflects a deficiency in social learning (see Chapter 9), vigorously disagrees (see also London, 1965).

The point is moot, as is the whole question of whether schizophrenia is a single or multiple entity with biological or psychological basis or bases. On the face of it, it seems reasonable to conclude that whatever biological dispositions are involved are reflected most clearly in simple or in process schizophrenia, while the learned dispositions are represented mostly in paranoid or in reactive cases. The biological *subject variables* may be more evident in the former and the influence of *stimulus situations* in the latter (see Chapter 9). To really understand any human behavior, as we have seen, it is necessary to examine both *susceptibility* (subject variables; behavioral dispositions; genetic, organic, structural characteristics) and *situation* (stimulus events, environment, learning, dynamics); it is their interaction, or *ecology*, which accounts for behavior, not their independent characteristics. A thorough understanding of this interaction is harder to come by for schizophrenia than for any other negative abnormality.

PERSONALITY (CHARACTER) DISORDERS

A thorough description of character disorders would require far more space than can be given here and would inevitably be even more puzzling to the thoughtful reader than the discussions of other negative abnormalities. The source of confusion would be the fact that the area of character disorders is the one where psychiatric classifications become most hopelessly muddled in the effort to straddle the fence between science and society (London, 1964; in press). Many of the disorders contained in this grouping involve profound personal miseries, but others may be no more than personal idiosyncrasies which happen to deviate from social mores and which have fallen into the province of psychiatry as much by historical accident as anything else. The purpose of this section is to identify the major character disorders and to delineate their overlapping social and personal features. The section does not attempt to describe their origins, symptoms, or dynamics, but uses them to illustrate the inordinate difficulty of distinguishing *deviation* from *disorder*, an inherent, and probably insoluble problem that arises from the statistical view of normality which dominates this volume.

There are two kinds of functional conditions contained in the diagnostic manual's four categories of personality (character) disorders: (1) personal disturbances of behavior, that is negative abnormalities which cannot easily be classified as neurotic, psychotic, or psychosomatic, and (2) social disturbances of behavior, where the only obvious thing wrong with a person may be that other people don't like his behavior. The manual fails to distinguish the very different implications these conditions have, though it does separate them to some extent.

Most of the conditions which the manual calls *special symptom reactions* involve only mild disorders, although they may cause a lot of misery to the people who have them. These include isolated symptoms like stuttering, enuresis, or sleepwalking. *Personality pattern disturbance* is a "wastebasket" term for people who look as if they might become psychotic but have not yet done so, and *personality trait disturbance* includes people who are immature, obnoxious, or otherwise troublesome but not psychotic and not exactly anything else. A compulsive personality in somebody who is not neurotic is one such trait. Another is a "passive-aggressive" personality, which means that the person doesn't commit crimes, become violent, or the like, but is continuously expressing aggression against others by passive means, such as *not* doing things he is supposed to do or that they demand of him. These too are considered relatively minor troubles, though both personality pattern and trait disturbances can be serious enough to result in discharge from military service, if not in hospitalization.

The really severe character disorders, which are both personal and social disturbances, are contained under what the manual calls *sociopathic personality disturbances*, a clumsy term meaning "nonconformity to prevailing social and ethical standards." There are really three categories of behavior which fall in this group (the manual lists four) and which are indeed very serious problems for the individual, for society, or for both: (1) *antisocial reaction*, especially aggression; (2) *addiction*, especially alcoholism; and (3) *sexual deviation*, especially homosexuality.

Antisocial reactions are primarily behavior that seems to be dominated almost entirely by pleasure-seeking impulses among people sometimes called *psychopaths* or *sociopaths* who are predominantly destructive in relation to society, like teenage hoodlums or the Hell's Angels, and professional criminals, who some psychiatrists would like to believe are mentally ill. Extreme psychopathy is quite a rare condition, although the term is colloquially used in relation to people who try always to gratify themselves without evident concern for others. Cleckley (1955) describes the condition dramatically and effectively: he believes that it is actually a rare form of psychosis. Psychopathy does not, in any case, create a large-scale social problem.

Extreme aggression and professional crime do, of course; crimes of violence in particular frequently seem to involve mental aberrations, and not merely deviations from conventional behavior. In Chapter 9 the learning of aggression is discussed at some length, but it is easier to understand how children learn aggression than it is to prevent or extinguish it in adolescents and adults. Professional crime does not typically involve violence as much as amateur crime does; an increasing number of violently aggressive crimes moreover, especially on the part of youths, seem to have no object except the expression of hostility. In some instances, of course, such acts are motivated by blatantly pathological desires, but it is clear that most of them are committed by youngsters who are bitterly antagonistic towards authority and towards "square" society but are not psychotic. Little systematic knowledge exists about the origins of this behavior or about its treatment, but the behavior itself is widely recognized as a mental health problem.

Addictions are serious personal as well as social problems. Of these, alcoholism is by far the most serious because if prolonged it prevents the individual from functioning effectively much of the time and eventually causes serious organic damage. As we shall see in Chapter 12, it is probably the most serious mental health problem in the United States. It is second only to schizophrenia in frequency of hospital admissions, and most alcoholics are never hospitalized at all.

There is a widespread belief that addiction to *psychedelic drugs* (drugs which affect mental processes) is far more serious and dangerous, if not more prevalent, than alcoholism. Some of these drugs, such as heroin, are physiologically addicting, meaning that discontinuing their use causes a number of distressing physical *withdrawal* symptoms, which are often more painful than harmful. Some drugs are toxic under some circumstances, like the barbiturates or, according to rumor, chemically impure ("green") LSD. And there is some evidence that some of them cause genetic damage (Cohen *et al.*, 1967; *Time*, 1967). On the other hand, alcohol is *always* toxic if used in large quantities (everybody knows that but doesn't think about it—we commonly call drunkenness *intoxication*) and will also produce withdrawal symptoms if its use is suddenly curtailed after a long period of excessive drinking (Godfrey *et al.*, 1958). Perhaps we are simply more accustomed to swilling drinks than to gulping pills, so that it is less shocking to contemplate people destroying themselves by one means than by the other.

Drugs probably have the same kind of reinforcing effects that alcohol has (see Chapter 9), which may be why people become so easily habituated even to those that are not addicting, as most of the popular ones (LSD, marijuana, amphetamines) are not. As with the psychoses, it is not entirely clear what the interaction of subject and situation variables is in the case of addictions; it is widely believed that some personality patterns predispose people to dependency on alcohol or drugs. On the other hand, the fact that addictions tend to occur most among young people and in lower socioeconomic strata suggests that they mainly serve the purpose of relieving the drudgery of miserable or anxiety-provoking life circumstances, like poverty or going to college.

In either case, it is important to realize that many psychedelic drugs, though generally not beneficial to health, are also not harmful in controlled and restricted amounts, perhaps even if they are taken over very long periods of time. This includes marijuana, LSD, and heroin. What makes this fact important is that, although the use of drugs is generally fostered and sustained by private personal unhappiness, there is a widespread public lunacy, currently very powerful in the United States, that turns the individual problem into a social nightmare by making the use of many drugs illegal even under the control of competent professional people. This has long been true in the United States in connection with marijuana and heroin, though in England a physician may legally administer heroin to an addict, and it is now becoming true for LSD, though there is no good evidence that controlled use of any of these drugs is itself harmful. A huge criminal industry has therefore been created for no good purpose: people who are habituated to drugs will go to great lengths to get them, and professional criminals have created a multibillion dollar industry that supplies them at fantastic prices, causing untold numbers of desperate people to commit thefts, assaults, or prostitution to get the money for drugs. The manufacturing cost of virtually all of them is very cheap. The cost to the public of suppression, which does not work, and of treatments, most of which are not successful, is simply astronomic.

Sexual deviations have much the same status as addictions except that nobody is deluded enough to think they are physically harmful and there is increasing public acceptance of them, which is gradually reducing the error of compounding these personal problems into criminal acts. There are about as many varieties of sexual activity as there are erogenous parts, orifices, and means of manipulation of the human body—maybe more. Anyway, the means by which sexual preferences are learned are probably the same or similar for all sex acts (see Chapter 9), and enough varieties of sexual activity are familiar to everyone that there is no need to belabor them here. Homosexuality is by far the most common sexual deviation, and it is reasonably typical of the problems of sex deviations. For many people who have learned these behaviors, their deviant tendencies provoke much anxiety and, in so far as they do, can be considered personality disorders. For others, however, unconventional sex behavior is an accepted part of their lives that provokes anxiety only to the extent that it arouses the contempt or disapproval of others and the retaliation of society. In such cases, it is doubtful that the notion of character *disorder* really applies.

SUMMARY

This chapter has been concerned with the major functional psychological disorders, the *psychoses* and *character disorders*. Neither "major" nor "functional" is a very precise term, but they are not meaningless either. In general, the major disorders tend either to disable the individual so that he cannot care for himself in society or else to create such large-scale social problems that society cannot permit the individual to go about his business without some peril to the general public. The disorders dealt with in the chapter are "functional" in the sense that they are not clearly "organic"; that is, they are not *known* to result from any specific physical deficiency. This does not mean, of course, that there are no genetic, constitutional, or other physical or medical aspects to them; a great deal of modern research on these disorders is actively trying to identify their physical determinants or correlates, but without very definite success thus far. The functional disorders therefore appear to be more directly the outcome of learning experiences than of biological events.

The American Psychiatric Association has published an official diagnostic manual of psychological disabilities, largely a modernized version of the classifications devised by Emil Kraepelin. Some of its categories are not very useful, however, either because they tend to be obsolete or to overlap with other kinds of disorder, and the divisions used in this chapter do not parallel the diagnostic manual very exactly.

Psychotic disorders are divided into two kinds, *affective* and *schizophrenic reactions*. The affective reactions are identified chiefly by extremes of mood, either of despair or of seeming elation; the former is called *depression*, the latter *mania*. Schizophrenic reactions are identified chiefly by extreme impairment of thought processes, generally accompanied by a strong tendency to withdraw emotionally from others. The most frequently encountered subtypes of schizophrenia are called *simple* and *paranoid*. The former is often mistaken for mental retardation and often goes undiagnosed, as many of its victims manage to sustain themselves in society by holding very low-level jobs and leading quietly isolated lives, usually in the anonymity of big cities. The latter is much like a very rare psychosis called *paranoia*, which is identified by its victim's insanely intelligent delusion that, for example, he is being persecuted or is a grand figure. Paranoid *schizophrenics* have such delusions, but also show the disturbance of thinking which is the main symptom of schizophrenia.

Delusions and hallucinations are important secondary symptoms that may occur with any psychosis. A delusion is a bizarre *idea* or *belief* about what is happening, while a hallucination is a bizarre *experience* of the senses, like hearing voices or seeing visions which are not evident to others. Because delusions and hallucinations tend to be dramatic events, most of us think of them as primary symptoms of psychosis, but they are not. People may have psychotic breakdowns without any of these experiences, and they may have transitory delusions or hallucinations without necessarily being psychotic. This is largely a question of the observer's judgment.

Three kinds of *character disorder* are briefly discussed: *antisocial reactions*, of which aggression is the most important; *addictions*, of which alcoholism is most critical; and *sexual deviations*, most important of which is homosexuality. The learning of these behaviors is discussed at some length in Chapter 9, and some statistics of their incidence follow in Chapter 12.

GLOSSARY

ACTION THERAPIES—therapies that concentrate on changing behavior (see Chapter 15).

ACUTE MANIA—a state of extreme extreme excitability and hyperactivity.

AFFECTIVE PSYCHOSES—psychotic disorders characterized by a tremendous change of mood.

AGITATED DEPRESSION—a depression characterized by tense and anxious excitement.

AGORAPHOBIA—fear of going outdoors.

AMBULATORY SCHIZOPHRENICS—unhospitalized and often undiagnosed schizophrenics.

ANHEDONIA—an apparent inability to derive pleasure from anything.

ANTISOCIAL REACTION—behavior which seems to be dominated almost entirely by pleasure seeking and, in relation to society, to be destructive.

ASTHENIC—Kretchmer's term for "lean and bony" body type; similar to Sheldon's *ectomorph*.

AUTISTIC THINKING—thought processes that are dominated by personal needs and desires; such thinking is so personal and apparently illogical that the thoughts have meaning only to the thinker.

BACK WARDS—wards in which relatively severe and chronic psychotics are housed.

BRAIN WAVE PATTERNS—patterns of electrical activity in the brain recorded from the surface of the head.

BREAKDOWN STAGE IN SCHIZOPHRENIA—the stage where the patient experiences anxiety and confusion about strange things happening to him, ranging from bodily ills to hallucinations, whose reality he may still doubt.

CATATONIC EXCITEMENT—an excited state in which the patient exhibits symptoms that look like delirious mania but are more dangerous.

CATATONIC SCHIZOPHRENIA—a psychosis marked by conspicuous motor symptoms, either generalized inhibition or excessive motor activity and excitement, or periods of alternation between both.

CATATONIC STUPORS—rigid or bizarre postures, often maintained for long periods of time.

CHRONIC UNDIFFERENTIATED SCHIZOPHRENIA—a psychotic disorder in which the onset is gradual and no single type of symptom predominates.

CONSENSUAL VALIDATION—agreement among observers about what a thing or event is or what it means.

CONSTITUTIONAL FACTORS—factors relating mainly to the chemistry and neurophysiology of the body.

DELIRIOUS MANIA—psychotic episodes of excitement, generally of short duration.

DELUSIONS—false beliefs.

DELUSIONS OF GRANDEUR—delusions in which the patient believes himself to be an extremely important person, with great wealth and power.

DELUSIONS OF PERSECUTION—delusions in which the patient believes that "others" (not necessarily human beings) intend to harm or kill him.

DEMENTIA PRAECOX—an obsolete term, used by Kraepelin, for schizophrenia; literally, a precocious insanity.

DENIAL—refusal to accept negative feelings about the self (see Chapter 4).

DEPENDENCY—reliance upon others for

the satisfaction of physical and psychological needs.

DEPRESSION—an emotional state of great sadness, often accompanied by guilt and anxiety, gloomy ruminations, lassitude, inability to respond to pleasant stimuli, and suicidal impulses.

DEPRESSIVE REACTION—a transient neurotic disorder usually precipitated by some personal loss or misfortune.

DEPRESSIVE STUPOR—a depressive disorder in which the patient may be so unresponsive that he has to be completely cared for and may look just like a catatonic schizophrenic.

DETERIORATING STAGE OF SCHIZOPHRENIA—the stage where the patient's more dramatic cognitive and perceptual symptoms may disappear along with most other signs of agitation and liveliness.

DEVIANT BEHAVIOR PATTERNS—see PSYCHOPATHIC BEHAVIOR.

DISSOCIATIVE HYSTERICAL CONDITION—see MULTIPLE PERSONALITY.

DYNAMIC DESCRIPTIONS—descriptions of the development of, and changes in, phenomena.

DYNAMIC VIEW OF PSYCHOPATHOLOGY—the view that the "major" mental disorders reflect primarily defects in learning and functioning rather than genetic and constitutional defects.

ECHOLALIA—the inclination to imitate meaninglessly the speech of other people.

ECOLOGY—as used here, the interaction of situation (environment) and susceptibility (personal characteristics) in the production of an ailment or disorder.

ECTOMORPHIC TYPE—Sheldon's term for slender and fragile body types; similar to Kretchmer's asthenic type.

ENDOMORPHIC TYPE—Sheldon's term for the soft, round body type; similar to Kretchmer's pyknic type.

ETIOLOGY—the study of causes, or origins.

FLATTENED AFFECT—a term used to describe the condition of individuals who appear neither to display nor to experience feelings about most things.

FLIGHT OF IDEAS—rush of ideas, generally fragmentary and minimally related to each other and to the issue at hand.

FUNCTIONAL PSYCHOSIS—a psychosis for which there is no known organic or structural origin.

GENERAL PARESIS—a progressive organic psychosis and paralysis resulting from a syphilitic infection of the brain.

GENETIC FACTORS—hereditary factors.

GRANDIOSE ELATION—frantic, elated behavior.

GUILT—the subjective feelings that result from doing something that is forbidden, or from the failure to perform some obligatory act (see Chapters 4 and 10).

HALLUCINATION—a false perception that has a compelling sense of reality, even though relevant and adequate stimuli for it are lacking.

HEBEPHRENIC SCHIZOPHRENIA—a psychotic disorder characterized by shallow and inappropriate affect and silly, inappropriate, or regressive behavior.

HOMOSEXUAL IMPULSES—sexual impulses directed towards a person of the same sex.

HYPOMANIA—mild episodes of excitement and elation.

IDEAS OF REFERENCE—highly personalized and irrational interpretations of events and experience in terms of one's own delusions.

INFANTILE AUTISM—a term used by some authors synonymously with childhood schizophrenia; note, however, that other theorists dispute this usage.

INTROJECTION—internalization; a defense mechanism involving the adoption of the attitudes and beliefs of powerful others, often after a period of resistance and hostility.

INVOLUTIONAL PSYCHOTIC REACTIONS—any functional psychosis that appears for the first time during middle age.

LIFE STYLE—characteristic mode of living.

LOSS OF CONTACT WITH REALITY—the loss of the ability to perceive objectively and respond to one's external environment.

MANIA—excitement manifested by mental and physical hyperactivity, disorganization of behavior, and elevation of mood.

MANIC DEPRESSIVE PSYCHOSES—a group of disorders characterized by states of overexcitement and elation (mania) or of sadness and hypoactivity (depression), or of oscillation between these.

MEGALOMANIA—a disorder characterized by delusions of grandeur, wealth, or power.

MENTAL RETARDATION—the *conservative* definition classifies as mentally retarded those who fall in the lowest 3 percent of the distribution of IQ scores; the definition established in the *Manual on Terminology and Classification in Men-*

tal Retardation includes all persons whose IQ falls below the population mean; the *social competence* definition classifies all those who are unable to meet minimal societal demands (see Chapter 14).

MESOMORPHIC TYPE—Sheldon's term for a strong, muscular, athletic body type.

MONOMANIA—persistent preoccupation with a single idea.

MORAL ANXIETY—a term used by Freud to describe feelings of guilt and apprehension that arise from actual or fantasied violation of conscience.

MULTIPLE PERSONALITY—a dissociative personality reaction characterized by the development of two or more personality subsystems within the same person.

MUTISM—a condition wherein a person refuses or is unable to speak because of psychological conflict.

NEOLOGISM—a word coined by the patient, commonly with private meaning.

NEUROSIS—a negative abnormality, ill-defined in character but milder than psychosis.

ORGANIC DISORDERS—mental disorders that arise from bodily malfunction.

ORGANIC VIEW OF PSYCHOPATHOLOGY—the view that mental disorders are attributable to one or another kind of hereditary misfortune, constitutional accident, or physical damage or disease.

OVERINCLUSION—a tendency to include in a concept all manner of objects and events that bear little or no relationship to it.

PARALOGICAL THINKING—thinking with a logic of its own which is not accessible to others.

PARANOIA—a psychological condition in which the person suffers from delusions which are organized into a tight logical and perceptual system around which his entire life revolves.

PARANOID REACTIONS—reactions that involve quite unwarranted feelings of personal significance, or the false belief that others are hostile and persecutory (see Chapter 10).

PARANOID SCHIZOPHRENIA—a psychosis characterized chiefly by autistic and unrealistic thinking, hallucinations, and most often highly elaborated and systematized delusions, particularly of persecution and grandeur.[1]

PARESIS—see GENERAL PARESIS.

PASSIVE AGGRESSIVE PERSONALITY—a disposition to continuously express aggression towards others by passive means, such as *not* doing things one is supposed to do.

PERSONAL DISTURBANCES OF BEHAVIOR—behavior that is abnormal in a negative way but cannot easily be classified as neurotic, psychotic, or psychosomatic.

PHYSICAL ASSAULT METHODS—methods devised for treating psychological disorders that involve the use of electrical, chemical, or other physical stimulation.

POSTPARTUM PSYCHOSIS—a psychotic condition precipitated by giving birth and usually predominated by feelings of depression.

PRECIPITATING FACTORS IN MENTAL DISORDERS—factors that actually bring about, or directly cause, mental disorders.

PREDISPOSING FACTORS IN MENTAL DISORDERS—factors that increase the probability of the occurrence of mental disorders, whether or not the disorders develop.

PREMORBID HISTORY—the history of an individual previous to his becoming mentally ill.

PREMORBID SOCIAL COMPETENCE—the disordered individual's ability to function in society previous to institutionalization or treatment.

PRIMARY PROCESS THINKING—a term used by Freud to describe thoughts, images, and the like which are dictated by internal states rather than by the nature of external reality.

PROCESS SCHIZOPHRENIA—schizophrenic psychosis whose symptoms develop slowly after years of poor social adjustment.

PROGNOSIS—informed opinion regarding the prospects of recovery from a mental or physical disorder.

PSYCHEDELIC DRUGS—drugs which affect mental processes, especially those that give an expanded sense of consciousness.

PSYCHIATRIC NOSOLOGY—a classification or list of nervous or mental disorders.

PSYCHIATRIST—a medical doctor who specializes in the diagnosis and treatment of nervous and mental disorders.

PSYCHODYNAMIC THEORY OF PERSONALITY

[1] This definition was taken from H. B. English and Ava C. English, *A Comprehensive Dictionary of Psychological and Psychoanalytical Terms*, New York: David McKay Company, Inc., 1958.

—those theories of human behavior, often derived from the work of Freud, that stress motives and drives as determinants of behavior.

PSYCHOLOGICAL VIEW OF PSYCHOPATHOLOGY —see DYNAMIC VIEW OF PSYCHOPATHOLOGY.

PSYCHOMOTOR RETARDATION—the slowing down of psychomotor responses.

PSYCHOPATHOLOGY—mental illness; negative psychological abnormalities (see Chapter 10).

PSYCHOSIS—an ill-defined term, generally meaning any severe negative psychological abnormality.

PSYCHOSOMATIC DISORDERS—physical symptoms resulting from psychological stress or conflict.

PSYCHOTIC DEPRESSIVE REACTION—a disorder marked by severe depression and gross misinterpretation of reality.

PUBERTY—the period of time in which the secondary sex characteristics appear.

PYKNIC TYPE—Kretchmer's term for the stocky and rotund body type; similar to Sheldon's endomorph.

REACTION FORMATION—a defense involving a behavioral display that is directly opposite to a presumed (unconscious) motive; thus, aggression may be a reaction formation to fear.

REACTIVE SCHIZOPHRENIA—a psychotic disorder wherein premorbid social functioning was good and where symptoms developed shortly after some stressful or traumatic experiences.

REGRESSIVE BEHAVIOR—childlike or infantile behavior.

RESIDUAL TYPE OF SCHIZOPHRENIA—the term applied to patients who were formerly severely disturbed and currently manifest mild symptoms of the disorder.

RETARDED DEPRESSION—a depression characterized by quiet, withdrawn behavior and passive, stuporous misery.

SCHIZO-AFFECTIVE SCHIZOPHRENIA—a disorder characterized by symptoms of an affective psychosis as well as of schizophrenia.

SCHIZOID CONDITIONS—a broad array of conditions, ranging in severity from mild to serious and characterized by tendencies to withdraw emotionally from others.

SCHIZOID PERSONALITY—a personality or character disorder; a diagnostic category which includes people who are relatively withdrawn, who avoid close relationships with others, and who have difficulty expressing feelings.

SCHIZOPHRENIA—a group of psychotic reactions characterized by fundamental disturbances in reality relationships, by a conceptual world determined largely by feeling, and by marked affective, intellectual, and overt behavioral disturbances.[1]

SECONDARY PROCESS THINKING—a term used by Freud to describe realistic thinking.

SELF-ESTEEM—the degree to which one values and appreciates one's self and characteristics.

SEPPUKU—dishonorable suicide in Japan.

SETTING-IN STAGE OF SCHIZOPHRENIA—the stage in which the patient comes to accept his symptoms as realities and to systematize them in relation to each other.

SEXUAL DEVIATION—sexual behavior that is considered abnormal in one's society.

SIMPLE SCHIZOPHRENIA—a psychosis marked chiefly by apathy, simplicity, reduced relatedness to the external world, and an impoverishment of human relationships.[1]

SOCIOPATHIC PERSONALITY DISTURBANCES—an ill-defined broad category that generally implies nonconformity to prevailing social and ethical standards.

SOMATIC DELUSIONS—delusions about one's own body.

SPONTANEOUS RECOVERY RATE—the rate at which symptoms of disorder disappear without therapy.

SYMPTOMATIC DESCRIPTIONS—groupings of disorders chiefly in terms of their superficial relations to each other, such as common symptoms.

TAXONOMIC SYSTEM—system of classification.

TAXONOMY—orderly classification of phenomena according to their presumed lawful relationships.

TOXIC—poisonous.

WAXY FLEXIBILITY—the condition of a patient whose limbs can be moved to strange and unusual positions and maintained in those positions like a wax statue.

WITHDRAWAL SYMPTOMS—painful physical symptoms caused by the abrupt cessation of drugs to which the body has become accustomed.

WORD SALAD—a jumble of words possessing no meaning for the listener.

REFERENCES

Becker, J. Achievement related characteristics of manic-depressives. *Journal of Abnormal and Social Psyschology*, 1960, **60**, 334–339.

Bockoven, J. S. Moral treatment in American psychiatry. *Journal of Nervous and Mental Diseases*, 1956, **124**, 167.

Bleuler, E. *Dementia praecox: Or the group of schizophrenias.* (Translated by J. Zinkin.) New York: International Universities Press, 1950. (Originally published, 1911.)

Buss, A. H. *Psychopathology*. New York: John Wiley & Sons, Inc., 1966.

Cameron, N. *The psychology of behavior disorders.* Boston: Houghton Mifflin Company, 1947.

———. *Personality development and psycopathology: A Dynamic Approach*. Boston: Houghton Mifflin Company, 1963.

Chapman, L. J., Dorothy Day, and A. Burstein. The process-reactive distinction and prognosis in schizophrenia. *Journal of Nervous and Mental Diseases*, 1961, **133**, 383–391.

Cleckley, H. *The mask of sanity: An attempt to clarify some issues about the so-called psychopathic personality.* St. Louis: The C. V. Mosby Company. 1955.

Cohen, M. M., Michele J. Marinello, and Nathan Back. Chromosomal damage in human leukocytes induced by lysergic acid diethylamide. *Science*, March, 1967, **155**, 1417–1419.

Delgado, J. M. R. Free behavior and brain stimulation. In *International review of neurobiology*. New York: Academic Press, Inc., 1964.

English, O. S., and G. H. J. Pearson. *Emotional problems of living: Avoiding the neurotic pattern.* New York: W. W. Norton & Company, Inc., 1963.

Erikson, K. T. Patient role and social uncertainty: A dilemma of the mentally ill. *Psychiatry*, 1957, **20**, 263–374.

Eysenck, H. J. Classification and the problem of diagnosis. In H. J. Eysenck (ed.), *Handbook of abnormal psychology*. London: Sir Isaac Pitman & Sons, Ltd., 1960.

Farberow, N. L., and T. L. McEvoy. Suicide among patients with diagnoses of anxiety reaction or depressive reaction in general medical and surgical hospitals. *Journal of Abnormal Psychology*, 1966, **71**, 287–299.

Ferster, C. B. Positive reinforcement and behavioral deficits of autistic children. *Child development*, 1961, **32**, 437–456.

Freud, S. *Gesammelte Werke*, Vol. VIII., London: Imago, 1940–1952. (Originally published, 1911.) As referred to by E. Jones in *The life and work of Sigmund Freud*, Vol. II. New York: Basic Books, Inc., 1955, pp. 268–273.

———. New introductory lectures on psychoanalysis (translated by J. H. Sprott). New York: W. W. Norton & Company, Inc., 1933.

Glueck, S., and Eleanor Glueck. *Physique and delinquency*. New York: Harper & Row, Publishers, 1956.

Godfrey, L., M. D. Kissen, and T. M. Downs. Treatment of the acute alcohol-withdrawal syndrome. *Quarterly Journal of Studies on Alcoholism*, 1958, **19**, 118–124.

Griesinger, W. *Mental pathology and therapeutics*, Ed. 2. London: New Sydenham Society, 1845.

Hinsie, L. E., and R. J. Campbell. *Psychiatric dictionary*, Ed. 3. New York: Oxford University Press, Inc., 1960.

Hoch, P. H., and J. Zubin (eds.). *Current problems in psychiatric-diagnosis*. New York: Grune & Stratton, Inc., 1953.

Humphreys, L. G. Characteristics of type concepts with special reference to Sheldon's typology. *Psychological Bulletin*, 1957, **54**, 218–228.

Jackson, D. D. (ed.). *The etiology of schizophrenia*. New York: Basic Books, Inc., 1960.

Joint Commission on Mental Illness and Health. *Action for mental health.* New York: Basic Books, Inc., 1961.

Kanner, A. Early infantile autism. *Journal of Pediatrics*. 1944, **25**, 211–217.

Kraepelin, E. *Clinical psychiatry* (translated by A. Ross Diefendorf). New York: Crowell-Collier and Macmillan, Inc., 1907.

Kety, S. S. Biochemical theories of schizophrenia: Part I. *Science*, 1959*a*, **129**, 1528–1532.

———. Biochemical theories of schizophrenia: Part II. *Science*, 1959*b*, **129**, 1590–1596.

Kretschmer, E. *Physique and character* (translated by W. J. H. Sprott). New

York: Harcourt, Brace & World, Inc., 1925.

Landis, C. *Varieties of psychopathological experience* (edited by F. A. Mettler). New York: Holt, Rinehart & Winston, 1964.

London, P. *The modes and morals of psychotherapy*. New York: Holt, Rinehart & Winston, 1964.

———. Discussion of papers for symposium: An experimental treatment program for childhood schizophrenia, American Psychological Association, Chicago, Illinois, September 4, 1965 (mimeographed).

———. Morals and mental health. In S. C. Plog and R. B. Edgerton (eds.), *Determinants of mental illness*. New York: Holt, Rinehart & Winston, in press.

Maher, B. A. Principles of *psychopathology*. New York: McGraw-Hill, Inc., 1966.

Meehl, P. Schizotaxia, schizotypy, schizophrenia. *American Psychologist*, 1962, **17**, 827–838.

Mental disorders: Diagnostic and statistical manual. Washington, D.C.: American Psychiatric Association, 1952.

Mowrer, O. H. *The crisis in psychiatry and religion*. Princeton, N.J.: D. Van Nostrand Company, Inc., 1961.

———. *The new group therapy*. Princeton, N. J.: D. Van Nostrand Company, Inc., 1964.

———. *Abnormal reactions or actions? An autobiographical answer*. Dubuque, Iowa: William C. Brown Company, Publishers, 1966*a*.

———. *New evidence concerning the nature of psychopathology*. To be published.

Munroe, Ruth L. *Schools of psychoanalytic thought: An exposition, critique, and attempt at integration*. New York: Holt, Rinehart & Winston, 1955.

Noyes, A. P., and L. C. Kolb. *Modern clinical psychiatry*. Philadelphia: W. B. Saunders Company, 1958.

Quay, H. *The psychoses*. In I. A. Berg, and L. A. Pennington (eds.), *An introduction to clinical psychology*, Ed. 3. New York: The Ronald Press Company, 1966.

Rees, L. Constitutional factors and abnormal behavior. In H. J. Eysenck (ed.), *Handbook of abnormal psychology*. New York: Basic Books, Inc., 1961.

Rimland, B. *Infantile autism*. New York: Appleton-Century, 1964.

Rosen, E., and I. Gregory. *Abnormal psychology*. Philadelphia: W. B. Saunders Company, 1965.

Selye, H. *The stress of life*. New York: McGraw-Hill, Inc., 1956.

Shagass, C., and M. Schwartz. Cerebral cortical reactivity in psychotic depressions. *Archives of General psychiatry*, 1962, **6**, 235–242.

Sheldon, W. H. *Varieties of temperament*. New York: Harper & Row, Publishers, 1942.

Shneidman, E. S., and N. L. Farberow. Suicide and death. In H. Feifel, *The meaning of death*. New York: McGraw-Hill, Inc., 1959.

Sourkes, T. *Biochemistry of mental disease*. New York: Paul B. Hoeber, Inc., 1962.

Sullivan, H. S. *The interpersonal theory of psychiatry*. New York: W. W. Norton & Company, Inc., 1963.

Szalita, A. B. Psychodynamics of disorders of the involutional age. In S. Arieti (ed.), *American handbook of psychiatry*. New York: Basic Books, Inc., 1966.

Szasz, T. S. The problem of psychiatric nosology: A contribution to a situational analysis of psychiatric operations. *American Journal of Psychiatry*, 1957, **114**, 405–413.

———. *The myth of mental illness*. New York: Paul B. Hoeber, Inc., 1961.

Time, September 15, 1967, **90**, No. 11, 84–85.

Vigotsky, L. S. Thought in schizophrenia. *A.M.A. Archives of Neurology and Psychiatry*, 1934, **31**, 1063–1077.

Wittman, P., W. H. Sheldon, and C. J. Katz. A study of the relationship between constitutional variations and fundamental psychotic behavior reactions. *Journal of Nervous and Mental Diseases*, 1948, **108**, 470–476.

Zigler, E., and L. Phillips. Psychiatric diagnosis: A critique. *Journal of Abnormal and Social Psychology*, 1961, **3**, 607–618.

SUGGESTED READINGS

1. Arieti, S. *Interpretation of schizophrenia*. New York: Brunner, 1955. A stimulating theoretical analysis of the origins of schizophrenia.
2. Beers, C. W. *A mind that found itself*. New York: Doubleday & Company, Inc., 1931. A classic both for its descriptions of mental hospitals and for its description of manic and depressive states.

3. Cameron, N. *The psychology of behavior disorders: A biosocial interpretation.* Boston: Houghton Mifflin Company, 1947. A magnificently stimulating treatise on behavior pathology, full of rich insights into origins and dynamics. The author's more recent book, *Personality development and psychopathology: A dynamic approach* (Boston: Houghton Mifflin Company, 1963) is more psychoanalytically oriented, and still provocative.
4. Eysenck, H. J. (ed.). *Handbook of abnormal psychology.* London: Sir Isaac Pitman & Sons, Ltd., 1960. A very valuable collection of papers that summarize the various literatures in this area.
5. Jackson, D. D. (ed.). *The etiology of schizophrenia.* New York: Basic Books, Inc., 1960. A collection of essays on the origins and dynamics of schizophrenia.
6. Joint Commission on Mental Illness and Health. *Action for mental health.* New York: Basic Books, Inc., 1961. A report of the results of a Congress-initiated survey of the incidence of mental illness in the United States and facilities and personnel for their treatment.
7. Kaplan, B. (ed.). *The inner world of mental illness.* New York: Harper & Row Publishers, 1963. Biographical reports, written by the patients themselves, of the experience of psychosis and severe neurosis.
8. Rosen, E., and I. Gregory. *Abnormal psychology.* Philadelphia: W. B. Saunders Company, 1965. An excellent treatment of the major psychological disorders.
9. Szasz, T. *The myth of mental illness.* New York: Paul B. Hoeber, Inc., 1961. A suggestion that psychological disorder is best viewed as a game or strategy rather than an illness.

12

A Social View of Psychopathology

LESLIE PHILLIPS

Pathological reactions are personal tragedies for their victims and their families, but they are also serious problems for society as a whole. The direct cost of mental illness in hospital and outpatient staffs and facilities is enormous, but the indirect cost in work loss, let alone in anguish, is simply staggering. There are no precise statistics of misery, but some idea of the social enormity of these problems can be gotten from the statistical information that does exist.

THE PREVALENCE OF PSYCHIATRIC DISORDERS

According to statistics released by the American Hospital Association, 51 percent of the 1,406,818 patients comprising the average daily census in all hospitals are patients in psychiatric care (*Hospitals,* 1963). Thus patients suffering from mental illnesses now occupy more hospital beds than the victims of polio, cancer, heart disease, tuberculosis, and all other diseases combined.

More than 98 percent of these patients are in *public* mental hospitals. Of all first admissions to state and county mental hospitals, the largest percentages are patients with schizophrenia (23 percent) and one or another kind of brain damage, such as cerebral arteriosclerosis and senile brain disease (23 percent). Because schizophrenic patients are relatively young on admission to hospitals and have a relatively low annual death rate, those who are not discharged tend to accumulate from year to year and to make up approximately half of the total resident populations of the public hospitals. Patients with circulatory and senile brain disease, on the other hand, have a high annual death rate and constitute only about 14 percent of the resident population of these mental hospitals.

Other causes of first admissions to state and county mental hospitals in-

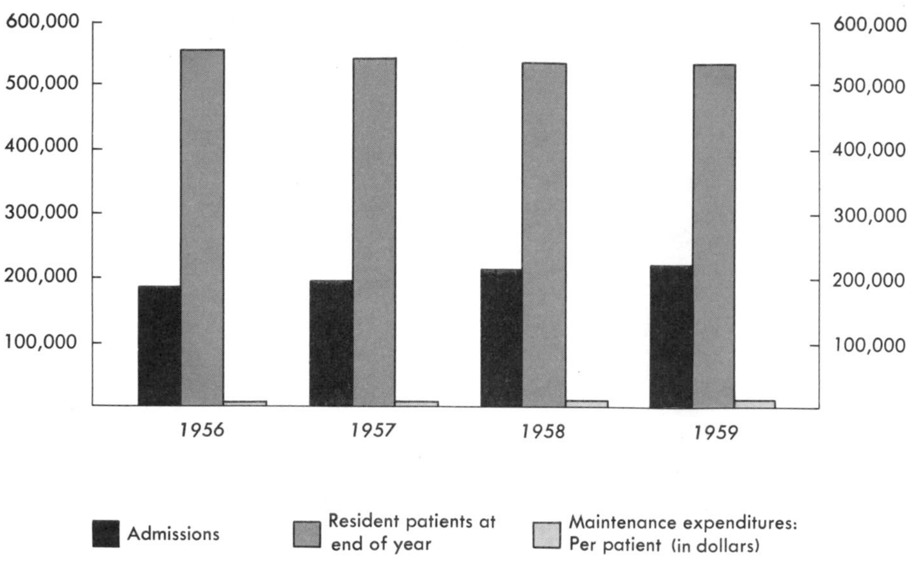

Figure 12.1 Statistics from public mental hospitals in the United States, 1956 to 1959. Data supplied by the Biometrics Branch, National Institute of Mental Health.

clude: alcoholism (15 percent), psychotic disorders other than schizophrenia (8 percent), personality disorders (7 percent), psychoneurotic reactions (7 percent), and mental deficiency (3 percent) (*Patients in mental institutions,* 1960). The various psychiatric disturbances affect different segments of the population and develop at different times of life. In the age range from fourteen to forty-four years, schizophrenia and personality disorders predominate. During the next decade of life, the involutional psychoses and alcoholic psychoses attain considerable importance. In the sixties, psychoses with cerebral arteriosclerosis and senile psychoses assume prominence, and the mental diseases specifically related to aging continue to rise until the end of the lifespan.

In addition to people hospitalized because of mental illness, approximately 741,000 patients per year receive psychiatric care in outpatient psychiatric clinics (*Fifteen indices,* 1964). At least 250,000 children with less serious disorders receive treatment each year at mental health clinics throughout the country. Further, it is estimated that there are 3,800,000 problem drinkers in the United States, of whom 950,000 are chronic and severe alcoholics. In addition, 50,000 persons are presumed to be addicted to narcotics (*Facts and figures about mental health and other personality disturbances,* 1952).

At the present time, it is estimated that the annual direct cost of mental illness is over four billion dollars (*What are the facts about mental illness in the United States?* 1964). This figure includes the total maintenance and operating expenditures of public and private mental hospitals, the cost of public assistance to mentally disordered and retarded persons, and the estimated income losses of patients in mental hospitals (see Figure 12.1).

These statistics are based on known, treated cases of mental disturbance. Various attempts have been made to ascertain the overall rate (including both treated and untreated cases) of psychiatric disorder in the general population, but the findings of different investigators have varied widely. This is strikingly demonstrated by the variation at army induction stations during World War II in rejection rates on grounds of psychiatric disability. These rates varied from a low of 0.5 percent to a high of 51 percent (Stouffer *et al.*, 1950).

In a study conducted in Baltimore during the early 1950's, it was estimated that about 11 percent of the noninstitutionalized population exhibited "obvious" mental illness (Commission on Chronic Illness, 1957). Another study of a rural county in Nova Scotia found that approximately 20 percent of the sampled residents had a "definite need for psychiatric help" (Leighton *et al.*, 1963). And in an intensive study of a population sample of a midtown section of Manhattan, also conducted during the early 1950's, 23 percent were rated as "seriously impaired" psychiatrically, while only 18 percent were considered psychiatrically "well," or essentially free of symptoms (Srole *et al.*, 1962). Of the seriously impaired, about 5 percent were being treated as outpatients, and more than 20 percent had been patients at some time in their previous history. Thus, about three-fourths of the seriously impaired had never come into psychiatric contact.

The more intensive the effort to discover psychiatric cases, the higher the resulting rates of mental disturbance become. Thus, in a 1930 survey (Brugger, 1938) carried out in Thuringia on psychotics, psychopathic personalities, neurasthenics, alcoholics, "eccentrics," and mental retardates, institution files yielded a rate of approximately 13 per 1000 population. In contrast, a house-to-house canvas increased the rate to nearly 60 per 1000. Similar increases of five or six times in prevalence rates have been reported by other authors as a result of an intensive search for unreported cases. Findings of this type have led many observers to draw the familiar "iceberg analogy": only a small proportion of persons in the community who are suffering from some form of psychiatric disorder have come to the attention of treatment agencies. A much larger group remains outside the purview of mental health services.

Antisocial Behavior

Increasingly interest has been centered on various kinds of sociopathic personality disorders, that is, behavior deviations from prevailing social standards. The growing frequency of these disorders may be linked to the increase in criminal and delinquent behaviors, one of the most serious social problems confronting this country today.

Each year more than two million crimes are reported in the United States (*Statistical abstracts of the United States*, 1965), of which more than 90 percent involve money or property (for example, burglaries, larcenies, auto thefts, and robberies), the remainder being directed against persons (aggravated assaults, forcible rapes, and murders). Annually, more than 750,000 children come before the juvenile courts because of alleged delinquent behavior. It is now estimated that one boy in every five is brought into court during his adolescence on a delinquency charge, including traffic violations (*Report to Congress on juvenile delinquency, February, 1960*). The cost of juvenile delinquency to this nation's economy is currently estimated at about four billion dollars a year (Fogarty, 1960).

Psychosomatic Disorders

Many people suffer from some form of psychosomatic ailment. Of all the patients annually admitted to general hospitals, about 6,000,000 have serious mental and emotional disorders which are partly responsible for their physical condition (*Facts about mental illness,* 1956). For example, in the ages from forty-five to sixty-four years, five of the twelve most common types of disabling illness are often considered to be psychosomatic diseases, including diseases of the heart, functional digestive disturbances, arthritis (combined with chronic rheumatism), hypertension (combined with arteriosclerosis), and headache. About 1 to 2 percent of the entire middle-aged population is disabled annually by one or more of these diseases (*Medical almanac,* 1961–1962).

In brief, pathological responses to adaptive failure can occur in any of the four spheres of function available to the human organism: the intropsychic and emotional (psychological disorders), the motoric (antisocial behaviors and addictions), and the somatic (psychosomatic diseases). Each of these types of maladaptive response is pervasively present in our society; combined, they represent a major dissonance between the ways of life which people, as individuals, want to lead and the communal expectations which encroach on them. That the lives of so large a proportion of the population can be touched in some degree by the effects of adaptive failure transforms the problem of pathology from an expression of personal tragedy, repeated endlessly in the lives of millions of individuals, to a social issue which only society through its institutional structures can attempt to resolve. To attempt this task requires a far more precise knowledge of the nature of pathology than we now possess.

THE QUESTION OF DEFINITION

Major differences of opinion still exist regarding the meaning and classification of the various forms of pathology, especially about the psychiatric disorders, which are defined for the most part in terms of the patient's psychological state. As we saw in Chapter 9, the major question at issue is whether these disorders are to be thought of as "disease" processes, analogous to physical diseases, or as the behavioral reactions of individuals who are pressured by events and experience into inappropriate and inadequate response patterns.

Logic demands that psychiatric symptoms be thought of simply as reaction patterns. Even if we assume that the onset of overt symptoms is the result of distortions in underlying psychological or somatic processes, the *hypothesized* presence of such distorted processes, as we saw in Chapter 9, cannot serve to define a disorder. Only when such causal factors have been demonstrated and measured can we relinquish *overt behavior* as the critical basis for psychiatric diagnosis.

Other difficulties beset the classification of psychiatric disorders. One finds with severe disorders, as indicated in Chapter 10 about the symptoms of neurosis, that diagnosis bears no one-to-one correspondence to symptom manifestation and that symptoms of considerable diversity are consistent with *all* diagnostic labels. Thus, hallucinations, delusions, blunted or inappropriate affect, seclusiveness, and suspicion are all common occurrences in cases diagnosed as schizophrenia, but the same diagnosis may be made on the basis of any one or more of these symptoms.

Alternatively, identical symptoms can appear in cases falling into different diagnostic syndromes. Zigler and Phillips (1961*a*) examined the psychiatric case records of 793 patients categorized as either manic-depressive, schizophrenic, neurotic, or having a character disorder. They investigated the frequency of occurrence of thirty-five common symptoms in each of these four groups and found sixty-seven relationships between individual symptoms and particular diagnostic categories, but the degree of relationship turned out to be quite small. In fact, the association between specific symptoms and diagnosis proved to be a highly unreliable guide to symptomatology and vice versa. These findings agree with those of earlier studies (Freudenberg and Robertson, 1956; Wittenborn *et al.*, 1953).

It is not surprising, then, to find that psychiatric classification is very unreliable. This may in part be blamed on inadequate professional technique, but much diagnostic variability has been traced to the obscurity and ambiguity inherent in the standard classification itself. Dayton (1940) reported on 89,190 patients with mental disorder admitted to the state hospitals of Massachusetts during the years 1917 to 1933. Great variability was found from one hospital to another, and within each of the participating hospitals, of cases assigned to broad diagnostic categories. In 1917, for example, 33 percent of Worcester State Hospital first admissions were classified as dementia praecox (schizophrenia). In this same category, Danvers State Hospital had a first admission rate of 21 percent. In 1925, the Northampton Hospital had 31 percent of such first admissions and Boston State, only 8 percent. In 1933, Northampton reported 35 percent, whereas at Boston State, the comparable figure was 3 percent. Over the period of the study, the dementia praecox rate increased at some hospitals and decreased at others.

In a study of the 1951 first admissions to state mental hospitals (Leighton *et al.*, 1957), it was found that the ratio of manic-depressive diagnoses to schizophrenic ones varied from 67:100 in Georgia to 6:100 in New York. There is no obvious reason for this striking discrepancy in the proportions of these two patient types, and the implication is that many patients diagnosed as manic-depressive in Georgia would have been classified as schizophrenic in New York.

Striking differences in diagnosis have also been found among men rejected by army induction stations because of psychiatric disorders. For example, the proportion of those classified as psychoneurotic varied across the country from 3 to 90 percent (Terris, 1959).

Consistency in psychiatric diagnosis was examined in a group of 794 enlisted men who were first seen by a psychiatric unit at a naval precommissioning installation and were subsequently transferred to a hospital for medical evaluation and separation from the navy (Hunt *et al.*, 1953). Diagnoses at the two installations were compared. Overall agreement on specific diagnoses was found in only 32 percent of these cases, while agreement increased to 54 percent for the broad classifications of psychosis, psychoneurosis, and personality disorder.

In a study of the basis for disagreements in classification, Ward *et al.* (1962) reported that one-third were caused by variability among diagnosticians, including contradictory decisions as to what should be considered the dominant pathology when there were mixed symptoms. Two-thirds of the disagreements, however, were ascribed to inadequacies in the classification system itself, including impractically narrow distinctions, the requirement of unnecessary decisions, as the forced choice between neurosis and personality disorder when symptoms of both were in evidence, and the lack of clear criteria for distinguishing between psychiatric categories.

Individual symptoms can be judged in a far more reliable fashion than global psychiatric diagnoses can. Ullmann and Gurel (1962) have reported a study in which different psychologists rated symptoms from 120 summaries of psychiatric admission notes. These assessments were in highly significant agreement. In addition, symptom ratings based on the admission reports were compared with those from face-to-face interviews carried out quite independently of the psychiatric admission procedures. Again, highly significant relationships were obtained from the two methods of symptom tabulation.

Whether one assumes that psychiatric disorder is some form of "disease" or "illness," or that it is a pattern of behavior adopted by the person to cope with the problems of his life, one can expect some consistency in the particular symptoms of any disorder. It is the ambiguous relation between symptoms and diagnosis which defeats the use of the present classification system of the American Psychiatric Association.

Various investigators have undertaken systematic analyses of the way in which symptoms tend to coincide among groups of patients. The kinds of questions which have been asked are: If a given patient hallucinates, will he also tend to be seclusive or euphoric? Studies of this sort are limited by the range of symptoms examined within any one investigation, by the variety of patient groups examined, and by the nature of the institution within which a study is carried out. The proportions of various types of disorder differ radically from a mental hospital to an outpatient psychiatric facility, a prison, or an institution for retardates.

Symptom factors of male psychiatric inpatients have been divided into three major clusters (Lorr *et al.*, 1955). These include (1) a set of affective factors, that is, manic-depressive or tense, agitated, depressive; (2) those indicative of social withdrawal and seclusiveness; and (3) a series of factors suggestive of resistiveness and belligerence. Another factor analytic study on 250 psychotic patients found three analogous clusterings: (1) depression with guilt, and hostility aimed at the self; (2) thought and personality disorganization with associated social withdrawal; and (3) a hostile belligerence or irritable combativeness (Lorr, 1957). These studies imply that a strong thread of disorganization in interpersonal relations characterizes psychotics, regardless of the specific diagnosis.

Leary and Coffey (1955) have also found that certain psychiatric syndromes, as measured by the Minnesota Multiphasic Personality Inventory (MMPI), correspond to certain consistent ways of viewing oneself and others and to patterns of interpersonal relationships. Obsessiveness was found to be associated with self-derogatory and passive attitudes, schizoid features with bitter, distrustful attitudes, and psychopathic tendencies with aggressiveness and rebelliousness.

Factor analytic studies of symptoms have also been undertaken among children. The symptoms of deviant behavior which brought a large number of children to a guidance clinic were analyzed by Lorr and Jenkins (1953), who found five common factors: (1) encephalitis or brain damage, (2) unsocialized aggression, (3) socialized delinquency, (4) overinhibition, and (5) schizoid character. The same factors were revealed for both sexes, although the symptom pictures were slightly different: boy socialized delinquents were likely to steal, girls to be untruthful, and among unsocialized aggressives, boys might be destructive, while girls were more likely to have tantrums. Notice that, apart from brain damage, three themes of interpersonal relationships somewhat similar to those observed among adult psychiatric cases emerge among these children. These are (1) aggression, delinquency, and rebellion; (2) schizoid (loss of social contact) and (3) overinhibition. This last differs, however, from the self-directed hostility, guilt, and depression characteristically found in adult psychiatric cases.

Two factors emerged for Peterson (1961) when he had teachers rate 831 kindergarten and elementary school children on fifty-eight clinically frequent problems. Remarkable consistency in symptom factors appeared across all age groups. The two factors were labeled "conduct problems" and "personality problems." The first factor implied a tendency to express impulses against society, the second suggested (1) low self-esteem and depressed mood and (2) social withdrawal. Here too, distorted interpersonal relationships are expressed symptomatically: either in a turning against others, a turning against the self, or a social withdrawal.

In short, many studies strongly suggest that symptomatic behaviors reflect a person's pattern or style of relating to other people. This interpretation receives explicit support from the findings of Phillips and Rabinovitch (1958) in a study of forty-six symptoms among 604 psychiatric patients. Thirty-nine of the original forty-six symptoms appeared at a sufficiently high frequency to warrant statistical analysis. Of these, thirty-one evidenced relationships with one or more other symptoms. Interpretation of these data led to the organization of twenty-five symptoms into three categories: Category 1 appears to imply a turning against the self, expressed either directly in action or thought (suicidal attempt, deprecatory ideas against the self) or in physical suffering (bodily complaints, insomnia). The second category involves turning against others (threatened assault, temper outbursts, robbery) or self-indulgent and socally disapproved behaviors (drinking, perversions). The last of three categories represents an avoidance of others, either directly (suspiciousness, withdrawal) or in distorted fantasy (hallucinations, sexual preoccupations, bizarre ideas). The idea that the symptom categories established in this study may be viewed as particular ways of relating to others is reminiscent of the "life style" proposed by a number of theorists, for example, "intropunitive" (Rosenzweig, 1945), "symbiotic relatedness" (Fromm, 1947), and "moving away from others" (Horney, 1945).

A different facet of "life style" may also be reflected in symptom manifestation, that is, whether the individual's preferred mode of self-expression is thought, affect, or action. Symptoms may appear primarily in one mode or another; in thought as suicidal ideas, sexual preoccupations, or hallucinations in affect as depression, tension, or temper outbursts; or in action as suicidal attempts, assault, or drinking.

A study by Phillips *et al.* (in press) first notes the paradox that individual symptoms show no substantial relation to assigned diagnosis and that, on the other hand, broad categories of diagnosis can be established among psychiatrists with modest reliability. Psychiatrists obviously make use of observed symptoms for their classification procedure, but they may also be systematically organizing the presenting symptoms into life-style categories in order to arrive at a diagnosis. Perhaps it is not so much the presence or absence of particular symptoms as the expression of symptoms predominantly in one life-style mode (thinking, affect, or action) that contributes to diagnosis. The authors also suggest that another aspect of life style in symptoms may contribute to diagnosis, namely, a patient's social role, that is, his attitudes toward himself and others. The hypothesis of their study was that both sphere dominance (mode of expression) and role orientation, as expressed in symptoms, account for the reliable part of psychiatric diagnosis. They examined the case histories of 762 patients, 455 males and 307 females. Sphere dominance scores were based on the relative dominance of thought, affect, or action symptoms:

- Thought symptoms
  - Bizarre ideas or delusions
  - Depersonalization
  - Feelings of going crazy
  - Fear of own hostile impulses
  - Feelings of perversion
  - Feelings of sexual inadequacy
  - Hallucinations
  - Obsessions
  - Perplexity
  - Phobias
  - Self-deprecation
  - Sexual preoccupations
  - Suicidal ideas
  - Suspiciousness
  - Threatened assault
- Action symptoms
  - Apathy
  - Depression
  - Euphoria
  - Maniacal outbursts
  - Mood swings
  - Temper outbursts
  - Tenseness
- Affect symptoms
  - All addictions except drinking
  - Assaultiveness
  - Murder
  - Compulsions
  - Refusal to eat
  - Drinking
  - Excessive eating
  - Fire setting
  - Homosexuality
  - Irresponsible behavior
  - Rape
  - Robbery
  - Sexual deviations, except homosexuality
  - Suicidal attempt

Symptoms were categorized into one of three role categories as follows: (1) turning against the self: suicidal ideas, self-deprecation, suicidal attempt, depression; (2) turning against others: threatened assault, robbery, temper outbursts; (3) avoidance of others: suspiciousness, perplexity, hallucinations, withdrawals, apathy.

Patients in this study were divided into four groups according to the diagnosis already made by the psychiatric staff. These categories were: (1) manic-depressive disorders (including involutional and depressive psychotic reactions); (2) schizophrenic disorders; (3) psychoneurotic disorders; and (4) personality disorders (including personality pattern disturbances, personality trait disturbances, and sociopathic personality disturbances).

The observed relationships were large enough to indicate that the style variable is an important component of the reliability of psychiatric diagnosis. The correlation between sphere dominance and diagnosis was 0.60, and the three role orientation groups correlated 0.71 across the four diagnostic categories. Indeed, the combined relation of sphere dominance and role orientation to diagnosis appeared to account for virtually all that is reliable in psychiatric diagnosis. Apparently, the diagnosis assigned by a clinician corresponds in substantial degree to the patient's life style.

LIFE STYLE AND PSYCHOPATHOLOGY

We have seen that the forms taken by psychopathology appear to reflect a characteristic style of behavior. The following propositions seem reasonable consequences from this observation: (1) individuals who share similar styles of life should tend to manifest similar patterns of pathology when it appears, and (2) individuals who differ in life styles should differ in their dominant forms of pathology.

Findings from three different sources tend to support these hypotheses. These include (1) studies which compare the forms of psychopathology in different societies and cultures; (2) changes over time in the dominant types of pathology within American society; and (3) differences in pathology which appear in American society according to social class, marital status, age, and sex.

Crosscultural Differences

What is the relation between the cultural forms of a society and its most frequent types of psychopathology? Many studies bear on this question, but they are comparatively unsystematic and do not provide an adequate basis for crosscultural comparisons. Much of the difficulty stems from uneven distribution of psychiatric facilities: where facilities do not exist, cases cannot be reported. Consequently, prevalence figures from one society to another must be viewed skeptically. In addition, the European and American system of diagnosis has been the dominant method of classification, but while it allows some comparisons of data collected in many studies, it does not clearly cover behavior deviations in cultures which differ widely from ours. Thus in nonliterate societies, one of the problems in detecting schizophrenia and other psychiatric disorders marked by severe disturbances in thought is the degree to which these societies distinguish between logical and illogical thought. Benedict (1958) has observed that technologically backward cultures are suffused with magical devices and supernaturalism which may reinforce the deluded thought of the psychotic. In such a world, the schizophrenic is often able to escape detection. In Brazilian rural society, for example, because it is considered possible to talk to God, religious zeal and psychosis might look alike. The contrasting emphasis in Western society on rational and objective thought makes it considerably more difficult for the psychotic individual to adjust and to escape detection. Nevertheless, Linton (1956) claimed that in no society does the "genuine psychotic" occupy a favored position.

As noted earlier, studies of psychiatric symptomatology in our own society have repeatedly indicated that deviant reactions tend to fall into three symptom clusters, indicative of different role orientations, that is, turning against the self, turning against others, and avoidance of others. Crosscultural studies suggest that these deviant role orientations bear some relation to the level of technological development in a society. In less developed societies, avoidance of others and a destructive turning against others are prominent symptoms, while in more advanced societies, symptoms of guilt and of turning against the self are more frequent. Further, in technologically less advanced societies, psychopathology tends to be oriented toward action, emotional symptoms are either explosive or apathetic, and thought symptoms typically are extremely disordered. In more advanced societies psychopathology is more often expressed in thought than in action, and the person is often depressed emotionally but relatively rational. For example, the psychoneuroses discussed in Chapter 10 are almost nonexistent in nonliterate societies although they are relatively common in more advanced cultures (Wittkower and Fried, 1959).

Benedict and Jacks (1954) have proposed that the high incidence in nonliterate societies of pathology marked by confused excitement and often combined with homicidal acts, and the contrasting rarity of depressive states, implies that in these societies psychotic hostility is typically directed outward, whereas in Western society this hostility is more often directed inward. As they have noted, Western culture presents a significant contrast to many nonliterate cultures in the mechanisms of conscience. In backward societies responsibility for one's fate tends to be shifted to supernatural powers to the virtual exclusion of ideas of free will and personal responsibility, so that the individual suffers from a minimum of self-reproach or feelings of guilt. Barbu (1960) likewise has observed that in advanced societies "the external function of society in preventing crime is partly handed over to the inner processes of guilt and atonement."

These observations suggest that in a technologically backward society, pathology is likely to correspond to an immature personality development with an emphasis on action disturbance, a profound disorganization in thought, and a self-centered tendency to blame others for one's difficulties. In contrast, pathology in technologically more advanced societies usually parallels a higher level of personality development. Action symptoms are inclined to be restricted, and pathology to be expressed in thought, which remains formally intact. The patient's preoccupations are apt to center on a feeling of personal guilt that is indicative of a pathologically exaggerated sense of moral responsibility for the welfare of others.

Changes over Time in Types of American Pathology

Consistent with the rapid evolution in the nature of our society, various investigators have noted changes in its dominant forms of psychiatric disorder. Thus Malzberg (1959) has reported a continuous decrease in first admission rates to New York State hospitals for manic-depressive psychoses in the period 1909 to 1951. Women are consistently more prone to this disorder, yet for both sexes the drop in rates is quite dramatic. During this period of forty-two years, the rate per 100,000 population decreased from 4.5 to 1.9 for men and for women from 7.4 to 3.1. During the period 1917 to 1933, however, a time which included both a major war and a depression for the United States, this general trend for the manic-depressive disorders was reversed. This finding conforms to data on the first admission rates for 1917 to 1933 in Massachusetts for manic-depressive psychoses (Dayton, 1940).

As indicated in Chapter 10, hysterical neuroses are another form of disorder which is becoming less frequent. Exact statistics are not generally available on the incidence of the milder forms of psychopathology, but there is general consensus that cases of hysteria, once the prime example of neurotic repression, are now rare. Wheelis (1958), Chodoff (1954), von Bertalanffy (1960), and Jackson (1960) concur in this observation.

In contrast, there is no doubt that criminal and delinquent behaviors have increased enormously. Juvenile delinquency, for instance, rose approximately 230 percent between 1940 and 1959, at a time when the number of ten- to seventeen-year-olds rose only 25 percent. During World War II, a particularly striking rise in delinquency rates took place, but they diminished again in the postwar period (*Uniform crime reports for the United States*, 1959). *General* crime rates also showed a significant rise of 70 percent from 1940 to 1959, but they slightly decreased during the war years. The number of arrests has risen correspondingly from 1940 to 1960: 102 percent for those under eighteen, and 53 percent for those eighteen years and over. World War II brought about a definite upsurge in arrests within the younger group and a decline in the older group (*Uniform crime reports for the United States*, 1960). Many of the latter were in the armed services while many younger persons lost a controlling father or older brothers. The inevitable disruption of home life in the absence of key family figures, a high proportion of working mothers absent from the home, and a growing trend for families to become migratory all contribute to juvenile crime.

While the population of the United States rose approximately 18.5 percent from 1950 to 1960, crimes rose between 60 and 90 percent, including crimes of theft and violence (*Uniform crime reports for the United States,* 1960). A similar increase in violations of the narcotic drug laws has taken place. In contrast, arrests for prostitution and rape have tended to decrease (*Uniform crime reports for the United States,* 1960). The indications are that violence and self-indulgent transgressions of traditional morality are on the increase; the decreased frequency of reported rape and arrests for prostitution suggest a widened range of sexual freedom among females, rather than a stricter observance of a moral code. In support of this notion, it should be noted that other sexual offenses, including sexual relations with girls below the legal age of consent, show no such drop in rate.

Malzberg (1959) has provided data on first admissions for schizophrenia to the New York State hospital system between 1909 and 1951. A consistent rise in first admission rates took place for both men and women. The increase was 10.8 to 31.5 per 1000 population for men, and 10.0 to 31.0 for women. Further, a marked shift has recently occurred in the proportions of cases which fall into the various subcategories of schizophrenia, that is, the hebephrenic, catatonic, and simple subtypes, all of which have almost disappeared. Of 500 cases of first admission for mental disorder at Worcester State Hospital from 1962 to 1965, there were no cases of hebephrenic or catatonic schizophrenia, and only a single case of simple schizophrenia.

On what basis have changes in types of psychiatric disorder come about? Partly, perhaps, they reflect changes in psychiatric diagnostic fads. But they also appear to reflect the extensive changes in personal values and attitudes in American life and an increased awareness and toleration of personal motives which would have been most severely disapproved a generation or two ago. Extension in the range of permissible personal experience corresponds to a decrease in the disorders that are manifestations of repression (hysteria) or of self-deprecatory attitudes toward one's achievements and sense of moral rectitude (manic-depressive disorders). The decrease in hysterical neuroses, which are considered in psychoanalytic theory to represent defensive measures against the overt expression of sexual wishes, is indicative of an increased societal and personal tolerance of sexual feelings, fantasies, and behaviors which previously were taboo. In contrast, this century has witnessed a general increase in both violence and self-indulgent pathologies expressed in rising rates of delinquency, crime, and addictions.

Differences within Present-Day American Society

Within our society major distinctions in expected behavior patterns are laid down according to social class, marital status, age, and sex. That is, we expect an upper class, older married woman to behave in a far different fashion from a lower class, young, single man. Either would be considered peculiar if he began to act in a manner which would be quite routine for the other. Corresponding differences in pathology have been noted in accordance with social class, marital status, age, and sex.

Social class. Myers and Roberts (1959) have reported on the specific types of symptoms shown by twenty-five neurotics and twenty-five schizophrenics drawn from different social classes. Even when they carried the same diagnosis, middle- and lower-class patients behaved in quite different ways. The symptoms of the middle-class group accented their chronic problems in social adjustment, which were expressed in inhibited actions. None of them was in trouble with the law. In contrast, lower-class patients were strikingly more nonverbal in behavior, tended to "act out," to be aggressive and rebellious, and to be violent and self-indulgent, as in drinking, in sexual indulgence and perversions, and in fighting. Sixty percent of this group were in legal trouble because of antisocial acts.

In the main, middle-class symptomatology among both neurotics and psychotics was expressed in self-deprecation and a pervasive sense of failure and guilt. In contrast, lower-class patients tended to blame others for their difficulties. They were suspicious of others and prone to threaten assault. In general, the pathological behaviors of the lower class expressed hostile and self-centered attitudes.

Marital status. Zigler and Phillips (1960) have examined the relation between marital status and symptomatology, classified explicitly according to the three role orientations described by Phillips and Rabinovitch (1958); (1) self-deprivation and turning against the self, (2) self-indulgence and turning against others, and (3) avoidance of others.

Married men and women alike tended to manifest symptoms of self-deprivation and turning against the self, including self-deprecation, depression, fear of their own hostile impulses, tension, insomnia, and headaches. Single persons showed more symptoms within the other two role categories, that is, (1) self-indulgence and turning against others (including robbery, assault, threatened assault, emotional outbursts, homosexuality, and, among women, maniacal and destructive outbursts), and (2) avoidance of others (including withdrawn, apathetic, bizarre ideas, hallucinations, sexual preoccupations, and, among women, suspiciousness). In general, married persons tended to show symptoms indicative of a tense and self-critical attitude, while single individuals tended either to turn destructively against others or towards a general withdrawal from social participation.

Age. Zigler and Phillips (1960) observed certain consistent relationships between age level and the type of symptom developed. Younger patients, for the most part, tended to manifest symptoms of self-indulgence and turning against others (for example, homosexuality, robbery, assault) or of avoidance of others, like withdrawal, perplexity, and hallucinations. Older patients were more likely to express pathology in symptoms indicative of self-deprivation and turning against the self, such as refusal to eat, depression, and tension.

Sex. Fairly consistent sex differences in pathological reactions have been observed among both children and adults. Males usually tend to manifest considerably more destructive behaviors, females to be inhibited and self-critical. First we shall review studies on behavior problems in childhood, and then adult deviations.

There is general agreement that more boys than girls are referred for treatment to child guidance clinics (Williams, 1933; Phillips, 1956; Gilbert, 1957; Levy, 1931), in an overall ratio of about 2½:1. With respect to aggressive or antisocial behavior in particular the ratio rises to 4:1 (Williams, 1933). Boys get involved in aggressive or delinquent behaviors more often than girls (Ackerson, 1938; Gilbert, 1957) and more often manifest "behavior" or "conduct" problems (Peterson, 1961; MacFarlane *et al.*, 1954; Beller and Neubauser, 1959; Hattwick, 1937; Terman and Tyler, 1954). Boys' symptoms typically include overactivity, competitiveness, lying, temper tantrums, stealing, truancy, and rudeness. Girls, on the other hand, predominantly tend to show "personality" rather than conduct problems (Terman and Tyler, 1954, MacFarlane *et al.*, 1954; Peterson, 1961). They more frequently report fears and worries; are shy, timid, overly sensitive, somber, or excessively reserved; feel inferior or lack self-confidence; suck their thumbs, bite their nails, or are fussy about food.

Freud (1927) posited that differences in superego formation are the basis for those "character traits for which women have always been criticized and reproached, that they have less sense of justice than men, less tendency to submit to the great necessities of life, and frequently permit themselves to be guided in their decisions by their affections or enmities." Yet empirical data on the occurrence of the various types of pathological behaviors contradict Freud's assumptions as to a deficient superego formation in women. In general, women tend to show higher rates of admissions for manic-depressive disorders. In contrast, men have far higher rates of arrests for criminal activity; they outnumber women here by 19:1 (Scheinfeld, 1943). In contrast, first admission rates for schizophrenia are relatively even between the sexes (Malzberg, 1959).

The sexes differ markedly in most types of symptoms. For men, deviant reactions are more frequently expressed in action; for women, they are commonly expressed in thought. The symptoms of men are also much more likely to reflect a destructive hostility toward others, as well as a pathological self-indulgence. The most common male delinquencies are burglary, larceny, embezzlement, and pathological self-gratifications like drunkenness, drug usage, gambling, and sex offenses. Women's symptoms, on the other hand, express a harsh, self-critical, self-depriving, and often self-destructive set of attitudes.

A study conducted by Zigler and Phillips (1960) compared the symptoms of male and female mental hospital patients and found male patients significantly more assaultive than females and more prone to indulge their impulses in socially deviant ways like robbery, rape, drinking, homosexuality, and other perversions. Female patients, on the other hand, were more often found to be self-deprecatory, depressed, perplexed, withdrawn, refusing to eat, suffering from thoughts of suicide, and making actual suicidal attempts.

Clearly, a person's characteristic behavior style influences the form his psychopathology may take. Behavior style itself, however, must of necessity be influenced by the social surroundings within which the individual lives out his life.

SOCIAL DISORGANIZATION AND PATHOLOGY

In order to participate effectively in society, a person must master mutually acceptable ways of relating to other people. Any change in the conditions of a person's existence which deprives him of the use of these "skills in living" threatens the stability of his adjustive patterns. In these circumstances, there is danger that he will resort to the inappropriate and nonconstructive responses we label pathological. In this section we shall review the effects that the breakdown of stable and familiar social structures has on the rate at which psychopathology appears. In turn we shall consider the pathological consequences associated with (1) breaking away from one's own cultural background, (2) disorganization in community living, (3) war and economic depression, and (4) stresses within the family.

Cultural Disorganization

It has been observed that societies in transition, and individuals in transition from one society to another, are fertile fields for anxiety and insecurity, with attendant consequences in psychiatric or somatic disorders. Wittkauer and Fried (1959) concluded from their review of available studies that a society's mental health problems increase to the extent that traditional bonds holding families and communities together are disrupted. They suggest that people socialized in well-knit families may suffer when estranged from the traditional system of security arrangements rooted in the family. Consonant with this belief, social scientists in Israel have observed that Yemenite and Bulgarian Jews, who emigrated to Israel as entire communities, adapted quickly and well to their new homeland, whereas Moroccans and members of other national groups who entered Israel as single individuals have suffered considerably more pathological reactions. Iraqi immigrants, for example, have developed bronchial asthma remarkably often. Wittkauer and Fried also report that persons drawn from the primitive rural communities of Peru to its urban coastal culture tend to develop psychosomatic symptoms, as did mainland Chinese who emigrated to Formosa.

A study on culture conflict and physical illness has been reported by Abramson (1961), who measured the incidence of physical symptoms in a group of Indian adolescent girls living in Durban, South Africa. Culture conflict was assessed in terms of the girls' appraisal of how traditional or modernistic women should be. Ill health was associated with a discrepancy between the traditionalism of the girl and her mother. In cases where the mother was relatively more traditional than other mothers, a higher incidence of symptoms occurred among modernistic daughters than among traditional ones. On the other hand, if the mother was relatively modern, a higher level of ill health was indicated among girls either more traditional or more modern than their mothers.

The impact of acculturation is often most intensely expressed in what is known as "second generation conflict." Lemert (1948), Thomas and Zaniecki (1958), and Stonequist (1937) have all stressed the conflicts between immigrant parents and their children. The children reject the old-fashioned practices of their parents and often become what Stonequist has called "marginal people" without secure roots or values. Among second generation Americans, high rates of delinquency, crime, venereal disease, divorce, and desertion appear, the result of too rapid acculturation and deficient ingroup support. Malzberg (1940) reported that children of mixed parents, one foreign born and one native American, have more commonly developed social psychoses, like alcoholism and general paresis, and generally higher rates of mental disorder than children of parents who are both either native or foreign born. This suggests that cultural conflict directly expressed within the family has an ominous potential for pathological consequences in the offspring.

Some consideration has been given to the degree of alienation of the immigrant from the dominant American culture and its consequences in mental health and disorder. Dunham (1961) has reported that persons residing in areas not primarily populated by their own ethnic group tend to show considerably higher rates of disorder than members of the dominant group. Dayton (1940), studying the hospitalization rates of the foreign born in Massachusetts from 1920 to 1930, found a higher rate of mental disorder among those who failed to become naturalized than among those who did.

A similar finding emerged in more detail when Srole *et al.* classified midtown Manhattan respondents as "attached" or "detached," with respect to cultural origins, according to relative preference for American or native cooking, celebration of ethnic get-togethers, and attitudes toward a child marrying outside the ethnic group. Ethnic affiliation decreased with an increasing number of generations in America, and as in Dayton's report, people who became acculturated to the American scene showed a lesser degree of psychiatric impairment.

Community Disorganization

In most cities certain areas are marked by social disorganization expressive of cultural conflict (Faris and Dunham, 1939). Slum dwellings, high population density, and high land values produce such disorganization, which in turn produces disorganized individuals, crime, delinquency, physical sickness, mental disorder, and suicide. Dohrenwend (1957) has stated that social disorganization infringes on the individual's needs for physical security, for love, and for status and creative expression, thus bringing on psychological stress and emotional disruption. A study by Belknap and Jaco (1953) indicated relatively high rates of schizophrenia in communities where people reported they had few friends and acquaintances, rented their homes, had little affiliation with organizations, and experienced high unemployment and job turnover rates. Jaco (1957) has related social isolation to schizophrenic and manic-depressive hospital admission rates and has found more schizophrenia in areas where people characteristically have little contact and communication with each other.

Clausen and Kohn (1954) set out to test the hypothesis that *externally imposed* social isolation plays a causal role in schizophrenia. They interviewed forty-five schizophrenic and thirteen manic-depressive first admission patients and a group of control subjects individually matched for age, sex, and occupation and found that approximately one-third of the schizophrenic and manic-depressive patients and none of the controls showed evidence of social isolation at thirteen to fourteen years. There was no evidence that this isolation was based on a lack of available playmates, parental restrictions, or severe illness, however, and Kohn and Clausen conclude that early social isolation is indicative of already existing difficulties in interpersonal relationships.

Similar findings are reported by Gerard and Houston (1953) in a study that attempts to explain Faris and Dunham's observation that cases of psychiatric disorder are not randomly distributed throughout a city but rather are concentrated in and around the central business district, and diminished in incidence toward the periphery of the city (Figure 12.2). In a study of 305 first admission cases of schizophrenia among men, Gerard and Houston found that the high rates in central districts were accounted for mostly by single, separated, or divorced men who were living alone. The majority of patients living with their families at the time of hospital admission did not live in central districts. Evidently, men who are isolated from their families tend to drift into the deteriorated central section of cities, but whether this drift precedes, accompanies, or follows the onset of schizophrenic disorder could not be answered by the study. Hare (1956) in Bristol, England, also found that high incidence rates for schizophrenia in the central areas of cities were related to living alone. Sainsbury (1956) found a high correlation between residence in a single room and suicide in different boroughs of London. Thus suicide, like other forms of social pathology, appears

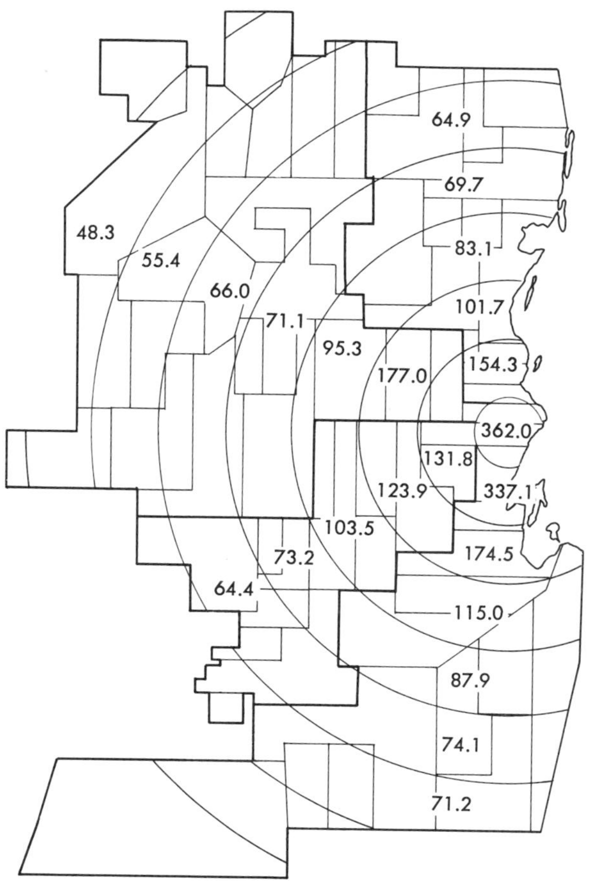

Figure 12.2 In a large city, the likelihood of mental illness increases as one approaches the center.

to be associated with disrupted relationships.

"Drift" alone is not an adequate explanation for the high rate of mental disorder in city centers; the incidence of commitment to mental hospitals is *fifteen times* greater in the center of the city than in the outskirts! The centers of cities are typically full of slums, which provide the largest proportion of all types of social pathology. The low socioeconomic status of most permanent residents of these areas also contributes greatly to the central urban concentration of mental disorder. In this connection, it may be noted that cases of manic-depressive disorder (primarily found in relatively competent people) are evenly distributed throughout large urban areas.

A number of writers (Fyvel, 1962; Tunley, 1962) suggest that the key factor in delinquency is the alienation of young people from society. The causes are several, but the outcome is the same. The home may have broken up; the family may have recently migrated, as have many Puerto Ricans to New York, or Deep South Negroes northwards. Style of life may have shifted with rising incomes, or both parents may work, leaving children unattended. Sometimes delinquency has been blamed on either poverty or affluence. It is probably neither directly; a more likely cause is sudden disruption of position in a coherent social structure.

The problem of teenage use of narcotics also typifies the relation between deviant behavior patterns and social disorganization. As reported by Leighton *et al.* (1957),

> Overwhelmingly, the teen-age narcotics users live in areas characterized by lowest socioeconomic status, high proportions of minority population groups, instability of family life, and high incidence of other social problems.

This concentration is evidenced by the fact that in Chicago, 91 percent of Narcotics Bureau cases and 96 percent of Boys' Court narcotics cases reside in areas which contain only 25 percent of the city's population. In each of the boroughs of New York City where drug use was high, the same pattern of concentration was found. In most census tracts of New York City, not a single teenaged resident was apprehended or treated for drug addiction in the period 1949 to 1952, while more than 10 percent of reported boys sixteen to twenty years old were apprehended or treated in the tracts of highest drug use. Rates of arrest for drug use or possession in Chicago revealed a high concentration among Negro males. Roughly 16 percent of Negro youths born in 1931 had been arrested for narcotics violations by 1952.

The increasing instability of Negro society may explain the disproportionately high crime rate of this largest minority group in the United States. Negroes are stigmatized and rejected in nearly all areas of the country, and they emigrate at high rates from the rural South to northern urban industrial centers. Systematic discrimination against the Negro, however, bars him from equal participation in the general culture. Prejudice largely restricts him to unskilled and underpaid jobs and to residence in slum settlements in which rents are excessively high. Life under these destructive social conditions sets the stage for an extreme expression of antisocial behaviors, most of which occur more in the slums than elsewhere. As a consequence, Negroes, who constitute approximately 10.5 percent of the population of the United States, are annually arrested for 30 percent of all offenses booked by the police. Further, they are yearly arrested for approximately 65 percent of the most violent crimes: murder, nonnegligent manslaughter, and aggravated assault.

War and Economic Depression

Certain major dislocations in established patterns of community living, such as those brought on by war or economic depression, influence the incidence of psychiatric and psychosomatic pathologies, although by no means always increase them. Lewis (1942) reports that in the week to ten days following bombing raids in England, there was a slight increase in neurotic complaints. Anxiety and depression were the most common symptoms and most often affected people who had suffered from neurotic symptomatology in the past. Stewart and Winser (1942) reported a sharp rise in the incidence of peptic ulcer perforations during periods of intensive air raids over London and Bristol. Illingworth *et al.* (1944) confirmed this finding but added that the rise in perforations antedated the raids and thus might have been caused by anticipatory tension and anxiety.

On the other hand, Hopkins (1943) reported a decrease of admissions to the mental hospitals of Liverpool during World War II, which he attributed to

> the strengthening of the community spirit, and a lessening of that conscious-

ness of mental isolation so favorable to the development of psychological abnormality. (Quoted in Reid, 1961.)

Coleman (1961), similarly, has observed that the morale of a combat unit before battle is a good predictor of the rates of neurotic and psychotic breakdown after (in Reid, 1961, p. 253).

Glass (1954) has reported that only 15 percent of psychiatric battle casualties evacuated from battle zones and treated intensively with traditional psychodynamic techniques could be salvaged for combat. In contrast, men maintained in combat zones who kept contact with their own outfits and who were treated only superficially, showed a much higher rate of return to combat. The incidence of neurotic reactions in World War II among London firemen and civil defense workers who were exposed to considerable danger also was quite low. Finally, Ødegaard (1954) concluded from his psychiatric studies in Scandinavia that there was an actual decrease in psychiatric disability during World War II, although some cases of psychotic reactions could be traced to traumatic war experiences. During World War II studies of psychiatric breakdown among the British armed forces revealed that, among Royal Air Force personnel, amount of flying hours bore no relation to breakdown rates, but a period of heavy casualties was strikingly related to increases in both breakdowns and venereal disease rates.

Hastings (1944) and other writers observed that most men exposed to combat never reported sick; Hastings found that 95 percent of 150 such men developed symptoms during their tour of duty and that one-third of these "had more severe disturbances" but never came under a psychiatrist's care. The increase in the workweek to more than seventy-five hours during wartime also was accompanied by a sharp rise in neurotic reactions, according to Fraser and Phelps (1947). Cameron (1946) believes that boring tasks, on the one hand, and undue responsibility, on the other, present psychological hazards in industry.

These studies provide too little evidence to give confidence about what factors may precipitate psychiatric disorder, but some tentative conclusions can be drawn: When people are actively engaged in what they are trained to do, even if the conditions are arduous or dangerous, psychiatric casualty rates are not particularly high; however, when they feel the pressure of undue responsibility, or when there is danger without the possibility of recourse or preventive action, psychiatric reactions soar.

Different pathological responses are possible under identical conditions of threat. In this brief survey alone, three patterns of trouble have appeared; psychiatric symptomatology, peptic ulcer perforation, and sexual promiscuity (expressed in an increased rate of venereal infection). The type of deviant response seems to be related both to the nature of the anticipated threat and the kind of person involved, but the precise role of each in determining the form of deviant response remains unclear.

Komora and Clark (1935) found no remarkable increase in mental hospital admission rates in the United States during the economic depression of the 1930's, although the economic situation was considered the precipitating factor in many individual instances. Nevertheless, as we noted earlier, both Dayton and Malzberg observed increased hospitalization rates for manic-depressive disorders during the depression. Similarly, Dublin and Bunzel (1933) found an inverse relationship between the suicide rate and an index of business activity, especially among white men. Swinscow (1951) also found a close relationship between the suicide rate for men in England and

Wales and the proportion of men employed in the same year. No such relation appeared for women. In England, among occupational groups most affected by economic depression, Halliday (1948) observed an increased suicide rate and a simultaneous drop in the birth rate. The ratio of men to women in suicide and peptic ulcer mortality rose during the depression, particularly within the worst affected occupations, such as mining and textiles. During 1931 to 1932 and 1935 to 1936, when Scotland was economically distressed, such disorders as peptic ulcer, gastritis, and "nervous debility" increased sharply, particularly in men under fifty-five years of age.

When we compare reactions to the dangers of bombing and combat with reactions to those of economic depression, certain differences in maladaptive response become evident. Somatic reactions like peptic ulcer are common responses to both, and neither situation seems to bring with it any general rise in psychiatric cases. In war, however, people seem to seek refuge in sexual escapades, which are not as easily found in depression, while in economically depressed states, we find a sharp rise in suicide rates and in chronic illnesses, reactions which do not increase in wartime. Why do these differences occur?

War, of course, is not of one's own making, and no sense of personal guilt need arise for its existence. The source of threat is external to oneself. In a depression, the subjective conditions can be quite different. Depression, like war, is the consequence of conditions beyond the control of any one man. Nevertheless, a man's failure to find work or to provide adequately for his family is inevitably seen as a failure in his own life. The question becomes one of where to assign the blame. In this context, one can see the rise in chronic illness as an indirect expression of a need to indicate that the failure is not a personal one; it has been forced on the man by physical disability. The increase in suicide rates perhaps states a different message: that economic failure is personal and that the suicidal act is a response to a traumatic sense of personal inadequacy. It will be noted that the increase in suicidal rates occurs particularly among white men. Negroes chronically have been deprived economically, so that a general economic depression need not confront them with a sense of either individual disaster or subjective failure.

Interpersonal Stresses

Most problems which beset adults are not the result of major social upheavals such as war, economic depression, or the alienation of ethnic or racial minorities from the wider society, but are rather results of the dilemmas, anxieties, and tragedies of individual lives. Relatively few studies concerned with the impact of these life crises have been undertaken. One was carried out in a slum of San Juan, Puerto Rico, on twenty married couples with at least one schizophrenic member and twenty couples with neither member diagnosed as schizophrenic (Rogler and Hollingshead, 1965).

It was found that the "schizophrenic couples" differed little from the control group in terms of their childhood and early adult experiences. The factors which distinguished between them appeared in the five-year period which immediately preceded the onset of disorder. During these years there was a disproportionately high occurrence of physical disease in either the patient or the spouse and a strikingly high number of deaths of children among families where the mother was schizophrenic. The year immediately preceding the onset of schizophrenia was particularly noteworthy for its high rate of trauma—sickness in the patient or the spouse, a complicated pregnancy, the illness or death of a child, unemployment with an attendant accumulation of debts and dependence on relatives or neighbors. Quarrels and threats between the spouses became unusually frequent and quarrels with neighbors also occurred, often over sexual adventures the husband became involved in during this period of stress.

Similar trauma have been noted to precede the onset of physical sickness. In a study of American working men and women, Hinkle and Wolff (1957) found that a high proportion of those with severe physical illness had experienced various kinds of social trauma, divorce, separation, conflicts with spouse, parents, or siblings, and unhappy living or working arrangements. In contrast, few of their healthiest subjects had suffered such experiences. In a similar vein, Pflanz *et al.* (1956) have observed that physically ill patients suffered a recurrence of symptoms if they became estranged or isolated from emotionally significant interpersonal relationships. A study by Minski and Desai (1955) of forty-five peptic ulcer patients found that for forty-three of them, the first symptoms started after isolation from a protective community. In a study of 152 cancer patients one important discriminator between them and a control group was that a relatively high proportion of the cancer patients had lost an important close personal relationship for which no satisfactory substitute had been found (LeShan and Worthington, 1955).

Holmes *et al.* (1957) have reviewed a number of studies on the onset and course of tuberculosis and made a similar observation. In many mays tuberculous subjects appeared as "marginal people." They tended to start life with an unfavorable social status and to grow in a crippling interpersonal environment. Their precarious social adjustment typically disintegrated in the two-year period preceding onset of TB or relapse into it. This period included a high frequency of broken marriages and changes in occupation and residence.

A relationship between changes in personal relationships, consequent feelings of depression, and the subsequent onset of a variety of physical diseases has also been observed (Schmale, 1958). Of forty-two medical patients studied, twenty-nine had suffered loss of a person close to them and had had feelings of helplessness and hopelessness immediately before the onset of symptoms, which often developed within a week after the loss. Only five patients reported feeling hopeless and helpless without a broken relationship, and the investigator believed that he observed some indirect evidence for actual, threatened, or symbolic loss and accompanying bad feelings in four of them.

It has been suggested that psychiatric symptoms

> represent transient responses by normal personalities to objective, stress-producing events, i.e., stressors in the immediate environment (Dohrenwend and Dohrenwend, 1965).

This often seems to be true of physical disease as well. The Dohrenwends suggests that the relatively high rate of psychiatric disorder in the lowest socioeconomic stratum is associated with the severe conditions of life in this segment of the population. They note the high death rate for children and young adults and the relatively short life expectancy for these people. They also point to their high unemployment rate and their frequent relocation by programs of urban development as stressful conditions which may initiate the symptoms of psychiatric disorder.

That stressful conditions in a person's life enhance the likelihood of disorder is supported by the work of Langner and Michael (1963), who reviewed the histories of a representative sample of individuals drawn from the general population. They examined the type and frequency of life stresses in relation to the severity of psychiatric impairment of the individual. Life stresses included things like broken home in childhood, quarreling between parents, poor physical health, and worries over work. They found that a simple sum of the number of stressful conditions to which the person had been exposed related more precisely to level of psychiatric impairment than did any specific type or combination of stresses. The greater the *number* of stresses, the greater the degree of psychiatric impairment.

Other findings by Langner and Michael do not support the Dohrenwend and Dohrenwend hypothesis very well. Langner and Michael found that the average number of reported life stresses did *not* differ appreciably among the various socioeconomic levels, although the degree of psychiatric impairment for any given number of stresses was greater among persons of low than among those of higher socioeconomic status. In other words, low status people tended to develop psychotic-like reactions while those of high status with the same number of stresses tended to respond with the less severe reactions of neurosis. At extreme stress levels, the lows were classified as 26.8 percent probable psychotics and 31.7 percent probable neurotics, while high status individuals were classed as only 4.3 percent probable psychotics and 43.5 percent probable neurotics.

This review of the relations between social disorganization and the incidence of pathology suggests the following conclusions: Threatening situations which permit a person to make use of his established skills, like conditions of war, may actually enhance his psychological well-being. On the other hand, any disruption of a person's life which renders his usual patterns of adaptation inoperative heightens the potential for pathological response. Further, individuals of low socioeconomic status who are deficient in educational and occupational competence tend to show a greater degree of psychiatric impairment in response to any given level of environmental stress than do those of higher socioeconomic competence.

SOCIAL COMPETENCE AND PSYCHOPATHOLOGY

In order to participate fully in society, a person must achieve competence both in the impersonal world of technological and socioeconomic activities, in which he acquires education and skills and ensures his physical welfare, and in the world of interpersonal relationships and intimate contact with others, which requires sensitivity and awareness of human motives and the subtleties of human relationships. These competencies are expressed in social participation and the acceptance of responsibility both for one's own fate and that of others, including one's immediate dependents and, more broadly, one's community.

People differ, of course, in the degree to which they learn to live effectively in society. Their potential for doing so has been called "social competence" (Phillips and Zigler, 1961), which connotes a person's range of skills and flexibility in meeting the vicissitudes of life. People's level of social competence is quite measurable. Some adults have failed to complete grade school; others attempt and complete graduate studies. Some become skilled machinists; others remain day laborers. Above and beyond these basic life tasks, there are even greater differences in individual competence in interpersonal interaction. For example, people differ considerably in the degree to which they show leadership and responsibility in social relationships; they differ in the age

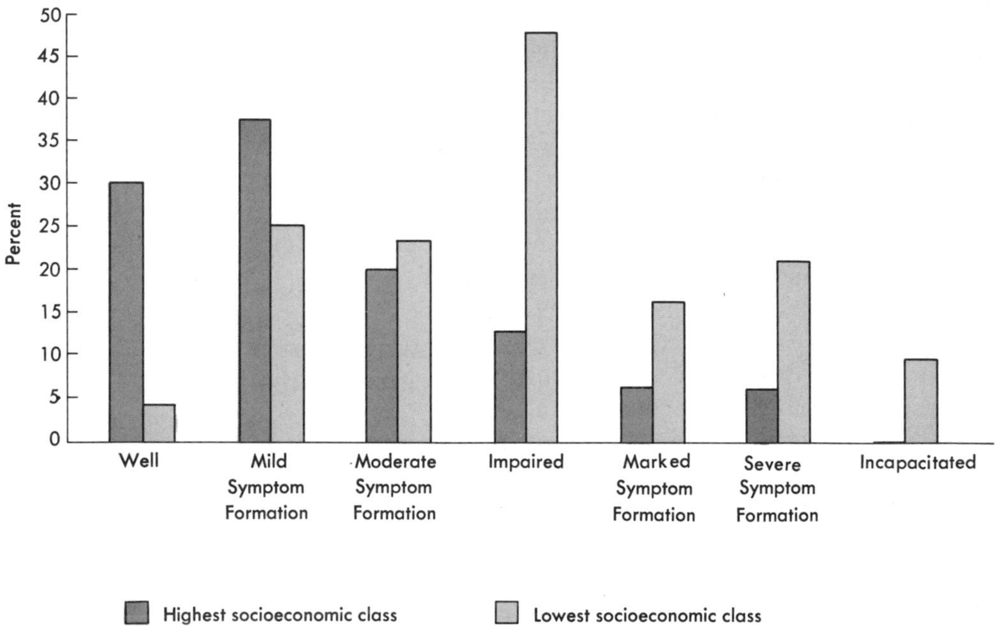

Figure 12.3 Bar graph showing Srole's results. *Impaired* includes *marked symptom formation, severe symptom formation,* and *incapacitated.* From *Mental Health in the Metropolis: The Midtown Manhattan Study,* Volume 1, edited by L. Srole, T. S. Langner, S. Michael, M. Opler, and T. Rennie. Copyright © 1962 McGraw-Hill, Inc. Used by permission of McGraw-Hill Book Company.

at which they achieve independence from parents; and they differ in the age at which they undertake marriage and in the maturity and responsibility they bring to it.

Individuals of lesser effectiveness in the skills of adult living are more likely than others to manifest pathological behavior patterns. We shall review in turn the consequences of (1) deficiencies in educational achievement and occupational skill and (2) immaturity and ineffectiveness in psychosexual relationships.

Educational and Occupational Achievement

Educational and occupational accomplishment have served as the two indices most often used to define social class (Hollingshead and Redlich, 1958). They are so efficient in doing so that, for our purposes, these variables are interchangeable. Most studies which have examined the relation of educational and occupational achievement to psychopathology have translated these measures into a combined index of social class called "socioeconomic status."

A survey conducted by Srole and his associates (1962) examined the relation of socioeconomic status (SES) to degree of psychiatric impairment. An interview of a representative sample of persons living in a community revealed a striking relationship between SES and impairment (Figure 12.3). In the highest stratum of SES, 67.5 percent of the samples either were well or showed only mild symptom formation. In contrast, only 29.6 percent of the lowest SES group were equally well. In the highest stratum, *no* cases appeared to be incapacitated by pathology, but nearly one person in ten from the bottom SES stratum was apparently functionally disabled by his symptoms.

Hollingshead and Redlich (1958) have provided us with data on the relative incidence of treated mental disorder in the various social classes. They found the proportion of cases inversely related to social class: the higher the class, the fewer the cases. An even more striking discrepancy was shown in the distribution of mild versus severe cases, that is, of neurosis and psychosis. Of the relatively few cases of mental disorder in Class I (the highest SES), 52.6 percent were of neurosis, 47.4 percent of psychosis. In contrast, in Class V, the neuroses constituted only 8.4 percent of the psychiatric population, the psychoses 91.6 percent. Both incidence rate and severity of disorder were strikingly higher in the lowest social class.

In a report on maladjusted families in Minneapolis, Buell *et al.* (1952) wrote that barely 6 percent of the community's economically deprived families absorbed more than half the resources of its casework, public welfare, mental health, and correctional agencies. A survey of the families receiving aid from these agencies indicated that they were involved in many kinds of difficulties. Because of the overlapping nature of their problems, they came to be designated as "multiple referral" families.

Poverty and the attendant experiences of lower class and slum living are associated with a wide range of social pathologies. A high prevalence of mental disorder coincides with high rates of crime and delinquency, promiscuity, and prostitution. Broken homes and child neglect are common. Chronic diseases such as tuberculosis and high rates of infant mortality are also frequent in slum areas, as are alcoholism, accidents, and suicide. Srole *et al.* (1962) have reported that cases of delinquency, tuberculosis, and infant mortality in the area of Manhattan covered by their study were concentrated overwhelmingly in city blocks of five- and six-story slum tenements.

The influence of the technological advancement of a nation on the proportion of individuals showing psychopathology is shown in a study by Rosen and Rizzo (1961), who compared scores on a personality test (MMPI) given to army recruits from different sections of Italy. The north is the most industrialized section of the country and has the highest per capita income and standard of living. The south is the least highly developed region, with the least dense population and fewest roads, automobiles, books, magazines, and newspapers. The authors found clear differences in scores between the northern and southern Italians: recruits drawn from the south showed the highest scoring in psychopathology, although those with a higher level of education showed less pathology.

Marital Status

The survey conducted by Srole and his associates on the psychiatric health of the community has also provided information on the relative degree of psychiatric impairment of groups differing in marital status. Their report compared the proportion of impaired respondents among married men and women who were equated for age. Among married people, the two sexes did not differ in the proportions rated psychiatrically impaired. In general, impairment rates among the widowed (data were available only on women) were about the same as among the married. In contrast, for higher rates of impairment were reported for divorced than for married people of both sexes.

The story was quite different for single men and women. Single women did not differ substantially from married women in the proportion of impaired individuals. In contrast, single men ranked consistently higher than married men in this regard. It is difficult to explain the relative psychiatric intactness of single women. It may be that women who feel self-reliant are as often inclined to remain single as to marry; findings by Martinson (1955) support this assumption. He reported that among fifty-nine pairs of single and married girls matched on many variables, the single girls showed better emotional adjustment, greater self-reliance, a greater sense of personal freedom, and fewer withdrawal tendencies.

Dayton's report (1940) on institutionalization for psychiatric disorder in Massachusetts from 1917 to 1933 suggests that married people have the least chance of developing mental disorders. The widowed, single, and divorced, in that order, have an increasing incidence of first admission rates to mental hospitals. Among women, the admission rates of widows are 45 percent higher than those of the married, of the single, 80 percent higher, and of the divorced, 230 percent higher.

Among males, the rates for the widowed are 130 percent higher than for the married, the single, 200 percent higher, and the divorced, 400 percent higher. Rates for married men and women are very nearly equal, but in the other groups, male first admission rates outnumber female by a considerable proportion. It appears that unmarried women are not the striking psychiatric risks that unmarried men are. Overall, the Dayton data on marital status and psychiatric impairment are remarkably similar to those revealed by the midtown Manhattan investigation. In the two studies, the married of both sexes have the lowest rate of psychopathology; the divorced, the highest.

Zigler and Phillips (1961*b*) also have reported on the relation of marital status to psychiatric diagnosis. Patients were classified as either single, married, or "other," which included divorced, separated, and widowed. The data on marital status were reported for six groups: (1) the general Massachusetts population, based on the 1950 census; (2) the total hospital population, which included a proportion of outpatient cases and a few people observed in jail; (3) manic-depressives; (4) schizophrenics; (5) psychoneurotics; and (6) people with character disorders.

The hospital group, as a totality, differed significantly in marital status from the general population. A disproportionately high number of patients were single, and for men, a greater proportion were separated, divorced, or widowed than was true for the general population. Within various diagnostic groups, a relatively low percentage of manic-depressive and psychoneurotic patients were single and a relatively high proportion married. In contrast, the character disorders and schizophrenia included the highest proportion of single people and the smallest proportion of marrieds.

Thus, consistent with findings in the midtown Manhattan and Dayton studies, Zigler and Phillips observed that unmarried people are disproportionately represented among the psychiatrically hospitalized. The discrepantly high ratio of unmarrieds occurs particularly among schizophrenics and people with character disorders, whose symptomatology emphasizes respectively social withdrawal and destructive hostility toward others. Manic-depressive conditions and neuroses, which imply self-critical attitudes and ideational pathology, are associated with higher proportions of married patients.

It is also of interest to compare marital status in relation to criminal activity. Data of this sort are difficult to obtain but Buell *et al.* (1952) have reported that only about one-third of the youths and men placed in reformatories, jailed, or imprisoned are married, in contrast to the approximately 70 percent of American men fourteen years of age or older who are married. As with cases of mental disorder, criminals appear to be drawn from a psychosexually less adequate segment of the total population; they also tend to be less educated and less occupationally skilled than average. Like psychopathology, criminality appears to be a response of individuals who fail to cope with societal expectations for their age and sex status.

As with the various disorders of psychopathology, arrests for various crimes are differentially related to marital status. For example, the pattern of marital status for violators of the liquor laws conforms closely to the distribution of marital status for the population as a whole. For those arrested for embezzlement and fraud, often called "white-collar" or middle-class crimes, distribution among the various types of marital status is also much like that in the general population. However, among those arrested on charges of "lower-class" crime like robbery or assault, a higher proportion are single. It must be recognized, on the other hand, that different types of crime are more frequently associated with certain age groups than with others. Thus, embezzlement and fraud tend to be committed at a later age than robbery and assault, and their perpetrators have therefore had more opportunity to marry. Nevertheless, the data presented on the relation of crime to marital status appear to support the idea that acting against the interests of others or to their injury is far more likely to be the behavior of the unmarried. The resulting inference, that criminal behavior is associated with psychosexual immaturity, appears reasonable. Since, in addition, most crimes are committeed by the less educated and skilled, criminal behavior appears to be characteristically the action of the generally less socially competent person in our society.

It seems reasonable to conclude that people best equipped in the skills of living, that is, those who are well educated, occupationally well placed, and psychosexually mature (as expressed in a stable marriage) are most immune to the vicissitudes of adult life. As we have seen, such individuals are less likely than the socially incompetent to develop some form of psychopathology or deviance. If competent people do manifest some form of disorder, it tends to be one of a lesser degree of severity than those which occur in less socially adequate persons.

SUMMARY

Sociologists have long been aware of the significance of social context in molding the dominant forms of human interaction. Mills (1960), for example, has noted that a person's biography and character cannot be explained entirely by his early family experiences or his current interpersonal setting. They are also influenced by the larger social context of his time, for man is a social and historical being whose life derives much of its meaning from specific social and historical structures. His way of life is a reflection of his culture, for much of human living consists of acting specified social roles, like worker, husband, and father, within established social contexts, like factory or family. Changes in economic and political conditions over the last century, as well as in family structure itself since Victorian days, have made for profound changes in the nature of social and personal relationships among people.

Adaptation in society depends to a substantial extent upon the clarity and general acceptance of a person's status. Certain positions in our social structure are poorly defined, such as that of aged parents, or the professionally trained woman, or the divorcee, so that considerable tension may arise for people occupying them. Other positions are simply disapproved, such as that of the poor, the occupationally unskilled, the school dropout, and until recently the ethnic or caste group—the Jew, Puerto Rican, and Negro. No amount of clarity as to one's place in the social framework will alleviate the difficulties faced by persons who occupy such niches in society. Strains are imposed on the personality of these people which may sometimes make it impossible for them to perform effectively. Every individual strives to establish types of relationships which provide an optimum balance between a sense of personal security and the fulfillment of his goals, values, and aspirations. What this balance will be is dependent on his past history and personal maturity. The immature adult, deficient in adaptive flexibility and skills of living, is likely to choose an unadventurous security. The mature person, confident of his powers of survival, may adopt a more vigorous and pioneering style of life. Environmental needs differ among persons of low and high maturity. Those of immature personality development require a stable, supportive, and cohesive environment. Those of higher personality development can flourish under less stable and less rigidly defined conditions.

Any circumstance which tends to disrupt the relationships a person has established is a source of threat. To less mature people, even relatively minor changes in interpersonal relationships may be profoundly disturbing. Leaving school and the loss of schoolmates with whom, in fact, contacts have been minimal, or the birth of a child to a distant relative, or any of a myriad of possible changes in the world in which they live may have severe effects on their patterns of adjustment. On the other hand, people who are adept at establishing personal ties are better able to weather unexpected disruption in their lives.

Psychopathology occurs when the complexities of a changing pattern of personal relationships or a change in one's social status imposes demands for effective response which are beyond the person's adaptive resources, that is, when the person is not sufficiently mature or socially skilled to devise the novel patterns of behavior which environmental change requires.

The response to failure in human adaptation can take any one of a number of forms. Sometimes failures in living are expressed in the ostensibly aimless, bizarre, and socially inappropriate behaviors of psychiatric disorder. Sometimes the difficulties of life are expressed in the distorted human relationships of delinquency and crime and at others, in the bodily dysfunctions known as psychosomatic disorders. There is increasing evidence that some proportion of the wide range of misfortunes seen in social welfare agencies—mental disorder, mental retardation, delinquency or crime, and physical disorders—may be regarded as diverse expressions of a deficiency in meeting societal expectations. Certainly, many forms of psychological, social, and physical pathology tend to cluster in one relatively small segment of the total population which fails to cope effectively with the complex problems of urban living.

The different forms of psychopathology are traditionally viewed as disease processes, that is, as some form of mental illness of which the person is an unwilling and often unwitting victim. They can, however, be understood in quite different terms. Rather than judge the symptoms of psychopathology as expressions of disease, we can see them simply as a person's ineffectual efforts to cope with problems unique to his life. His symptoms *are* the person caught in difficulties beyond his capabilities for mastery. Their natures express that particular person's circumstances, his values and place in society, as well as the values of his time and culture. Regularities in symptomatology, which we recognize as conventional diagnoses, can then be seen to express common elements of human experience which mark a particular historical period and society.

GLOSSARY

ACCULTURATION—the process whereby children learn the behavior patterns characteristic of their social group especially of the larger social group or culture.

ACTING OUT—a defense mechanism in which aggressive, sexual, or self-damaging behavior is performed as a means of reducing anxiety; for example, an adolescent with hostile feelings toward authority may deface the statue of a general.

ADDICTION, NARCOTICS—reliance upon the effects of a narcotic drug with the results that progressively stronger doses are required to obtain these effects and that there is both psychological and physiological distress when the drug is withdrawn.

AGGRESSION—behavior intended to injure or distress another person (see Chapters 3 and 4).

ALCOHOLIC PSYCHOSIS—a disturbance caused by chronic excessive drinking of alcohol and manifested by impairment of brain tissue.

ALCOHOLISM—prolonged use of alcohol in excessive amounts.

ALIENATION—psychological separation of the individual from his society; the failure to find meaning in society's norms, goals, or conventions.

BEHAVIOR PROBLEMS—a general term for antisocial behavior: truancy, rudeness, stealing, lying, temper tantrums, overactivity.

BEHAVIOR STYLE—see LIFE STYLE.

BLUNTED AFFECT—emotional responses that are weaker than those normally produced by a given situation.

CASE HISTORY (RECORD)—a collection of all available evidence—social, psychological, physiological, biographical, environmental, vocational—that promises to help explain an individual.

CATATONIA—catatonic schizophrenia; a pathological disorder characterized by either generalized inhibition of overt response or excessive activity or excitement (see Chapter 11).

CEREBRAL ARTERIOSCLEROSIS—a thickening of the arterial walls in the brain causing destruction of brain tissue.

CHARACTER DISORDER—a condition with symptomatic behaviors including antisociality, aggression, dishonesty, and deception (see Chapter 11).

CHARACTER TRAITS—attributes or features that make up or distinguish an individual and that persist over time (see Chapter 8).

COMPULSION—an irrational, repetitive act.

CONDUCT PROBLEMS—see BEHAVIOR PROBLEMS.

CONTROL SUBJECTS GROUP—in an experiment, persons who are not exposed to the experimental variable but are exposed to as many as possible (and ideally all) of the other conditions in the experiment, the purpose being to ensure that the obtained effects are not the result of irrelevant or unnoticed considerations.

CORRELATION—a relationship between two things such that a change in one is accompanied by a corresponding change in the other.

CULTURAL DISORGANIZATION—a disruption in traditional cultural bonds, values, and so forth resulting from transition within a society or transition of an individual from one society to another.

CULTURE CONFLICT—conflict that arises from the simultaneous influence of two irreconcilable cultures on the individual.

DELINQUENCY, JUVENILE—generally, minor violations of laws by children or adolescents that bring them into conflict with law enforcement officials.

DELUSIONS—false beliefs that resist all argument and evidence; they tend variously to make the believer feel more important, enable him to rationalize his behavior, provide a target for hostility, or explain events which he finds otherwise inexplicable.

DEMENTIA PRAECOX—obsolescent term for schizophrenia.

DEPERSONALIZATION—a state in which a person loses the sense of his own reality, or feels his own body to be unreal.

DEPRESSION—an emotional state of great sadness, often accompanied by guilt and anxiety, gloomy ruminations, lassitude, inability to respond to pleasant stimuli, and suicidal impulses.

ENCEPHALITIS—an infectious disease of the brain, known also as sleeping sickness.

ETHNIC GROUP—a group of people related nationally, linguistically, or religiously.

FACTOR ANALYTIC STUDIES—studies that attempt to extract the underlying relationships within a complex of correlations.

GENERAL PARESIS—a progressive organic psychosis resulting from a syphilitic infection of the brain.

GUILT—the subjective feelings that result from doing something forbidden, or from failure to perform some obligatory act (see Chapters 4, 8, and 11).

HALLUCINATION—a false sensory perception which has a compelling sense of reality, even though relevant and adequate stimuli for it are lacking.

HEBEPHRENIA—hebephrenic schizophrenia; a form of schizophrenia characterized by giggly, silly behavior, hallucinations, delusions, and inappropriate affect.

HOMOSEXUALITY—a tendency to find sexual or erotic gratification with a person of the same sex.

HOSTILITY—a motivational state that may lead to aggressive behavior.

IMPULSE—an act performed without delay, reflection, or voluntary direction.

INAPPROPRIATE AFFECT—emotions or emotional responses that are incongruent with what is ordinarily expected in a given situation.

INTROPUNITIVE BEHAVIOR—aggression directed to the self.

INVOLUTIONAL PSYCHOSIS—a disturbance, sometimes developed during menopause, characterized by depression, insomnia, guilt feelings, and anxiety.

LIFE STYLE—characteristic mode of living.

MANIC DEPRESSIVE PSYCHOSES—a group of severe disorders characterized by states of overexcitement and elation (mania) or of sadness and hypoactivity (depression) or of oscillation between these.

MENTAL DEFICIENCY—a generic term for subnormal intellectual development (see Chapter 13).

MENTAL RETARDATES—conservatively, those who fall in the lower 3 percent of the distribution of IQ scores; according to the *Manual on Terminology and Classification in Mental Retardation*,[1] all persons whose IQ falls below the population mean; the *social* competence definition includes all those who are unable to meet minimal societal demands (see Chapter 14).

MINNESOTA MULTIPHASIC PERSONALITY INVENTORY (MMPI)—a personality questionnaire used primarily for assessing psychopathology.

MULTIPLE REFERRAL FAMILIES—families whose members have been referred to a variety of social agencies.

NEURASTHENIA—a neurotic syndrome involving constant feelings of weakness and fatigue that are without apparent physiological basis.

NEUROSIS—a negative abnormality, ill-defined in character, but milder than psychosis.

OBSESSION—an irrational, repetitive thought.

OUTPATIENT—a person receiving treatment from a hospital or a clinic but not residing there.

OVERINHIBITION—inability to give spontaneous expression to feelings and thoughts even when social conditions are facilitating.

PERSONALITY DISORDERS—a disorder of behavior that is manifested chiefly in motivation and by social maladjustment, rather than primarily emotional or intellectual disturbances.[2]

PERVERSIONS—usually, socially condemned sexual behavior, such as exhibitionism, fetishism, homosexuality.

PHOBIA—abnormal anxiety or fear.

PREJUDICE—a denigrating judgment or attitude, formed on the basis of minimal and overgeneralized evidence.

PREVALENCE RATES—statistics describing the degree to which particular phe-

[1] This definition is taken from H. B. English and Ava C. English, *A Comprehensive Dictionary of Psychological and Psychoanalytical Terms*, New York: David McKay Company, Inc., 1958.

nomena are prevalent in a society or locale.

PSYCHOANALYTIC THEORY—a theory of personality set forth by Freud and modified by his disciples.

PSYCHODYNAMIC—describing theories of behavior or therapeutic techniques addressed to motives and drives and commonly based on the work of Freud.

PSYCHOPATHIC PERSONALITY—a disordered personality as evidenced by criminal acts, sexual perversion, or general inability to delay gratification.

PSYCHOPATHOLOGY—negative psychological abnormalities.

PSYCHOSEXUAL IMMATURITY—the inability to participate in age-appropriate sexual behavior.

PSYCHOSOMATIC DISORDERS—persistent physiological symptoms or impairments that originate in psychological distress.

PSYCHOTICS—an ill-defined term, generally meaning a person with any severe negative psychological abnormality.

RELIABILITY—accuracy; the degree to which one is able to obtain identical results on repeated measurement.

REPRESSION—the exclusion of psychological contents (like memories and feelings) from awareness, commonly because they provoke anxiety.

SCHIZOID—describing a broad array of conditions ranging in severity from mild to serious and characterized by tendencies to withdraw and inability to express feelings openly.

SCHIZOPHRENIA—a group of psychotic reactions characterized by fundamental disturbances in reality relationships, by a conceptual world determined largely by feeling, and by marked affective, intellectual, and overt behavioral disturbances.[2]

SELF-ESTEEM—the degree to which one values himself or his characteristics.

SENILE BRAIN DISEASE—brain disease resulting from natural aging processes.

SEXUAL DEVIATIONS—sexual behavior that is considered abnormal in one's society.

SIMPLE SCHIZOPHRENIA—a psychosis marked chiefly by apathy, simplicity, reduced relatedness to the external world, and an impoverishment of human relationships.[2]

SOCIAL COMPETENCE—a person's potential for learning to live effectively in his society; the range of skills and flexibility necessary for this learning.

SOCIAL DISORGANIZATION—changes in the conditions of a person's environment which deprives him of the use of his "skills in living" and threaten the stability of his adjustment patterns.

SOCIAL WITHDRAWAL—a defense mechanism characterized by a lessening of social response patterns and narrowing of interests and activities.

SOCIOPATHIC PERSONALITY—a broad category of disorders in one's relationship with society and with the cultural milieu.

SUPEREGO—in Freudian theory, one of the three major dynamic systems of personality; the learned and internalized demands of parents and society.

SYMBIOTIC RELATEDNESS—a condition in which a person depends upon others, not for cooperative mutual support and affection, but for exploitation and the satisfaction of neurotic needs.

SYMPTOM—a behavior regarded by psychologists and psychiatrists as socially undesirable, statistically deviant, and the product of anxiety and conflict.

SYMPTOMATOLOGY—the systematic study of observable behavioral or structural traits that are characteristic of disorders.

SYNDROME—a pattern of symptoms.

TRADITIONAL PYSCHODYNAMIC TECHNIQUES—techniques set forth by Freud and his disciples for the treatment of psychological disorders.

TRAUMATIC EVENT—any experience that inflicts serious damage upon the organism.

TURNING AGAINST THE SELF—a defensive action which results in punishing the self (with anxiety, depression, and feelings of low self-esteem) for real or imagined guilt.

VALUE—an abstract concept, often merely implicit, that defines for an individual or for a social unit what ends or means to an end are desirable.[2]

VENEREAL DISEASE—a disease usually transmitted through sexual intercourse.

REFERENCES

Abramson, J. H. Observations of the health of adolescent girls in relation to cultural change. *Psychosomatic Medicine*, 1961, **23.**

Ackerson, L. *Children's behavior problems.* Chicago: University of Chicago Press, 1938.

Barbu, Z. *Problems of historical psychology.* New York: Grove Press, Inc., 1960.

Belknap, I., and E. G. Jaco. The epidemiology of mental disorders in a political-type city (based on 1949 population of 129,500). In *Interrelations between the social environment and psychiatric disorders.* New York: Milbank Medical Fund, 1953, p. 237.

Beller, E. K., and P. B. Neubauer. Patterning of symptoms in early childhood. Paper presented at the 115th Annual Meeting of the American Psychiatric Association in Philadelphia, 1959.

Benedict, P. K. Socio-cultural factors in schizophrenia. In L. Bellak (ed.), *Schizophrenia: A review of the syndrome.* New York: Logos Press, 1958.

——— and I. Jacks. Mental illness in primitive societies. *Psychiatry,* 1954, **17,** 377–389.

Bertalanffy, L. von. Some biological considerations of the problem of mental illness. In L. Appleby *et al.* (eds.), *Chronic schizophrenia.* New York: The Free Press of Glencoe, 1960.

Brugger, C. Psychiatrische Bestandesaufnahme im Geblete eines medizinsch-anthropologischen Zenus in der Nahe von Rosenheim. In A. H. Leighton *et al.* (eds.), *Explorations in social psychiatry.* New York: Basic Books, Inc., 1957. (Originally published, 1938.)

Buell, B., *et al. Community planning for human services.* New York: Columbia University Press, 1952.

Cameron, D. E. Psychologically hazardous occupations. *Industrial Medicine,* 1946, **15,** 332–335.

Chodoff, P. A reexamination of some aspects of conversion hysteria. *Psychiatry,* 1954, **17,** 75.

Clausen, J. A. Social patterns, personality, and adolescent drug use. In A. H. Leighton *et al* (eds.), *Explorations in social psychiatry.* New York: Basic Books, Inc., 1957.

——— and M. L. Kohn. The ecological approach in social psychiatry. *American Journal of Sociology,* 1954, **60,** 140–149.

Coleman, J. Discussion of D. Reid. Precipitating proximal factors in the occurrence of mental disorders: Epidemiological evidence. *Milbank Memorial Fund Quarterly,* 1961, **39,** 253.

Commission on Chronic Illness. *Chronic illness in a large city: The Baltimore Study.* Cambridge, Mass.: Harvard University Press, 1957.

Dayton, M. A. *New facts on mental disorders.* Springfield, Ill.: Charles C Thomas, Publisher, 1940.

Dohrenwend, B. P. The Stirling County study. *American Psychologist,* 1957, **12.**

——— and B. S. Dohrenwend. The problem of validity in field studies of psychological disorder. *Journal of Abnormal Psychology,* 1965, **70,** 1.

Dublin, L. I., and B. Bunzel. *To be or not to be: A study of suicide.* New York: Harrison Smith and Robert Hayes, 1933.

Dunham, H. W. Social structures and mental disorder: Competency hypothesis of explanation. *Milbank Memorial Fund Quarterly,* 1961, **39,** 257–311.

Facts about mental illness. Washington, D.C.: National Association for Mental Health, January, 1956.

Facts and figures about mental illness and other personality disturbances. Washington, D.C.: National Association for Mental Health, April, 1952.

Faris, R. E. L., and H. W. Dunham. *Mental disorders in urban areas.* Chicago: University of Chicago Press, 1939.

Fifteen indices. Washington, D.C.: Joint Information Service of the American Psychiatric Association and the National Association for Mental Health, 1964.

Fogarty, J. E. Statement at U. S. House of Representatives Appropriations Subcommittee for Departments of Labor and Health, Education, and Welfare opening special hearing on juvenile delinquency, March, 1960.

Fraser, R., and Phelps. The incidence of neurosis among factory workers. Medical Research Council, Industrial Research Board, Report No. 90. London: His Majesty's Stationery Office, 1947.

Freud, S. Some psychological consequences of the anatomical distinction between the sexes. *International Journal of Psychoanalysis,* 1927, **8.**

Freudenberg, R. K., and J. P. S. Robertson. Symptoms in relation to psychiatric diagnosis and treatment. *Archives of Neurology and Psychiatry,* 1956, **76,** 14–22.

Fromm, E. *Man for himself.* New York: Holt, Rinehart & Winston, 1947.

Fyvel, T. R. *Troublemakers: Rebellious youth in an affluent society.* New York: Schocken Books, 1962.

Gerard, D. L., and L. G. Houston. Family

setting and the social ecology of schizophrenia. *Psychiatric Quarterly*, 1953, **27**, 90–101.

Gilbert, G. M. A survey of "referral problems" in metropolitan child guidance centers. *Journal of Clinical Psychology*, 1957, **13**, 37–42.

Glass, A. J. Psychotherapy in the combat zone. *American Journal of Psychiatry*, 1954, **110.**

Halliday, J. L. *Psychological medicine: A study of the sick society*. New York: W. W. Norton & Co., Inc., 1948.

Hare, E. H. Mental illness and social conditions in Bristol. *Journal of Mental Science*, 1956, **102**, 349.

Hastings, D. W. Psychiatry in the Eighth Air Force. *Air Surgeon's Bulletin*, 1944, **8**, 4–5.

Hattwick, L. A. Sex differences in behavior of nursery school children. *Child Development*, 1937, **8**, 343–355.

Hinkle, L. E., Jr., and H. G. Wolff. Health and the social environment: Experimental investigations. In A. H. Leighton *et al.* (eds.), *Explorations in social psychiatry*. New York: Basic Books, Inc., 1957.

Hollingshead, A. B., and F. C. Redlich. *Social class and mental illness*. New York: John Wiley & Sons, Inc., 1958.

Holmes, T. H., *et al.* Psychological and psychophysiologic studies of tuberculosis. *Psychosomatic Medicine*, 1957, **19.**

Hopkins, F. Decrease in admissions to mental observation wards during war. *British Medical Journal*, March 20, 1943, **1**, 358.

Horney, Karen. *Our inner conflicts*. New York: W. W. Norton & Co., Inc., 1945.

Hospitals, August 1, 1963, guide issue.

Hunt, W., *et al.* A theoretical and practical analysis of the diagnostic process. In P. Hoch and J. Zubin (eds.), *Current problems in psychiatric diagnosis*. New York: Grune & Stratton, Inc., 1953, pp. 53–65.

Illingworth, C. F. W., *et al.* Acute perforated peptic ulcer: Frequency and incidence in West of Scotland. *British Medical Journal*, November 11, 1944, **2**, 617.

Jackson, D. D. (ed.). *The etiology of schizophrenia*. New York: Basic Books, Inc., 1960.

Jaco, E. G. Social factors in mental disorders in Texas. *Social Problems*, April, 1957, **4**, 322–328.

Komora, P. O., and M. A. Clark. Mental disease in the crisis. *Mental Hygiene*, April, 1935, **19**, 289–301.

Langner, T. S., and S. T. Michael. *Life stress and mental health*. New York: The Free Press of Glencoe, 1963.

Leary, T., and H. Coffey. Interpersonal diagnosis: Some problems of methodology and validation. *Journal of Abnormal and Social Psychology*, 1955, **50**, 110–126.

Leighton, A. H., *et al.* (eds.). Some issues reexamined. In A. H. Leighton *et al.* (eds.), *Explorations in social psychiatry*, New York: Basic Books, Inc, 1957.

Leighton, D. C. *et al. The character of danger: Psychiatric symptoms in selected communities*, Vol. III: *The Stirling County study of psychiatric disorder and sociocultural environment*. New York: Basic Books, Inc., 1963.

Lemert, E. M. Exploratory study of mental disorders in a rural problem area. *Rural Sociology*, 1948, **48**, 13.

LeShan, L., and R. Worthington. *Journal of Clinical Experimental Psychopathology*, 1955, **16**, 281–288.

Levy, J. A quantitative study of behavioral problems in relation to family constellation. *American Journal of Psychiatry*, 1931, **10**, 237.

Lewis, A. Incidence of neurosis in England under war conditions. *Lancet*, August, 1942, **2**, 175–183.

Linton, R. *Culture and mental disorders*. Springfield, Ill.: Charles C Thomas, Publisher, 1956.

Lorr, M. The Wittenborn psychiatric syndromes: An oblique rotation *Journal of Consulting Psychology*, 1957, **21**, 6.

——— and R. L. Jenkins. Patterns of maladjustment in children. *Journal of Clinical Psychology*, 1953.

——— *et al.* Factors descriptive of psychopathology and behavior of hospitalized psychotics. *Journal of Abnormal and Social Psychology*, 1955, **50**, 78–86.

MacFarlane, Jean W., *et al. A developmental study of the behavior problems of normal children between twenty-one months and fourteen years*. Berkeley, Calif.: University of California Press, 1954.

Malzberg, B. *Social and biological aspects of disease*. New York: State Hospital Press, 1940.

———. Important statistical data about mental illness. In S. Arieti (ed.), *Ameri-*

can handbook of psychiatry, Vol. 1. New York: Basic Books, Inc., 1959, pp. 161–174.

Martinson, F. M. Ego deficiency as a factor in marriage. *American Sociological Revue*, 1955, **20**, 161–164.

Medical almanac. Compiled by Peter S. Nagan. Philadelphia: W. B. Saunders Company, 1961–1962.

Mills, C. W. *The sociological imagination*. New York: Grove Press, Inc., 1960.

Minski, L., and M. M. Desai. *British Journal of Medical Psychology*, 1955, **28**, 113–134.

Myers, J. K., and B. H. Roberts. *Family and class dynamics in mental illness*. New York: John Wiley & Sons, Inc., 1959.

Odegaard, O. Incidence of mental disease in Norway during World War II. *Acta Psychiatrica et Neurologica Scandinavica*, 1954, **29**, 333–353.

Patients in mental institutions, 1960, Part II. Bethesda, Md.: Biometrics Branch, National Institute of Mental Health.

Peterson, D. R. Behavior problems of middle childhood. *Journal of Consulting Psychology*, 1961, **25**, 205–209.

Pflanz, M., *et al. Journal of Psychosomatic Medicine*, 1956, **1**, 68–74.

Phillips, L. Cultural versus intropsychic factors in childhood behavior problem referrals. *Journal of Clinical Psychology*, 1956, **12**, 400–401.

——— *et al.* Sphere dominance, role orientation and diagnosis. *Journal of Abnormal Psychology*, in press.

——— and M. S. Rabinovitch. Social role and patterns of symptomatic behavior. *Journal of Abnormal and Social Psychology*, 1958, **57**, 181–186.

——— and E. Zigler. Social competence, the action-thought parameter and vicariousness in normal and pathological behaviors. *Journal of Abnormal and Social Psychology*, 1961, **63**, 137–146.

Reid, D. Precipitating proximal factors in the occurrence of mental disorders: Epidemiological evidence. *Milbank Memorial Fund Quarterly*, 1961, **39**, 229–258.

Report to Congress on juvenile delinquency, February, 1960. Washington, D.C.: Department of Health, Education, and Welfare.

Rogler, L. H., and A. B. Hollingshead. *Trapped: Families and schizophrenia*. New York: John Wiley & Sons, Inc., 1965.

Rosen, E., and G. B. Rizzo. Preliminary standardization of the MMPI for use in Italy: A case study of intercultural and intracultural differences. *Educational and Psychological Measurement*, 1961, **21**, 629–636.

Rosenzweig, S. An outline of frustration theory. In J. McV. Hunt (ed.), *Personality and the behavior disorders*, Vol. 1. New York: The Ronald Press Company, 1945.

Sainsbury, P. *Suicide in London: An ecological study*. New York: Basic Books, Inc., 1956.

Scheinfeld, A. *Women and men*. New York: Harcourt, Brace & World, Inc. 1943.

Schmale, A. H., Jr. Relationship of separation and depression to disease. *Psychosomatic Medicine*, 1958, **20**.

Srole, L., *et al. Mental health in the metropolis: Midtown Manhattan study*, Vol. 1. New York: McGraw-Hill, Inc., 1962.

Statistical abstracts of the United States, Ed. 86. Washington, D.C.: U.S. Bureau of the Census, 1965.

Stewart, D. N., and D. M. Winser. Incidence of perforated peptic ulcer: Effect of heavy air-raids. *Lancet*, 1942, **1**, 259–261.

Stonequist, E. V. *The marginal man*. New York: Charles Scribner's Sons, 1937.

Stouffer, S., *et al. The American soldier*, Vol. IV; *Measurement and prediction*, Princeton, N.J.: Princeton University Press, 1950.

Swinscrow, D. Some suicide statistics. *British Medical Journal*, 1951, **1**, 1417–1423.

Terman, L. M., and Leona E. Tyler. Psychological sex differences. In L. Carmichael (ed.), *Manual of child psychology*, New York: John Wiley & Sons, Inc., 1954.

Terris, M. Discussion of A. M. Macmillan, A survey technique for estimating the prevalence of psychoneurotic and related types of disorders in communities. In B. Pasamanick (ed.), *Epidemiology of mental disorder*. Washington, D.C.: American Association for the Advancement of Science, 1959.

Thomas, W. I., and F. Zaniecki. *The Polish*

peasant in Europe and America. New York: Alfred A. Knopf, Inc., 1958.

Tunley, R. *Kids, crime, and chaos*. New York: Harper & Row, Publishers, 1962.

Ullman, L., and L. Gurell. Validity of symptom rating from psychiatric records. *Archives of General Psychiatry*, 1962, 7 (8), 130–134.

Uniform crime reports for the United States. Washington, D.C.: Federal Bureau of Investigation, 1959.

Uniform crime reports for the United States, Washington, D.C.: Federal Bureau of Investigation, 1960.

Ward, C. H., *et al*. The psychiatric nomenclature. *Archives of General Psychiatry*, 1962, 7, 198–205.

What are the facts about mental illness in the United States? Washington, D.C.: National Committee Against Mental Illness, Inc., 1964.

Wheelis, A. *The quest for identity*. New York: W. W. Norton & Company, Inc., 1958.

Williams, H. D. A survey of predelinquent children in ten midwestern cities. *Journal of Juvenile Research*, 1933, **17**, 163–174.

Wittenborn, J., *et al*. Symptom correlates for descriptive diagnosis. *Genetic Psychology Monographs*, 1953, **47**, 237–301.

Wittkower, E. D., and J. Fried. Some problems of transcultural psychiatry. In M. K. Opler (ed), *Culture and mental health*. New York: Crowell-Collier and Macmillan, Inc., 1959, pp. 489–500.

Zigler, E., and L. Phillips. Social effectiveness and symptomatic behaviors. *Journal of Abnormal and Social Psychology*, 1960, **61**, 231–238.

——— and ———. Psychiatric diagnosis and symptomatology. *Journal of Abnormal and Social Psychology*, 1961*a*, **63**, 69–75.

——— and ———. Social competence and outcome in psychiatric disorder. *Journal of Abnormal and Social Psychology*, 1961*b*, **63**, 264–271.

SUGGESTED READINGS

1. Faris, R. E. L., and H. W. Dunham. *Mental disorders in urban areas*. Chicago: University of Chicago Press, 1939. One of the first studies in the ecology of psychiatric disorder. The authors found that the rate of mental disorder increased as a function of proximity to the center of the city.
2. Zigler, E., and L. Phillips. Social effectiveness and symptomatic behaviors. *Journal of Abnormal and Social Psychology*, 1960, **61**, 231–238. A report on a large study that examined the relationship between social competence and various symptoms and defenses in a psychiatric population.

13

Mind, Body, and Behavior: Control Systems and Their Disturbances

MICHEL TREISMAN

BODY AND MIND

It is common to make a sharp distinction between the "body" and the "mind." On the one hand we have feelings, fears, hopes, and ambitions; on the other we know that our bodies consist of bones and muscles, heart, lungs, and brain, and it may seem very difficult to relate these two areas of interest. We also make this distinction when our health is disturbed. For example, some diseases, like measles, seem to be purely physical events happening in our bodies; on the other hand, depressions, anxieties, and other disturbances seem to be purely "mental" events. But in many cases we find that "mind" and "body" seem to be closely connected. When we drink alcohol it produces changes in the body; but it can also have a very pleasant effect on our state of mind. The temper of a harassed executive may be frayed by the worries of his job; he may also develop a stomach ulcer. Complaints like this are sometimes called "psychosomatic," meaning that the "psyche," or mind, has affected the "soma," or body. But this leaves us with the fascinating problem of what the link between the two may be.

How are our behavior and our thoughts, feelings, and emotions related to the events that go on in our bodies? This is still partly an unsolved problem, especially when we have to explain the more complex achievements of human beings. But we may get some insight if we look at the simpler bodily structures and see how they produce elementary behavior, such as reflexes. Perhaps we will find principles which we can apply to more complicated behavior. This may seem impossible to people who feel that "mind" and "body" are completely different. They might say that features of behavior or personality, like forethought or kindliness, are too different from bodily functions to be explained by studying the brain or glands.

This is not a very good argument, as we can see if we consider a far-fetched example. A Martian arrives on earth and for the first time in his life sees an automobile, something completely new to him. He is puzzled by it. He watches how it performs and finds that automobiles hold the road well or poorly, have high or low maximum speeds, travel downhill better than uphill, prefer smooth roads, and never fly or swim. But when he opens the hood and looks inside, all he sees is bits of metal, various wires, and a tank of smelly fluid. There is nothing that looks like the maximum speed, or the road-holding ability. He concludes that the automobile's behavior cannot be explained in terms of what lies under the hood, and he gives up in despair.

Now this is obviously wrong of him. The behavior of a complex system may seem very different from its structure. It is useless to look at the automobile engine without knowing how its parts function, the laws that determine how they work together. It is like a primitive person who has found a wireless set, but has never heard of electricity. However much he puzzles, he will never make sense of the collection of wires he finds inside the box. Indeed he is likely to focus on the wrong aspects of what he sees and decide that what matters is the colors of the components.

Our position is similar when we want to explain the behavior of a human being, in health or disease. We need to understand a complex system which is not a product of our own technology, so that we have no idea of the principles it is built on. We have to try to discover what its structure is and the laws which govern its functioning. Not until we have got these straight can we see how far they explain human behavior.

What is the basic structure of a human being? Like most other living organisms he is made up of a vast assemblage of cells. A cell is a particle of living matter equipped to keep itself alive. It consists of cytoplasm, which contains a nucleus, and is surrounded by a membrane. The cytoplasm has a number of different parts. It builds up the structure of the cell and obtains energy from food substances that are absorbed by the cell. The master plan for the structure of the cell itself is stored in the genes in the nucleus. The membrane, or cell wall, keeps the cell together and protects it from the environment. Simple organisms, like bacteria, have only one cell each. To reproduce itself this single cell divides into two new cells. More complex organisms, like plants or men, consist of a large number of cells organized together. Growth occurs by division of cells to give more cells.

Cells vary greatly in size. They can be quite large. A hen's egg starts as a single cell, and if it is kept warm and does not land on somebody's breakfast table, it will divide again and again until it ends up as a chicken of about the same total size but consisting of a very large number of cells. The cells in a chicken or a man are so small that they are measured in a special unit, the micron, which is equal to one thousandth of a millimeter; about twenty-five thousand microns would make one inch. In man most cell bodies would be between 5 and 100 microns across.

In the body similar cells may group together as tissues, such as muscle, bone, or nerve tissue. Cells may lie in an intercellular substance which can be watery, like blood, or solid, like bone, but is usually jelly-like or fibrous. The tissues are organized together to form the various organs of the body.

Now we saw that the Martian did not get very far by looking at the automobile without knowing how the parts worked. In the same way, we need to understand how the cells and tissues work together. The needs of an individual cell are simple: it must move away from harmful or poisonous conditions, and it must approach points in the environment which offer food substances and oxygen. A single cell can affect its environment in three main ways: it can alter its shape and thus move itself from one place to another, it can take in or excrete substances, and it may produce electrical effects. When cells unite together they still have the same needs, but there is now a division of labor in satisfying them. Muscle cells specialize in the power of changing their shape: when they all shorten together the muscle contracts, and so it can move a whole limb. Certain cells develop the ability to secrete special substances, and groups of such cells are known as glands. Examples are the salivary glands, which produce saliva in order to start digestion of food, and the sweat glands, whose secretion helps to cool the body.

For this division of labor to benefit all the many millions of cells, their activities must be coordinated with one another; and this is a tremendous problem of communication. All or most of the cells in a muscle must shorten or lengthen together, or the muscle as a whole will not contract or relax. If different parts of the body try to move in different directions at the same time the animal may tear itself to pieces. The chest must expand and contract as a whole, so that fresh oxygen is drawn into the lungs and waste gases are got rid of. The different parts of the heart must contract and relax in the correct sequence so that it will act as a pump and make the blood carry oxygen around the body to all the cells that need it. In some ways the problem is like that of coordinating the activities of a nation in time of war, or organizing production in a factory. A great many individuals or sections have to be made to work together so that a common end can be achieved. There are problems of planning, of control, and of communication between all the parts.

The science which studies the control and direction of complex systems is known as "cybernetics," and it has thrown a good deal of light on how the human body functions. We will consider some of the basic principles of cybernetics and then discuss how these apply to the organization of human behavior.

In physical terms, doing any job involves the use of energy. "Energy" is the power of doing work. When energy is expended it can produce movements, or warmth, or chemical changes, and it is often stored as an electric potential or in chemical form. For example when coal burns it combines chemically with oxygen and releases stored energy in the form of heat. In body cells food substances combine with oxygen at a controlled rate; the energy released keeps the body warm, and it is used to cause the changes in muscle cells which result in their contracting. Similarly, energy released when gasoline combines with oxygen in the motor of an automobile warms it up and also provides the power which turns the wheels.

Any industrial process, or other activity, depends on the transportation of energy and its use to change the positions and shapes of objects, or to produce heat or chemical changes. But energy transfer is not all that is necessary. To construct an automobile energy is needed to power the machines that stamp out the bodies and make the engine parts, but the machines would be no good if they stamped out the wrong shapes or put the engine together in the wrong arrangement. Not only energy, but also the order and pattern of the changes produced are important. This is also true of human behavior. An automobile driver transfers energy to the steering wheel. But two drivers may use the same amount of energy, and one will drive his automobile off the edge of a cliff, while the other keeps his on the road. The difference is not in the amount of energy used, but the pattern and order of the movements energized.

The orders and instructions that control the use of energy are known as "information." For example, on a battlefield soldiers have guns or other weapons which allow energy to be used destructively. But they also need to know who they are fighting, and where to find the enemy. A soldier may fire in the correct direction because his commanding officer tells him what to do, or because a scout reports where the enemy are, or because he sees the smoke of their campfire. In each case he receives information and uses it to control the application of energy. Technically we define *information* in terms of the choices or alternatives that are open to the soldier (or anyone else). Before he received information he might have fired in any direction. Once he has received it he chooses the correct direction. We say that information has been transfered from a source (his commanding officer, or the scene before him) when it determines his choice of direction. If he gets the message but doesn't understand it, or fires at random anyway, then, in the scientific sense, no information has been transfered.

In the factory, information may be embodied in the design of the machines, so that they stamp out parts of the correct shape. It is also essential for the day-by-day running of the factory: when an executive speaks to a foreman on the telephone the purpose is to transfer information in one or both directions. The executive may be the "source" and the foreman the "receiver." The telephone cable joining them is known as the "channel" which transmits the information. Any complex organization needs a system of communication channels to organize its use of energy; this is especially true of the vast collection of cells that make up the human body.

Energy and information are both transfered in every human action, and there are channels for each of them. For example, to kick a football the player uses energy which comes from the food he eats. This is digested and glucose and other substances enter the bloodstream. The glucose travels to the muscles, where, by combining with oxygen, it frees chemical energy, which powers a movement of the leg. This movement transfers the energy to the football, so that it moves through the air. But to get this result the right muscles had to contract in the right order and to the right extent. The instructions or information that arranged this came from the nervous system along the nerves. In this case the channel for energy was the bloodstream, and the nerves were the channel for information.

Once a ball has been kicked or a gun fired we can see where the ball or the bullet goes, but we can't affect their course any further. Here information travels along a simple direct route, from the nervous system, which decides the original aim, to the point where the ball or the bullet lands. By the time we can see that the ball is going in the wrong direction it is too late to do anything to correct our aim. But this is not always the case. Some processes take enough time so that an indication of the result can be seen before the process is complete. A good example is a man trying to swim towards a goal, say a buoy in the sea. If he notices that it is over to his left he knows he is aiming too far to the right, and he shifts his course so that the buoy is again directly ahead. Here his eyes provide him with information about the result of his actions, and he uses this to alter the information his nervous system sends to his muscles. This means that the information is traveling along a loop: it is generated in the nervous system and dispatched to the

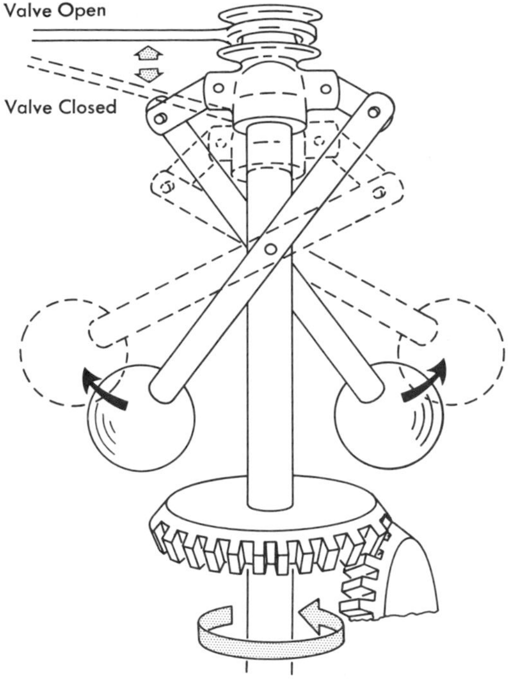

Figure 13.1 The flyball governor invented by James Watt as a means of automatically controlling the output of a steam engine.

muscles, and information about the resulting movements travels back to the nervous system and modifies the instructions it is giving. This sort of system, where information about the output, the movements, is "fed back" to the source, where it modifies the further generation of information, is sometimes called a "closed loop." In contrast, there is no "feedback" of information when a man fires a single shot from a gun, and this may be called an "open loop" (Bayliss, 1966; Guilbaud, 1959).

The principle of feeding back information in a closed loop had to be discovered before the first steam engine could be developed. In the steam engine coal is burned and heats water, which is converted into steam. The pressure of the hot steam is used to turn the wheels. The difficulty is to control engine speed. If more coal is thrown into the boiler the engine will go quickly, and if coal is taken out the heat will be reduced and the engine will go more slowly. But this is a clumsy and inefficient way of controlling speed. A partial solution is to have a valve in the pipe which takes the steam to the engine. The valve can be closed so that no steam gets through, and the engine will slow down. If the valve is opened steam gets through again and the engine speeds up. But if the valve is left at a fixed setting the engine will still speed up or slow down when fuel is added or used up.

To overcome this difficulty James Watt invented the steam engine "governor" in 1788 (Figure 13.1). This keeps the engine speed constant despite variations in the heat produced by the boiler. The governor consists of a shaft geared to the engine, so that it turns at the same rate, and it has "flyballs" attached to it. These are rotating balls which swing further and further out as the engine speeds up and centrifugal force increases. They are attached to the valve which lets steam into the engine, so that when they are thrown out by the centrifugal force they close the valve, and the engine slows down. If this happens the shaft will turn more slowly, the flyballs will not swing out so far, and the valve opens again and lets steam through. Consequently the engine speed will remain fairly constant, since the "governor" will correct it whenever it gets too fast or too slow (Piel *et al.*, 1955).

The boiler and engine transfer the energy of the coal to the wheels, and the governor generates information which controls this process by closing or opening the valve which lets the steam through from the boiler to the engine. In order to do this properly, it has to know what the engine is doing; it needs a "sensor" or sense organ which can measure whether the engine's output is high or low. The flyballs do this, because they are *sensitive* to the centrifugal force produced by the engine, so that their position is a measure of it. This information determines the next "instruction" to the engine. If the output speed is higher than the optimum speed "aimed at," the error is positive, and it is compensated for by a negative correction: the valve is closed. If the output speed is too slow, the error is negative, and a positive correction will increase the input of steam into the engine.

This sort of control is called "negative feedback" because the correction is in the opposite direction to the error. Because a device which can solve logical or mathematical problems is called a "computer," we can describe the governor as a simple computer linked to a simple sensor. This is a very simple control system, but most control problems are complex. In most complex organizations, many sorts of information affect each decision and more complicated computers are needed.

The governor is an *analogue computer*: It is based on a physical process which gives the right output to solve a particular problem. We are more accustomed to solving mathematical problems by working with numbers, and computers which operate in this way are known as *digital computers*. They are very flexible and can be used in many different ways, depending on how we set them up. The set of instructions that will make a computer operate in a particular way is known as its "program."

We have discussed the traditional sharp distinction between "mind" and "body." We tend to talk about our behavior in terms of our thoughts, feelings, hopes, intentions, and, in general, the contents of our minds. On the other hand our bodies, with organs such as brains, bones, and muscles, seem very different from the mind. Traditional ideas about their relations have not gone much beyond beliefs such as that the heart is the seat of affection or the guts of courage, which are not very helpful. But there are also difficulties in separating mind and body completely, since so many changes occur in parallel in both of them. For example, when people are afraid, their skins may pale, and they sweat and tremble; harassment and anxiety may be accompanied by the development of an ulcer.

But even though the behavior of a complex system may look very different from its components, it may still be caused by them. To see what the relations are we need to study the working of the components and how it produces behavior. Man is the complex system the behavioral scientist must study. The components of the body are cells, which are regulated to work together for the common end of survival. How they interact depends on their biochemical constitution and the needs that follow from it—requirements for energy and for materials to build up their structures—and is governed by the principles of cybernetics. We have considered *information transfer, loops*, and *communication channels*, as well as the *computational processes* which use information to select the best behavior. In the next section we shall consider the structure and functioning of the particular control mechanisms found in the human body.

THE MECHANISMS THAT CONTROL THE BODY

Human beings have evolved from very primitive ancestors over the course of millions of years. At one time the most complicated animal was the solitary free-living cell. Then cells grouped together to form small multicellular organisms, and these became more elaborate. The biochemical mechanisms of the cell reached a high degree of development at

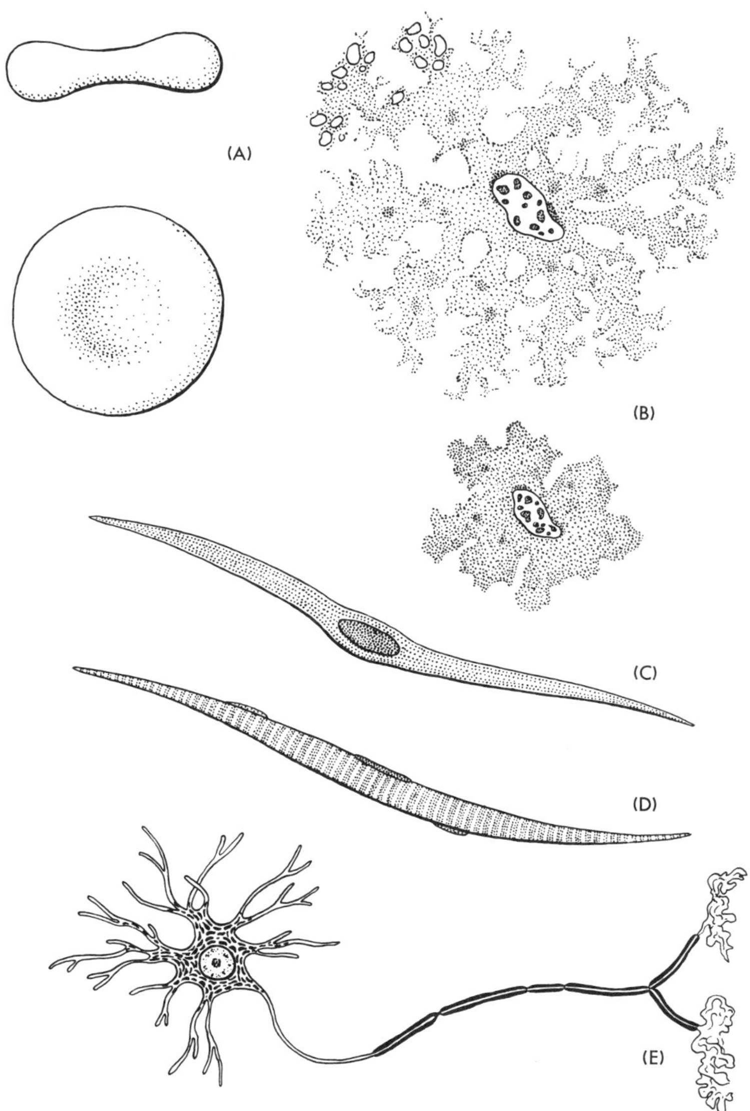

Figure 13.2 Animal cells of different shape: (*A*) human red blood cells, front and side views; (*B*) melanocyte containing pigment, expanded and contracted; (C) smooth muscle cell; (*D*) striated muscle cell; (*E*) nerve cell with axon (long branch) and dendrites (the finer, small branches). From Carl P. Swanson, *The Cell, Ed. 2,* © 1964. Reproduced by permission of Prentice-Hall, Inc., Englewood Cliffs, New Jersey.

an early stage (Figure 13.2) and the main changes in later evolution were in the form and control of the parts of the body. The cells of a fish and a man are much more similar at the chemical level than the structures of their bodies are.

The first organisms worked with fairly simple mechanisms of control. Later on, more complex mechanisms were added to the simple ones so that our bodies contain a hierarchy of mechanisms; remnants of the simple and more ancient ones are acted on and controlled by more efficient and specialized ones. For this reason, some of the mechanisms in our bodies are quick and efficient, others, usually the older ones, are relatively slow and crude.

If a sore or cut on the hand is infected, the surrounding skin becomes red and swollen. We say it is inflamed. This illustrates the simplest way in which one cell can influence its neighbors: damaged cells release substances which diffuse away from them and, when they reach nearby cells, prepare them to deal with the invading bacteria. But this way of achieving bodily coordination has marked limitations: it is slow, it affects only a few neighboring cells, and it does not distinguish between different causes of inflammation. A big improvement became possible when *blood circulation* evolved.

In very primitive animals food gets to the cells, and wastes are got rid of, by diffusion. This is slow and inefficient, and blood circulation developed as a means of distributing substances rapidly throughout the body. But once it had appeared its use was extended. One way in which multicellular animals protect themselves from invasion by hostile organisms, such as bacteria, is by producing substances which will attack and destroy the invaders. Vertebrate animals produce *antibodies*, which combine with and destroy particular substances, known as antigens, in the attacking organisms and so kill them. The antibodies are disturbed by the bloodstream and so can reach invaders throughout the body. Production of antibodies by *the immunity system* (the spleen, lymph nodes, and bone marrow) depends on initial exposure to the antigens. Thus a first attack of measles or mumps results in a long-lasting production of antibodies effective against the viruses responsible for these diseases, and if at a later time, the body is again attacked by these viruses, they will be destroyed by the antibodies before any signs of disease are produced. This accounts for the immunity against reinfection which follows an initial attack of many diseases. To operate effectively, the immunity system must have two complementary abilities: on the one hand, it must detect foreign substances in the body and develop antibodies against them; on the other, it must be able to recognize that other circulating substances come from its own cells, and it must refrain from self-destructively producing antibodies against these substances (Glynn and Holborow, 1965). As well as distributing energy and structural substances for building up the cells, and antibodies, the bloodstream can also help to coordinate the cells by carrying messages that can change the behavior of all or some of the cells in the body. These messages are carried by chemical messengers known as *hormones*, which are released into the bloodstream. Hormones can correlate the responses of the different parts of the body to an external situation, like a sudden emergency, or they can coordinate processes of growth and development in the body, such as the numerous bodily changes that accompany sexual development at puberty.

This control is exercised by cells which are specialized to produce the hormones; these cells are grouped into special structures called endocrine (meaning "secreting into the body") glands. One of the most important is the *thyroid gland.* It is a shield-shaped structure at the base of the neck, and it produces a hormone, *thyroxin*, which is essential for proper growth and development. If the thyroid is absent at birth the nerve cells in the brain do not develop properly; the child is mentally retarded and is known as a *cretin* (Figure 13.3). He learns to walk

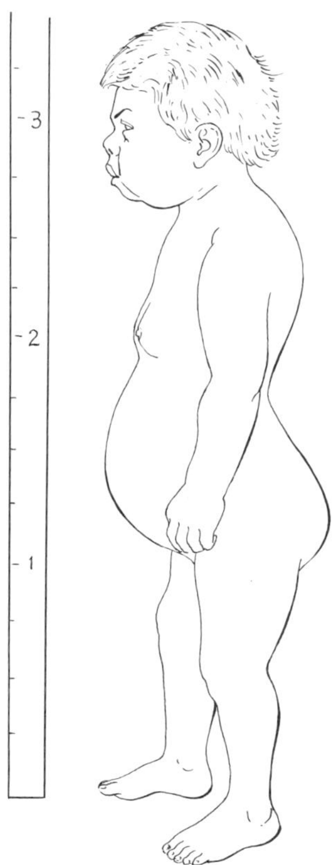

Figure 13.3 A cretin.

and to talk late and poorly, and he is stunted and dwarfish and does not grow normally. Thyroxin is also important for maintaining the rate of activity of the cells. If there is too much of it, the body uses energy too quickly, if there is too little, it slows down.

Another important gland is the *adrenal*. The name means "next to the kidney," and there is one above each kidney. Each adrenal gland has two separate parts with different functions. The core or "medulla" of the gland produces hormones known as adrenaline (sometimes called epinephrine) and noradrenaline, which adjust the body to meet states of alarm or emergency. When they are released into the bloodstream, they make the heart beat more strongly and quickly, they contract the blood vessels to the organs in the abdomen, so that less blood goes there, and they stop the movements of the gut. In a state of alarm, digestion is not essential, and the abdominal organs can get along for a while with less blood than usual. But our lives may depend on seeing clearly and thinking and acting quickly, so adrenaline in the blood maintains and improves the blood supply to the muscles and the brain and dilates the pupil of the eye.

The outer part of the adrenal gland, the "cortex," is also concerned with emergency situations involving stress. It mainly affects biochemical mechanisms at a cellular level and increases resistance to inflammation.

Another important pair of endocrine glands are the *gonads*, that is, the testes or ovaries. They are necessary for coordinated sexual development. The testes become active at puberty—about ten to twelve years—when they start to secrete *testosterone*. This hormone stimulates the growth of the sex organs, so that the penis gets larger and the secondary sex characteristics appear: hair grows on the face and trunk, pubic hair develops, the larynx grows larger and the voice breaks, the muscles develop, and interest in girls increases. Similarly, in the woman the ovary regulates sexual development by producing a hormone known as *estrogen*. At puberty the uterus enlarges and the breasts grow, pubic hair develops, and the body becomes more rounded. The female has a complicated sexual cycle, taking about a month, which is regulated hormonally. During an initial period of about two weeks, estrogen is produced, and this makes the lining of the uterus develop. Then ovulation occurs, and an egg is freed by one of the ovaries. It enters the uterus, and if it is fertilized, it implants in the lining of the uterus and starts to grow. The ovary now starts to produce a hormone, *progesterone*, which prepares the uterine lining for pregnancy.

If the ovum is not fertilized, the production of progesterone stops after about twelve days, and the thickened uterine lining strips away, causing menstruation. The uterus is then ready to start a new cycle.

This hormonal sequence can repeat itself month after month with great regularity. It is not controlled primarily from the ovary, but from a gland at the base of the brain known as the *pituitary*. The anterior (front) part of the pituitary produces *gonadotropic hormones*, which are so called because they stimulate the testis and ovary to produce their hormones. The pituitary starts puberty and controls the sexual cycle. It produces two gonadotropic hormones, one which stimulates the production of estrogen and a second which causes the production of progesterone. The correct level of gonad activity is maintained by a negative feedback cycle acting on the pituitary. When there is too much estrogen, the amount of gonadotropic hormone released is cut down. If the level of estrogen falls too low, the pituitary increases its production of gonadotropic hormone. In this way the pituitary controls the blood level of estrogen or progesterone.

The gonads are not the only glands under the control of the anterior pituitary. Similar feedback cycles control the activity of the thyroid and adrenal cortex, operating through *thyrotropic hormone* and *adrenocorticotropic hormone* (ACTH). Thus control of the main glands regulating the activity of body cells is centralized in the anterior pituitary. This lies directly below the base of the brain and, as we shall see, is partly controlled by it.

But though endocrine control is partly unified by the pituitary, it is still a very primitive system. It is slow; because the chemical messengers must be spread by the blood, the quickest responses are measured in minutes. And it is not very selective: the hormones affect sensitive cells throughout the body. Thyroxin affects most cells, and estrogen or testosterone affect cells in sensitive organs like the external genitalia or the breasts. A control system with these features would not be good enough to operate a set of muscles because it could never make a tissue of only one sort work in a number of different patterns at high speeds. For problems like that of muscular control a new type of element was needed, and the *neuron* or nerve cell was developed.

The great advantage of the neuron is that it provides a new sort of channel for information instead of relying on the bloodstream. It is specialized to release a small quantity of chemical transmitter at the exact point where it is required, and it is to the bloodstream what a telephone system is to a megaphone. As with other cells in man, the soma, or body, of the nerve cell is very small, and it is surrounded by a membrane, which not only keeps the contents of the cell inside and deleterious substances outside, but also maintains an electric charge. The body fluids consist of water containing many dissolved substances. Some of the atoms or molecules of these dissolved substances become electrically charged, and are then known as ions. The membrane of a cell tends to keep positive ions outside and negative ions inside, causing a difference in the electrical charge on the two sides of the membrane, the cell contents being negative with respect to the fluid between the cells. This is called "polarization."

The nerve cell has two special advantages. Firstly, although its body is small, it has developed thin fibers which extend away from the cell and can be extremely long. A single fiber may reach from the base of the spine to the foot, starting from a cell body in the spinal cord which is only a few thousandths of a millimeter wide. In the foot this fiber can deliver

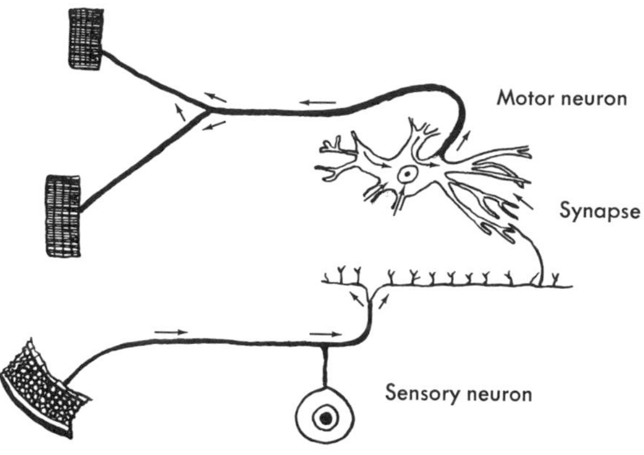

Figure 13.4 A sensory neuron synapsing with a motor neuron, forming a reflex arc. The arrows show the direction of conduction. From Ranson-Clark, *Anatomy of the Nervous System*, 10th edition. Philadelphia, W. B. Saunders Co., 1959.

a small quantity of a chemical transmitter, *acetylcholine*, to a selected muscle cell, which then contracts. This is vastly more precise than pouring acetylcholine into the blood and contracting all the muscle cells in the body would be.

Secondly, as well as developing a new sort of channel for information, the nerve cell has developed a new sort of message. The chemical transmitter does not travel all the way down the fiber: this would be a very slow process. Instead it is stored at the end of the fiber, and an *electrical impulse* travels down the fiber at high speed and liberates the transmitter when it reaches the end. What is an impulse? We saw that the membrane is electrically polarized, with positive charges outside and negative charges inside. When certain substances act on the surface of the nerve cell they let the positive ions flow into the cell, and the cell membrane becomes depolarized. One spot on the cell will recover quickly from this, but meanwhile it will trigger depolarization of the neighboring area of membrane. This recovers quickly too, but not before the next area on the fiber has been triggered, and in this way a wave of depolarization will travel all the way down the fiber. This is known as an impulse, and the great advantages of using it to convey messages are that it can travel very quickly and that the fiber recovers from the depolarization very quickly, so that a rapid sequence of impulses is possible, up to rates of about 1000 per second. Impulses travel at rates ranging from 2 to 200 miles per hour, the higher rates occurring in the thicker fibers, so that nerve cells can convey information quickly and precisely.

The development of neurons gave a big bonus: they can be linked together to form complex devices for handling information. Some fibers mainly affect muscle or gland cells, others connect with sensory receptors. For example, some fibers end at the bases of hairs in the skin. When the hair is moved impulses are set up in the fiber, so that the fiber conveys sensory information when the hair is touched. The retina of the eye has sensory receptors for light. These are specialized cells known as rods or cones, and they are in contact with nerve cells. When a rod or cone absorbs light it sets up impulses in the associated nerve cell.

The information arriving from a sense receptor can be passed on to another neuron. The fiber that carries impulses away from the nerve cell body (it is called an "axon") can end on another nerve cell and can set up impulses in it (Figure 13.4). (The junction where a fiber meets another cell which it can excite is called a "synapse.") This gives three classes of nerve cells: *sensory neurons*, which receive information from sensory receptors; *motor neurons*, which excite muscles or glands; and *interneurons*, which lie between them. These neurons can perform basic logical operations like those done by a digital computer. For example, if a neuron, A, is fired (that is, impulses are set up in it) by neurons *B* and *C*, it can respond in a number of ways. A may fire only if *B* and *C* both excite it at the same time, in which case either alone has no effect and an impulse down A's axon means that *B* and *C* were firing; A functions as an "adder." If either *B* or *C* alone can fire A, then an impulse from A would mean that *B or C* was firing. Some neurons also have the opposite effect: instead of exciting impulses in other neurons, they inhibit them so that they do not fire. They do this by making it more difficult to depolarize the membrane. If *B* is an excitatory neuron and *C* is an inhibitory neuron, then the output from A would represent *B* minus *C*. These are like the operations performed in a high speed digital computer. When a large number of such operations are carried out in the order specified by a program (a set of instructions to the computer), very complicated logical and mathematical problems can be solved. Thus the evolution of the neuron provided a component which could be used to build "biological computers" for dealing with the control problems of the living body.

The simplest arrangements of nerve cells in the human body are little groups closely associated with organs which they control. These groups are known as "ganglia." For example, a series of ganglia are associated with the gut. The gut contains muscle fibers to aid digestion and move food along. To do this they have to contract in the right sequence, so that sometimes food is mashed up and at other times it is moved down the gut. If there is an irritant poison in the stomach, the muscle fibers will reverse their order of contraction so that it is vomited up. These different patterns are organized by the ganglia associated with the gut. The ganglia which lie close to organs such as the heart, lungs, and gut and are responsible for their spontaneous activities when they are undisturbed were introduced in Chapter 3 as the "parasympathetic nervous system" (see Plate 3). They tend to be independent of one another and concentrated on the local control needs of individual organs.

In contrast is a second set of ganglia which lie alongside the spine and are known as the "sympathetic nervous system." Their axons travel out to the organs they affect and are important in their control in situations of alarm or emergency. They suppress digestive movements of the gut, dilate the pupils of the eyes and open up the air passages (bronchi), increase the blood pressure, and divert blood from the internal organs to the muscles. They also control the sweat glands. "Emotional" stimuli produce sweating in the "emotional sweating areas," the palms and soles, armpits, groin, and forehead. This effect on the palms and soles may be inherited from the time when the best defense against a beast of prey was climbing a tree: a moist palm gives a better grip on a slippery object. In animals with a hairy coat the sympathetic system contracts small muscles in the skin which set the hairs on end; this serves either to make the animal look bigger and more threatening when it is in a combat situation or to conserve body heat in conditions of cold. In man the hairy coat is vestigial, but we still possess these erector muscles and they may cause "goose pimples" in conditions of fear or cold (Kuntz, 1953).

The sympathetic ganglia are much more closely interconnected than the parasympathetic ganglia so that the system can operate as a whole. Unlike the parasympathetic system and other nerves acting on the organs and muscles of the body, which release acetylocholine as their transmitter, the sympathetic fibers release noradrenaline. Adrenaline and noradrenaline are also released by the medulla of the adrenal gland, and the sympathetic nervous system and

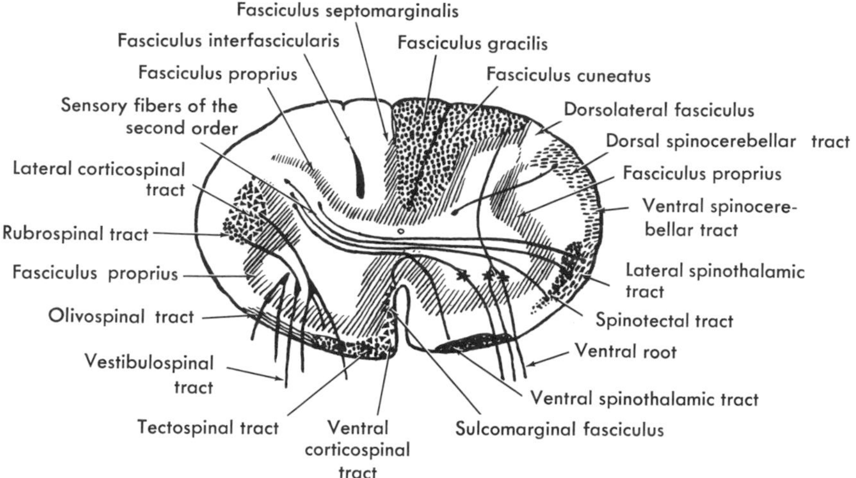

Figure 13.5 A cross section of the spinal cord showing the bundles of nerve fibers which travel up and down it. Those which travel up are marked on the right, those traveling down on the left. From Ranson-Clark, *Anatomy of the Nervous System*, 10th edition. Philadelphia, W. B. Saunders Co., 1959.

the adrenal medulla work together. The sympathetic system is a more advanced system for doing a similar job. Its advantage is that it can operate more quickly, and that when necessary it can be selectively active. For example, it dilates the blood vessels going to a contracting muscle.

The sympathetic and parasympathetic systems together are known as the "autonomic nervous system." "Autonomic" means "self-governing," but this system is not truly independent, because it has come under the control of the more advanced *central nervous system*—the brain and spinal cord. The central system has some control of the organs and blood vessels through its connections with the autonomic system, but it has evolved mainly to solve the complex problem of controlling the skeletal muscular system. This is the system of muscles that moves the limbs, the body, and the head. We would be helpless without them, but to use them properly we need a control system that is precise and graduated and that makes rapid decisions on the basis of all the available sensory information. It must be precise so that muscles and parts of muscles can move independently and in the right order. An action as simple as walking requires that each limb be bent and straightened at all its joints in the right order and to the right extent. Even standing upright requires the use of information from all parts of the body. In fact, standing upright is a complex achievement. In order to stand still, a man must really make very small movements all the time. The position of each of his limbs, and the tension in all his muscles is continually recorded by special sense receptors in the muscles and joints. When a limb starts to sag, or his trunk starts to sway to one side, this is reported by the sensory fibers, and muscles contract which will straighten him up again. If he stretches his hand out in front of him, his spine will arch backwards slightly to prevent his weight from throwing him forward. Little unnoticed adjustments like this have to be made all the time to prevent falling down.

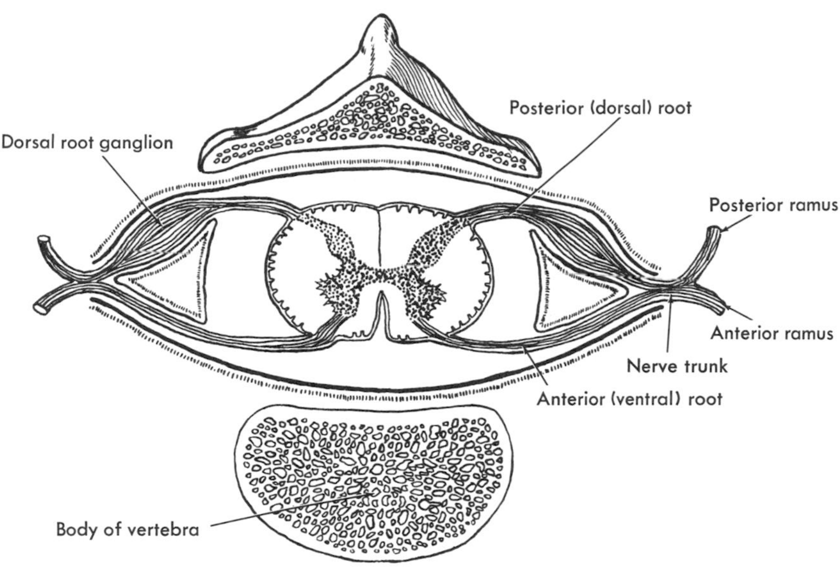

Figure 13.6 A cross section of the spinal cord, with sensory nerve fibers entering it and motor nerve fibers leaving it. From T. A. Rogers, *Elementary Human Physiology*, John Wiley & Sons, Inc., 1961.

Control of the skeletal muscles not only uses all the sensory information coming in, both from inside and outside the body, but it also uses information from the past. You can see this if you give someone a heavy case to lift, then give him one which looks just as heavy but is really empty: when he starts to lift it he will stagger backwards. He has stored information about how heavy to expect the case to be, and his program of movements for lifting it is based on this information. So he uses too much force for an empty case and falls backwards.

Our early wormlike ancestors were made up of a series of segments, and this design still shows in the way some parts of the body are constructed: each vertebra in the back-bone corresponds to an original segment, and some of the segments are still represented by a pair of ribs. The spinal cord is a midline structure looking rather like a length of cord or rope running down the center of the backbone. It is made up of nerve cells and their axons. The nerve cell bodies lie in the center of the cord, and the axons run up and down on the surface (Figure 13.5). A mass of nerve cell bodies looks gray, and a mass of axons looks white; therefore, the inside of the spinal cord is gray and the outside white. The cord began as a neural organization for each segment, and these later linked together. The original segments are still represented by a pair of motor and sensory nerve roots on each side (Figure 13.6). The motor nerve roots consist of bundles of axons from motor neurons which leave the front surface of the cord and travel out in the nerves to the muscles. The nerves also contain fibers which come from sensory receptors in the skin, muscles, and other places. Most of the neurons in the spinal cord are interneurons—there are thirty for every motor neuron. They receive most of the sensory information coming into the cord, and they organize the motor output: they decide which motor neurons shall fire and, therefore, which muscles will contract.

This system allows each segment to receive information and to use it to organize a response. Everyone has had his knee tapped as part of a medical examination. The doctor does this to test how the nervous system is working at the segmental level. By tapping the tendon below the kneecap he suddenly stretches the muscle which normally straightens the leg at the knee. This stimulates the sensory receptors in the muscle that signal stretching—they are known as "muscle spindles" because of their shape—so that they fire rapidly. Their sensory fibers enter the spinal cord and end on the motor neurons in the muscle; the sudden input from these stretch receptors excites the motor neurons so that they make the muscle contract. We see the sudden muscle twitch as a knee jerk.

This looks like a very simple piece of behavior, an "open loop" in which information goes straight through, but in fact it is more complicated. It results from a negative feedback system which keeps the muscle length constant. The feedback counteracts slight shortenings or lengthenings of the muscle which alter the stretch on the muscle spindles. When the muscle is at the right length, the steady firing of the spindles keeps the motor neuron output at the right level to maintain that length. But if for some reason the motor neurons fire too slowly and the muscle starts to stretch, the spindles also stretch and therefore fire more quickly. This higher rate of firing speeds the motor neurons up, and the muscle shortens again. If it shortens too much the stretch is taken off the spindle, which then fires more slowly, and the muscle slackens. In this way the muscle is kept oscillating at about its right length. This is the "stretch reflex," and when we tap the tendon we are just getting an exaggerated oscillation out of it.

Most of the behavior programmed in the spinal cord involves more than one segment and more than a single feedback loop. For example, a single movement of the leg in walking depends upon a number of segments working together to make the muscles contract and relax in the right sequence. Because stretch reflexes tend to take the limb back to where it was, they must be reset to maintain the new muscle lengths. The cooperation between segments is mediated by interneurons, which take information from one segment to another. They also help to coordinate different programs. For example, if one leg is lifted, then the other must be kept down. The cord also organizes other programs, such as withdrawing a leg if it gets hurt, or scratching, but it cannot produce behavior much more complicated than this or make extensive use of memory and learning. To meet these needs the *brain* has developed.

The head end of a simple creature is what gets into danger first, so that it is an advantage to have the distance receptors, the nose, eyes, and ears, at the head. With the neural segments of the head receiving all this specialized information, they needed to be more complicated than the spinal cord and thus developed into the brain. The brain is divided into three parts: the hind-, mid-, and forebrains (Figure 13.7).

The *hindbrain* receives information from the ear, one part of which, the cochlea, is sensitive to sound, and another part, the labyrinth, to the position of the head in space. The hindbrain lies immediately above the spinal cord, and it solves complicated problems of positioning the body in space.

If a cat is dropped, it twists in midair so that it lands on its feet. Information about the position of its limbs in space and about the position of its head has

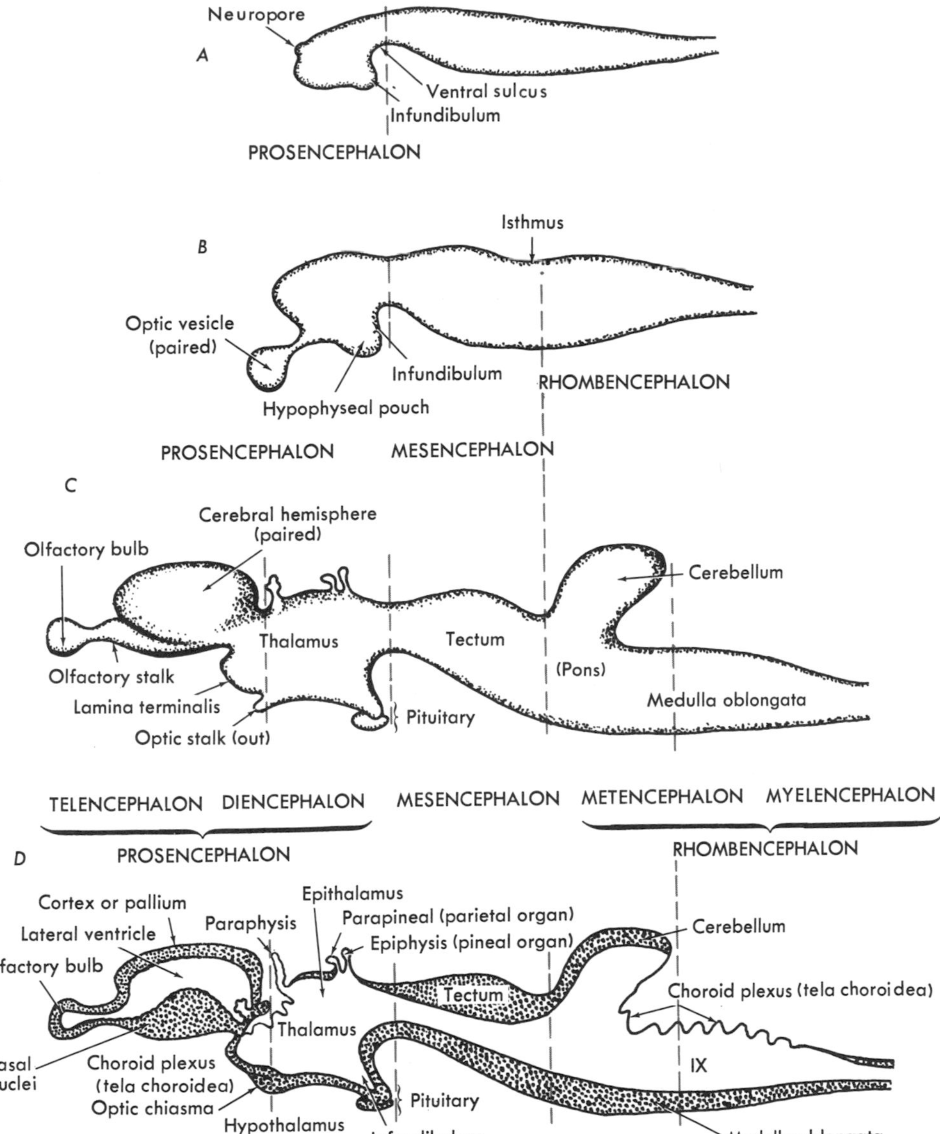

Figure 13.7 Some early stages in the development of the brain in the embryo. *A*, only the forebrain is distinct from the rest of the neural tube. *B*, three main divisions are established: forebrain (prosencephalon), midbrain (mesencephalon), and hindbrain (rhombencephalon). *C*, more mature stage (side view). *D*, the same in median section. From A. S. Romer, *The Vertebrate Body*, 3rd edition. Philadelphia, W. B. Saunders Co., 1962.

been put together, and it has chosen the right movements to bring its body upright. A special part of the hindbrain called the *cerebellum* received the position information from the spinal cord and combined it with information from the labyrinths on each side. This information is acted on by interneurons in the hind- and midbrains arranged in a loose network called the reticular system, which

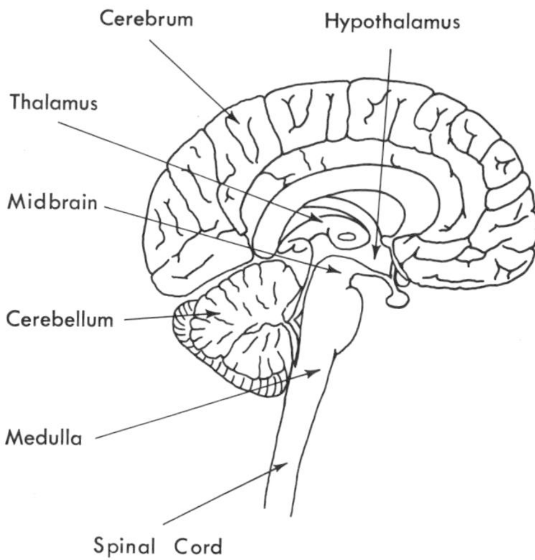

Figure 13.8 The medial aspect of the human brain as it would be seen if a midline cut were made from the nose (on the *right*) to the back of the head.

controls muscle tension throughout the body, mainly by making the muscle spindles fire slowly or quickly.

The hindbrain also produces chewing and swallowing when food is in the mouth, controls the heart rate, and organizes respiration. The control of breathing is governed by negative feedback. When the cells use oxygen, carbon dioxide accumulates in the blood and makes the hindbrain speed up breathing; the excess carbon dioxide is lost in the air breathed out from the lungs. If there is too little carbon dioxide in the blood, breathing slows down or stops until the carbon dioxide returns to the optimum level. Many important constituents of the body are kept at the optimum levels for life by this use of negative feedback, which is known as homeostasis.

In primitive animals the *midbrain* dealt with information from the eye, but in man most of this information goes straight on to the *forebrain*, which is the largest and most noticeable part of the brain in man, in whom it is better developed than in any other animal (Figure 13.8). Originally it dealt mainly with information from the organ of smell, and the oldest part of it is still known as the "smell brain" or rhinencephalon, but it has developed many other functions as well. It has a hollow central core, with a floor known as the *hypothalamus*, and two big outgrowths, one on each side, which are known as the *cerebral hemispheres* (Brewer, 1961; Morgan and Stellar, 1965; Deutsch and Deutsch, 1966).

We have seen how the organization of behavior becomes more complex as we go from the spinal cord to the hindbrain and midbrain. The cord produces walking, and the hindbrain organizes chewing and swallowing and can run simple homeostatic systems. But to keep alive we have to do more than this: for example, we need to get hungry, that is, we must know when we need food, and when this happens we must be able to find food and eat it. Food-seeking behavior is organized from the *hypothalamus*. It has been studied mainly in animals such as rats and dogs, but because there is a lot of similarity between men and rats, we can learn a lot about human beings from experiments on animals. These show that the hypothalamus contains a hunger center and a satiety center. The hunger center produces eating, but activity of the satiety center suppresses it. When the hunger center has been damaged rats will starve themselves to death rather than eat, but when the satiety center is out of action they eat excessively and become grossly fat (Anand, 1961; McCleary and Moore, 1965; Marler and Hamilton, 1966).

Systems that organize behavior that serves essential needs like eating, drinking, and sexual activity are known as drive systems (sometimes they are called "instincts"). The control of many drives appears to be centered in the hypothalamus, which acts on the motor centers at lower levels, producing behavior in the right sequence. The periodic behavior of eating is produced by the hunger center, which lies in the lateral hypothalamus (that is, toward the side of the hypothalamus), and the satiety center in the ventromedial (towards the midline) nucleus, acting in combination (Plate 4). There is some evidence that other drives which produce intermittent effects on behavior may be controlled in a similar way by hypothalamic mechanisms located in areas which partly overlap those determining eating. Damage to the lateral hypothalamus may suppress drinking as well as eating. Electrical stimulation of this area, which may simulate the effects of high drive, may produce eating or drinking in satiated animals, or may result in release of the hormone which preserves the body's supply of water by reducing urine production by the kidneys. Damage in the area of the ventromedial nucleus may not only reduce the inhibitory activity of the satiety center and thereby cause excessive eating; it may also cause excessive drinking, aggressive behavior, and sleep (which should also be considered an effect of a drive mechanism). As well as becoming hungry and thirsty, rats with lesions of the ventromedial nucleus may be sleepy and vicious (Herberg, 1967).

Some animals show a drive to hoard food. Rats, for example, collect food pellets and store them in neat heaps in their nests. The occurrence of this behavior depends on whether the animal is well or poorly fed, but not on his state of hunger. However, electrical stimulation of the same area in the lateral hypothalamus produces both hoarding and feeding. It appears that the act of feeding does not result in inhibition of all other activity in the feeding-and-hoarding center, but instead blocks the connections which allow the center to organize eating behavior. But since the connections subserving hoarding do not come under the inhibitory control of the satiety center, the lateral hypothalamic center may produce hoarding when the animal does not appear hungry; in this case the satiety center blocks feeding but not hoarding (Herberg, 1967).

Many "secondary drives" which lead men to work for esthetic or material rewards or pleasures are not obviously related to these basic physiological cycles. It is possible, however, that they are related to the physiological drives in that their ultimate motivation comes from primary drive centers in the lateral hypothalamus but that they are not subject to the inhibitory effects of satiety and other mechanisms in the ventromedial nucleus, so that they are more or less continuously active (Herberg, 1967).

An important function of the hypothalamus affects the endocrine system through its control of the pituitary gland and the production of hormones by certain specialized cells of the hypothalamus itself. For example, on the one hand it controls eating through the hunger center, producing sequences like searching for food, finding it, and eating it, and on the other, it can directly affect the rate at which energy is used by controlling the amount of thyrotropic hormone released by the anterior pituitary. Similarly, it has centers for drinking, and there are cells in the hypothalamus which produce a hormone to control the rate at which the kidneys lose water (Cannon, 1932; Hess, 1957). The hypothalamus also controls many visceral functions, such as the activity of the heart and blood vessels, acting through the autonomic nervous system; hypothalamic activity may determine whether sympathetic or parasympathetic effects are dominant, where these oppose each other (Hess, 1957).

At all the levels we have discussed, sensory information is used rather crudely. The spinal cord uses only enough information to distinguish between a firm surface the foot can walk on and a painful stimulus it must be withdrawn from. The midbrain level is not much better. We can see its deficiencies in animals with little cerebral cortex, whose behavior is organized mainly by the structures we have described. For example, robins fight other male robins to preserve individual nesting territories. But what the robin attacks is the red breast: it will ignore a male robin without a red breast but will launch a ferocious assault on a bundle of red feathers. It sees the world in a very primitive way, selecting a clear detail, like a splash of red, which is easy to pick out, and using that alone. The information about the red breast is not related to the rest of the sensory information it might use, such as the presence or absence of the robin itself.

In man the development of the *cerebral hemispheres* allows us to avoid behaving in this "bird-brained" way. These are the highest centers for processing the sensory information entering the nervous system. Most of the sensory input to lower levels is routed on to the cerebral cortex, which analyzes it, stores it, and uses it to plan skilled and learned behavior. The cortex consists of a sheet of nerve cell bodies lying on the outer surface of the cerebral hemispheres, which are grooved and folded to make room for more cells. The cortex on each side is divided into four main areas: the frontal lobe at front, the parietal lobe at the side, the occipital lobe at the back, and the temporal lobe lying under the temple.

The occipital lobes receive messages from the eyes (Plate 5). Information about sound goes to the temporal lobes, and messages from the skin and muscles go to the front part of the parietal cortex (Plate 6). Each lobe also includes areas which organize and compare the information further. For example, the left parietal lobe is particularly concerned with the comprehension of language (in right-handed people), the right parietal lobe is important for visual orientation in space, and the temporal lobe governs memory.

When information has been processed and it becomes necessary to take action, control passes to the posterior part of the *frontal lobe*, which sends axons down to the lower motor centers (Plate 7). These centers use the sensory information analyzed in the cortex to control skilled learned behaviors. This part of the brain is the latest development in evolution and, in animals, it works mainly through the lower levels. If the frontal lobe is cut in a cat, we will notice hardly any difference in the cat's ordinary behavior: it walks about as well as before. But the difference becomes obvious if we make it walk along a horizontal ladder and compare it with a normal cat. The latter walks along the ladder easily, but the operated cat clings to it, frozen, and falls off if it tries to move. Without information processed by the cortex to guide its movements, it is helpless when the task needs skill. In man the frontal cortex plays an even more important role, and it has taken the place of the lower centers to a much greater extent. If the motor outflow from the frontal cortex is damaged in a man, unlike the cat, he is paralyzed and has very little chance of recovering.

Messages from the sense organs go to the cortex, which builds up a picture of the environment from them. Behavior which is mainly organized at lower levels may be guided by information from the cortex. This is illustrated by the effects of brain lesions on the cat's aggressive behavior (Plate 8). A cat whose cortex has been removed is easily provoked to produce attacks which look just like rage. They are organized by the hypothalamus and the centers under its control. But although the animal bites and claws, its behavior is undirected; it hits out at the empty air. These attacks are sometimes called "sham rage." In a cat whose cortex has not been damaged, rage can be evoked by stimulating the hypothalamus with an implanted electrode, but now the attacks will be aimed directly at anyone within reach. The presence of the cortex allows the cat to use the sensory input it receives to direct its behavior to an appropriate goal.

The temporal lobes may be especially important for providing sensory guidance to the drive mechanisms. If the temporal lobes are removed in monkeys, their drives are disturbed in a number of ways. They become very placid, and as they do not show normal flight and attack reactions, they appear very tame. They will eat anything, even meat, which normally they abhor. They may make sexual approaches to animals of the same sex, or even to animals of other species, such as cats. Their social responses are disrupted: they treat other monkeys like physical objects.

Man is a social animal who lives in groups, and this fact underlies many important features of human behavior. Many of the social interactions of animals are built in physically; they may involve the production of special signs or actions, which function as recognizable signals for members of the species, when they are engaged in mating approaches, conflicts, or other interactions. Examples of such unlearned signals are the peacock's display of its tail feathers to the peahen and the wolf's snarl. Similarly, human social behavior has built-in bases, to which a great deal of learned behavior is added. Smiling is universal among humans and is probably built in; shaking hands is not. We have seen that some basic drives, like eating and drinking, are organized by the hypothalamus. We do not know much in detail about the neural organization underlying the important social drives, such as parents' care of their infants, but it is likely that in man the cortex has an important role. The elaboration of human social life depends on the detailed communication that language makes possible, and the ability to understand and use language depends on the cortex, especially the parietal lobe. Social rank and status in humans are paralleled by dominance hierarchies in some social animals. For example, a band of monkeys has a social order, and each monkey is submissive to those above him and dominating to those below. But removal of a monkey's frontal lobe produces disastrous effects on its social life. It no longer takes account of the hierarchy, with the result that it is repeatedly punished for its impertinence by its superiors. In man, damage to the frontal lobes is often marked by a loss of sensitivity to social pressures and expectations, together with loss of initiative and the ability to make long-term plans and carry them out.

We have seen that human behavior is produced by a hierarchy of mechanisms, from the endocrine glands to the cerebral cortex and that each higher level handles more complicated control problems. These levels developed successively in the course of evolution, the later mechanisms controlling and working through the earlier, so as to make more skillful and complicated behavior possible. The interdependence goes both ways, since later levels developed in the active presence of earlier ones and may be dependent on them for proper functioning. For example, certain neural mechanisms are disturbed if the proper hormonal balance is not maintained. Aggressive behavior in many male animals depends on the presence of adequate testosterone and is reduced if they are castrated, and most features of sexual and maternal behavior are affected by the balance of the sexual hormones. Excessive production of thyroid

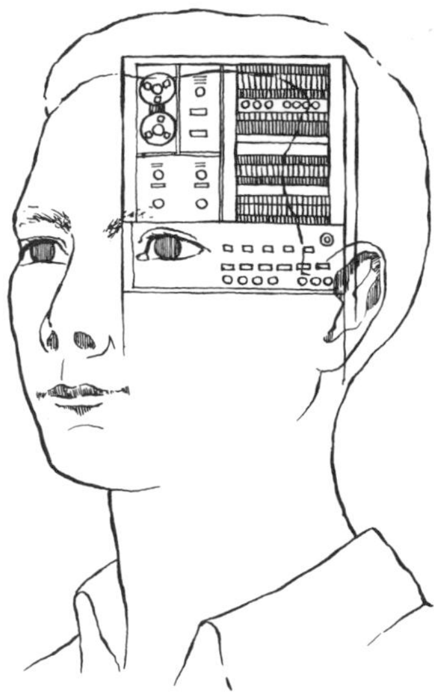

Figure 13.9 The cortex as a "neural computer."

hormone may cause increased irritability and anxiety. At a higher level, the reticular system in the hind- and midbrain, which controls the general level of muscle tone produced by the spinal mechanisms, has also come to have a controlling effect on the cortex. It can arouse the cortex, causing a high degree of activity, or depress it. The level of cortical arousal is important for the behavior governed by many of the "drive systems"; high arousal may be desirable when sensory information has to be processed and acted on rapidly, as in hunting, fighting, or fleeing, but falling asleep requires a reduction in arousal. Thus complex behavior depends on coordinated activity at all levels of the control hierarchy. In the cycle of hunger and eating, for example, mechanisms such as the hunger and satiety centers must select the appropriate behavior for the animal's state, whether this is hunting, eating, or withdrawal from food; sensory information must be processed; the level of arousal must be adjusted in accordance with the level of activity. The autonomic system also helps to adjust the body to the amount and type of activity required of it, whether this is hunting prey or digesting a meal; and the hormonal mechanisms also play a varying role, increasing the level of insulin when the blood sugar rises after a meal, or releasing blood sugar from storage depots when the body needs it.

With its vast number of nerve cells, which store past information and handle a continuous input of fresh sensory information, we can think of the cortex as a "neural computer," although it probably functions in different ways from any manmade digital computer (Figure 13.9). The ability to reason and solve problems must depend on the operation of this computer. The basis of our feelings and emotions is not well understood. We have seen that hunger and thirst are associated with the operation of the control mechanisms for eating and drinking in the hypothalamus. In a similar way, feelings and emotions, like affection, depression, and friendliness, may be associated with the activity of mechanisms that govern our social behavior. Every time we see the word *restaurant* on a sign and head toward it because we are hungry, sensory information has been processed by the cortex and used to guide behavior produced by a drive center. Sensory information, and the logical operations performed on it, which correspond to "thinking," may also be used to arouse and guide the mechanisms that organize our social behavior and that may perhaps determine whether we feel anxious or friendly, depressed or hopeful. However, in this area our knowledge is still scant, and much work remains to be done.

DISTURBANCES OF THE CONTROL SYSTEMS

It is common to distinguish between "mental diseases," in which disturbance is limited to behavior, mood, and thought and no major physical changes are present, and "physical diseases," such as pneumonia. But in some cases, observation suggests that physical symptoms may result from or be closely linked to emotional disturbances, and the term *psychosomatic* is sometimes used to describe this relation. It is not a very good term, since it reflects a belief that the "psyche" or mind acts on the "soma" or body to produce disease, and it suggests that this is a clearly understood relation between two different levels. But we have seen that control of the body is better described in terms of a hierarchy of physiological control mechanisms, the highest levels underlying such "mental" processes as thought. These mechanisms have many interrelationships, and not all disturbances of them fit easily into one of the three classes, "mental," "physical," and "psychosomatic." If Alan A. has pneumonia, he may seem to have a simple physical disease. We understand that he coughs blood and has a pain in his chest because of damage done by the pneumococci invading his lungs. We might suppose that his headache is also due to the toxins produced by these bacteria. In fact, the expression on his doctor's face may have made Alan feel that he was likely to die, and the anxiety generated contributed to the headache, so that his symptoms were partly due to "mental" causes.

A "psychosomatic" component of this sort is frequently present in physical diseases. But the term "psychosomatic" is usually restricted to diseases where it is felt that a disturbance of emotion or mood plays a fundamental causal role and that bodily changes accompanying the emotional disturbance underlie the development of the physical symptoms (Wolff *et al.*, 1950; Wolff, 1953). In fact the relations between the different levels of control are complex; it is rare that a single system is disturbed and that the causation can be clearly seen. In almost every case a number of factors may contribute to a "psychosomatic" breakdown. The environment may contain factors that put an emotional strain on an individual, such as responsibility for a difficult job, but the way in which he responds, whether with anxiety or with determination, and the degree of pressure experienced and the reaction to it will vary from person to person, depending on previous experience, training, and personality. Even if two people perceive the environment in the same way and show the same type and duration of emotional response, the physical effects of this emotion may differ. For example, the pattern of autonomic adjustments that accompany a particular emotional response varies somewhat among people; in one man fear may mainly affect the control of heart rate, causing his heart to beat violently, while another may show only a moderate rise in pulse rate but may suffer marked disturbances in the control of the stomach and intestines, perhaps causing cramps and diarrhea. But even if the response to stress of the autonomic and other control systems is similar in two cases, the pathological effects of the response may differ. Differences in physical factors in the environment, such as the diet eaten and the constitution inherited, may cause a breakdown, such as an ulcer, in one person but not in another. Thus many factors besides emotional stress may contribute to "psychosomatic" disturbances, and it may be very difficult to disentangle the parts played by each and to discover in any particular case whether emotional strain was an important or a negligible factor in the final physical breakdown.

The emotions a person typically experiences depend to some extent on his personality. Physicians have often noted that certain types of personality appear more common in certain diseases. But we must be very cautious not to jump to the conclusion that the personality "causes" the disease. Many factors interact in causing a breakdown, and it is difficult to assess the role of personality in each case. A first difficulty is that clinical impressions may be wrong: the clinician may be impressed by a few notable cases and overlook other contradictory ones. Only objective statistical studies can determine whether there is a correlation between personality features and medical disorders, and not many such studies have been made. However some associations have been noted independently by many physicians and can be regarded as established. But there are a number of possible interpretations when such a relation is found. It may be a result of self-selection by the patients: for example, people who readily seek help for minor difficulties are more likely to go to the doctor than those with more robust personalities; in the extreme, we have the *hypochondriac* who seeks help and is concerned about very minor disorders indeed. But this explanation could not account for many of the distinctive associations recorded. Another possibility is that both personality features and physical symptoms may be independent results of the same environmental factor: for example, early deprivation and hunger might affect an individual's personality and also weaken his resistance against certain physical disorders. Constitutional factors may play a similar role: a person may have weakness of a particular organ or system and at the same time might show particular personality features, both being independent effects of the same hereditary factor. The type of mental retardation known as mongolism illustrates this relation: children with this condition have happy and pleasant natures, and they also have various physical defects, both of which are consequences of an abnormality of their chromosomes, the structures in the cell which carry genetic information (see Chapter 2). Features of personality might also develop as a consequence of a physical disorder: for example, a disease producing prolonged invalidism and hospitalization in childhood might result in a tendency to feel isolated and dependent in later life. Finally, the personality may contribute causally to the development of the physical disorder. For example, a patient may develop a pattern of emotion which throws repeated stress on a particular organ or control system, and this may contribute to a breakdown of the latter when other factors favoring this, such as a constitutional weakness of the organ or control system, are also present. It is interesting to look for the possibility of this "psychosomatic" relation when an association between personality and physical symptoms is found, but the relation is difficult to prove since so many alternative relations are possible and more than one may apply at the same time.

To illustrate the interrelations between different control systems and the emotional and physical symptoms which may result from their disturbance, a number of cases will be described and possible interpretations suggested. These accounts are mainly based on real case histories, but names, dates, and other details have been altered, and in some cases several histories have been combined together. Although a number of control systems are almost always affected because they interact, the cases will be grouped according to the level of the main sites of disturbance: (1) endocrinological (hormonal), (2) autonomic, (3) spinal, hind- and midbrain, and hypothalamic, and (4) cortical.

Allergic and Hormonal Disturbances

A case of hives. Anna A., a twenty-seven-year-old nurse, was engaged to be married and was somewhat anxious and uncertain about this adventure. A week before her wedding day she developed a severe attack of urticaria (hives): most of her body was covered with raised white, intensely itchy wheals. However, she continued with the preparations for the wedding. Two weeks after her marriage, she reappeared at the hospital, radiantly happy and with quite clear skin.

Urticaria is usually an allergic condition. One way the body defends itself against invasion by foreign organisms is by producing antibodies, which serve as the basis for establishing immunity to them. In some cases, abnormal immune responses are mediated by a special type of antibody known as a reagin, which provokes excessively intense reactions known as allergic responses. These mainly affect particular organs, such as the skin, causing urticaria, or the lining of the nose, causing hay fever. In some cases a patient's responsiveness to an allergen varies from time to time. What may have happened in Anna A.'s case was that her mood of apprehension and anxiety before marriage was accompanied by changes in the skin (probably mediated by the autonomic nervous system) which allowed an extensive allergic reaction to develop; her change of mood during her honeymoon altered the state of her skin so as to make it resist the effects of the disturbed immunity responses, and her urticaria disappeared. That activity at a high level in the nervous system can effect an allergic response in the skin has also been demonstrated in experiments which use hypnosis. Although the basis of hypnosis is not well understood, we can consider it as a procedure that induces a state in which information given verbally to the subject produces effects on his behavior more readily than it would in the unhypnotized state, perhaps because the trains of thought set up by the hynotic suggestion are not opposed by competing mental activities normally occurring in the waking state. A young child may find it difficult to refrain from acting on his impulses or accompanying his thoughts with corresponding actions; when he learns to read, he finds it easier to read aloud than silently, and he has to learn to inhibit his lip movements. It is possible that in hypnosis this sort of block is reduced. In experiments on allergic subjects allergens, such as pollen extract, were inoculated into the skin of the forearm when the subject was in the normal waking condition, and again under hypnosis, and the two reactions were compared. The hypnotic suggestions included statements such as: "You will have the same injection again, but this time there will be no response; there will be no heat, no redness, no swelling, no itching, no reaction. Your arm will no longer respond to the fluid as it did before. It will be just as if water had been pricked in." It was found that the allergic response, as measured by swelling of the skin and an increase in its temperature, could be reduced by the hypnotic suggestion. In further experiments, the allergic response was made to occur in the skin of a nonallergic subject by injecting both allergen and serum containing skin-sensitizing antibodies from an allergic patient; this transferred allergic response could also be inhibited by hypnotic suggestion (Black, 1963*a*, 1963*b*; Black *et al.*, 1963).

A false pregnancy. Betty B. was born in a small country town in Oklahoma, the second of four children. Her mother was aggressive and demanding, her father mild and passive. She feared her mother and resented her domination, but was warmly attached to her father. She grew up as a sheltered child and became a shy, insecure girl who was disgusted and embarrassed by sex. At the age of thirteen she developed diabetes, which made her feel inferior to and different from other children.

She married when she was eighteen years old and was sexually frigid. After a year she became pregnant, and the baby was delivered by Caesarian section. Her first husband divorced her, and a year later she married again. She very much wanted another child, and against her doctor's advice, she conceived again. But the fetus died, an operation was necessary, and her uterus was removed.

After the operation Betty felt deeply depressed, with no interest in life, and she felt inadequate and guilty. Her housework was neglected, and she spent most of her time playing with her daughter and wanted to adopt another child. This made her husband resentful and hostile, and he became interested in another woman. She felt inadequate as a woman and wished she could be pregnant again.

Soon after, Betty began feeling sick and vomiting in the morning. She noticed that her breasts were increasing in size and becoming pigmented, and her abdomen was getting larger. In the following month there was a milky discharge from the breast, and her weight increased. She also felt "quickening" and urinary frequency. She was certain she was pregnant and began wearing maternity clothes and planning for the delivery.

Her relatives became alarmed, and she was admitted to a psychiatric ward. Although restless and tense, she was cooperative and friendly. She was preoccupied with her domestic difficulties. When she was examined she said at one point, "I *know* I'm not pregnant; I *know* I don't have a uterus"; yet a few minutes later she felt quickening and remarked, "This pregnancy is no different from my others." During the course of psychotherapy she discussed her resentment of her mother, the shame and guilt she felt about sex, and her feelings of sexual inadequacy following the removal of her uterus. She made a good recovery and returned to live with her husband.

A number of factors acting together had produced a situation of great emotional difficulty for Betty. Feelings of inferiority derived from her poor relationship with her mother and her diabetes, her inability to enjoy her sexual role, and her feeling that she was only half a woman since the loss of her uterus, together with the fear that her second husband would leave her as her first had done, created a situation for which another pregnancy would have been a solution. She had always been very fond of children and interested in having them, and pregnancy would again make her the center of attention, establish her in her feminine role, and attract her husband back. It is no wonder that she had persistent thoughts and fantasies of having another child. But as well as these thoughts, the bodily symptoms and signs of pregnancy developed, and she eagerly used them as evidence that the fantasy was being realized. Her appreciation of reality in general was good, yet she chose to wear maternity clothes and would alternate between admitting that she could not be pregnant and knitting tiny garments (Greaves *et al.*, 1960).

The breast changes, with the production of milk, indicate that the hormonal balance had altered. The persistent desire for pregnancy activated neural mechanisms that control the anterior pituitary, making the gonadotropic hormone and estrogen in the blood rise, so that the hormonal state was similar to that of pregnancy. Along with endocrine changes there were autonomic effects, such as nausea and vomiting, and the abdomen was held permanently puffed out so that it seemed enlarged. Normal sensory stimuli were misinterpreted to support the fantasy: the "quickening" was probably an abnormal interpretation of normal bowel movements.

It is interesting that Betty's knowledge that she had no uterus and that therefore it was quite impossible for her to be pregnant was ineffective in preventing her obsessive desires from leading to these changes. Symptoms of pregnancy may occur in husbands when their wives are pregnant, and among some peoples there is a formalized ritual known as the "couvade" (from the French *couver*, meaning to brood or hatch): the father-to-be takes to his bed at the time of his wife's confinement, where he appears to suffer the pangs of childbirth and receives the attention usually given to women at this time. The complete false pregnancy syndrome has also been described in a male patient (Knight, 1960).

Betty's emotional disturbance produced far-reaching changes in the system controlling sex hormone function and in other control systems. Though we are far from a precise knowledge of the neural mechanisms responsible for this, we are all familiar with the fact that physiological changes may occur as a consequence of thought processes. For example, a mother may read a letter containing the news that her son is seriously ill; cortical mechanisms analyze the visual input, and the sad news which it conveys sets up thought processes whose end result is the emotional state of grief. She turns pale, she feels faint, her heart beats rapidly, and her eyes fill with tears —effects produced through the autonomic nervous system; if the grief is persistent, it may also disturb the hormonal cycle, so that menstruation is suppressed. Betty's emotional state and the obsessive thinking about pregnancy accompanying it produced physiological changes which were not randomly assorted; they combined to mimic pregnancy and so partly satisfied her emotional needs. They were not caused by conscious pretense or malingering. We know too little at present about the relations between the cortical mechanisms active in thinking and the hypothalamic and other systems on which they act to be able to explain in detail how this disturbance was produced. However there are experimental observations which may help to throw light on this sort of case, although no complete explanation is available.

You recall from Chapter 3 how the Russian physiologist, Pavlov, showed that if the ringing of a bell repeatedly preceded the presentation of food to a dog, the bell's ring would come to evoke salivation. This showed that information about the environment which may be extracted by cortical mechanisms, in this case the information that the bell had rung, can come to have a reliable effect on a function controlled by the autonomic nervous system, salivation. Other experiments have shown that autonomic effects such as changes in heart rate or blood pressure level may also be classically conditioned in humans (Smith, 1966). Conditioning of this sort may be common; it is illustrated by the following report by a doctor who regularly used breathing exercises to produce sleep at night (Taylor, 1962).

> Whilst breathing—and concentrating the mind on this to the exclusion of all else—I became faintly aware of the rhythm of my heart beat. I was concentrating as follows: one—breathe in, two —pause, three—breathe out, four—pause, making four distinct operations. In my mind I imagined this to constitute four sides of a rectangle and I decided to make the exercise even more regular by timing the breathing so that a heartbeat fell on each of the corners.
>
> Within a week or two I was beginning to get frequent extrasystoles [extra heartbeats] which I had never experienced before, but I did not connect the fact with the exercise. Shortly these became very frequent and then extended periods of complete irregularity of the heartbeat occurred. Being quite fit physically and not many years past thirty I thought, well, that's the way the cookie crumbles. My previous health had been excellent. However, I soon noticed that the arrhythmia [irregularity of the heart] was brought on by a combination of tiredness and emotional stress, and so I

> was able to connect it directly with the exercise. The heart was beginning to respond directly to the thinking, so that whenever this was disturbed it beat irregularly. By assuming one mind state or another (troubled or calm) I could bring on or stop the irregularity, and I demonstrated to myself that I could beat extrasystoles at will. . . . In the exercises I found I was no longer tagging the breathing on to the heartbeats but was rather causing the heart to beat with a resounding thump on each corner, as if pacing a square and deliberately stamping the corners. Not caring much for the consequences I stopped the practice of involving the heart in the exercise and the irregularities ceased forthwith, and haven't been back in the nine months or so since. I have a feeling that the heart knows its own business best and should be left in peace to attend to it.

Here the heart action may have come under control by being conditioned to stimuli produced by the subject, such as stimuli arising during breathing. Betty had experienced a previous pregnancy, in which thoughts about the pregnancy occurred in association with the symptoms of it, and it is possible that repeated thoughts about her desire for a child may have acted like the bell in the conditioning experiment, producing some of the associated symptoms. However this would not account for all the effects; for example, it would not explain Betty's puffed-out abdomen, which was produced by muscular action. In true pregnancy, the abdomen gets larger because of passive distension.

Many of Betty's symptoms seem "directed" to an end, that of mimicking pregnancy. We can compare this with the effect of hypnosis on allergic responses, which was described earlier. The hypnotic suggestion did not randomly disturb autonomic control; apparently the effects produced were those which would tend to reduce the inflammatory reaction normally provoked by the allergen. These "directed" effects suggest that in some people cortical activity corresponding to particular thought processes may be able to influence the activity of the autonomic and other control systems, perhaps by altering the levels which the homeostatic systems attempt to maintain, although these people may not be aware of, and are not normally able to use, this ability.

Disturbances such as Betty's nausea and vomiting, or her distended abdomen, are sometimes said to "symbolize" an underlying need, in this case her desire for pregnancy. This description does not imply that the patient is consciously or deliberately "acting." It refers to the meaningful relation between the form of the disturbance and the emotional problems leading to it, but it does not explain how this relation comes about. It is interesting to compare the development of these "directed" symptoms with the learning of goal-directed behavior. In the learning process known as operant conditioning or instrumental learning, an animal or human learns to maintain responses that lead to reward and to eliminate unsuccessful responses (see Chapter 5). For example, if a hungry rat learns to run a maze for food, it gradually ceases to enter the blind alleys and finally only runs along the direct path to the goal. A pigeon in a Skinner box may have to learn to peck a button to receive food; other responses, such as grooming, turning, or other movements, gradually drop out, and in the end it produces a high rate of pecks instead. To train the pigeon to do this a procedure known as "shaping" is sometimes employed. When it is first put in the box the untrained bird will perform a variety of responses, and it is not particularly likely to peck the button. At this stage the experimenter may reward any movement in the direction of the button. When these movements become frequent, he will reward only those movements followed by a peck. When the bird is pecking reasonably often, only pecks at the button will result in food being delivered to it; in this way the pigeon is brought to perform the required response.

Human subjects can be trained to perform a variety of responses by operant conditioning in a similar way. For example, a reward such as a smile, or "Mmm," or "Good," delivered by the experimenter according to an appropriate schedule, can cause a human subject to perform responses such as producing plural nouns in conversation, slapping his ankle, touching his chin, and many others, at a high rate. His behavior can also be "shaped" to the desired response: for example, if the experimenter wants him to take the top off his pen and replace it, he may at first reward the subject for any movement; when movements are occurring frequently, he rewards him for movements of the right hand only; then only when he touches his pen; then for lifting it; and finally only for taking the cap off and putting it on again (Verplanck, 1956). In this precedure many subjects may be unaware that they are being conditioned, what the response is, and that it is increasing in frequency (Verplanck, 1956; Sasmor, 1966).

These responses are motor responses. But it is also possible to produce operant conditioning of responses controlled by the autonomic system, such as heart rate in humans (Shearn, 1962) and rats, salivation in dogs, and dilation of the blood vessels and intestinal contractions in rats (Miller, 1966). This makes it seem that it may be possible to draw a parallel between the development of many of Betty's symptoms and the results of operant conditioning. Slight changes in the operation of the homeostatic control mechanisms might have produced effects similar to those she had experienced in her previous pregnancy or associated with this state. Because of her desire for a child pregnancy would have been rewarding (not necessarily consciously), and this fact would have tended to maintain the alterations in the control systems. So by a process similar to experimental "shaping" she would finally have come to the state in which she suffered symptoms such as nausea and vomiting, her abdomen was permanently distended, and her condition mimicked pregnancy in other ways. Because she was not consciously aware of this process, the symptoms seemed all the more convincing to her.

In the present state of our knowledge, this sort of explanation can be considered only as a possibility. But it suggests that the principles which are needed to explain the processes of learning may also help us eventually to explain how "psychosomatic" symptoms develop in forms that "symbolize" the patient's underlying emotional needs.

The results of a shock. Clara C. had a rigid moralistic mother who disliked her baby and gave it away at birth. After three years, her father insisted that Clara be brought back. Clara's mother was restrictive and unkind to her, and predicted that she would turn out to be a prostitute. Clara tried desperately to gain her mother's affection and to prove that she was the only child her mother could rely on. She was an outstanding scholar at school, became a teacher, and drove herself to exhaustion to win approval from her principal. But her mother continued to reject her, and she left home and became intimate with a crippled war veteran, not knowing that he was already married. She learned of his marriage, to her shock and horror, when his wife accosted them in public, calling Clara degrading names and striking her. But she found herself unable to give him up, and she felt that her mother's prediction had come true: she was no better than a prostitute and would never be able to face her mother again.

Following this shock, Clara was thrown into an anxious turmoil. Some weeks later she visited her doctor, complaining that she was extremely restless and irritable, weeping over small annoyances and easily depressed. She also felt hot and had palpitations. The doctor found that she had a rapid pulse and tremor of the fingers. Her eyes had become prominent and staring, she had lost weight, and her thyroid gland was enlarged. He diagnosed hyperthyroidism. An operation was performed to remove part of the thyroid gland. Following this, Clara's mood improved and the symptoms subsided.

Clara was suffering from excessive activity of the thyroid gland, a condition known as *hyperthyroidism* or thyrotoxicosis. Clinical observation suggests that in some cases it may follow severe or prolonged emotional stress, that patients often have marked feelings of personal insecurity and a strong sense of responsibility, and that they tend to assume a dependent role in relation to others. The emotional shock is often caused by a sudden threat to this dependent relationship, such as the death of a parent (Alexander, 1950; Lidz and Whitehorn, 1950; Kaplan and Hetrick, 1962). Hyperthyroidism is more common in women than in men, and it usually occurs between the ages of ten and thirty.

In this condition, the thyroid gland increases the output of its hormone, *thyroxin,* which normally stimulates the metabolism, increasing the rate of cell activity. When it is present in excess, the rate at which the body uses energy rises, resulting in loss of weight as fat stores are drawn on, increased appetite, and increased liberation of heat by the body. Thyroxin also makes the body more sensitive to adrenaline, and it produces more rapid heart action, which is felt as "palpitations," and a fine tremor of the hands. The overactive thyroid gland enlarges.

Thyroxin affects brain mechanisms controlling mood, and its presence in excess has marked effects on personality and behavior. The patients become restless and irritable, they are emotional and easily startled. Occasionally profound mental changes develop; the patient might develop symptoms like those of schizophrenia or manic-depressive psychosis (Cobb, 1960). Since the patient's final emotional state may reflect both an original stress and emotional effects produced by the excess thyroxin, the disease may have both "psychosomatic" and "somatopsychic" aspects.

Overactivity of the thyroid probably arises from malfunction of the immunity system. At an early stage in an individual's development, his immunity system learns to "recognize" the protein components of his body, so that in later life it will not treat them as antigens and will not produce antibodies against them. But in some cases, perhaps for constitutional reasons, this "self-recognition" may break down or be imperfect, and an "autoimmune" response against tissues of the person's own body may develop. In thyrotoxicosis, a substance known as "long-acting thyroid stimulator" is found in the blood. This appears to be an autoantibody against a component of the thyroid gland, and it has the effect of stimulating thyroid gland activity (Anderson *et al.*, 1964; Meek *et al.*, 1964; Adams, 1965; Hartog, 1966). When a stress appears to precipitate thyrotoxicosis, it is probable that the autoimmune reaction was already present but under control and that this control breaks down as a result of the stress. How this happens is not known. A shock or strain usually has the effect of increasing the output of adrenocorticotropic hormone and reducing the output of thyrotropic hormone from the pituitary gland (Brown-Grant, 1956; Brown-Grant and Pethes, 1960; Docommun *et al.*, 1966). Perhaps because of a fluctuation in the control of the thyroid gland, or in some other way, the emotional stress might reduce resistance to the autoimmune reaction, just as a patient's emotional condition may affect his sensitivity to an allergic reaction.

Other endocrine systems may also show secondary effects of disturbances which arise elsewhere, or they may themselves interfere with other levels of control. "Psychosomatic" and "somatopsychic" effects are often shown by the system controlling blood sugar (glucose) level. This system is of particular importance to the body because blood sugar is a major source of energy, especially for the brain cells. When the glucose level in the blood is too low, fresh glucose is mobilized by adrenaline from storage sites such as the liver; and the hormone insulin, which is produced by the pancreas, makes it move from the blood into the cells, where it is utilized. Physiological stress, such as infection, injury, surgery, or emotional shocks may greatly increase the body's need for insulin. However, sufferers from diabetes are unable to produce sufficient insulin for their needs and must be given regular injections of it. If a diabetic suffers a physical or emotional shock, his need for insulin may increase rapidly, and if his daily dose of insulin is not increased at the same time, an emotional shock such as the death of a relative may be followed in a few hours by *diabetic coma,* a state of unconsciousness resulting from the body's inability to metabolize glucose normally.

The opposite effect may occur if a tumor of the pancreas known as an insulinoma develops; this tumor may produce large quantities of insulin without reference to the body's needs. As a result blood glucose falls to a level at which the energy needs of the brain cells cannot be met, and mental symptoms develop. A fifty-six-year-old housewife with an insulinoma developed bouts of confusion, trancelike states, and spells of depression (Todd *et al.,* 1962). Her first attack came when walking home from work. Although her recollection of the attack was blurred, she remembered that she became confused and bewildered. The goods in the store windows seemed distorted in shape. When she got home she wandered around in a state of increasing bewilderment, "seeing" herself surrounded by the entire contents of her five-room apartment. She recovered when her husband gave her tea *with sugar.* Her husband described another attack:

> She seemed to be laughing all the time. You could not understand what she said, her words were so slurred. She behaved like a little baby; she sat with her legs over the arms of a chair holding her little dog. She suddenly threw it from her, saying "I don't like you, you look horrible." She had spasms of jerking her legs.

She always awoke from these states with a throbbing headache and a mood of deep depression. It was found that she had a tumor of the pancreas, and her attacks ceased after an operation to remove the tumor. On the basis of such cases, one wonders how many of the clinical depressions and manias described in Chapter 11 may actually involve hormonal imbalances.

Autonomic Nervous System Disturbances

The autonomic nervous system (see Plate 3) is the lowest level of nervous control. It consists of ganglia, collections of nerve cells which control the organs and blood vessels of the body. As we saw in chapter 3, these constitute two systems, the sympathetic and parasympathetic, which tend to have opposed actions. The sympathetic system acts to adjust the body to states of alarm or emergency, and the main role of the parasympathetic nervous system is to organize the normal activity of the body's organs.

But the two systems are not simply opposed; in many instances, they act in a coordinated pattern peculiar to the drive. For example, if a corrosive poison is swallowed, there is sympathetic arousal, with dilation of the pupils and sweating, together with vomiting, which is organized by the parasympathetic system.

The nerves from the spinal cord have branches to the sympathetic ganglia, which they control; the parasympathetic ganglia are controlled by branch nerves at the lower end of the spinal cord and by a nerve from the medulla (the lowest part of the brain) known as the vagus ("wandering") nerve because it connects with most of the organs of the body, including the heart, lungs, liver, stomach, and much of the digestive tract.

Interest in the relations between personality and disease has led to a number of studies of the autonomic system, partly because a number of indices of its activity can be measured quite readily (Ax, 1964). As indicated in Chapter 3, these include the heart rate (speeded by the sympathetic system, slowed by vagal activity); the electric resistance of the skin (the "galvanic skin response" or "electrodermal response"); the temperature of the skin; and the blood pressure.

The pattern of bodily changes produced by the autonomic system in response to stress, you recall, varies in accordance with the subject's emotional response (see Chapter 3). As Ax (1953) found when he induced fear or anger experimentally, a different pattern of physiological changes tended to occur in each case: The changes in fear resembled those produced by the injection of adrenaline, but the effects which occurred in anger were like those produced by the combined action of adrenaline and noradrenaline. Also, Funkenstein *et al.* (1957) distinguished between anger directed outwards (rage) and anger directed against oneself (depression). Anger directed against the self showed patterns of physiological response which corresponded to the predominant secretion of adrenaline, but if anger was mainly turned outwards, the physiological changes suggested that the main increase was in the secretion of noradrenaline (Chapter 3). Hoagland (1961) examined the secretion of these hormones. If the subject was tense and anxious, a big increase in adrenaline, largely produced by the adrenal medulla, was found. But active aggressive behavior, such as boxing, openly expressed anger, or just competitive activity, such as a strenuous ice hockey game, caused a proportionately greater rise in noradrenaline, the hormone liberated at the sympathetic nerve endings.

Other differences between patterns of autonomic response have been found. The pattern is affected by the stimulus or situation evoking the response; for example, an electric shock may make the heart accelerate, but an auditory or visual stimulus of moderate intensity may slow it down. The response pattern also depends on the individual; some people may show predominately cardiovascular changes, others mainly gastrointestinal responses to a variety of stimuli (Lacey *et al.*, 1962; Graham and Clifton, 1966; Sternbach, 1966). *This suggests that the attitudes or emotional reactions typical of different personality types may be associated with corresponding patterns of autonomic response. These in turn might favor particular physiological disturbances.* Interviews with patients suffering from particular "psychosomatic" diseases provide some evidence that certain diseases are associated with particular attitudes. For example, the *patient with hives* may characteristically feel that he is taking a beating and is helpless to do anything about it, while the typical *hypertensive* patient may feel that he has to be constantly on guard against assault from outside (Graham *et al.*, 1962). In some cases there may be an association between a disease and a pattern of physiological response. Malmo and Shagass (1949) examined psychiatric patients who had a history either of cardiovascular complaints or of head and neck pains, then subjected them to painful stimuli. The responses of the first group gave greater heart rate scores and respiratory variability scores, while the second group showed greater responsiveness in the muscular system. Engel and Bickford (1961) found that a much greater proportion of hypertensives than of normals showed a rise in blood pressure as the main response to a variety of stimuli.

These findings could have a number of explanations. The patient's disease, his attitudes and perceptions, and his typical pattern of response could all arise from common causes lying either in his constitution or his previous experience. Experiments on animals show that environmental factors can affect both later behavior and physiological features. For example, the effect on rats of being handled daily as infants by the experimenter has been studied. The adult behavior of these rats is different from that of controls who were not handled: when placed in a novel environment they explore more freely and are less fearful than the controls. In the novel situation, the output of hormones from the adrenal cortex (an increase in this output is part of the response to stress) is only moderately increased, but they show a near maximum output if given an electric shock. Rats which have not been handled in infancy are not so flexibly adaptive to the situation, giving a near maximum hormonal response both to shock and to novelty (Levine and Mullins, 1966). Other studies have shown that early experience with toys, maze running, and exploration makes rats more efficient at solving problems in later life and also increases the size of the brain cortex as compared with controls (Rosenzweig, 1966).

Another possibility is that a pattern of autonomic response *results* from the strains imposed by a disease, but this possibility has not been much studied. There is some evidence that attitudes directly determine the patterns of autonomic response associated with them (Stern *et al.*, 1961). Graham *et al.* (1962) used hypnotic suggestion to induce attitudes in normal subjects which clinical observation had suggested were typical of hives or hypertension. They then measured the physiological response to a threat and found that when the "hives attitude" was induced, a greater rise in skin temperature and a smaller rise in diastolic blood pressure took place than if the "hypertension attitude" had been suggested. Thus it seems possible that a patient's habitual emotional reactions may throw a repeated strain on a particular control system, such as autonomic control of blood pressure. If other factors are present which work in the same direction, such as a hereditary weakness in the system, the repeated failure to maintain homeostasis might result in a physical breakdown. Some of the following cases illustrate this possibility, but it must be remembered that we do not yet know enough to come to a final conclusion about the weight to be given to this possible mechanism.

Raised blood pressure. Doris D. was the oldest of four children. She had a warm attachment to her father, whom she greatly admired, but felt that her mother did not understand her. She got married at the age of twenty and soon after that her father died. Her husband kept a store with not much success. They had three children. Her relation to her husband was not altogether happy. She felt that he made errors in running the store, but although she grumbled, she was not assertive and accepted his decisions. She spent much of her time keeping the store and their apartment in order, although she did not do this particularly efficiently. She was conscientious and hardworking, rarely acting on impulse, and she gave much careful thought even to minor decisions or purchases. She tended to suppress feelings of anger or hostility and to make excuses for her husband when she came into conflict with him.

When she was forty-five her husband had a mild stroke, and some weeks later she visited her doctor, complaining of headaches and dizziness, and he found that her blood pressure was raised. She expressed many anxieties. She was afraid that she and her husband would not be able to continue to make a living. She was worried that she might have cancer. She felt that she had not made the best of her life and that she had failed her children, although she had lavished much care on them. Her oldest son had not completed his course at college and she felt that this was in some way her fault. She had attacks of depression and often missed her late father.

The blood pressure is controlled by the autonomic nervous system, the adrenal medulla, and centers in the hindbrain and medulla. Sensory information about the level of blood pressure comes from the main arteries, especially from a structure called the carotid sinus, part of the internal carotid artery in the neck which is the main source of blood for the brain. This pressure information is fed back to a center in the hindbrain which controls the level of blood pressure, raising it if it is below the optimum, lowering it if it is too high. It operates through the sympathetic system, whose fibers control the caliber of individual arteries. These can also be affected by the release of adrenaline and noradrenaline by the adrenal medulla. This feedback system can be overriden: for example, in anger or fear or any emergency, messages from higher centers will temporarily set the blood pressure at a high level. Other independent systems can also affect the blood pressure level; a particularly important influence arises from the kidney. If a kidney gets insufficient blood because of a damaged artery, for example, it releases a substance which raises the blood pressure so that its blood supply is restored to an adequate level.

A number of physical causes, such as disease of arteries or the kidney, can cause sustained hypertension, but in many cases no clear physical reason can be found. Clinical observation suggests that many hypertensives have personalities like that of Doris D. They tend to be unassertive, dependent on others, anxious to placate them and keep the peace, but often having underlying hostile and critical feelings. They are anxious about and anticipate pain and suffering, while feeling helpless to do much to prevent it. This may find expression in compulsive behavior, such as repeatedly checking that the doors have been locked before going to bed at night, or in fears about their bodily health, which often center on the raised blood pressure itself, once they find out about it (Saslow *et al.*, 1950). There is a strong hereditary factor in hypertension, which appears to be due to effects of a number of different genes, and it is likely that environmental factors are also important (Miall and Oldham, 1963; Pickering, 1965). There is no conclusive evidence that personality plays a part in determining the development of hypertension, but it is possible that people who usually keep their angers and conflicts from open expression may do so at the cost of repeatedly provoking rises in blood pressure, and this might eventually adjust to a permanently raised level. A raised blood pressure throws a strain on the blood vessels and other organs such as the kidneys. This may gradually produce changes in them which cause the raised pressure to be maintained for physical reasons, even if the original emotional causes no longer operate.

Experiments on animals provide some support for this account. Rats and cats have been repeatedly exposed to frightening stimuli, each exposure causing arousal of the sympathetic system, with an accompanying rise in blood pressure, for several months. The stimuli were loud noises for the rats, and exposure to barking dogs for the cats. The animals varied considerably in individual susceptibility, but in some of them the result was a maintained rise in blood pressure (Gellhorn and Loofbourrow, 1963).

However, it has not been shown that such stress activates any important mechanism in human hypertension. It is quite possible that its association with personality might be due to common environmental or genetic factors. An underlying difference in the way the sympathetic system functions is suggested by the observation that children of hypertensives, even though they themselves may have normal blood pressure, may be more sensitive than controls to noradrenaline injected into the arteries.

Sudden death at the railroad station. At the railroad station, Edna E., a nineteen-year-old girl, was saying goodbye to her fiancé, a soldier, who was leaving for the front. He kissed her farewell and she fell dead on the platform.

We have seen that blood pressure is controlled by a feedback cycle which detects and corrects departures from the optimal level of pressure. If a feedback loop overcorrects it will cause a swing in the opposite direction. Anyone who has ever learned to ride a bicycle will have gone through a stage in which he overcorrected for errors, so that each time he began to lose balance in one direction, he corrected violently in the opposite direction in a series of increasing wobbles ending in a fall. This was not a disaster, but it can be disastrous if a physiological feedback loop overcorrects. When blood pressure is too high, the autonomic system may slow down by vagal action to help the heart restore normal pressure. When Edna's boyfriend kissed her, he pressed the carotid sinus in her neck, and this pressure caused a sudden sensory input from the sinus, such as would have been caused by a sharp rise in blood pressure. Her autonomic system overcorrected, not merely slowing the heart down, but causing it to stop completely for long enough to cause death. In most people, this feedback loop is not so dangerously oversensitive, so that tragedies of this sort are rare. It is possible that in Edna its sensitivity was increased by her high state of emotional excitement and accompanying sympathetic arousal.

In addition to the blood vessels, the autonomic nervous system also controls the caliber of the air passages (bronchi). If these are excessively constricted, there there may be difficulty in expelling air from the lungs, a condition known as asthma.

Difficulty in breathing. Flora F. was the second of three daughters in a Negro family. From her first year of life, she suffered from attacks of bronchial asthma. When she was six she was sent to a tuberculosis preventorium for eighteen months. She felt this separation from her family keenly. While growing up, she suffered a number of losses. In her early adolescence, her younger sister died, then a favorite cousin, then a school teacher of whom she was very fond, and finally, when she was nineteen, her mother. She had been very much attached to her mother, who had given her close and loving care, and she was also warmly attached to her father.

After her mother died, she married and had a son, but she separated from her husband and returned to live with her father. Her customary mood was one of sadness, dominated by longings for her mother. She was extremely sensitive to loss, or the threat of it, which often precipitated her asthmatic attacks. One severe attack occurred when she learned that her doctor, social worker, and nurse on the asthma project were all about to leave. Another major attack followed a visit to an aunt who had shown her a picture of her dead mother. She was distressed by separations from her psychotherapist and also by reunions with him, and both situations could precipitate attacks. During an asthmatic attack she usually felt sad and hopeless.

The parasympathetic and sympathetic nervous systems control the air passages of the nose and lungs. In weeping, the parasympathetic system causes secretion of tears by the eyes, and it dilates small blood vessels in the nose, which becomes congested; in the lungs, parasympathetic activity contracts the bronchi. The sympathetic system dilates the bronchi and also constricts the small blood vessels in the lining of the nose.

The nose is the first line of defense against irritant dust in the air. In people who are particularly sensitive to irritation by dust, or are allergic to pollen, the irritating substance may cause a parasympathetic reaction, with dilation of the vessels and excessive secretion of the membranes in the nose, giving the blocked, running nose of hay fever, sometimes accompanied by congestion of the sinuses, which causes headache. If these substances reach the lungs, they may cause a similar reaction in the bronchi, which constrict, and the same effect may be produced if the patient eats food which he is allergic to. This constriction of the bronchi prevents the patient from breathing out freely, which is the main difficulty in an asthma attack.

In some people, a parasympathetic reaction producing asthma can occur in the absence of airborne irritants, or their sensitivity to pollen and dust may vary from time to time, depending on their emotional state (Funkenstein, 1950; Holmes *et al.*, 1950; Rees, 1959). In most cases of asthma, allergic and infective factors are present, and a psychological factor is often present too. Clinical observation suggests that people who are dependent on others but also have feelings of hopeless resentment and frustration may be particularly susceptible. As with Flora, their attacks are often precipitated by loss of or separation from someone they love or need, or they may occur in situations which arouse fears, or after a marked increase in job responsibility. Anger provoked by someone they need, following unfair criticism by the patient's doctor, for example, may also provoke an attack. Note the similarity to the onset of depressions (Chapter 11).

A state of tension, with feelings of fear and irritability, may precede an attack, although asthma may sometimes follow a period of elation. During the attack, feelings of depression, hopelessness, and helplessness are often present, and patients may feel the desire to weep (Knapp, 1960; Knapp and Nemetz, 1960).

In situations of loss or frustration, or in the aftermath of excessive elation, there may be feelings of depression which might cause some of the parasympathetic changes associated with weeping. In the asthmatic, these effects may be sufficiently marked to cause physical symptoms; it has been suggested that the asthma attack may be regarded as a "suppressed cry for the mother." It is probably not just loss of someone loved but also conflicts and uncertainty in the relationship that are of particular importance. When some asthmatic children are completely separated from their parents, by being sent to a hospital or boarding school, they may improve dramatically.

Spinal Cord and Brain Stem Disturbances

We shall now consider some features of breakdowns occurring in the central nervous system, in the spinal cord, and at one of the immediately higher levels of control.

Results of a war wound. George G., a twenty-three-year-old soldier in good physical condition, was struck by a shell splinter in the small of the back, slightly to the right of the midline. He was removed to the hospital. On examination, after he had recovered from the immediate effects of the wound, it was noted that he could not move his right leg, which was *spastic*; that is, the muscles were taut and resisted movment when the doctor manipulated his leg. There was a marked knee jerk when his knee was tapped. He was also unable to detect changes in the position of his toes, leg, and thigh when the doctor moved his right leg about, although the skin was still sensitive to touch and to warmth and cold, and he felt pain when pricked. On the other hand, he could move his left leg perfectly well, and if the doctor altered its position while George kept his eyes shut, he could tell what was being done to it. But he could not tell the difference between being pricked with the point of a pin or touched with its blunt end on the left leg. Nor could he tell whether a probe touching this leg had been warmed or cooled, or whether it was at body temperature.

At first sight these disturbances seem bizarre and hysterical (see Chapter 10), but they all make sense if we consider them in relation to the "wiring diagram" of the spinal cord, which was injured by the splinter. The cord carries sensory information upwards to the brain and carries motor instructions down from higher centers, through bundles of fibers whose course through the cord is known.

In George's case, communication of information along the spinal cord was disrupted by the shell splinter, which cut all the pathways on the right side of the cord, and the effects of the wound are explained by the loss of information. When the splinter cut the right half of the cord, it interrupted the fibers from the motor area of the frontal cortex, which travel down on the right side and convey instructions to the motor nerve cells, which go to the muscles, thus allowing voluntary movement of the right leg. It also cut paths from the hind- and midbrain, which control and modulate the spinal motor mechanisms responsible for muscle tension and the postural reflexes. When these paths are cut, there is little residual ability in the spinal motor mechanisms in man. Freed from higher control, the feedback loops governing muscle tension maintain a greater degree of tone than is normal, so that although the limb is paralyzed, it feels stiff and rigid if someone tries to move it. The overactivity of the postural reflexes is also shown by the exaggerated knee jerk. Postural information from sensory receptors in the muscles and joints activates these reflexes, yet George had no idea what was happening if his eyes were shut when the doctor altered the position of his right leg. The reason is that when the fibers conveying postural information enter the spinal cord, they branch, one branch supplying the reflex center and the other traveling up the same side of the cord to the higher centers; the splinter had cut these ascending branches. Fibers conveying pain and temperature information cross to the opposite side of the cord before they travel upwards so that these fibers from the right escaped damage and George could tell temperature and feel pain in his right leg. The fibers with touch information from the skin are divided, some traveling upwards on the same side of the cord and some on the opposite side, so that some touch information from the right leg arrived centrally.

For the same reason, touch information from the left leg also arrived centrally, and so did postural information from the left side, since it traveled in the left half of the cord. But fibers conveying pain and temperature information from the left leg had crossed to the right and were cut at the site of the injury. Voluntary movement and normal reflexes were retained on the left, since the motor pathways, traveling down on the left, were not injured.

This case illustrates the effects of sharply localized damage to the spinal cord which interrupted communication with higher neural levels, causing disordered action of the spinal motor control mechanisms and loss of sensory information which could no longer be transmitted upwards. Above this level, in the hind- and midbrain, lie centers for controlling functions like respiration and maintenance of normal blood pressure. At this level, the cerebellum exercises overall control of posture at rest and elaborates the adjustments of body position that accompany voluntary movement.

A case of clumsiness. Harold H. was thirty-eight years old, married, and the father of two children. For some months he found himself getting increasingly irritable and anxious, and he had trouble doing his work as a carpenter, although he had always been a skilled workman. Syphilis had been diagnosed and treated when he was twenty. His wife did not know of this, and he was worried that the disease might not have been cured and was recurring. He saw his doctor and complained that he was suffering from headaches and that his work was deteriorating. He found it difficult to draw a straight line and to pick up screws and small objects, and when he walked, he was told, he sometimes looked as though he was drunk. He first noticed his unsteadiness of gait when he was teased by his friends, but it had been slowly increasing, and his arm movements had also become unsteady and irregular. When he was examined by his doctor, he had difficulty picking up a coin from the table quickly; the more he tried, the more he fumbled before he could get hold of it.

The headache was mainly at the back of the head, and recently he had two attacks of vomiting and several fits of giddiness. When he looked to one side, his eyes showed a succession of regular horizontal jerking movements, known as nystagmus. When he tried to touch an object with his index finger, his hand showed a coarse, irregular, to-and-fro jerky movement which became worse as his finger approached the object, and he frequently overshot the target. His walk was irregular and staggering. He spoke in a slow and drawling fashion, pronouncing each syllable separately. Harold was admitted to the hospital, where it was found that he had a tumor of the cerebellum.

Anxieties were the cause of Harold's impatience and irritability, and his anxieties were aroused by his symptoms, but then were due to a physical disturbance, a tumor, in the cerebellum. The tumor produced the headaches and the vomiting and giddiness. It also interfered with the proper functioning of the cerebellum and thus caused Harold's other symptoms. The cerebellum processes *position information* from all sources and uses it to maintain posture and to guide active movements. When Harold tried to touch an object or pick up a screw, the feedback loops which normally correct for small errors in the direction of movement were slowed down, with the result that the corrections were made late and his hand wobbled to-and-fro in an "intention tremor." The information that his hand had reached its goal, implying that the approach movement should be charged to grasping, was also delayed, and this delay caused overshooting. Similar effects made his walk irregular and uncertain. (Alcohol probably affects the gait by causing a similar physical impairment in cerebellar function; see Chapter 11).

The nystagmus of the eyes is explained in the same way: when eyes try to focus on a target, impairment of the feedback loops results in a jerky to-and-fro movement. Feedback is also involved in speech: we monitor the sounds we produce as we talk, and it was probably delays in this process that led to the slowing down and breakup of words in Harold's speech.

Like the previous case, this story illustrates the effects of a physical breakdown at an intermediate level of control, with secondary emotional effects due to the patient's anxiety about his condition. It would have been an unfortunate mistake to suppose that the anxiety and irritability were primary and that the bizarre symptoms were consequences only of an "anxiety state."

The cerebellum allows smooth performance of individual movements. Sequences of movements that may be necessary to achieve aims such as satisfying a need for food depend on the guidance of drive centers like the hunger center in the hypothalamus.

Refusal to eat. Irma I. was admitted to the hospital at the age of fourteen because of refusal to eat. Over the course of several months, she had lost thirty pounds, and she expressed anxiety about getting too fat and felt that she needed to diet. She was constantly active in the ward, helping to feed other patients, and she had fantasies about preparing and eating food, but she was afraid to eat and felt unhappy if she did so.

Irma's difficulties had started at puberty. Her sexual attitudes were dominated by anxiety and shame, and she had felt embarrassed and conspicuous when her breasts began to increase in size. Her sexual ideas were infantile, and she felt unable to discuss them with her mother. She equated getting fat with being pregnant and was very much afraid of this. She had first refused to eat after her classmates had teased her about getting too fat, suggesting that she had a baby inside.

Irma's refusal to eat was accompanied by cessation of menstruation. For three months in the hospital she continued to lose weight and was removed from the hospital by her parents against the doctors' advice. Some months later she died.

The control of eating involves hunger and satiety centers in the hypothalamus, and disturbance in eating behavior can result if this system is damaged. Activity of the hunger center is normally produced by a need for food. When food is eaten and digested, the glucose in the blood rises and is absorbed by body cells. This activates the satiety center, which is sensitive to the rate at which glucose is absorbed, so that eating is terminated. This mechanism can be affected by disturbances at the biochemical level. For example, in diabetes there is a deficiency of the hormone insulin, which is necessary for glucose to pass from the blood into body cells. Therefore, although blood sugar (glucose) is high, the rate at which it is absorbed into the cells is low. Consequently, the satiety center does not become properly active, and diabetics eat excessively. But Irma's difficulties arose at a higher level, as a consequence of severe anxieties and mistaken thought processes. In some way, cortical activity, because of her sexual fears and misconceptions about eating, began to interfere with drive mechanisms in the hypothalamus, suppressing the sexual cycle and menstruation and reducing eating. It is likely that the hunger center was active, since fantasies about eating and interest in food were still present, but that the cortex blocked its usual effect, perhaps by activating the satiety center.

"Anorexia nervosa," as this disorder is called, is a serious disease which can be fatal. It usually occurs during puberty and adolescence in girls who refuse to eat despite marked loss of weight, and who often have anxieties and distorted beliefs about sex and eating. They have an unrealistic attitude to their illness, insisting that they are too fat even when they are obviously emaciated. It may also occur in boys and in childhood (Blitzer *et al.*, 1961), and occasionally in adults. In one case during World War II a girl of ten stopped eating. She had a Teutonic name and had been ostracized by the other children at her British school, who called her "the fat German." She could do nothing about her name, but she was no longer fat. Her difficulties were discussed and her anorexia explained to her, and she started to eat again (Wright, 1945).

Fears and anxieties are important in suppressing eating in this condition, and anorexia often responds well to treatment with chlorpromazine, a tranquilizer which suppresses fear. During or after recovery, some patients pass through a phase of compulsive overeating and become overweight. Some may show compulsive stealing (kleptomania), mainly to get food (Dally and Sargant, 1966).

A duodenal ulcer. John J. was the second of three children, and his family lived in a small country town where his father was the butcher. His mother died when he was twelve. He was a good student at high school and he helped his father, but after graduation he left home because he wanted to travel and see the world. Shortly after, he was drafted and spent some time in Europe. When he was released from the army, he got a job in a garage as a general mechanic. He was hard working and very dependable. He always did his best and was proud of his achievements. If he had any free time, he looked around the shop for things to do.

For two nights a week John attended the local university, where he was taking three courses with the hope of getting a degree in engineering in four to six years. To get to his classes on time, he had to rush there straight from work, and he had no supper until he got home at ten o'clock. Often in class he had hunger pains and heartburn. He lived alone in an apartment, and he cooked, shopped and kept the apartment in order for himself.

At twenty-five, John was a modest, dependable young man with a somewhat bashful manner. He was ambitious, wanting to get a university degree, design machinery himself, and have a well-paid job. But he was doing well in only two of his three courses and he was worried about this. In order to get the degree, he would have to take six courses. But the program was rigorous, and he had been warned that there were many failures. He also very much wanted to get married but seldom had time for a date. If he took more courses, he felt, he would have no social life at all. Thus he was in a state of considerable indecision about taking the engineering course. He was also troubled by the feeling that he ought to be at home helping his father, a quiet, distant man to whom he had never felt close. His father had no sympathy with his desire for travel and education and strongly urged him to settle down as a butcher in his home town.

For three days John had been troubled by this conflict and had felt in an unusual state of mind, depressed and with no ambition. A letter came from his father asking when he would be returning home, and in the evening, after a hasty supper, he sat down to try to write a cheerful reply that would evade the question, when he was struck by sudden agonizing abdominal pain. He felt it might be indigestion and waited some hours, but it was so severe that eventually he had to be taken to the hospital, where it was found he had a perforated duodenal ulcer which required immediate surgery.

John illustrates many of the features found in the typical ulcer patient: they are hard working and conscientious, ambitious and always active, yet with self-doubts and underlying feelings of inadequacy. Often they are the youngest or middle children in the family, in rivalry with older and younger children, and the relationship with their fathers has not been close. They have difficulty relaxing or resting, and the strains produced by this mode of life may be felt most sharply by the delicately balanced system controlling the production of the digestive juices (Castelnuovo-Tedesco, 1962).

The stomach secretes acid and enzymes in order to digest the food arriving there. The cells lining the walls of the stomach and the duodenum (the first part of the small gut, which arises from the stomach) are protected from this digestive action by a layer of mucus. It has been found that people who produce gastric juice rich in hydrochloric acid and pepsin (the digestive enzyme) are more likely than others to develop ulcers. It is unlikely that strong digestive juices ever damage the wall of a normal stomach or duodenum, but if some minor damage exposes the tissues beneath the lining of the duodenum, the strong juices may impair healing and make the damage more likely to persist; this damaged area is then known as an ulcer. If damage to the wall continues at a high rate, the ulcer may perforate and the stomach contents escape into the abdominal cavity. Many other physical factors may also contribute to the development of an ulcer, although their mode of action is often not well understood; for example, blood of type O predisposes to duodenal ulcer (Cowan, 1962).

The level of gastric acid is readily affected by the emotional state, particularly in situations producing tension and anxiety. A classical case is that of Dr. Hoelzel, a scientist who studied the physiology of the stomach and analyzed his own gastric juices regularly every morning. In 1928 he was living in Chicago, and in January of that year his landlady was shot dead during an attempted robbery. He was responsible for the arrest of the culprits, and during the following ten days he was acutely anxious that he would be killed in revenge. On the morning of the shooting, his gastric acid was 100 percent higher than the highest level it reached normally, and it remained more than 30 percent above the normal level until he moved to a safer place (Wright, 1945).

The relation between the occurrence of ulcers and the level of stress is illustrated by some wartime figures. Before World War II, the incidence of ulcers in the U. S. Army was 1.6 per 1000 soldiers. In 1941, it rose to 3.2, and in 1942, after the beginning of the war, it was 5.8 per 1000. It was the sixth most important cause of invalidism in the Navy, despite special efforts to exclude ulcer patients before induction (compare Chapter 12).

As we have seen, the hunger center lies in the hypothalamus, an area also involved in elaborating rage and flight responses. Through its control over the autonomic system, this area can affect features of bodily functioning such as motility of the gut or supply of blood to the muscles. There are interrelations between these drive systems: we tend to be irritable when hungry, perhaps because a hungry animal must be prepared to hunt and fight for its food, and we are more placid when well fed. In fear and anger, hunger is often suppressed, there is sympathetic activation and general arousal, and the motility of the gut is reduced. When hunger has been satisfied, parasympathetic activity is marked, the digestive organs are active, and vigilance is reduced; perhaps we sleep.

The pattern of autonomic functioning varies from one drive state to another, and there are also big, individual differences—one man becomes red with anger, another turns pale, depending on whether blood vessels to the skin dilate or contract. The sympathetic system is active in both anxiety and aggression, but the proportions of adrenaline and noradrenaline produced are different in each case. The first direct observations on the changes that may occur in the secretion, movement, and appearance of the stomach lining were made by an early nineteenth century physician, Dr. W. Beaumont, whose patient, Alexis St. Martin, a Canadian trapper, had had the misfortune to wound himself in the stomach and abdomen by accidentally firing a shotgun. In the process of healing, the stomach wound became attached to the abdominal wall, creating a permanent opening from the outside of the body into the stomach cavity known as a fistula. A fold of the stomach lining lay in such a position that it normally did not permit food to escape from the fistula, and Alexis St. Martin was restored to perfect health, enabling his physician to make many pioneering observations on the physiology of digestion and the behavior of the stomach. More recently Wolf and Wolff (1947) have studied the effects on the stomach of emotions such as fear and anger in a patient, Tom, whose stomach also opened directly onto the abdominal wall as the result of an accident. Tom was employed as a laboratory assistant, and they were able to observe his stomach directly while he was in various emotional states. When Tom was afraid, the lining of his stomach went pale; the sympathetic system reduced the blood supply to the abdominal organs and it also reduced the motility of his gut. When he was angry or resentful, a parasympathetic effect could be seen: the stomach lining flushed red, becoming engorged with blood, and it secreted strongly, pouring out digestive enzymes and acid.

As well as showing short-term autonomic responses to fear or anger, the digestive tract may be affected by hormonal changes caused by stress. In a situation of physical or emotional difficulty the anterior pituitary gland secretes adrenocorticotropic hormone, which acts on the adrenal cortex to make it increase its output of hormones. These increase the resistance of body tissues in general, and they also make the stomach secrete more acid.

Rage or flight responses can be evoked by electrically stimulating the hypothalamus or neighboring areas. It has also been shown that regular stimulation of the hypothalamus by implanted electrodes can produce ulcers in animals and that fearful situations may produce ulcers in rats (Sawrey, 1961; Sawrey and Sawrey, 1964). Since a severe stress or conflict can increase acid secretion both by activating the parasympathetic system and by increasing the output of adrenal cortical hormones, it will favor the development of ulceration. Considerable emotional conflict preceded the perforation of John's ulcer. Accidents are another source of unexpected and severe physical and emotional stresses. In severe accidental burning there may be considerable pain, anxiety, and shock, and in some cases there is rapid development of a duodenal ulcer, which may perforate and cause death.

John's ulcer was probably present for some time before it perforated. Like many ulcer patients he was hard working and conscientious and had a number of problems. What were the particular features of the way he conducted his life that favored development of an ulcer? This question has been studied with the use of monkeys as subjects. An experimental monkey was paired with a control monkey, each being kept in restraining

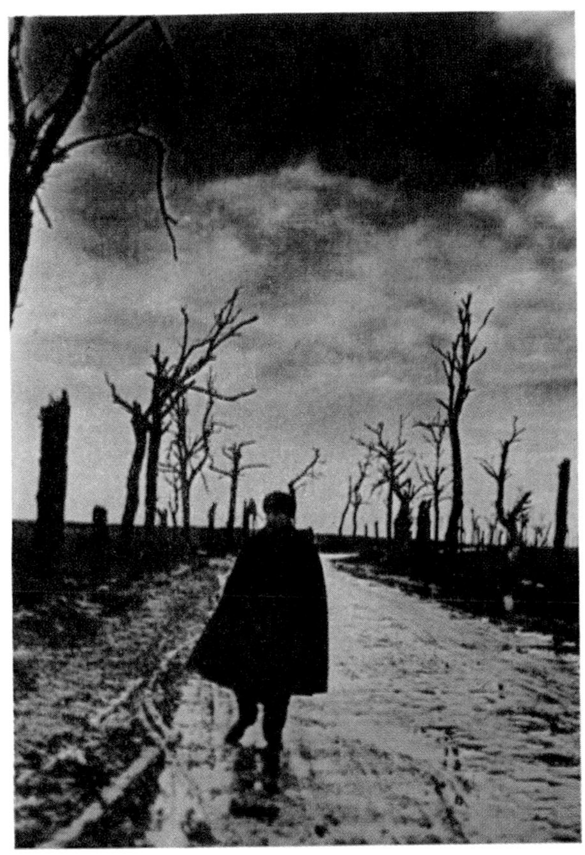

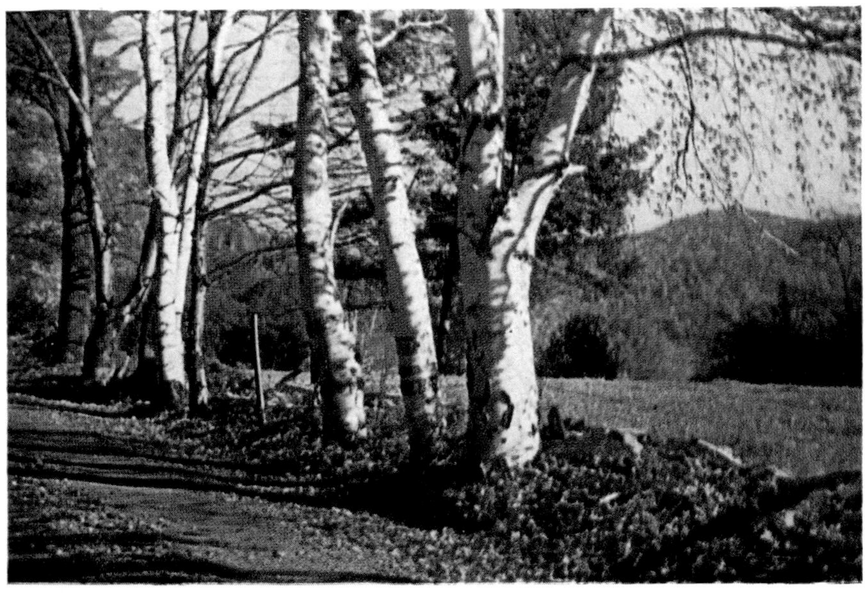

Plate 1 Examples of high tension and low tension pictures used in studying avoidance responses in visual viewing. Average viewing times: high tension, 3.4 seconds; low tension, 10.0 seconds.

orange red green blue orange red blue green orange green blue

orange green orange green red orange red red orange red orange

green orange blue red blue green blue orange green orange green

orange red blue red red orange red blue green orange red

blue green red orange red blue red blue green blue green

green blue red blue red orange red orange blue red orange

blue green red green blue green orange blue orange red green

red red blue red green orange green green green blue orange

green blue blue green red blue red orange orange blue green

green red blue red orange orange red red orange green red

blue blue blue orange green orange red orange green orange green

blue orange green orange blue green red red orange orange red

blue blue green red blue red orange green orange green green

blue red blue green red blue orange blue red orange blue

red orange red green blue orange green orange blue red red

red blue green red orange blue green orange red orange blue

Plate 2 The Stroop test.

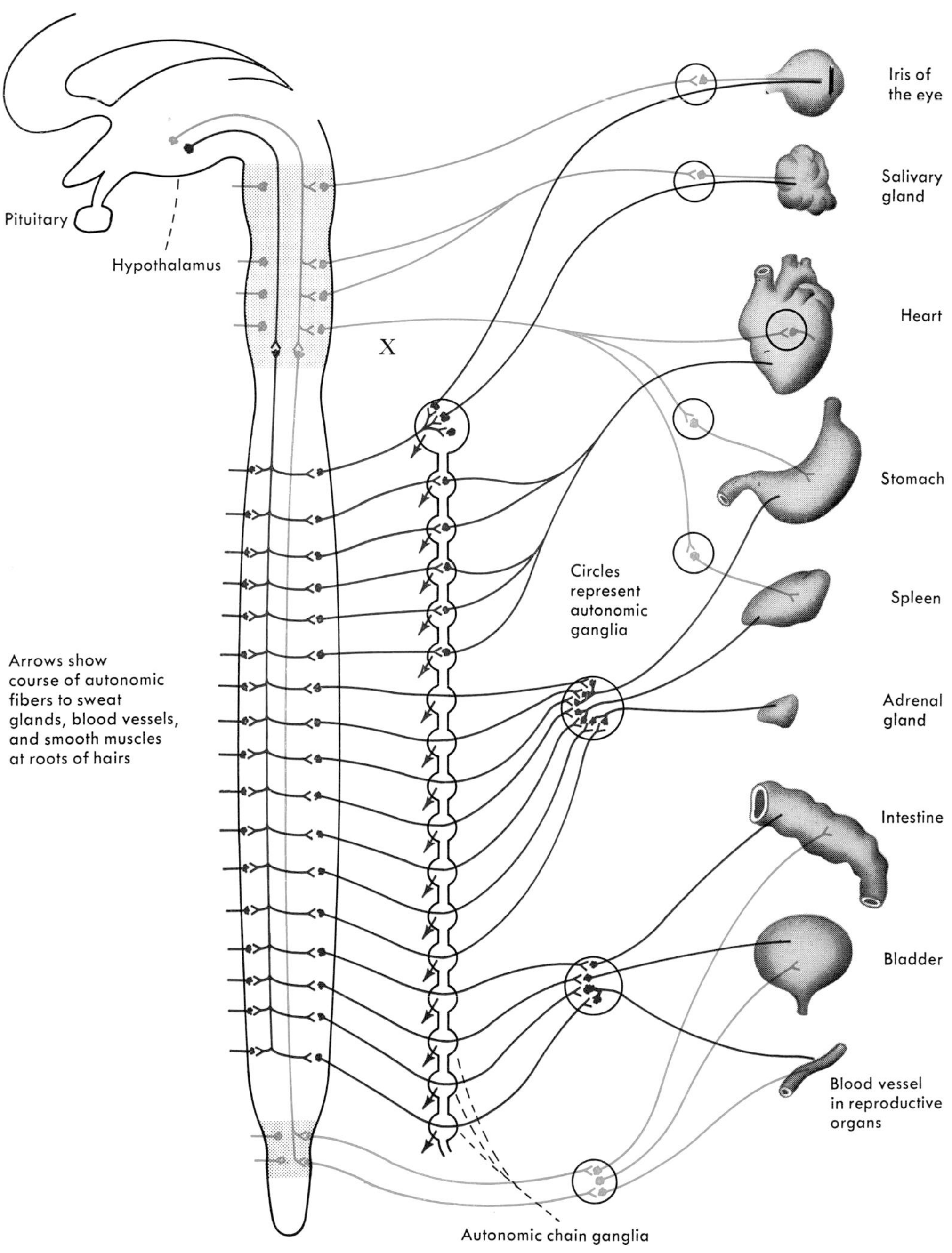

Plate 3 A systematic diagram of the autonomic nervous system.

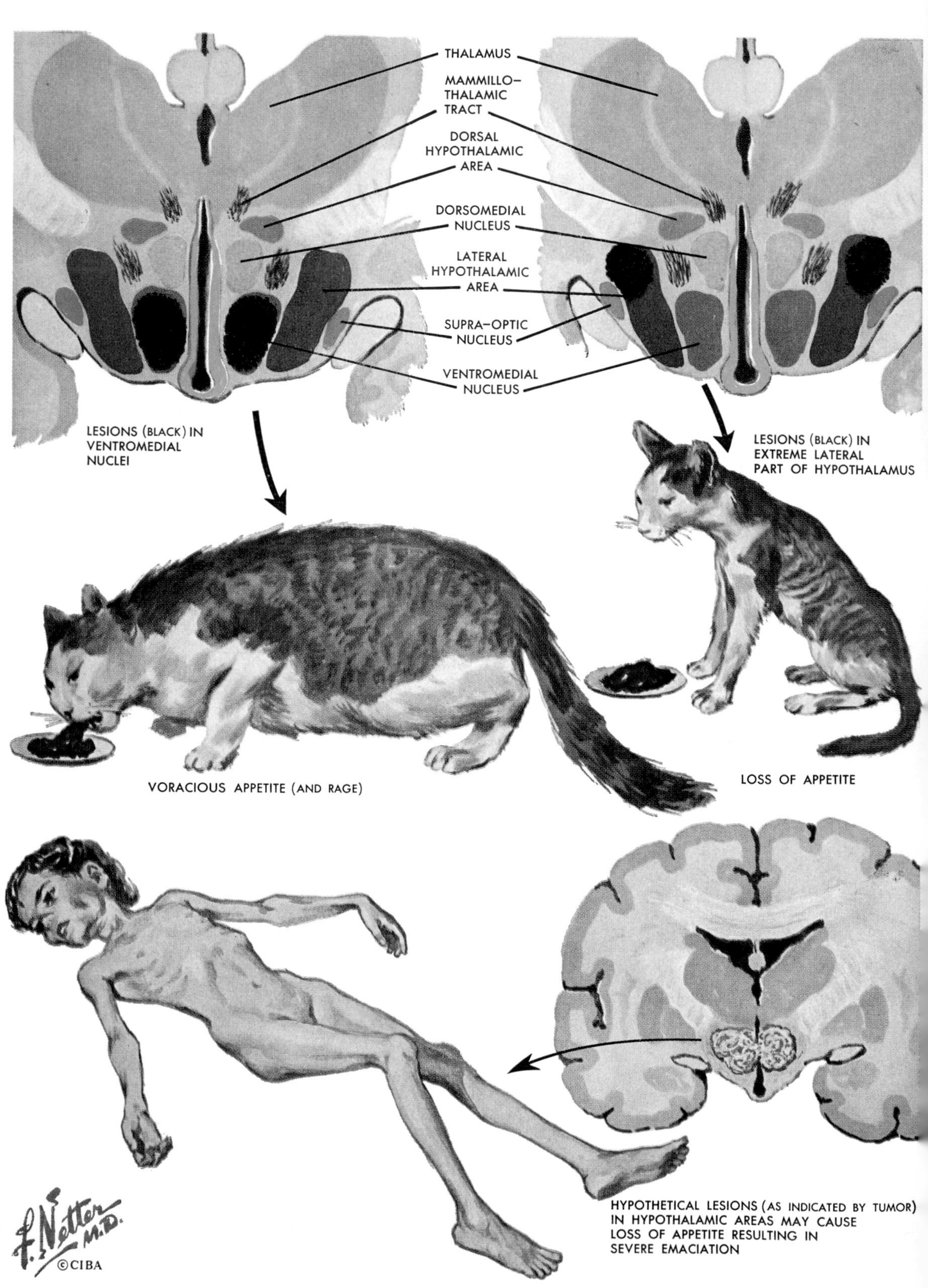

Plate 4 The control of eating by the hypothalamus. Copyright *The Ciba Collection of Medical Illustrations* by Frank H. Netter, M.D.

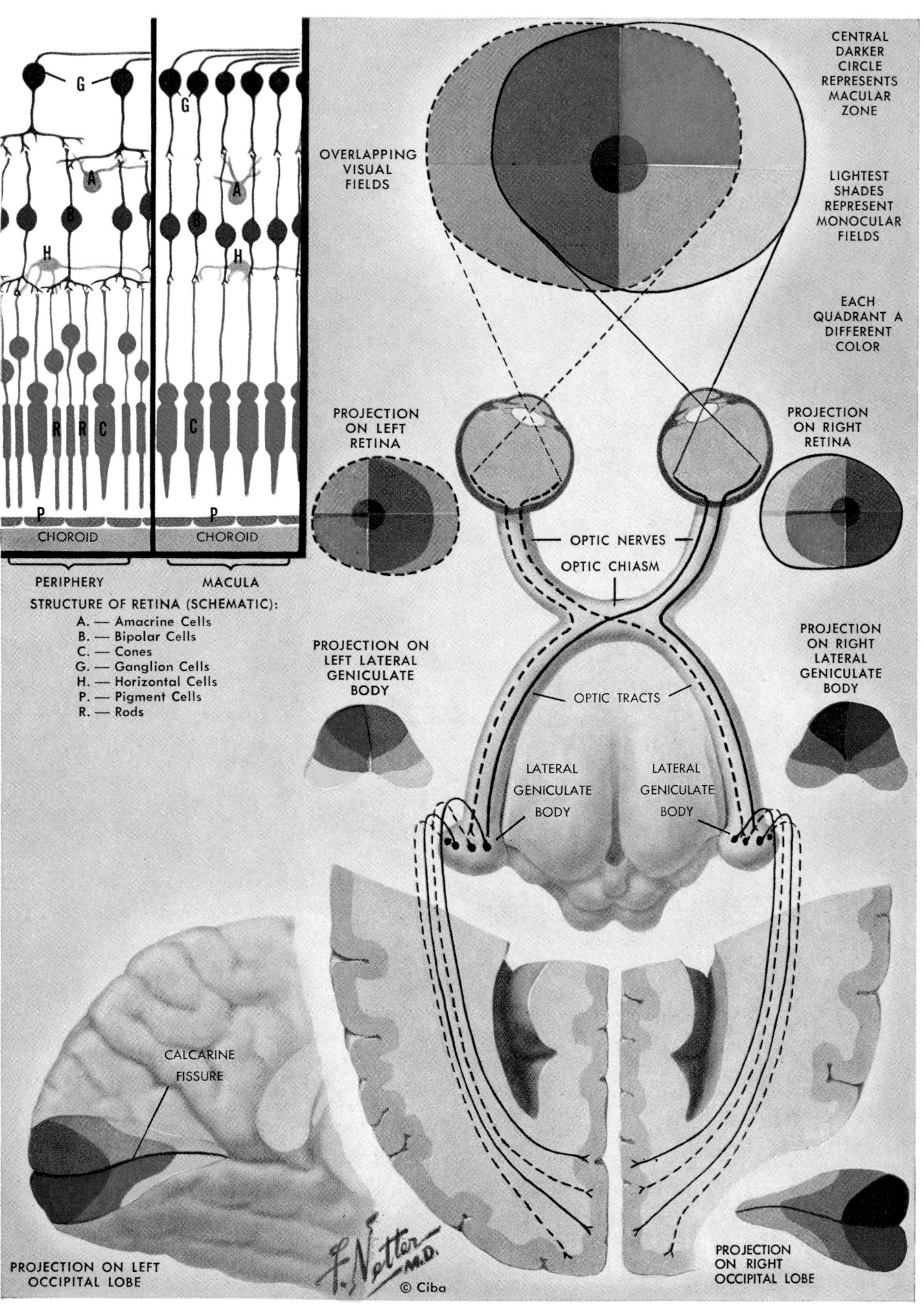

Plate 5 The visual system. An enlargement of the retina is shown, and also the pathways leading to the visual cortex, at the posterior part of the brain. Copyright *The Ciba Collection of Medical Illustrations* by Frank H. Netter, M.D.

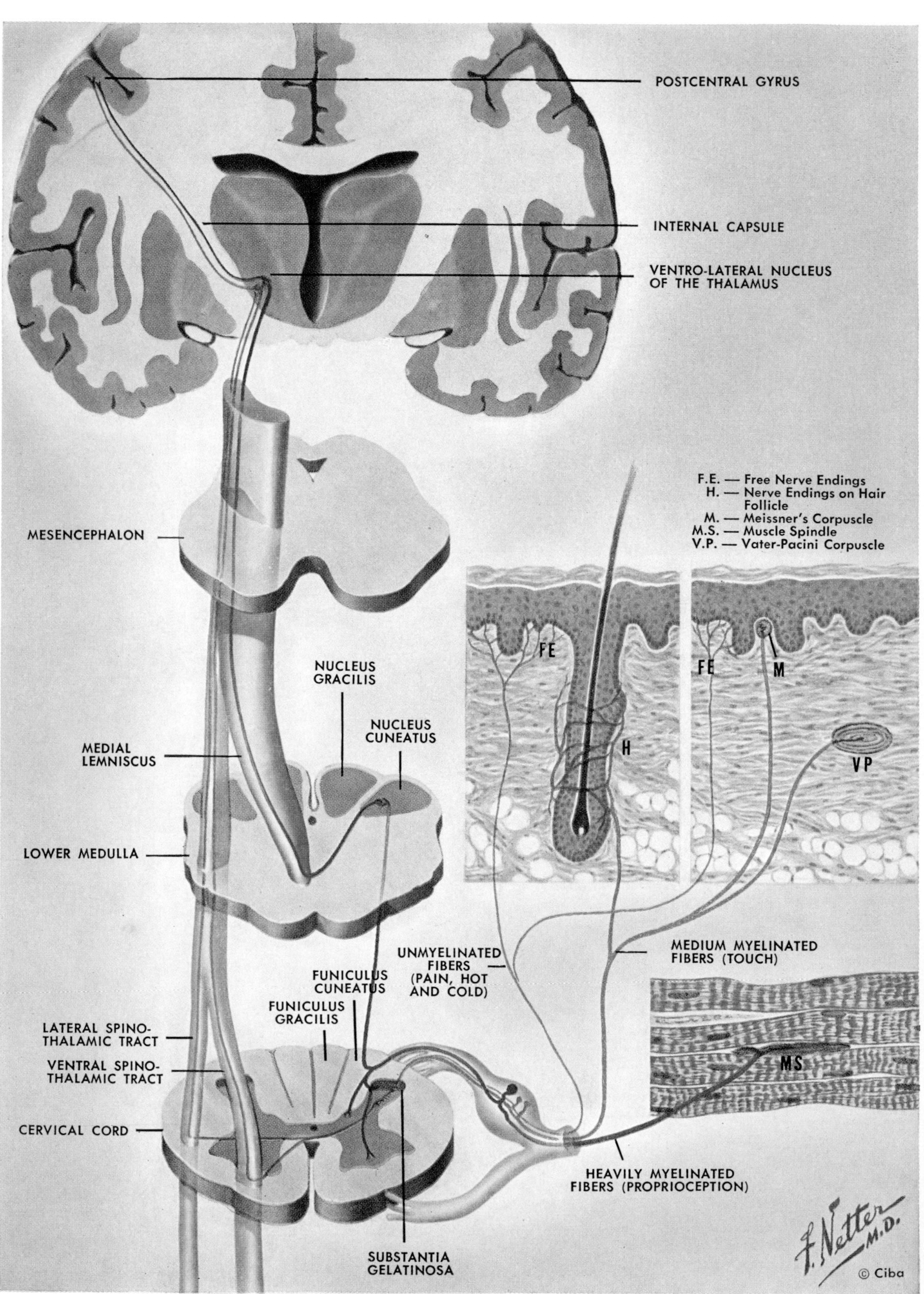

Plate 6 The pathways for sensory messages from the skin or muscle to the brain. Copyright *The Ciba Collection of Medical Illustrations* by Frank H. Netter, M.D.

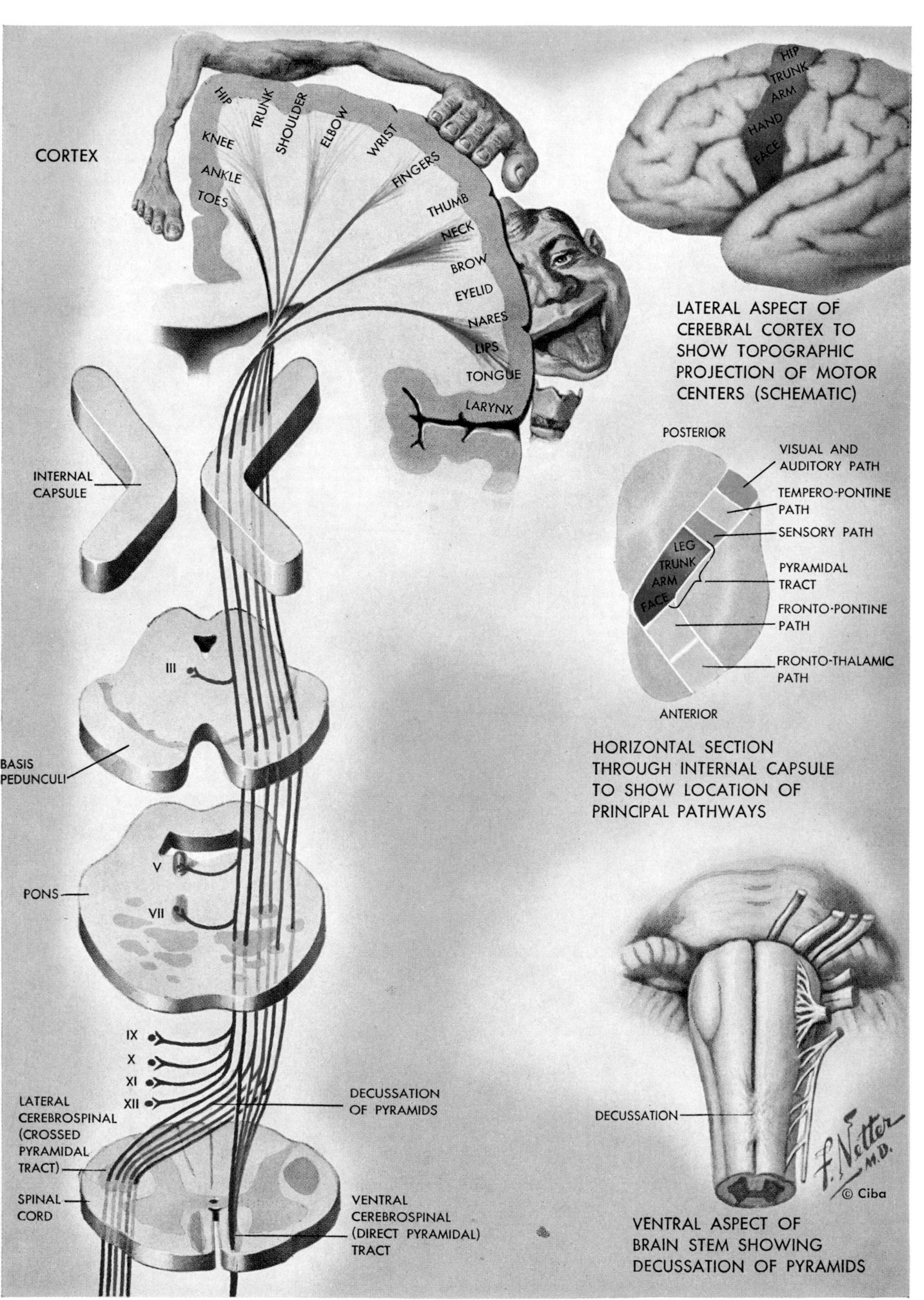

Plate 7 The pathways for motor messages from the brain to the motor centers in the spinal cord. Copyright *The Ciba Collection of Medical Illustrations* by Frank H. Netter, M.D.

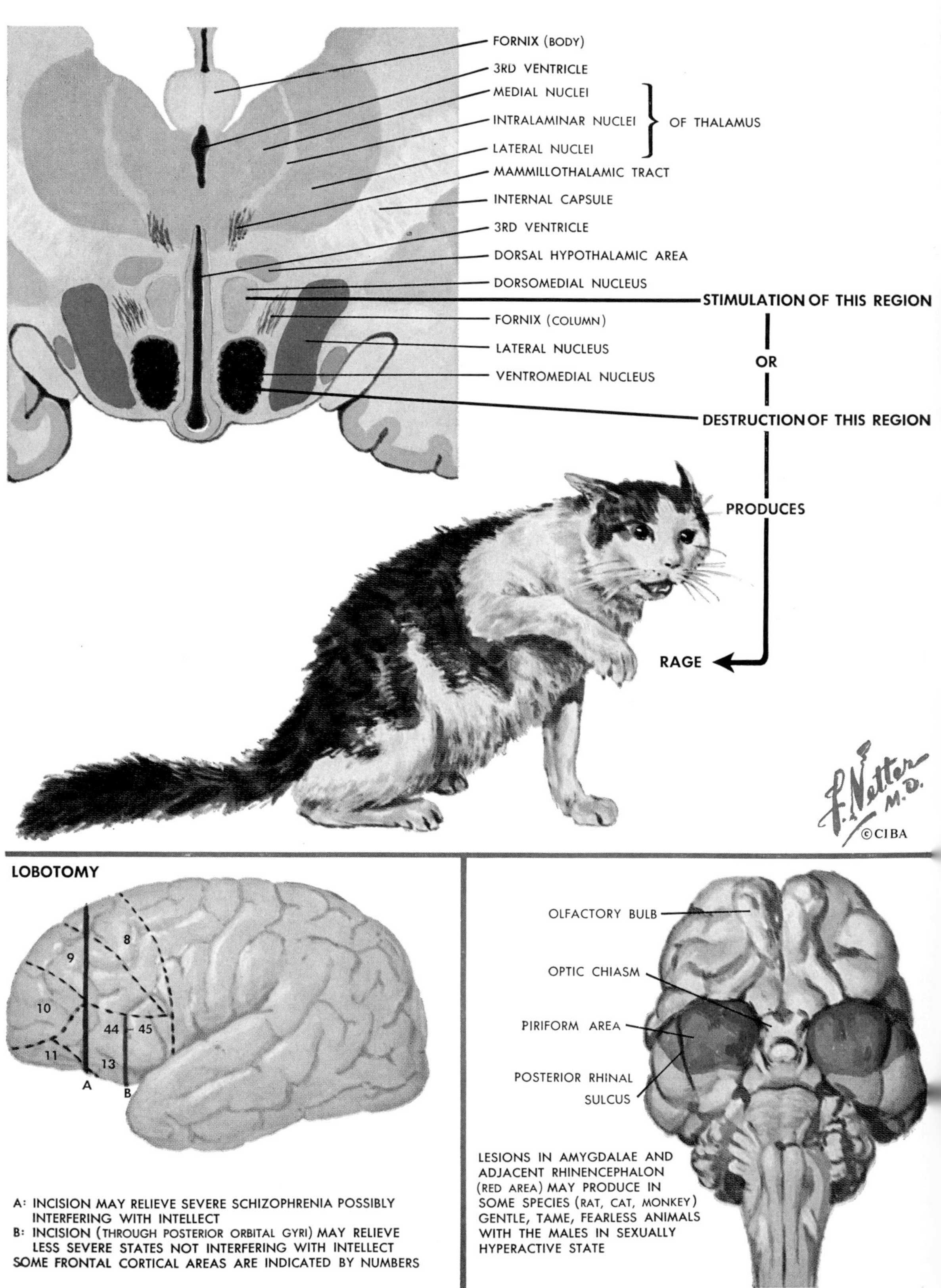

Plate 8 The control of aggression by the hypothalamus and cortex. Copyright *The Ciba Collection of Medical Illustrations* by Frank H. Netter, M.D.

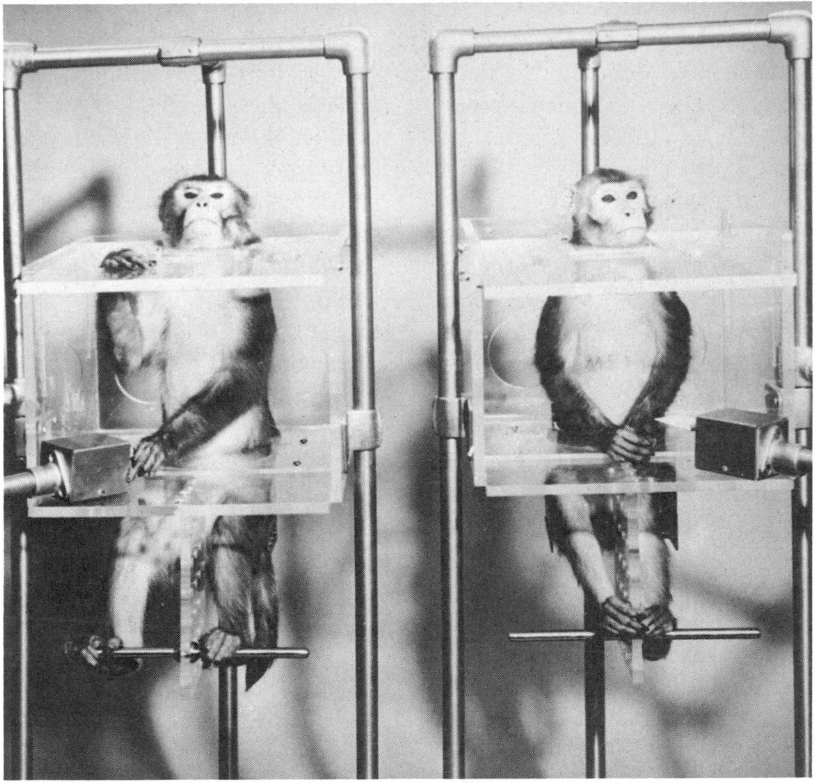

Figure 13.10 Conditioning experiment involves training monkeys in restraining chairs. Both animals receive brief electric shocks at regular intervals. The "executive" monkey (*left*) has learned to press the lever in its left hand, which prevents shocks to both animals. The control monkey (*right*) has lost interest in its lever, which is a dummy. Only executive monkeys developed ulcers. Photo courtesy of the Medical Audio Visual Department, Walter Reed Army Institute of Research, Washington, D.C.

chairs which they could not leave, although they could move their limbs freely (Figure 13.10). For six hours of every twelve, the monkeys were given a brief electric shock to the feet every twenty seconds. The experimental monkey could prevent the shock by pressing a lever within the twenty seconds before the shock was due. The control monkey had a dummy lever which it could press but without effect. However, each time the experimental monkey avoided a shock, the control monkey was not shocked either. Thus each monkey had the same number of shocks and the same degree of restraint. The experimental monkey became quite adept at avoiding shocks by pressing the lever, so that both monkeys got relatively few shocks. However, within a few weeks the experimental monkey had died of perforating ulcers, while the control monkey was perfectly healthy (Brady, 1958).

From this experiment, it seems that it was not discomfort or restraint that resulted in ulceration, *but the necessity of repeatedly making decisions and taking action to prevent unpleasant occurrences.* This suggests that it was not the discomforts in John's life, but the anxieties involved in making and being responsible for decisions that predisposed to the ulcer.

But along with the immediate stressful situation, and the patient's personality, physical factors are important in determining the occurrence of duodenal ulcers. The interaction of these variables has been studied in army inductees (Weiner *et al.*, 1957). Sixty-three inductees with the highest, and fifty-seven with the lowest, levels of gastric secretion in a group of 2073 inductees were examined at the beginning of their basic training and again after eight to sixteen weeks. Four draftees had duodenal ulcers to start with and five more had developed an ulcer by the second examination. The basic training was a stressful situation, but it did not induce ulcers in all 2073 draftees. What distinguished the nine patients with ulcers from the rest was that they were all in the group with the highest rates of gastric secretion. However, not all members of this group developed an ulcer. Psychological testing suggested that the draftees with ulcers had strong underlying needs to be fed and supported; they felt anxiety about expressing hostility for fear that they would lose desired support. When support was not given, they were not able to express the anger they felt. These observations suggest that personality, stress, and level of gastric secretion are related to the development of duodenal ulceration, but further work is needed to clarify the relations between these factors.

Migraine. Migraine is a condition in which severe, often incapacitating attacks of headache recur at regular or irregular intervals. The sufferers often have a characteristic personality; they are strongly motivated, ambitious and perfectionist, and often show much persistence in activities such as stamp collecting. The headache typically affects one side of the head (*migraine* comes from the Greek for "half head"), and there may be various accompanying symptoms. In the initial phase, which precedes the headache there may be visual disturbances such as a temporary "blind spot," and "battlement figures" may be seen. Sometimes the patient feels thirsty or hungry at this stage, and frequently the body retains water, producing less urine than usual. Irritability and aggressive behavior sometimes precede the attack by several hours, and deep sleep may occur immediately before. In the second phase, when the headache develops, many of these symptoms may reverse. Excess urine is now produced, there may be a loss of appetite and nausea and vomiting, and the earlier irritability and sleepiness are replaced by ebullience and wakefulness when the attack is over (Wolff, 1953).

There is evidence that this disorder results from an imbalance between the inhibitory and excitatory drive mechanisms in the lateral hypothalamus. Herberg (1967) suggests that in migraine patients there is chronic overactivity of the excitatory drive mechanisms, which normally are restrained by the inhibitory mechanisms so that, for example, normal cycles of eating and drinking occur. But an exacerbation of this overactivity may escape inhibitory control and may cause symptoms similar to those produced in animals by lesions to the ventromedial nucleus, such as hunger, thirst, water retention, sleep, and aggressiveness. The lateral hypothalamic area, which contains the feeding and drinking centers, overlaps the area from which autonomic stress responses may be obtained (Hess, 1957); this control system is involved in the overactivity and produces widespread constriction of blood vessels. One consequence is that the blood supply to the area of the cortex responsible for higher levels of visual organization is reduced and there are visual disturbances (Wolff, 1953).

The second phase of the attack occurs when the hypothalamic excitatory mechanisms are exhausted or inhibitory control is reestablished. The blood vessels now dilate, and excessive distension of vessels in the scalp produces the headache. Hunger and thirst and water retention are replaced by anorexia and excessive production of urine, and the aggressiveness and sleepiness cease. Herberg (1967) also suggests a link between the chronic overactivity of the excitatory mechanisms and the characteristic migraine personality. If many human complex behaviors produced by "secondary drives" are ultimately motivated by the hypothalamic excitatory centers but are not subject to inhibitory control, then in these patients they would tend to occur at a high and persistent level, producing persevering, hard-working, and meticulous people.

A case of cyclical disturbances of mood. Karen K. a married woman aged twenty-seven, sought treatment from her physician for recurrent headaches. She had been married seven years and had four children. Since the birth of her first child she had been troubled by headaches during the week preceding her menstrual period. At these times she also suffered from bouts of depression, tension, and irritability. Although normally placid, she would readily fly into rages, and she was afraid she might hurt her children. Also during the week preceding menstruation, there would be swelling of her face, hands, and feet, and she would get rheumatic pains in her shoulders. Sometimes there were also excessive eating and increased sexual desire. All her symptoms subsided rapidly once menstruation began. She was given the hormone progesterone, with considerable improvement in her symptoms.

This condition is known as "premenstrual tension," and it is sometimes attributed to a disturbance in the production of the hormones controlling the female sexual cycle. These hormones come from the ovary, and the rate at which they are secreted is governed by the anterior pituitary gland. This gland is situated at the base of the brain, where it is under nervous control, and it may be affected by emotional disturbances. In some women, for example, periods of excitement or stress, such as may be caused by taking up a new job in a strange city, or anxiety, such as fear of an unwanted pregnancy, may cause a temporary disturbance or suppression of the cycle, and menstruation may be irregular or even absent for a few months. But premenstrual tension is probably not caused by emotional factors but arises as a primary disturbance in the control of the sex hormone balance, resulting in too low a proportion of progesterone to estrogen production in the premenstrual period. The disturbance may be in the hypothalamus, which controls the anterior pituitary and is responsible for the occurrence of the sexual cycle.

Estrogen and progesterone have important effects on many systems of the body. During the monthly cycle the balance between them changes. The uterus is first prepared to receive the fertilized ovum, and then it is prepared for pregnancy. If no fertilized ovum implants in the uterus, the second phase comes to an end in menstruation, when the thickened uterine lining strips away and the uterus prepares for a new cycle. Not much is known about the hypothalamic mechanisms which control this changing balance, but some of Karen's other symptoms suggest that the primary disturbance was at this level. We have seen that the hypothalamus contains excitatory drive mechanisms and, in some cases, corresponding inhibitory mechanisms; for example, the lateral hypothalamus has a feeding center whose effect may be suppressed by a satiety center in the ventromedial nucleus of the hypothalamus. The different excitatory mechanisms, such as those for eating and drinking, overlap to some extent in the lateral hypothalamus; they also overlap other mechanisms, such as those which activate the sympathetic nervous system in response to stress, or retain water in the body by reducing the production of urine. The corresponding inhibitory mechanisms, where they exist, appear to overlap too; in animals, destruction of the area of the ventromedial nucleus may release not only excessive eating and drinking but also aggressive behavior and sleepiness.

Herberg (1967) has shown that the occurrence of migraine may be explained by the development of bouts of excessive activity in the excitatory mechanisms, which the inhibitory mechanisms are unable to suppress, and the same explanation may apply here. It seems likely that in Karen's case the hypothalamic mechanism determining the sex hormone balance used to become excessively active in the premenstrual period. It then either communicated this activity to other excitatory mechanisms, or suppressed the corresponding inhibitory mechanisms, disturbing the balance between them. Release of the excitatory mechanism for feeding would account for the excessive eating. Similar overactivity of the excitatory mechanisms would explain the increased sexual desire and the tendency to fly into rages. Increased production of antidiuretic hormone, which leads to retention of water in the body, caused the swelling of her face and limbs. Swelling of soft tissues due to the water retention resulted in the "rheumatic" pains. Disturbed functioning of the lateral hypothalamic mechanisms controlling the blood vessels, and the strain on them resulting from the increased volume of blood, may have caused dilatation of blood vessels in the scalp, causing the headaches. Giving Karen progesterone may have reduced excessive activity in the hypothalamic mechanism controlling the menstrual cycle and may thus have diminished her symptoms.

Herberg (1967) suggests that secondary drives may derive to some extent from hypothalamic excitatory centers. If so the increased activation of the mechanisms responsible for aggressiveness in this condition would have some effect on social behavior. Some degree of premenstrual disturbance has been found to occur in about 40 percent of women, and it has been noted that during the premenstrual and menstrual periods the work and behavior of schoolgirls is worse than at other times, and that an excessive proportion of automobile accidents involving women drivers, suicides of women, and criminal offenses by women occur during these parts of the cycle (Dalton, 1959, 1960).

It is interesting to compare Karen K. with Irma I. It seems likely that anorexia nervosa is brought about by excessive activity in the inhibitory hypothalamic mechanisms, perhaps extending from the satiety center to other inhibitory mechanisms, and it is thus not surprising that many of the symptoms in these two conditions appear opposed. Karen K. had bouts of overeating, Irma I. would not eat. Karen was depressed and irritable; Irma was active and helpful and seemed unrealistically unconcerned with the seriousness of her condition, and menstruation was suppressed. In keeping with the suggestion that the satiety center inhibits the output from the feeding center, which produces eating, but does not suppress activity in the center itself, Irma had fantasies about eating and food, despite her refusal to consume any. The compulsive eating and stealing (mainly to get food) which may occur after recovery from anorexia nervosa (Dally and Sargant, 1966) suggest that recovery from hypothalamic inhibitory dominance may sometimes produce a temporary excitatory dominance, with effects on both "primary" and "secondary" motivation.

Cortical Disturbances

A human weasel. Leon L., a boy of thirteen, was brought to a clinic by his mother. For the previous two years he had done poorly at school and frequently played truant. He had no friends, and spent most of his time on his own in the woods. At home he was quiet and uncommunicative, but he suffered from a distressing habit of repeatedly throwing his head upward in a sudden sharp jerk. He might do this twenty times in a quarter of an hour. He also fidgeted with his hands and grimaced. The jerking increased when he was excited or emotionally distressed; it decreased if he was distracted by something, and it disappeared altogether when he was asleep. He was a slight, undersized boy who had been ill for long periods during his childhood.

Leon was given psychotherapy, and it became clear that he felt very much alone. Because he was smaller and clumsier than the other children in his class they frequently teased him. He was also picked on by his father, who was alcoholic. He felt that he could save himself only by constant watchfulness, and he thought of himself as a silent, quick, ferocious wild animal, like a weasel or mink, small but dangerous and cunning and anything but clumsy. His head jerks were movements made by the weasel, looking around for enemies and preparing to strike back. Leon responded to therapy; he gained more confidence and ceased to need this fantasy, and the head jerking became less frequent and finally stopped.

Leon continually repeated a sequence of thought which involved feelings of being under attack and culminated in the idea of looking around and striking back. A young child's thoughts are closely related to and accompanied by movements. The information-processing operations in his cortex that correspond to a train of thought tend to activate the motor output that produces the corresponding movements. Later he learns to suppress the movements: for example, he learns to read without moving his lips. But under strain, such as reading under difficult and distracting conditions, this accomplishment may break down, and he will go back to the easier procedure of letting the movements occur. Similarly, under continual emotional stress, Leon's repetitive thought sequence was manifested as a repeated output from the motor cortex, resulting in the disorder known as a *tic*.

Children with tics are often found to be restless, sensitive, quick-tempered, anxious, lacking in self-confidence, stubborn, and excitable. The tic is sometimes precipitated by a sudden conflict at home. The great majority of children eventually recover from tics, although they may continue for four to six years. As well as the psychological factor, physical factors may also play a part in the genesis of tics, since they tend to occur more frequently in children who have suffered slight neurological damage at or before birth. Tics are frequently found in close relatives of these children, indicating that a genetic factor as well as an effect of learning or imitation may be involved.

As well as being the source of the motor output from the cortex, the frontal lobes are also important in organizing social relations and behavior, and for long-term planning and initiative. Much of what we know about its functions in man comes from reports on the effects of accidental or operative damage to parts of the frontal cortex, such as the classical description by Dr. Harlow of Massachusetts, in 1868, of *The Case of Phineas Gage.*

Phineas Gage, an efficient and capable foreman, was engaged one day in tamping dynamite when it exploded, blowing the large iron tamping rod through his upper jaw and left eye socket and out through the top of his head. Though his frontal lobes were damaged, he was not killed; in fact, he retained sufficient vigor to walk to the surgeon's office. The bar was removed and the wound healed. Afterwards, in Dr. Harlow's words,

> His physical health is good, and I am inclined to say that he has recovered. Has no pain in head, but says it has a queer feeling which he is not able to describe. Applied for his situation as foreman, but is undecided whether to work or travel. His contractors, who regarded him as the most efficient and capable foreman in their employ previous to his injury, considered the change in his mind so marked that they could not give him his place again. The equilibrium or balance, so to speak, between his intellectual faculties and animal propensities, seems to have been destroyed. He is fitful, irreverent, indulging at times in the grossest profanity (which was not previously his custom), manifesting but little deference for his fellows, impatient of restraint or advice when it conflicts with his desires, at times pertinaciously obstinate, yet capricious and vacillating, devising many plans of future operation, which are no sooner arranged than they are abandoned in turn for others appearing more feasible. A child in his intellectual capacity and manifestations, he has the animal passions of a strong man. Previous to his injury, though untrained in the schools, he possessed a well balanced mind, and was looked upon by those who knew him as a shrewd, smart business man, very energetic and persistent in executing all his plans of operation. In this regard his mind was radically changed, so decidedly that his friends and acquaintances said he was "no longer Gage."

No longer the sober workman of before, Phineas Gage now worked only intermittently and was frequently drunk (Fulton, 1949).

This deterioration in social relations and in richness of character has frequently been seen after damage to the frontal lobes, which may be operated on to remove a tumor, to relieve severe pain, or to treat obsessive anxieties that do not respond to any other treatment. In cases of intractible pain, the sensory information still arrives at the higher centers, and the patient recognizes that the pain is still there, but the apprehensive anticipation of pain and the misery that formerly accompanied it are no longer shown after the operation; in fact, the patient appears relatively indifferent to the pain. After removal of part of the frontal lobes, many patients become tactless and their emotional state is changeable. Relatives feel that they are shallow and do not shoulder their share of responsibilities. They lose their sense of the value of money, buying things without concern for the price. Their more intellectual interests are often lost, and they may say that they feel neither real happiness nor deep sorrow. After operation, a woman who previously had been a clever cook now had difficulty using new recipes and made ridiculous mistakes with them, although she could still follow her old recipes faultlessly. If she went out to buy food, she might meet a friend, forget her duties, and go off with her, disappearing for half a day.

Experiments on monkeys have shown that removing the frontal lobes impairs their performance when information given to them at one time needs to be applied later on. It appears that for storing information in memory, the temporal lobes have special importance. In operations on them for the cure of tumors or epilepsy, it is sometimes necessary to stimulate the temporal cortex electrically, and in some cases this may repeatedly evoke complicated memories in the patient. He might, for example, see himself standing on a certain street corner listening to a melody, and the whole scene may run through his mind each time the surgeon stimulates a certain spot on his temporal cortex (Penfield and Rasmussen, 1950).

Loss of recent memory. Michael M., a twenty-nine-year-old motor winder, had suffered from epileptic fits since the age of ten. He had a placid, pleasant temperament, and despite his epilepsy he managed to graduate from high school. As the fits increased in severity and frequency and could not be controlled medically, it was decided to remove parts of the temporal lobe on each side. After Michael recovered from the operation, it was found that his personality was unchanged but that he suffered from a major disturbance of memory. He could give minute details of his early life, but he did not remember that he had had a brain operation. He could not recognize the hospital staff or find his way to the bathroom. He could not learn the doctor's name, however often he was told it.

He returned home to his family, who moved to a new house. Ten months later he had still not learned the new address, though he knew the old one perfectly, nor could he find his way around the new house. He could not remember from day to day where articles in common use, such as the lawnmower, were kept; he would do the same jigsaw puzzles day after day without showing the effect of practice, and he would read the same magazines over and over again without finding them familiar. He did not improve with time.

This case demonstrates the important part played by the temporal lobes in storing information for future use (Scoville and Milner, 1957). But the temporal lobes are not the only parts of the brain that are important for this. Much of the information that allows us to understand and use language appears to be stored in the left parietal cortex (in right-handed people), and damage here may cause a disturbance in the ability to produce and understand speech known as *aphasia* (Penfield and Roberts, 1959). The use and comprehension of language may be disturbed in a number of different ways, and other disturbances such as difficulty in reading may be associated with it. Aphasic patients may have difficulty finding the right words, or getting them into the proper syntactical order, or understanding spoken speech when they are addressed. For example, an officer who had been kicked in the left side of the head by a horse and had sustained a fractured skull and brain injury was asked to name colors shown to him. His replies were, for black —"what you do for the dead"; for blue—"my arm" (he had a blue band on his arm); for green—"what is out there" (pointing to the trees through the window); for white—"what you wear" (the doctor's white coat); for yellow—"this one" (holding his yellow tie). A soldier whose parietal lobe had been damaged by a fragment of a mortar bomb spoke in "jumbled" speech, using wrong words or phrases, when he could not find the right ones. A month after his injury he wrote the following letter:

> Dear John,
>
> Many thanks for your letter. Am afraid it will be very long time for O.K. again. I have fractured skull and cannot read properly yet. Added to which by left arm is pretty U/S. I speech is getting on pretty stupid still. This is my 2nd letter which is you can see is pretty haywire. (Head, 1926.)

The parietal lobes also contain the cortical receiving areas for sensory information from the skin, muscles, and joints.

Loss of sensation in the hand: Hysteria revisited. As a child, Norman N. was always "very nervous" of his father, a brutal disciplinarian who sometimes thrashed him every day for a week and put him on bread and water. When Norman reached the age of five, his father made him work in the garden every day from 4:30 A.M. until school began. He wanted to be an engineer, but his father would not allow it, and he became a clerk and was fairly successful. He was very ambitious and eager to do well.

At the age of twenty, he became engaged and needed to get promoted so that he could get married. Soon after his engagement, he was transferred to work under a different superior, a very difficult man who could not keep assistants. Norman found he was given more and more work and was falling behind. His boss was domineering and unpleasant, and Norman disliked him but found himself unable to protest. Even in the mornings he felt exhausted, and the burden increased when his father had a stroke and Norman had to make a special journey each day to shave him.

A month later, Norman caught his hand in some office machinery and cut his wrist. The wound healed, but he found that he was unable to use his hand, which as well as being paralyzed was also completely insensitive. On medical examination, there was no atrophy (wasting) of the muscles, as there would have been had a motor nerve been damaged. The loss of sensation was complete—pins could be driven into his hand without his noticing—and it affected the whole of his hand but stopped sharply at the wrist. He was helpful and cooperative when examined, and seemed to accept his disability with placid indifference. The diagnosis was: *hysterical anesthesia and paralysis*. Norman was given psychotherapy and the anesthesia and paralysis disappeared.

Norman's disorder was not due to damaged nerves; there was no break in the physical pathways conveying sensory information from the hand or motor instructions to it. Three different nerves carry sensory information from the hand, and damage to any one of them produces a characteristic pattern of sensory loss; for example, damage to the ulnar nerve causes anesthesia in the little finger and the neighboring half of the fourth finger, but not in the other fingers. No injury to a nerve in the arm would destroy sensation in the area exactly corresponding to what people commonly think of as the "hand," ending sharply at the wrist. This "glove anesthesia" was not produced by the injury but came from the higher level, where sensory information is organized and motor instructions elaborated, and the unit affected, the hand, was what a naive patient might expect to be damaged by the injury.

Norman was faced with what was for him an insoluable problem. Because of his desire for success and his need for promotion, he had to do well. But he had more work than he could cope with, and on top of that, the burden of his father's illness; moreover, a timid and hesitant attitude towards his superiors, which derived from his childhood relations with his father, kept him from making any effective protest at the way he was being treated on the job. In this situation he could not satisfy his needs. The paralysis and anesthesia of his hand provided an excuse for giving up work and failing to achieve promotion, it attracted the sympathy and support of his girl friend, and it allowed him to leave his unpleasant boss without getting into open conflict with him.

This disorder, as we saw in Chapter 9, is known as conversion hysteria. Symptoms include many sorts of paralyses or disturbances of sensation. They tend to vary from one examination to another and are susceptible to suggestion; they can often be removed or modified under hypnosis. Their form reflects the patient's expectations and problems and because it plays a role in solving an emotional problem, these patients often show a calm and placid absence of real concern about the awful disabilities from which they appear to suffer.

It should be reemphasized (as in Chapter 9) that these patients are not malingering or pretending. They genuinely believe in their illness. Norman can be compared with Irma I., who refused to eat. Irma's disturbed thought processes, corresponding to activity of the "neural computer" in the cortex, interfered with the mechanisms that guide eating. In

Norman's case, they interfered with the processing of sensory information. The level of this interference must be high, since it can be shown that in hysterical anesthesias, sensory information is still available for certain purposes. For example, if a patient with hysterical blindness is told to walk by himself, he will stumble along with a hesitant shuffling gait, but he will not trip over obstacles placed in his path. It is likely that the interference is at the level of the cortex, since symptoms very similar to those of conversion hysteria are sometimes produced by tumors or damage of the right parietal cortex (Critchley, 1953). This brain area is involved in the use of sensory information for complex tasks, such as continuously identifying the parts of the body. When it is damaged, a patient may sometimes deny that part of his body belongs to him. He may claim that his left arm is not his but belongs to someone else, and he may even give it a nickname, such as "Toby." One patient was shown that the rejected hand was attached by way of the arm to her own body, but she continued to deny it was hers, saying, "But my eyes and my feelings don't agree, and I must believe my feelings. I know they look like mine but I can feel that they're not, and I can't believe my eyes."

Even more complex recognition tasks may be affected by damage in the parietal and occipital regions of the brain (Critchley, 1953; Bornstein and Kidron, 1959; Pevzner *et al.*, 1962).

Unrecognizable faces. Otto O. was a merchant who had completed high school. He could read, write, and speak five languages, and he was married and had two children. One night when he was sixty-four years old he woke up with a severe headache. It got somewhat better in the next few hours, and he got up and caught a bus in order to keep an appointment. On the way, the headache got worse, and he decided to turn back home. He got off the bus, and on the way to another bus stop, on a familiar road, he suddenly felt that the whole area was strange, though he knew where he was. He got on the bus home and found that the route was now strange. He guessed when to get off according to the time the bus had taken. He gave some passersby his address, and they told him how to reach his home. When he got there, it also seemed strange; inside, the room, furniture, and pictures looked different. He looked in a mirror and saw a strange face. After a rest, he went to find his doctor, an old friend who lived across the street, but he could not find the house until he noticed the doctor's nameplate on one of the doors. A woman opened the door. Only when she said, "Come in Mr. O.," did he realize that she was the doctor's wife.

On the way to the hospital, he noted that though the route was a familiar one, it *seemed* strange. He knew from memory what landmarks lay along the way, but when he passed them, they looked different from what he expected. In the hospital, he had great difficulty recognizing faces. He learned to distinguish his three doctors by the fact that one was very tall, another had glasses and a moustache, and the third had neither. He could also tell them apart by their voices, and at first he could only recognize his own son by his voice, though after a few days he learned to recognize his walk as well.

He could read, write, and speak easily and correctly. He could recognize pictures of animals, national costumes, stamps, road signs, and so on, but he had great difficulty with pictures showing action. For example, when he was shown a picture of a policeman directing traffic, he could not make out the meaning of the picture. He recognized the policeman, noted a child crossing the road, observed the number of cars, but did not realize what the theme of the picture was.

He recovered from most of his symptoms during the course of a few months, except for some residual difficulty in recognizing faces.

Otto O. had a thrombosis in an artery to the brain, resulting in damage to the right occipital cortex and interference with processing of complex sensory information. Although after the stroke he could still recognize the individual parts of a face, he could not tell different faces apart, probably because he was failing to detect the details by which we distinguish one face from another.

SUMMARY

We have now seen some of the ways in which the control mechanisms of the body can be disturbed. These mechanisms range from the coarse controls provided by the distribution of hormones in the blood to the complex computations by which the cortex analyzes the scene around us and plans and adjusts our behavior to fit in with it. The control mechanisms are sometimes disturbed at a single level only, but this is probably rare. More commonly, a disturbance at one level causes disturbances at others. Lower levels may affect higher, as when endocrine changes cause changes of mood in hyperthyroidism or premenstrual tension; or disturbances at a high level can affect lower levels, as we saw in Betty's false pregnancy. In many cases the effects and interactions are complex: numerous factors work together to cause a breakdown, as in hypertension or duodenal ulcer. In some cases, we know some of the more important factors: warts cannot occur unless there is infection with a virus, but they are also dependent on the resistance of the skin, which may change markedly as a result of emotional factors that, perhaps, work through the autonomic nervous system (Yalom, 1964); in bronchial asthma, allergy and infection have been identified as two important factors. But in many cases, the underlying factors are difficult to identify and have not been adequately studied. Failure to use control groups may produce difficulties of interpretation. For example, emotional states may be recorded to frequently precede a given illness, but the importance of this observation is difficult to assess if no comparison has been made with the rate at which such stresses occur in a control group; some stressful events occur in most people's lives. Murphy *et al.* (1962) interviewed women who were in the hospital for the normal delivery of a baby and found an average of 2.8 events that might be considered stressful (divorce, death of a relative, change of job, a court appearance, and so on) for each woman during the previous year. Similarly, observations on the personality of patients are difficult to evaluate if no comparison is made with control groups.

When coordinated changes in different systems are found, we are still far from understanding their relationships. For example, many factors, both genetic and environmental, may affect the resistance of organs to disease, their mode of functioning, and also features of personality; lack of sufficient food in childhood might have such effects. Or a change in one system may be the result of a disturbance in another. An added source of complexity arises from the possibility that the mechanisms of learning may play a part in altering the normal functioning of systems at different levels, without the patient's knowledge.

A traditional view is that "body" and "mind" are separately subject to physical and mental illnesses, but that they may interact to produce a third category of "psychosomatic" complaints. This interaction then seems to present a special problem. As Francis Bacon (1561–1626) put it:

> For the consideration is double, either how, and how farre the humours and affects of the bodie doe alter or work upon the minde; or againe, how and how farre the passions, or apprehensions of the mind doe alter or work upon the bodie.

But when we consider the whole range of disorders in terms of the control systems involved, we see that this traditional form of the problem is misleading. Instead we find that there are many levels of control, which can interact in many ways, and that purely "physical" and purely "mental" diseases are just two extremes of the range of possible kinds of disorders.

GLOSSARY

ACETYLCHOLINE—a chemical, released by a nerve fiber, that contracts a muscle.

ADRENAL MEDULLA—the central portion of the adrenal gland that produces the hormones, adrenaline and noradrenaline.

ADRENALINE (EPINEPHRINE)—a substance secreted by the adrenal gland that, among other things, causes heart rate to speed up, the peripheral blood vessels to constrict, the bronchia of the lungs to dilate, the mucus of the nose to dry, and the pupil of the eye to enlarge.

ADRENOCORTICOTROPIC HORMONE (ACTH)—a hormone secreted by the pituitary gland.

ANOREXIA NERVOSA—self-induced food aversion and loss of appetite which serves as a solution to psychic conflicts.

ANTERIOR PITUITARY GLAND—a gland that reacts to physical or emotional difficulty by secreting a hormone, adrenocorticotrophic hormone, which, in turn, stimulates the adrenal cortex to increase its output of hormones.

ANTIBODIES—substances, produced by the spleen, lymph nodes, or bone marrow, that attack foreign organisms in the body by destroying their antigens.

ANTIDIURETIC HORMONE—a hormone that causes water retention in the body.

ANTIGEN—a substance in an attacking organism present in the bloodstream of another organism.

APHASIA—a disturbance in the ability to produce and understand speech.

ARTERIES—blood vessels that carry blood *away* from the heart.

AUTOIMMUNE RESPONSE—the production of antibodies that are harmful to the organism's own tissues.

AUTONOMIC NERVOUS SYSTEM—a major division of the nervous system, concerned chiefly with the regulation of the glands and internal muscles.

AXON—the extension on a nerve cell that carries impulses away from the cell body.

BLOOD PRESSURE—the pressure exerted by the blood on the walls of the blood vessels.

BLOOD SUGAR LEVEL—the amount of glucose in the blood.

BRAIN STEM—the portion of the brain nearest the spinal column; the part of the brain that remains when the cerebrum and the cerebellum are removed.

BRONCHI—the vessels in the lung that allow the passage of air.

BRONCHIAL ASTHMA—asthma resulting from the spasmodic contraction of the bronchial muscles.

CARDIOVASCULAR—pertaining to the heart and blood vessels.

CAROTID ARTERY—artery in the neck which is the main source of blood for the brain.

CAROTID SINUS—a structure that is part of the carotid artery.

CELL—a particle of living matter equipped to keep itself alive.

CELL MEMBRANE—the outer portion, or covering, of a cell.

CENTRAL NERVOUS SYSTEM—the brain and spinal cord.

CEREBELLUM—a part of the hindbrain responsible for coordination.

CEREBRAL HEMISPHERES—the two halves of the cerebrum, which are mainly responsible for man's "higher" behaviors.

CHLORPROMAZINE—a strong tranquilizer.

CHROMOSOMES—rodlike bodies in the nucleus that are considered to be the seat of the genes.

CLASSICAL CONDITIONING—the process of establishing "connections" between a neutral stimulus (such as a bell) and a meaningful one (such as delicious food which makes one salivate) such that the neutral stimulus evokes the meaningful response (salivation).

COCHLEA—the spiral bony tube in the inner ear which contains the hearing mechanism.

COMMUNICATION CHANNEL—the means or mode of communicating information between a "speaker" and a receiver.

COMPULSIVE BEHAVIOR—irrational, repetitive actions.

CONDITIONING—the learning of a particular response as a consequence of specific stimuli which either elicit or reward it.

CONE—a specialized cell in the retina of the eye that enables light and color differentiation.

CONTROL MECHANISM—in this context, a mechanism by which some aspect of the inner environment is regulated; for example, a reduction in blood-sugar affects some specialized cells (the "mechanism"), which, in turn, "tell" us that we are hungry.

CONTROL SYSTEM—a means by which some aspect of the inner environment is regulated; oxygen level, blood sugar level, and so on are all regulated by control systems.

CONVERSION HYSTERIA—a form of neurotic behavior involving both the belief that one is physically ill and the manifestation of symptoms of illness, which may consist of paralysis, blindness, deafness, and such; to be distinguished from malingering, which consists primarily of simulation of physical illness without the belief that one is ill.

CORRELATION—a relationship between two things such that a change in one is accompanied by a corresponding change in the other.

CORTEX—the covering, or outer layer, of a (brain) structure; sometimes used interchangeably with cerebral cortex.

CRETINISM—physical and mental retardation caused by an absence of thyroid at birth.

CYBERNETICS—the science which studies the control and direction of complex systems.

CYTOPLASM—the amorphous substance of a cell, excluding the nucleus.

DEPOLARIZATION—the movement of positive ions through the cell membrane and into a neuron, allowing information, in the form of electrical impulses, to be transmitted.

DEPRESSION—an emotional state of great sadness, often accompanied by guilt and anxiety, gloomy ruminations, lassitude, inability to respond to pleasant stimuli, and suicidal impulses.

DIABETES—a disease manifested by the body's failure to transmit blood glucose to the cells, caused by an insufficiency of insulin.

DIABETIC COMA—a state of unconsciousness resulting from the body's inability to metabolize glucose normally.

DIASTOLIC BLOOD PRESSURE—the blood pressure obtained during the period in which the heart cavities fill with blood.

DIGITAL COMPUTER—a computer that operates on a numerical system.

DUODENAL ULCER—a damaged area in the lining of the duodenum.

DUODENUM—the first part of the small gut, which arises from the stomach.

DRIVES—predisposing forces in the individual, both biological (primary) and learned (secondary), that sensitize him to certain classes of stimuli within the environment.

ELECTRIC RESISTANCE OF THE SKIN—see GALVANIC SKIN RESPONSE.

ELECTRODERMAL RESPONSE—see GALVANIC SKIN RESPONSE.

ENDOCRINE GLANDS—glands that secrete hormones directly into the blood system; the *endocrine system* is a group of endocrine glands that have an integrated function.

ENZYME—a substance secreted by the body cells that induces chemical changes in other substances; enzymes secreted by the stomach aid in digesting food.

EPILEPSY—the name given to a group of nervous diseases marked primarily by convulsions.

ESTROGEN—a hormone, produced by the ovaries, that regulates female sexual development and the menstrual cycle.

EXCITATORY DRIVE MECHANISM—nervous or hormonal mechanisms which produce drive-related activity.

FALSE PREGNANCY—a condition in which the characteristics of pregnancy occur when there is no physiological basis for them.

FEEDBACK—the return, in the form of information, to the input of a part of the output of a system.

FEEDBACK, NEGATIVE—information regarding the relative absence of a necessary substance in the system; negative feedback leads to a correction that is in the opposite direction of the error.

FISTULA—an abnormal passage leading from an abscess or hollow organ to the body surface or from one hollow organ to another.

FOREBRAIN—the largest and most noticeable part of the brain in man; it has a hollow central core, with a floor known as the hypothalamus, and two big outgrowths, one on either side, known as the cerebral hemispheres.

FRONTAL CORTEX—the outer layer of the frontal lobes.

FRONTAL LOBE—the most frontal division of the cerebral cortex, presumed to be responsible for skilled motor behaviors, social sensitivity, initiative, and long-term planning.

GALVANIC SKIN RESPONSE—electrical reactions of the skin, detected by a galvanometer.

GANGLIA—bundles of nerves.

GENE—an inferred submicroscopic structure in the chromosomes which is the physical unit of heredity.

GENITALIA—the organs of the reproductive system, especially the external ones.

GLANDS—groups of cells that develop the ability to secrete special substances.

GLOVE ANESTHESIA—a condition in which a person cannot move or feel the part of the arm and hand that a glove would normally cover.

GLUCOSE—sugar.

GONAD—a primary sex gland; ovary, testis.

GONADOTROPIC HORMONES—hormones that stimulate, or act upon, the gonads.

HEREDITARY—logically determined by transmission through the parents.

HINDBRAIN—the part of the brain that lies immediately above the spinal cord; it controls body positioning in space, produces chewing and swallowing when food is in the mouth, controls the heart rate, and organizes respiration.

HOMEOSTASIS—the process of maintaining the equilibrium of body substances (fluids, salts, sugars, and so forth); it is controlled by negative feedback.

HOMEOSTATIC SYSTEMS—systems whereby homeostasis is maintained; when there is a deficiency of some body substance in the bloodstream, a homeostatic system triggers off processes whereby more of that substance is either manufactured in the body or procured from the environment (negative feedback).

HORMONES—a chemical substance produced by the endocrine glands.

HYDROCHLORIC ACID—a strong acid, normally present in very dilute form in gastric juices.

HYPERTENSION—high blood pressure.

HYPERTHYROIDISM—a disorder caused by overactivity of the thyroid gland; characterized by loss of weight, nervousness, irritability, and enlargement of the thyroid gland.

HYPNOTIC SUGGESTION—the heightened receptivity of a person under hypnosis to suggestion from the hypnotist.

HYPOCHONDRIAC—a person who is overly concerned about, and pained by, very minor body ailments.

HYPOTHALAMUS—the "floor" of the forebrain, situated beneath the cerebral hemispheres; it is involved mainly in emotional and "drive" behavior, and in homeostatic regulation of the body.

HYSTERICAL ANESTHESIA—a psychogenic disorder in which some part or parts of the body become anesthetized.

HYSTERICAL PARALYSIS—a psychogenic disorder in which some part or parts of the body are paralyzed, entirely without organic basis.

IMMUNITY SYSTEM—the spleen, lymph nodes, and bone marrow, which produce antibodies that provide immunity to certain diseases.

IMPULSE—in the context of neural transmission, the outcome of the process of depolarization of the nerve cell membrane and axon; it transmits the cell's "message."

INFORMATION TRANSFER—the passage of information from a source to a receiver.

INSTINCTS—in this context, systems that organize behavior to serve essential needs such at eating, drinking, and sexual activity.

INSTRUMENTAL LEARNING—learning of a behavior that effects an alteration in the environment.

INSULIN—a hormone, produced by the pancreas, that makes blood sugar move from the blood into the cells; insufficient quantities of insulin cause diabetes.

INSULINOMA—a tumor in the pancreas that may force it to produce large quantities of insulin without reference to the body's needs.

IONS—atoms or molecules in solution that have an electrical (either positive or negative) charge.

Kleptomania—a disorder involving the obsessive impulse to steal.

Labyrinth—that part of the ear which is sensitive to the position of the head in space.

Lateral hypothalamus—the side of the hypothalamus, which elicits food-related activity or arousal (hunger drive).

Mania—excitement manifested by mental and physical hyperactivity, disorganization of behavior, and elevation of mood.

Manic-depressive psychosis—a group of disorders characterized by states of overexcitement and elation (mania) or of sadness and hypoactivity (depression), or of oscillations between these.

Medulla—the lowest portion of the brain.

Midbrain—the portion of the brain between the fore- and the hindbrain, it contributes to the general level of muscle tone produced by spinal mechanisms.

Migraine—a severe, often incapacitating headache that recurs at regular or irregular intervals.

Mongolism—a hereditary form of mental retardation.

Muscle spindles—sensory receptors in the muscle that are activated when a muscle is stretched.

Neurons—nerve cells; sensory neurons receive messages from sensory receptors, motor neurons excite muscles or glands, and interneurons carry messages to the motor neurons or away from the sensory neurons.

Noradrenaline—a substance secreted by the adrenal medulla that produces the variety of body reactions that characterize the anxious state.

Nucleus—the central part in a cell which contains the genes; it is essential to the life of that cell.

Nystagmus—rapid, uncontrollable, back-and-forth movements of the eyes under certain conditions.

Occipital lobe—the portion of a cerebral hemisphere that is critical for visual processes.

Operant conditioning—the process of learning to "operate" on the environment in order to gain reward.

Ovaries—the female endocrine glands that produce estrogen (a hormone) and ova (eggs).

Ovulation—the release of an ovum by an ovary.

Ovum—the egg produced by an ovary.

Pancreas—a large gland that secretes digestive enzymes and the hormone insulin.

Parietal lobe—the lobe of the cerebral cortex that is on the side of the cerebral hemisphere.

Pathological—altered or caused by disease.

Pepsin—a digestive enzyme produced by the pancreas.

Pituitary gland—an important gland at the base of the brain necessary to sexual development (in the female) the sexual cycle; it regulates endocrine control and is, in turn, controlled by the hypothalamus.

Polarization—the maintenance of a positive charge outside the neuron and a negative charge inside the neuron.

Premenstrual tension—disturbances of mood preceding menstruation, probably caused by an irregularity of hormone production.

Progesterone—a hormone produced by the ovaries, which prepares the lining of the uterus for pregnancy.

Program—as used here, a set of instructions (for the computer).

Psychosomatic symptoms — persistent physiological symptoms or impairments that originate in psychological distress.

Puberty—the period of time in which secondary sex characteristics appear.

Reagin—an antibody that in some cases provokes excessively intense reactions known as allergic responses.

Reflex—a very simple act in which there is no element of choice or premeditation and no variability save in intensity or time.[1]

Reticular system—a network of interneurons in the hind- and midbrains that controls muscle tension throughout the body.

Retina—the sensory membrane of the eye that receives the image formed by the lens; it is the immediate instrument of vision.

Rhinencephalon—the chiefly olfactory part of the forebrain.

Rod—a rod-shaped structure in the retina believed to enable achromatic vision.

[1] This definition is taken from H. B. English and Ava C. English, *A Comprehensive Dictionary of Psychological and Psychoanalytical Terms*, New York: David McKay Company, Inc., 1958.

SCHIZOPHRENIA—a group of psychotic reactions characterized by fundamental disturbances in reality relationships, by a conceptual world determined largely by feeling, and by marked affective, intellectual, and overt behavioral disturbances.[1]

SENSOR—a receptor or sense organ.

SENSORY INFORMATION—information about the environment obtained by the sensory receptors.

SENSORY RECEPTORS—neurons capable of responding to the physical conditions of the environment.

SHAPING—a Skinnerian procedure in which a desired response is obtained by rewarding successive approximations to that response.

SKINNER BOX—a device for studying learning used primarily with animals.

SOMATOPHYSIC—pertaining to a mental condition which has a somatic basis.

SPASTIC—pertaining to a condition in which the muscles are taut and resist movement.

SPINAL CORD—the long bundle of nerve tissue that extends down the back.

STRETCH REFLEX—the immediate subcortical response produced by stretching the muscle spindles (as in the "knee jerk").

SYMPATHETIC NERVOUS SYSTEM—that part of the nervous system that helps regulate the functions of the heart, lungs, blood vessels, and various internal organs.

SYNAPSE—the junction where an impulse from one neuron passes to another.

TEMPORAL LOBE—the portion of the cerebral hemisphere lying under the temple; it is implicated in hearing, memory, and drive-regulated behavior.

TESTES—the male reproductive gland responsible for the secretion of testosterone.

TESTOSTERONE—the hormone responsible for the growth and development of sex characteristics in the male.

THROMBOSIS—formation of a blood clot.

THYROID GLAND—a shield-shaped structure at the base of the neck that produces thyroxin, a hormone essential for proper growth and development.

THYROPTIC HORMONE—the hormone released by the anterior pituitary gland and capable of controlling the activity of the thyroid.

TIC—a nervous twitch that cannot be voluntarily controlled.

TISSUES—the groupings of similar cells in the body, such as muscle, bone, and nerve.

ULNAR NERVE—an afferent (sensory) nerve in the hand.

VAGUS NERVE—a nerve from the medulla that connects with most of the organs of the body, including the heart, lungs, liver, stomach, and much of the digestive tract.

VENTROMEDIAL NUCLEUS OF THE HYPOTHALAMUS—a portion of the hypothalamus important for the control of eating, known as the satiety center; lesions in this area produce overeating.

REFERENCES

Adams, D. D. Pathogenesis of the hyperthyroidism of Graves' disease. *British Medical Journal*, 1965, **1**, 1015–1019.

Alexander, F. *Psychosomatic medicine: Its principles and applications*. New York: W. W. Norton & Company, Inc., 1950.

Anand, B. K. Nervous regulation of food intake. *Physiological Review*, 1961, **41**, 677–708.

Anderson, J. R., D. G. Gray, D. G. Middleton, and J. A. Young. Autoimmunity and thyrotoxicosis. *British Medical Journal*, 1964, **2**, 1630–1632.

Ax, A. F. The physiological differentiation between fear and anger in humans. *Psychosomatic Medicine*, 1953, **15**, 433–442.

———. Goals and methods of psychophysiology. *Psychophysiology*, 1964, **1**, 8–25.

Bayliss, L. E. *Living control systems*. London: English Universities Press, 1966.

Blitzer, J. R., N. Rollins, and A. Blackwell. Children who starve themselves: Anorexia nervosa. *Psychosomatic Medicine*, 1961, **23**, 369–383.

Black, S. Inhibition of immediate-type hypersensitivity response by direct suggestion under hypnosis. *British Medical Journal*, 1963*a*, **1**, 925–929.

———. Shift in dose-response curve of Prausnitz-Kustner reactions by direct suggestion under hypnosis. *British Medical Journal*, 1963*b*, **1**, 990–992.

———, J. H. Humphrey, and J. S. F. Niven. Inhibition of Mantoux reaction by direct suggestion under hypnosis. *British Medical Journal*, 1963, **1**, 1649–1652.

Bornstein, B., and D. P. Kidron. Prosopagnosia. *Journal of Neurology, Neurosurgery and Psychiatry*, 1959, **22**, 124–131.

Brady, J. V. Ulcers in "executive" monkeys. *Scientific American*, 1958, **199**, No. 4, 95–100.

Brewer, C. V. *The organization of the central nervous system*. London: William Heinemann, Ltd., 1961.

Brown-Grant, K. The effect of ACTH and adrenal steroids on thyroid activity, with observations on the adrenal-thyroid relationship. *Journal of Physiology*, 1956, **131**, 58–69.

——— and G. Pethis. The response of the thyroid gland of the guinea-pig to stress. *Journal of Physiology*, 1960, **151**, 40–50.

Cannon, W. B. *The wisdom of the body*. New York: W. W. Norton & Company, Inc., 1932.

Castelnuovo-Tedesco, P. Emotional antecedents of perforation of ulcers of the stomach and duodenum. *Psychosomatic Medicine*, 1962, **24**, 398–416.

Cobb, S. Some clinical changes in behavior accompanying endocrine disorders. *Journal of Nervous and Mental Diseases*, 1960, **130**, 97–106.

Cowan, W. K. Blood groups and disease. ABH antigens on human duodenal cells. *British Medical Journal*, 1962, **2**, 946–948.

Critchley, M. *The parietal lobes*. London: Edward Arnold & Co., 1953.

Dally, P. and W. Sargent. Treatment and outcome of anorexia nervosa. *British Medical Journal*, 1966, **2**, 793–795.

Dalton, K. Menstruation and acute psychiatric illnesses. *British Medical Journal*, 1959, **1**, 148–149.

———. Schoolgirls' behavior and menstruation. *British Medical Journal*, 1960, **2**, 1647–1649.

Deutsch, J. A., and D. Deutsch. *Physiological psychology*. Homewood, Ill.: Dorsey Press, 1966.

Docommun, P., E. Sakiz, and R. Guillemin. Dissociation of the acute secretions of thyrotropin and adrenocorticotropin. *American Journal of Physiology*, 1966, **210**, 1257–1259.

Dunbar, F. *Emotions and bodily changes*. New York: Columbia University Press, 1954.

Engel, B. T., and A. F. Bickford. Response-specificity: Stimulus-response and individual-response specificity in essential hypertensives. *Archives of General Psychiatry*, 1961, **5**, 478–489.

Fulton, J. F. *Functional localization in the frontal lobes and cerebellum*. New York: Oxford University Press, 1949.

Funkenstein, D. H. Variations in response to standard amounts of chemical agents during lacerations in feeling states in relation to occurrence of asthma. *Research Publications of the Association of Nervous and Mental Diseases*, 1950, **29**, 566–582.

———S. H. King and M. E. Drolette. *Mastery of stress*. Cambridge, Mass.: Harvard University Press, 1957.

Gellhorn, E., and G. N. Loofbourrow. *Emotions and emotional disorders*. New York: Harper & Row, Publishers, 1963.

Glynn, L. E., and E. J. Holborow. *Autoimmunity and disease*. Oxford: Blackwell Scientific Publications, 1965.

Graham, D. T., J. D. Kabler, and F. K. Graham. Physiological response to the suggestion of attitudes specific for hives and hypertension. *Psychosomatic Medicine*, 1962, **24**, 159–169.

———, R. M. Lundy, L. S. Benjamin, J. D. Kabler, W. C. Lewis, N. O. Kunish, and F. K. Graham. Specific attitudes in initial interviews with patients having different "psychosomatic" diseases. *Psychosomatic Medicine*, 1962, **24**, 257–266.

Graham, F. E., and R. K. Clifton. Heart-rate change as a component of the orienting response. *Psychological Bulletin*, 1966, **65**, 305–320.

Greaves, D. D., P. E. Green, and L. J. West. Psychodynamic and psychophysiological aspects of pseudocyesis. *Psychosomatic Medicine*, 1960, **22**, 25–31.

Guilbaud, C. T. *What is cybernetics?* London: William Heinemann, Ltd., 1959.

Hartog, M. Hormones and the endocrine system. *British Medical Journal*, 1966, **1**, 225–227.

Head, H. *Aphasia and kindred disorders of speech*. New York: Crowell-Collier and Macmillan, Inc., 1926.

Herberg, L. J. The hypothalamus and the aetiology of migraine. *Proceedings of First Migraine Trust Symposium*. London: William Heinemann, Ltd., 1967.

Hess, W. R. *The functional organization of the diencephalon*. New York: Grune & Stratton, Inc., 1957.

Hoagland, H. Some endocrine stress responses in man. In A. Simon, C. C. Herbert, and R. Straus (eds.), *The physiology of emotions*. Springfield, Ill.: Charles C Thomas, Publisher, 1961.

Holmes, T. H., T. Treuting, and H. G. Wolff. Life situations, emotions and nasal disease: Evidence on summative effects exhibited in patients with "hay-fever." *Research Publications of the Association of Nervous and Mental Diseases,* 1959, **29,** 445–457.

Kaplan, S. M., and E. D. Hetrick. Thyrotoxicosis, traumatic neurosis, and the dangerous environment. *Psychosomatic Medicine,* 1962, **24,** 240–248.

Knapp, P. H. Acute bronchial asthma: II. Psychoanalytic observations on fantasy, emotional arousal, and partial discharge. *Psychosomatic Medicine,* 1960, **22,** 88–105.

——— and S. J. Nemetz. Acute bronchial asthma: I. Concommitant depression and excitement, and varied antecedent patterns in 406 attacks. *Psychosomatic Medicine,* 1960, **22,** 25–31.

Knight, J. A. False pregnancy in a male. *Psychosomatic Medicine,* 1960, **22,** 260–266.

Kuntz, A. *The autonomic nervous system.* Philadelphia: Lea & Febiger, 1953.

Lacey, J. I., J. Kagan, B. C. Lacey, and H. A. Moss. The visceral level: Situational determinants and behavioral correlates of autonomic response patterns. In P. Knapp (ed.), *Expression of the emotions in man.* New York: International Universities Press, Inc., 1962.

Levine, S., and R. F. Mullins. Hormonal influences on brain organization in infant rats. *Science,* 1966, **152,** 1585–1592.

Lidz, T., and J. C. Whitehorn. Life situations, emotions and Graves' disease. *Research Publications of the Association of Nervous and Mental Diseases,* 1950, **29,** 445–457.

Malmo, R. B., and C. Shagass. Physiologic study of symptom mechanisms in psychiatric patients under stress. *Psychosomatic Medicine,* 1949, **11,** 25–29.

Marler, P., and W. J. Hamilton. Mechanisms of animal behavior. New York: John Wiley & Sons, Inc., 1966.

McCleary, R. A., and R. Y. Moore. *Subcortical mechanisms of behavior: The psychological functions of primitive parts of the brain.* New York: Basic Books, Inc., 1965.

Meek, J. C., A. E. Jones, U. J. Lewis, and W. P. VanderLaan. Characterization of the long-acting thyroid stimulator of Graves' disease. *Proceedings of the National Academy of Science,* 1964, **52,** 342–349.

Miall, W. E., and P. D. Oldham. The hereditary factor in arterial blood pressure. *British Medical Journal,* 1963, **1,** 75–80.

Miller, N. W. Extending the domain of learning. *Science,* 1966, **152,** 676.

Morgan, C. T., and E. Stellar. *Physiological psychology,* Ed. 3. New York: McGraw-Hill, Inc., 1965.

Murphy, G. E., N. O. Kuhn, R. F. Christensen, and E. Robins. "Life stress" in a normal population: A study of 101 women hospitalized for normal delivery. *Journal of Nervous and Mental Diseases,* 1962, **134,** 150–161.

Penfield, W., and T. Rasmussen. *The cerebral cortex of man.* New York: Crowell-Collier and Macmillan, Inc., 1950.

——— and L. Roberts. *Speech and brain mechanisms.* Princeton, N.J.: Princeton University Press, 1959.

Pevzner, S., B. Bornstein, and M. Lowenthal. Prosopagnosia. *Journal of Neurology, Neurosurgery and Psychiatry,* 1962, **25,** 336–338.

Pickering, G. Hyperpiesis: High blood pressure without evident cause—essential hypertension. *British Medical Journal,* 1965, **2,** 959–968, 1021–1026.

Piel, G., D. Flanagan, L. Svirsky, G. A. W. Boehm, R. W. Ginna, J. Le Corbeiller, J. R. Newman, E. P. Rosenbaum, and J. Grunbaum (eds.), *Automatic control.* London: G. Bell & Sons, Ltd., 1955.

Rees, L. The role of emotional and allergic factors in hay fever. *Psychosomatic Research,* 1959, **3,** 234–241.

Rosenzweig, M. R. Environmental complexity, cerebral change, and behavior. *American Psychologist,* 1966, **21,** 321, 332.

Saslow, G., G. C. Gressel, F. O. Shobe, P. H. DuBois, and H. A. Schroeder. The possible etiological relevance of personality factors in arteria hypertension. *Research Publications of the Association for Research in Nervous and Mental Diseases,* 1950, **29,** 881–897.

Sasmor, R. M. Operant conditioning of a small scale muscle response. *Journal of Experimental Analysis of Behavior.* 1966, **9,** 69–85.

Sawrey, W. L.. Conditioned responses of

fear in relationship to ulceration. *Journal of Comparative and Physiological Psychology*, 1961, **54**, 347–348.

——— and J. M. Sawrey. Conditioned fear and restraint in ulceration. *Journal of Comparative Physiological Psychology*, 1964, **57**, 150–151.

Scoville, W. B., and B. Milner. Loss of recent memory after bilateral hippocampal lesions. *Journal of Neurology, Neurosurgery and Psychiatry*, 1957, **20**, 11–21.

Shearn, D. W. Operant conditioning of heart rate. *Science*, 1962, **137**, 530–531.

Smith, R. W. Discriminative heart rate conditioning with sustained inspiration as respiratory control. *Journal of Comparative Physiological Psychology*, 1966, **61**, 221–226.

Stern, J. A., G. Winokur, D. T. Graham, and F. K. Graham. Alterations in physiological measures during experimentally induced attitudes. *Journal of Psychosomatic Research*, 1961, **5**, 73–82.

Sternbach, R. A. *Principles of psychophysiology*. New York: Academic Press, Inc., 1966.

Taylor, S. W. Wooing sleep. *British Medical Journal*, 1962, **1**, 879.

Todd, J., A. D. Collins, F. R. R. Martin, and K. E. Dewhurst. Mental symptoms due to insulinomata. Report on two cases. *British Medical Journal*, 1962, **2**, 828–831.

Verplanck, W. S. The operant conditioning of human motor behavior. *Psychological Bulletin*, 1956, **53**, 70–83.

Weiner, H., M. Thaler, M. R. Reiser, and I. A. Mirsky. Etiology of duodenal ulcer: I. Relation of specific psychological characteristics to rate of gastric secretion (serum pepsinogen). *Psychosomatic Medicine*, 1957, **19**, 1–10.

Wolf, S., and H. G. Wolff. *Human gastric function: An experimental study of a man and his stomach*. New York: Oxford University Press, 1947.

Wolff, H. G. *Stress and disease*. Springfield, Ill.: Charles C Thomas, Publisher, 1953.

———, S. G. Wolf, and C. C. Hare (eds.), *Life stress and bodily disease. Research Publications of the Association for Research in Nervous and Mental Diseases*, 1950, **29**.

Wright, S. *Applied physiology*, Ed. 8. New York: Oxford University Press, 1945.

Yalom, I. D. Plantar warts: A case study. *Journal of Nervous and Mental Diseases*, 1964, **138**, 163–171.

SUGGESTED READINGS

1. Brady, J. V. Ulcers in "executive" monkeys. *Scientific American*, 1958, **199**, No. 4, 95–100. A report of an experiment showing that monkeys who were able to *terminate* shock after its onset (by pressing a lever) developed ulcers, while monkeys who received the same amount of shock, but were not able to terminate it, did not develop ulcers.
2. Brewer, C. V. *The organization of the central nervous system*. London: William Heinemann, Ltd., 1961. A text of neuroanatomy and neurological function.
3. Guilbaud, C. T. *What is cybernetics?* London: William Heinemann, Ltd., 1959. An introductory text on feedback theory and cybernetics.
4. Hebb, D. O. *The organization of behavior*. New York: John Wiley & Sons, Inc., 1949. A significant speculative treatise on the relations between brain and behavior.
5. Morgan, C. T., and E. Stellar. *Physiological psychology*, Ed. 3. New York: McGraw-Hill, Inc., 1965. A general text in physiological psychology.
6. Wolf, S., and H. G. Wolff. *Human gastric function: An experimental study of a man and his stomach*. New York: Oxford University Press, 1947. The classic study of Tom, who had a fistula in his stomach through which his physicians could observe the effects of his emotional state on the state of his stomach lining.

14

EDWARD ZIGLER

Mental Retardation

Mental retardation is a problem of serious social concern, a concern justified by the large number of persons in our society who are considered mentally retarded. The conventional assumption is that 3 percent of the population is retarded, and on this basis the President's Panel on Mental Retardation (1962) estimated that almost 5½ million children and adults in the United States are mentally retarded. The criterion for mental retardation established in the *Manual on Terminology and Classification in Mental Retardation* (Heber, 1959) and adopted by the American Association on Mental Deficiency as well as the Biometrics Branch of the National Institute of Mental Health the mean IQ of the population: is all persons whose IQ's fall one standard deviation below the population mean are considered retarded. If one accepts this criterion (and many do not, such as Garfield and Wittson, 1960), there are almost 30 million mental retardates in the United States. According to the more conservative 3 percent estimate, mental retardation is twice as prevalent as blindness, polio, cerebral palsy, and rheumatic heart conditions combined (Doll, 1962)!

The typical textbook pictures the distribution of intelligence as *normal* or Gaussian in nature, with approximately the lowest 3 percent of the distribution encompassing the mentally retarded (see Chapter 1). A common class of persons is thus constructed, a class defined by intelligence test performance which results in a score between 0 and 70. This schema has misled many laymen and students and has subtly but harmfully influenced

Preparation of this article was facilitated by Research Grant MH-06809 from the National Institute of Mental Health, United States Public Health Service, and the Gunnar Dybwad Award of the National Association for Retarded Children. The author is deeply indebted to Susan Harter for her help in organizing this paper and for her assistance in clarifying many of the ideas presented. Thanks are also extended to Frances Capobianco for her critical reading of the manuscript.

the approach of experienced workers in the area. For if one fails to appreciate the *arbitrary nature* of the 70 IQ cutoff point, it is but a short step to the false belief that all those falling below this point compose a homogeneous class of "subnormals." Since the conceptual distance between "subnormal" and "abnormal," with its age-old connotation of disease and defect, is minimal, the final false step is to regard retardates as a homogeneous group of defective organisms, immutably different from persons with higher IQ's.

The idea that mental retardates are a homogeneous group is seen in numerous research studies that make comparisons between retardates and normals solely on the basis of IQ. The view that mental retardates, as a group, are "different" is most vividly encountered in comparative studies that put mental retardates in a position on the phylogenetic scale somewhere between monkeys and children of average intellect. It is of some interest to note that people whose performance on intelligence tests is deficient are usually not called mental *deficients* but rather mental *defectives*.

The defect orientation to mental retardation originally included the notion of moral defect, which stemmed anywhere from the belief that retardates, like other deviants, were possessed by devils to the empirical fact of the higher than average incidence of socially unacceptable behaviors, such as crime and illegitimacy, among them. More recently, the notion of defect has meant defects in either physical or cognitive structures, and this approach has a clearly valid component. A sizable group of retardates suffer from a variety of known physical defects. Mental retardation may be due to a dominant gene, as in epiloia, to a single recessive gene, as in gargoylism, phenylketonuria, and amaurotic idiocy (see Chapter 2), to infections, like congenital syphilis, encephalitis, or rubella in the mother, to chromosomal defects, as in mongolism, to toxic agents such as radiation during intrauterine life or lead poisoning, and to Rh incompatibility or cerebral trauma. (For a complete list of the many types of mental retardation, see Heber, 1959.)

The diverse causes or etiologies noted above have one factor in common: in every instance, examination reveals an abnormal physiological process, that is, specific defects in physiological functioning. Such persons *are* abnormal in the orthodox sense of being disordered since they suffer from a known physiological defect. However, in addition to this group, which forms a minority of all retardates, is the group labeled "familial," or more recently "undifferentiated," which comprises approximately 75 percent of all retardates. This group presents the greatest mystery and has been the object of the most heated disputes in the study of mental retardation. Familial retardation is diagnosed when examination fails to reveal any of the physiological manifestations noted above and when retardation exists among parents, siblings, or other relatives. As will be seen in a later section, several writers have extended the notion of defect to this type of retardate. On the basis of differences in performance between retardates and normals on some experimental task, rather than on physiological evidence, they have advanced the view that *all* retardates suffer from some specifiable defect over and above their general intellectual retardation. These theoreticians differ, as to the specific nature of the defect. It is helpful to an understanding of mental retardation if a distinction is maintained between *physiologically defective* retardates with known etiologies and *familial retardates* whose etiology is unknown. For the most part, work with physically defective retardates involves investigation into the exact nature of the underlying physiological processes with the goals of removing or ameliorating the physical and intellectual symptoms. Jervis (1959) has suggested that such "pathological" mental deficiency is primarily the domain of medical sciences, whereas familial retardation represents a problem for behavioral scientists, including educators and behavioral geneticists. Diagnostic and incidence studies of these two types of retardates have disclosed certain striking differences between them. The retardate with an extremely low IQ (below 40) is almost invariably of the defective type, though one can find defective retardates at every level of retardation. Familial retardates, on the other hand, are almost invariably mildly retarded; their IQ's are usually above 50.

The belief that the familial retardate must suffer from a defect analogous to that found in other retardates dates back to the early history of psychiatry. When one mental disorder, paresis, was found to be a result of a specific disease entity (syphilis), Kraepelin (1912) and the *organically oriented* psychiatrists who followed him insisted that every mental disorder was the result of a disease or a biochemical defect. Whatever the ontogenesis (the origin of the condition in an individual), the defect position emphasized the innate, if not immutable, difference between retarded and normal intellects.

THE PROBLEM OF DEFINITION

The decision as to whether a person is retarded is often based, not upon his intellectual characteristics, but upon legal and occupational factors and on his general level of social adjustment. The matter has been put most succinctly by Maher (1963), who stated:

> What constitutes mentally retarded behavior depends to a large extent upon the society which happens to be making the judgment. An individual who does not create a problem for others in his social environment and who manages to become self-supporting is usually not defined as mentally retarded no matter what his test IQ may be. Mental retardation is primarily a socially defined phenomenon, and it is in large part meaningless to speak of mental retardation without this criterion in mind. (P. 238.)

This emphasis on social factors in defining mental retardation may produce more confusion than clarity, as indicated by the discrepancies found among various surveys of its prevalence. The data of Table 14.1 imply that the prevalence fluctuates not only across age groups but

Table 14.1

Percentage of Persons Classified as Mentally Retarded

Age	Locality		
	England[1]	Baltimore, Maryland[2]	Syracuse, New York[3]
Under 5	0.12	0.07	0.45
5–9	1.55	1.18	3.94
10–14	2.56	4.36	7.76
15–19	1.08	3.02	4.49

[1] Report of the Mental Deficiency Committee, 1929.
[2] Lemkay *et al.*, 1941.
[3] New York State Technical Report, 1955.

also across localities and even across dates at which data are collected. If mental retardation is defined strictly in terms of IQ, and if we assume a certain constancy of IQ score, we would expect no difference in the prevalence of mental retardation at different ages.

The prevalence reported in Table 14.1 is understandable if one realizes that they reflect diagnoses based on some combination of IQ and success in meeting social demands. For example, the extremely low prevalence under five years of age may reflect the minimal demands which society makes on young children. The highest prevalence, at the ten to fourteen age level, occurs when the child is faced with school and more demanding intellectual tasks. It is probably in this age range that the correspondence between IQ scores and ability to meet societal expectancies, that is, successful school performance, is greatest. Stated somewhat differently, it is probably in this age range that *either* IQ *or* success in meeting social demands would classify a child as mentally retarded or not. A "test-score orientation" to mental retardation results in the view that approximately 3 percent of the population is mentally retarded. The "social competence viewpoint," however, yields a much smaller incidence: data obtained by surveying representative samples of large populations, or the entire population of certain limited regions in England and Scandinavia, indicate that about 1 percent or less of adults are classified as mentally retarded by this means (Dahlberg, 1937; Fremming, 1951; Lewis, 1929; Sjögren, 1948; Strömgren, 1938).

Armed with the information that a person's social adequacy has much to do with whether or not he is considered retarded, we begin to get some inkling of the arbitrariness involved in such a classification. As A. M. Clarke (1958) stated,

> To the extent that mental deficiency is a social concept, with fluctuating thresholds of community tolerance, classification is bound to be somewhat arbitrary, and no system is likely to be either comprehensive or permanent. (P. 64.)

THE NATURE OF INTELLIGENCE

Whether mental retardation is defined by an intelligence test score or by social competence, which many claim reflects intelligence, the essence of mental retardation is still lower intelligence than that displayed by the model member of an appropriate reference group. There is little agreement, however, when the question precipitated by this statement is raised, namely: What is the nature of intelligence? We cannot answer this question by saying that "intelligence is what an intelligence test measures" since it is obvious that the IQ test constructor must have some definition of intelligence in mind before he can select test items. However, some consensus can probably be found for the view that intelligence is a hypothetical construct that ultimately refers to the cognitive processes of the individual, that is, to the caliber of his memory, perceptual discriminations, concept formation, and abstract reasoning. Given this, we still do not know whether intelligence represents a single cognitive process which permeates all other cognitive processes, or whether it represents a variety of relatively discrete cognitive processes which can be sampled and then summated to yield an indication of a person's total intelligence.

In either case, the more important questions are exactly how do such cognitive processes develop over the life-span, and exactly how do genetic and environmental factors interact to influence their development? Approached in this way, the problem of defining intelligence becomes one with the problem of the nature of cognition and its development.

Cognitive and Psychometric Approaches

The implication in the above discussion is that if we are to understand the nature of intelligence, we must consult workers investigating the nature and development of cognitive processes, rather than the work of test constructors and psychometricians. There has been little exchange between these two groups, which have approached the investigation of intellective functioning quite differently.

The former group utilizes a variety of techniques and, through extremely detailed analyses, tries to tease out the intricacies of human cognitive functioning. These scholars have tried to evolve a theory of human cognition and its development. If they had developed intelligence tests, psychology might have avoided the perplexing state of affairs now encountered when one tries to define intelligence. Tests devised by such a group would, of necessity, be indicators of the formal features of the cognitive structure at various times in the life cycle. Recently, workers within this framework (Laurendeau and Pinard, 1962; Woodward, 1963) have taken an interest in the problem of assessment. Although the task of providing an acceptable theory of the development of cognition is far from finished, Laurendeau and Pinard have taken the first step toward the construction of an intelligence test based on the formal features of cognition isolated by Piaget. (See Flavell, 1963, for a review of Piaget's work.)

From a historical point of view, the practical demands of society for a test which would measure intellectual functioning meant that intelligence became the province of the second group, namely, the testers and psychometricians. Furthermore, for a variety of reasons, American thinking has not been receptive to the approach of the cognitive theorists. The practical orientation of the testers can be seen in the efforts of Binet, whose intent was not to investigate the nature of intelligence but rather to discover what test items would discriminate between successful and unsuccessful school performance. As Tuddenham (1962) has pointed out, Binet viewed his empirically selected tests as a social screening device, rather than as a theoretical attack on the nature of intelligence. The success of Binet's test in predicting school achievement led workers to the belief that such tests were inextricably bound to intelligence or cognitive functioning.

For the psychometricians, it then became clear that the nature of intelligence could be understood by examining the nature of the tests employed to measure it. By discovering correlations between tests, it was felt, the structure of intellect would be revealed. However, despite the statistical rigor involved, no very satisfactory theory of intelligence has come out of these correlational or factor analytic methods. There is, in fact, little agreement among workers even on the one constant theoretical issue throughout this body of work, namely, the global versus the specific nature of intelligent behavior—that is, whether intelligence involves a *general ability* which is manifested on all kinds of tasks or a set of *specific abilities* reflected in greater or lesser degree on different kinds of tests.

It should be emphasized that the weakness of current theories of intelligence has led to a conceptual impasse in the area of mental retardation. Without a satisfactory theory of intelligence, the essential aspect of mental retardation must escape us, and we must be content with superficial approaches to this complex problem. We do not necessarily have to await a complete theory of intelligence, however, to cut through much of the complexity, disputation, and confusion in the study of mental retardation. Some clarification appears possible through the simple process of reorienting our approach to the subject. A rather sizable step forward is taken if a simple IQ test approach is abandoned in favor of a concern with cognitive processes.

The Process-Content Distinction

The plea is not that we abandon tests, for every cognitive theorist must eventually employ tests, or devices which can broadly be defined as tests. What is needed is for workers in the field to turn their attention from the superficial content of tests, that is, the right or wrong answer, and come to grips with the problem of the cognitive structures and processes that give rise to content. The distinction between *structure* and *content* has too long escaped most workers in mental retardation. (See Werner, 1937, for further arguments that such a distinction is essential.)

How conventional tests are viewed by process-oriented cognitive theorists can be seen in the following statement by Laurendeau and Pinard (1962):

> Their analytic and artificial character has been emphasized too often to require further reiteration. As Piaget and Inhelder, for instance, pointed out on several occasions, these tests measure only the end product of intellectual activity, but they completely disregard the internal dynamics of mental operation. One would be ill-advised to draw definite conclusions, on the basis of test results, about the quality of the reasoning process or about the fundamental nature of intellectual maturity. (P. 48.)

In general, however, Piaget's approach, with its developmental and normative emphasis, has had very little appeal to students of mental retardation, who are usually committed to the study of *individual* differences, the technical term for conventional measurement practices. In this context, the efforts of Laurendeau and Pinard to construct tests appear very promising since these followers of Piaget have formulated the stages of cognitive development in terms of the cognitive operations achieved, thus emphasizing the nature of the cognitive structure and its processes. In their work we see a bridge between a truly cognitive approach to intelligence and the need, as in the area of mental retardation, for an instrument with which to make comparisons.

The conventional focus on the *content* of test behavior has been carried over to many nontest situations, and often an insufficient distinction is made between intelligence and intelligent behavior. It is my view that "intelligence" must refer to the formal characteristics of the cognitive structure and its processes, whereas "intelligent behavior" should refer to the content of behavior, specifically to the appropriateness, however arbitrarily defined, with which an organism carries out an act. (See Maher, 1963, for another discussion of the distinction between intelligence and intelligent behavior.) Some years ago, for example, we all marveled at Skinner's ping-pong-playing pigeons (Skinner). These pigeons certainly evinced much more intelligent behavior than one would expect to be within their capacity. However, would we want to assert that the cognitive structures of these pigeons had changed, or that these structures were analogous to those of the human adult who evinces similar ping-pong-playing responses? The animals are still only pigeons, and what has been demonstrated is that, *given their cognitive structure*, one can gradually shape their behavior to produce what we might call very intelligent behavior *for a pigeon*.

This shaping phenomenon can also take place among the mentally retarded. In a sheltered workshop, I recently encountered a retardate working with a surprisingly complex piece of machinery. His ability to use this machinery defied knowledge then current about the capabilities of the retarded. The director of the workshop explained that the retardate had been taught to operate the machine through a shaping process like that Skinner used in training his pigeons. It was also learned that the retardate could handle the machine quite adequately provided its position was not changed. When the machine was rotated about 90 degrees, the retardate became somewhat agitated and was no longer able to operate it. (Piaget has also observed that remarkable intellectual feats performed by children in a task cannot be repeated after relatively minor alterations in the task stimuli.) Ordinarily, however, the retardate behaved just as intelligently with the machine as an operator with a normal IQ. This accomplishment does not indicate that his intelligence had become normal. Presumably he used a more primitive cognitive process to achieve intelligent behavior than the normal person does. These examples should also make it clear that process analyses require a more careful analysis of content than that provided by a superficial "product" criterion of correctness.

Social Competence and Mental Retardation

An emphasis on the contents of behavior, rather than on the underlying cognitive processes which govern it, may also be seen in the definition of mental retardation which emphasizes social competence. We do not know what the intellectual demands of social competence are, and very little effort is made to discover what they might be. In mental retardation, social competence usually means ability to maintain oneself without frequent involvement with state schools, state hospitals, welfare agencies, and police officers. Although social competence defined in this way reflects certain cognitive abilities, it may also reflect other factors reminiscent of important *non*intellectual aspects of intelligence test performance, such as social values, attitudes toward other people, emotional needs, and luck. Thus, existing intelligence tests may predict social competence better than an ideal intelligence test would because of their nonintellectual components.

Social competence does not inevitably reflect normal intellectual functioning any more than its absence in the emotionally unstable, the criminal, or the social misfit reflects intellectual subnormality. It is much too heterogeneous a phenomenon and reflects too many nonintellectual factors to be of great value in understanding mental retardation. The basic problem is that the concept of social competence is so laden with value and its definition so vague that it has little empirical utility. Windle (1962) has pointed out that the social competence definition of mental retardation is applicable only to institutionalized people, whereas quite different criteria must be employed with noninstitutionalized retardates. The only clear and acceptable operational definition of social competence would appear to be related to whether the individual has managed to function outside of an institutional setting.

The need to separate the psychological from the environmental aspects of social adequacy has been noted by Tredgold (1952), who stated,

> To constitute abnormality and defect, the failure must be due to psychological and not to economic and social causes; and there is usually little difficulty in distinguishing between the two.

A. M. Clarke (1958) has pointed out that Tredgold provides no criteria for making such a distinction and correctly points out that

> social criteria (particularly those which are not operationally defined) are just as arbitrary as the IQ, if not more so, and have not even the advantage of being based on norms for an entire population.

The inadequacy of the social competence idea as a part of the definition of retardation has been noted by other investigators as well. Even Heber (1962), who has made the strongest case for employing social competence, has admitted that objective measures of it are presently unavailable and that the social competence construct is so ambiguous that, in practice, intelligence test performance must remain "the most important and heavily weighted of the criteria used."

A further problem with social competence is related to a fallacy which has permeated much of our thinking about retardation. We have somehow come to believe that it is impossible for anyone who is truly retarded to meet the complex demands of our society. But the bulk of retardates with mental ages (MA's) in the nine to twelve range (a MA of sixteen is the upper limit for an individual of average IQ) have the intellectual wherewithal to meet the minimal demands of our society. This becomes immediately apparent if one considers how little intellectual ability is really required to arise in the morning, dress oneself, catch a bus or walk to work, perform some simple labor, and return home. In the 1920's and 30's it was discovered that there were no less than 118 occupations in our society suitable for individuals with mental ages from five to twelve (Beckham, 1930; Burr, 1925). As late as 1956, DeProspo (Whitney, 1956) noted that 54 percent of jobs require no schooling beyond the elementary level.

Another major aspect of social competence is the ability of the individual to abide by the values of the society, that is, to obey laws and so forth. While the incidence of crime among the retarded is higher than among others, it is not terribly great, especially if one controls a study for the social class factor. Here again it is an error to view obedience to the law as something beyond the ability of the retarded, especially if one considers the stages of moral development found by Piaget (1948) and Kohlberg (in press), who discovered that fairly young children are capable of a morality based on absolutism; that is, the rules inhere in the very fabric of existence and are not to be broken under any circumstances. Individuals who never achieve a higher state of moral development are certainly not developmentally adequate, but neither are they likely to break many laws.

If social competence is to be a useful indicator of cognitive functioning, we must abandon any simplistic notion of it in favor of a complex scheme theoretically based upon the cognitive demands society makes of individuals. Such indices could then be considered independent indicators of intellectual functioning. Empirical efforts of this sort may be seen in the Vineland Social Maturity Scale and the Worcester Scale of Social Attainment. A more theoretical effort may be found in the work of Phillips and Zigler (1961, 1964) in which both intelligence test scores and conventional social competence indices are combined into an index of developmental or maturational level.

RETARDATION AND NATURE-NURTURE

It is now possible to turn our attention to the role of cognitive capacity in mental retardation. Maher (1963) believes that the concept of capacity has considerable empirical value for workers in the area of mental retardation. By *intellectual capacity,* we mean something akin to what Hebb (1949) calls "intelligence A," that is, an *innate potential for the development of intellectual functions.* Those who argue that the intellectual capacity notion is a relatively useless one, like Chein (1945), Ferguson (1954, 1956), Liverant (1960), Spiker and McCandless (1954), appear to be invariably committed to an environmentalistic or learning orientation.

Maher's position (1963) is that the capacity concept has value as related to

> the differences between individuals in rate of acquisition of responses under similar learning conditions. Such a concept necessarily implies the existence of structural differences between individuals and is compatible with a psychology of the empty organism. (P. 250.)

It is in this last sentence that we see the theoretical value of the capacity concept; it forces us to view individuals as biological organisms differing innately in their potential manifestation of many traits. Thus the concept of capacity is intimately related to the biological concept of the genotype (see Chapter 2).

The environmentalistic view, while sometimes giving lip serve to the importance of biological capacity, treats human behavior essentially as the outgrowth of experience. One environmentally oriented theorist, McCandless (1964), has argued that, although heredity and environment interact in the production of intelligent behavior, we need only concern ourselves with environment since "we can do something about environment." This approach implies that the manipulations of environments are expected to have constant results. It also ignores the possibility that children with particular capacities will need specific environmental events for maximum cognitive development. The one group that has seriously considered the nature of the interaction between genotype and experiences in producing behavior (phenotypes) has been the behavior geneticists, who, as we saw in Chapter 2, have presented evidence that the effects of particular experiences and the behavior to which they give rise depend upon the biological nature of the organism (Fuller and Thompson, 1960; Gottesman, 1963; Hirsch, 1963).

The attempt to determine the proportion of variance attributable to heredity or to environment is full of difficulties, as we have seen. Jones (1954) has enumerated some of these:

> (1) The proportional contribution of heredity and environment does not refer to the make-up of individual IQ's or to the general level of intelligence, but either to average effects upon individual differences or to differences between groups. (2) Existing studies are based on fallible and incomplete measures both of intelligence and of the environment; this fact should be remembered when the data are being manipulated to yield an apparently highly exact result. (3) Even if it is ever logically feasible to seek a single value for the effect of environment, the particular value reported in a given study may not apply in samples involving (*a*) a different environmental level, (*b*) a different hereditary selection, (*c*) a change in variability of either of the above factors, or (*d*) a change in any special conditions which may affect the interaction of these factors. (P. 633.)

Despite the shortcomings of the nature-nurture work on intelligence, it is still possible to derive certain conclusions. (In addition to Chapter 2, the reader is referred to reviews by Anastasi, 1958; Fuller, 1954; Jones, 1954; McCandless, 1964; McClearn, 1964; Tyler, 1956; Woodworth, 1941.) Studies of parent-child resemblances in intelligence, sibling resemblances, a variety of twin studies, and studies on children in foster homes have made it clear that inherited intellectual endowment is a much more important factor in intelligence than those who are environmentally oriented would have us believe.

At the same time one must not forget the importance of environmental factors on manifest intelligence. The role of environment is evident even where a known genetic defect is the cause of mental retardation. In the case of genetically determined phenylketonuria, subnormal intelligence occurs only in an environment which provides phenylamine in the diet of the affected individual. A specific change in the environment, withholding phenylalanine from the diet, will prevent the occurence of subnormal intelligence. Some thirty years ago Hogben (1933) stated the matter well when he asserted,

> No statement about a genetic difference has any scientific meaning unless it includes or implies a specification of the environment in which it manifests itself in a particular manner (P. 14.)

The importance of genetic factors in intelligence has been stressed by Erlenmeyer-Kimling and Jarvik (1963), who concluded that

> Individual differences in behavioral potential reflect genotypic differences; individual differences in behavioral performance result from the nonuniform recording of environmental stimuli by intrinsically nonuniform organisms. (P. 1478.)

An issue in the nature-nurture controversy of special pertinence to mental retardation concerns the degree to which the environment may produce individual differences in intelligence in contrast to affecting the absolute achievement level of man. It is one thing to assert that the environment plays a role in determining the range of individual differences and quite another to say that environmental events can cause the individual born with a normal intellect to be retarded, or that they can prevent retardation.

This distinction was made by Thorndike (1905), who warned us against confusing two totally different things:

> (1) the power of environment—for instance, of schools, laws, books, and social ideals—to produce differences in the relative achievements of men, and (2) the power of the environment to produce differences in absolute achievement. It has been shown that the relative differences in certain mental traits which were found in . . . one hundred children are due almost entirely to differences in ancestry, not in training; but this does not in the least deny that better methods of training might improve all their achievements fifty percent, or that the absence of training, say in spelling and arithmetic, might decrease the corresponding achievements to zero. (P. 11.)

Different environments as defined, for example, by rural or urban setting, racial and cultural situation, and social class are associated with differences in intelligence. To what extent such differences reflect environmental as opposed to inherited factors remains an open issue. Most students are nurture oriented, and the prevailing argument is that social class or cultural environment produces retardation. To state the matter more simply, the extreme hereditarian asserts that one is in a lower socioeconomic class because one is less intelligent, whereas the extreme environmentalist asserts that one is less intelligent because one is in a lower socioeconomic class. More specifically, mental retardation is sometimes seen as a major consequence of social deprivation. Such a view assumes that children are capable of "normal" intellectual functioning if we expose them to enough "cultural enrichment."

Environmental Factors and Changes in IQ

A question of considerable importance in testing such hypotheses is: how great are the changes that could be effected in IQ as a result of changes in the environment? Many investigators have been relatively pessimistic in their conclusions. Woodworth (1941) has noted certain conclusions that relatively large differences in environment are required to produce any substantial change in IQ. McClearn (1962) has also pointed out that the size of IQ changes attributable to environmental factors, although statistically significant, has been so minute as to be practically negligible. Burks (1928), in a classic study bearing on the nature-nurture controversy, reports findings later confirmed by Leahy (1935):

> Home environment in the most favorable circumstances may suffice to bring a child just under the borderline of dullness up over the threshold of normality, and to make a slightly superior child out of a normal one; but it cannot account for the enormous mental differences to be found among human beings. (P. 308.)

In support of the environmental position, however, rather marked improvements in IQ have sometimes been reported to follow some type of environmental manipulation. McCandless (1964) makes perhaps the strongest statement in favor of the environmentalistic position. The Iowa studies of Coffey and Wellman (1936–1937), Skeels *et al.* (1938), and Wellman (1932–1933, 1934–1935, 1937–1938, 1938*a*) have also reported rather sizable changes in IQ.

Other studies (Smith, 1942; Wheeler, 1942) have indicated that when schools and communication in an area improve, there is a tendency for the IQ's of all the inhabitants to rise. Wheeler's study of Tennessee mountain children is of considerable interest. Testing over 3000 subjects in 1930, he found that IQ's ranged from a mean of 95 among six-year-olds to a mean of 74 at age sixteen. Testing a new sample ten years later, he found a mean increase in IQ of approximately 10 points at every age level! However, he again found a steady decline with age, from a mean of 103 at age six to a mean of 80 at age sixteen, despite the general increase. Jones (1954) has remarked in relation to these findings, "It is a little surprising, however, that the rate of decline in IQ is not affected by the changes which have produced a generally higher level" (P. 658).

There has been a certain inconsistency in studies that have attempted to relate IQ changes to environmental factors. In some instances, significant correlations have been found between subjective ratings of the "goodness" of the environment and increase in IQ (Newman *et al.*, 1937; Thorpe, 1946). But in other instances no environmental correlates could be found to account for changes in the IQ (Bradway, 1945; Jones, 1954). Jones has given some especially striking case histories of children who have manifested marked changes in IQ without the apparent involvement of environmental factors.

A continuing problem has been that of specifying just what constitutes a good environment for optimal intellectual development. The dominant implicit view is that the American middle-class home represents some sort of standard. A related matter, of course, is the problem of defining cultural or social deprivation. The social deprivation concept has been loosely applied to certain events in early childhood which are supposed to be important in the development of certain social behaviors, but there is little agreement as to what either the early events or the resultant behaviors are. Clarke and Clarke (1960) have suggested that the major dimensions of childhood deprivations are: social isolation; cruelty and neglect; institutional upbringing; adverse child-rearing practices; and separation experiences of varying severity. These factors all need much further definition and clarification.

The view that it is extremely difficult to improve the quality of cognitive functioning in a fairly standard environment reflects the bulk of findings resulting from efforts to improve children's performance on Piaget-type tasks (Smedslund, 1961; Wohlwill and Lowe, 1962). Of course, familial retardates do not come from what we consider standard environments. But even with these children, there is considerable evidence that no great intellectual improvement is produced through environmental manipulation with a variety of techniques (Doll, 1962). Binet, with a concept called "mental orthopedics," and Itard, with similarly great faith in the possibility of improving the quality of intellect, were responsible for the philosophy underlying early work with retardates in this country. After several years of using a variety of techniques, many of which are today being rediscovered, it became apparent that their optimism was unwarranted. In the early days, training schools in this country were just what the name implies. They became custodial institutions only when it became apparent that many retardates could not be trained to a level that would make them self-sustaining in society. A reaction appears to have set in at this time, and the view prevailed that we could do nothing for retardates except provide them with a comfortable domicile. There is much for contemporary workers to learn from this marked swing in attitude toward the retarded. It suggests that undue optimism is dangerous since it eventually breeds undue pessimism. Improving both the cognitive functioning and the behavioral adequacy of retardates is not a hopeless task. The last decade has witnessed renewed concern and investigation in the area of cognitive development. Theoreticians like Hunt (1961) and Bruner (1964) have turned their attention to this field and have devised provocative frameworks within which research on improving cognitive functioning is now being conducted. Although these efforts are relatively recent, they may have major implications for the training of the retarded. At a more applied level, we find encouraging efforts in the work of such educators as Kephart (1960) and Kirk (1961).

The conclusion that may be reached concerning the relevance of the heredity and environment controversy for mental retardation has been well stated by Penrose (1963), who, after a lifetime of work with the retarded, wrote:

> The most important work carried out in the field of training defectives is unspectacular. It is not highly technical but requires unlimited patience, good will and common sense. The reward is to be expected not so much in scholastic improvement of the patient as in his personal adjustment to social life. Occupations are found for patients of all grades so that they can take part as fully and usefully as possible in human affairs. This process, which has been termed socialization, contributes greatly to the happiness not only of the patients themselves but also of those who are responsible for their care. (P. 282.)

It is perhaps within the area of socialization that we can do most to enhance the everyday effectiveness of the retarded. Both Burks (1939) and Leahy (1935) discovered that personality and character traits were more influenced by environment than intellectual level was. Such findings bolster the argument that many factors important in the determination of social adjustment can be modified. It is not rare to encounter different individuals with the same intellectual ability demonstrating quite disparate social adjustments. Perhaps the question is not how to improve the cognitive functioning of familial retardates, but rather how to maximize their adjustment whatever their intellectual capacity may be. Considerable change in performance can result from the manipulation of nonintellective, motivational factors, as will be made clear in the final section of this paper.

A Two-Group Approach to Mental Retardation

Hirsch (1963) has asserted that we will make little headway in understanding individual differences in intelligence and many other traits unless we incorporate into our thinking the fact that such differences largely reflect inherent biological properties of man. As we saw in Chapter 2, no genotype spells itself out in a vacuum; the phenotypic expression is finally the result of environment interacting with the genotype. However, as Hirsch has noted, we can no longer make the

> gratuitous uniformity assumption that all genetic combinations are equally plastic and respond in like fashion to environmental influences. . . . Without an appreciation of the genotypic structure of populations, the behavioral sciences have no basis for distinguishing individual differences that are attributable to differences in previous history from those that are not, and no basis for understanding any differences whatsoever where there is a common history. (P. 1442.)

Work in population genetics appears capable of bringing considerable order to the area of mental retardation. From the polygenic model advanced by geneticists (see Chapter 2), we would deduce that the distribution of intelligence is normal, that is, characterized by the bisymmetrical bell-shaped curve described in Chapter 1. This theoretical distribution is a fairly good approximation of what is actually encountered in the observed distribution of intelligence. In the polygenic model of intelligence (see also Gottesman, 1963; Hirsch, 1963; Penrose, 1963), the genetic foundation of intelligence is not viewed as dependent upon a single gene, but as the result of a number of discrete genetic units. (This does not mean, of course, that single gene effects are never to be encountered in mental retardation. As noted earlier, certain relatively rare types of mental retardation are the product of such simple genetic effects.)

Several specific polygenic models propose theoretical distributions of intelligence that are congruent with observed distributions (Burt and Howard, 1956, 1957; Gottesman, 1963; Hurst, 1932; Pickford, 1949). Again, caution is in order. An environmentalistic model positing five environmental factors acting additively would also generate an approximation to a normal curve. However, such a model appears much less capable of encompassing the data encountered in investigations of intelligence. An aspect of polygenic models of special interest for mental retardation is that they generate IQ distributions of approximately 50 to 150. Since an IQ of approximately 50 appears to be the lower limit for familial retardates, it has been concluded (Allen, 1958; Burt, 1958; Burt and Howard, 1956; Penrose, 1963) that the etiology of familial retardation involves the same factors that determine "normal" intelligence. Approached in this way, the familial retardate can be seen as normal, where *normal* is defined as in Chapter 1, that is, representing an integral part of the statistical distribution which goes by that name. Within such a framework, it is possible to refer to the familial retardate as less intelligent, but he is just as integral a part of the normal distribution as the 3 percent of the population who are considered superior or that still more numerous group of individuals that we consider average (McClearn, 1962).

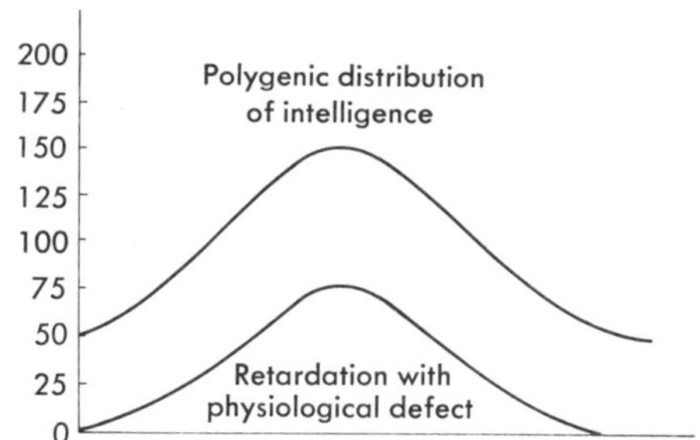

Figure 14.1 The empirical distribution of intelligence.

The two-group approach to mental retardation (familial and defective) calls attention to the fact that the second group, with known physiological defects, represents a distribution of intelligence which is considerably lower (the IQ is usually below 50), on the average, than that of the familial retardates. Thus, the empirical distribution of intelligence may best be represented by two curves (Figure 14.1). Considerable clarity could be brought to the field if we were to stop thinking of the intelligence distribution as a single continuous normal curve. The more appropriate representation is to depict the intelligence of the bulk of the population, including the familial retarded, as a normal distribution with a mean of 100 and lower and upper limits of about 50 and 150 respectively. Superimposed on this curve would be a second somewhat normal distribution with a mean of approximately 35 and a range from 0 to 70. The first curve would represent the polygenic distribution of intelligence; the second would represent the distribution of intelligence among people whose intellectual functioning reflects factors other than the normal polygenic expression, that is, among retardates in whom there is an identifiable physiological defect.

This two-group approach to the problem of mental retardation has been supported by Penrose (1963), Roberts (1952), and Lewis (1933). The very nature of the empirical distribution of IQ's below 100, especially those in the 0 to 50 range (Penrose, 1963), seems to demand such an approach. The resulting total distribution is exactly what we would expect if we combined the two distributions discussed above, as is the general practice.

Once we adopt the position that the familial mental retardate is not defective or pathological but essentially a normal individual of low intelligence, the problem of familial retardation becomes part of the general problem of developmental psychology. In terms of cognitive development, the familial retardate would then be viewed as progressing from one intellectual stage to the next in the same sequence that other children follow. He would, of course, progress at a slower rate than other children, and the final stage achieved would be lower than that achieved by more intelligent members of the population. In terms of cognitive functioning alone, a ten-year-old familial retardate with an MA of seven would be similar, that is, at the same developmental level intellectually, as a seven-year-old child with an IQ of 100. (The reader must remember that the mental age, which is invariably based on the IQ, can be considered only a very rough indicator of the cognitive or developmental level; however, to date it is the best measure available).

It is no surprise that groups of 70 IQ and 100 IQ children of the same chronological age (CA) differ on a variety of tasks. These children are at different developmental levels, and such differences are to be expected. What is surprising is the repeated demonstration that even when groups are matched for mental age, the retardate does less well, or at least behaves differently, than the "normal" child. Two distinctly different explanations for this phenomenon have been advanced. One view is that the performance differences reflect experiential or motivational differences. The second is that the familial retardate is really not a normal individual developing at a slower rate, but an inherently different type of organism who, at every level of development, is suffering from some defect in his physiological or cognitive structure. These hypothesized defects presumably could produce differences in behavior between the groups even where the mental age is the same. The next section will consider this defect orientation, and the motivational position will be discussed in the final section.

RETARDATION AS A DEFECT

In this section we shall deal with theoretical and empirical efforts that have advanced the view that *all* retardates, including the familial, suffer from some specifiable defect. This idea opposes the view that the familial retardate suffers only from a slower and more limited rate of cognitive development. The evidence typically offered by the defect theorist is that even when groups of normals and retardates are matched on MA, the two groups behave differently, suggesting that some physiological or cognitive defect is responsible for the slower rate of development. Where the hypothesized defect is an explicitly physiological one, it would appear to be a simple matter to obtain direct validation for its existence from biochemical and physiological analyses and from pathological studies of familial retardates. A number of such studies have, of course, been carried out. Although there is an occasional report of some physical anomaly, the bulk of the evidence has indicated that the familial retardate does not suffer from gross physiological defects. Indeed, if evidence that he does were readily available, the defect theorist would not have to rely on the ambiguous data provided by studies of molar behavior. The failure to find direct evidence for the existence of a physiological defect in the familial retarded should not, however, deter theorists from postulating such defects.

Spitz (1963) and Masland (1959) maintain that our failure to discover physical defects in the familial retarded is due to the relatively primitive nature of contemporary diagnostic techniques. It is perfectly legitimate to assert that, although it is presently not observable, the physical defect that causes familial retardates to behave differently than normals of the same MA will someday be seen. Physicists of a not-too-distant era asserted that the electron existed even though it was not directly observable. Analogously, defect theorists of mental retardation validate the existence of a defect by first asserting that it should manifest itself in particular behaviors of the retarded and secondly devising experiments in which, if the predicted behavior occurs, the existence of the defect is confirmed.

Most theories of mental retardation are basically defect theories, but these differ among themselves. One difference involves the theoretician's effort to relate the postulated defect to some specific physiological structure. The language of some defect theories is explicitly physiological, that of others is nonphysiological, and that of others is vague. Particular defects that have been attributed to the retarded include: relative impermeability of the boundaries between regions in the cognitive structure (Kounin, 1941*a*, 1941*b*; Lewin, 1936); primary and secondary rigidity caused by subcortical and cortical malformations, respectively (Goldstein, 1942–1943); inadequate neural satiation related to brain modifiability or cortical conductivity (Spitz, 1963); malfunctioning disinhibitory mechanisms (Siegel and Foshee, 1960); improper development of the verbal system resulting in a dissociation between verbal and motor systems (Luria, 1963; O'Connor and Hermelin, 1959); and relative brevity in the persistence of the stimulus trace (Ellis, 1963).

Luria and Verbal Mediation Theory

One of the best known defect positions has been offered by the Russian investigator, A. R. Luria, whose work has influenced investigators in England and the United States. As in the United States, the Soviets divide the retarded into three groups, although they use the older terms, *idiot*, *imbecile*, and *debile*. The generic term for mental retardation is *oliogophrenia*. They do not distinguish, however, between retardates having known organic impairments and the larger group having unknown etiologies.

In the United States, there is considerable consensus that the larger group (familial) is the product of complex genetic determinants and cultural deprivation. In contrast, as Pevsner (1961) and the subcommittee of the President's Panel, which recently visited the U.S.S.R., have noted (Mental retardation in the Soviet Union, 1964), Soviet workers do not consider mental retardation as determined either by genetic or by cultural factors. They attribute all grades of mental retardation to central nervous system damage, suggesting that it occurs initially during the intrauterine period or during early childhood and produces a disturbance of the child's subsequent mental development.

In the Soviet Union, the diagnosis of mental retardation involves the specification of a defect in some neurophysiological system. In fact professional researchers and teachers working with the retarded are called "defectologists." Knowledgeable visitors such at Kety (see Mental retardation in the Soviet Union, 1964) have pointed out that, given such an approach, diagnosticians may be predisposed to "discover" some possible indication of organicity. He also noted that pupils in the Soviet schools for the debile (mildly retarded) are primarily retardates who would be diagnosed as familial in the United States. With rare exceptions, these were the children of unskilled workers and in some instances were actually children of graduates of such schools.

General intelligence tests are not used in Russia. Diagnosis in mental retardation is made by neurologists and psychophysiologists who rely heavily on gross pathological signs, in the case of the severely retarded, and minor physical defects, minute examinations of electroencephalographic patterns, and certain qualitative (nonstandardized) tests of perception, conditioning, and concept formulation (with special emphasis on the identification of specific types of language disorders), in the case of the more mildly retarded.

Luria's orientation toward mental retardation is an outgrowth of his work on verbal mediation, which demonstrated that the behavior of retardates resembles that of younger normal children in that verbal instructions do not produce smooth regulation of motor behavior. On all of his tasks requiring verbal mediation, the retarded subjects have considerable difficulty. In light of these behavioral data, Luria has inferred that the major defect in the retarded child involves both an underdevelopment or a general "inertness" of the verbal (nervous) system, and a dissociation of this system from the motor or action system of the brain. The general effect of this dissociation, vaguely conceptualized as a disturbance in normal cortical activity, is that a verbal response cannot serve as an adequate regulator of voluntary behavior.

Unfortunately, Luria's data do not throw any light on the issue of whether the cognitive processes of familial retardates differ from those of normal children of the same mental age. As noted earlier, a Russian defectologist would not consider this a legitimate question. Since there is no concern with the intelligence quotient in Russia, there is no way to determine the mental ages of the retardates and normals compared in Luria's work. Furthermore, the question of whether his retarded subjects are what we would call the physiologically impaired or the familial-cultural type remains unanswered. However, Luria's discussion of "profound atrophic changes . . . expressed in the underdevelopment of the complex neuron structures of the first and third strata of the cortex" and his classification of these retardates as imbeciles rather than debiles makes it sound as if his subjects suffer from gross physiological impairment.

It must be concluded, then, that these data have extremely limited relevance to the issue of whether familial retardates suffer from some physiological defect, and we must look to English and American workers for more adequate tests even of the proposition that all retardates differ from normals in the degree to which they employ verbal cues in regulating voluntary behavior. For example, O'Connor and Hermelin (1959) have found no significant difference between normals and retardates in the number of trials required to learn a size discrimination. However, their finding that retardates required significantly fewer trials to learn a reversal was interpreted as supporting Luria's position. They reasoned that, on the original learning task, the normal child uses both motor and verbal mediational responses in his learning, while the retarded child relies primarily on motor response. When the reversal is introduced, the normal child must unlearn both the original motor and verbal responses. The retardate, having to unlearn only the motor response, would thus be expected to learn the reversal problem more easily. The findings of O'Connor and Hermelin are inconsistent, however, with earlier studies (Plenderleith, 1956; Stevenson and Zigler, 1957) in which mental retardates were not found to be superior on a discrimination reversal task. In an effort to resolve this discrepancy, Balla and Zigler (1964) ran a reversal-learning study involving several different reversal tasks and different types of retardates at different MA levels. Their results provided no support for the Luria position.

Milgram and Furth (1963) compared retarded and normal children of the same MA on concept tasks which varied in the degree to which language might facilitate performance. Their findings were consistent with expectations derived from Luria's position. However, in an experiment comparing retardates and normals of the same MA on their ability to employ verbal mediators, Riber (1964) obtained results inconsistent with those that would be derived from Luria's theory. In sum, the evidence mustered to date to support Luria remains equivocal.

Spitz and Cortical Satiation Theory

Another major defect position is that of Herman Spitz (1963), who has extended the Köhler-Wallach (1944) cortical satiation theory to the area of mental retardation. Spitz argues that all retardates suffer from inadequate neural satiation, which is related to the modifiability of the brain or cortical conductivity; he has tested this position by comparing normals and retardates of the same ages. Again, it should be noted that no direct physiological evidence has been presented that familial retardates suffer from inadequate neural or cortical functioning. Furthermore, there *is* direct physiological evidence which calls into question the validity of the entire Köhler-Wallach position (Lashley *et al.*, 1951).

Like the earlier Gestalt workers, Spitz has primarily employed perceptual tasks to test his position. His extensive program of research has now been summarized (Spitz, 1963), and any complete review would be beyond the scope of this chapter. Spitz's most convincing evidence has been obtained on those perceptual tasks, such as figural aftereffects and Necker cube reversals, that are thought to be sensitive to possible cortical satiation effects.

The empirical value of Spitz's position can be seen in his recent efforts to extend his postulates beyond the area of visual perception to generate specific predictions about learning, transposition, generalization, and problem solving. Spitz (1963) has noted a number of studies in these areas which lend credence to his basic position. He has also been quite explicit in noting the limitations of his view. He has pointed out that, contrary to his theory, cortical satiation as measured by his perceptual indices does not in general correlate with IQ, but rather only differentiates the average performance of two distinct groups." The extensive overlap between normals and retardates on his tests of satiation led him to conclude "that the satiation variable must be only a very small one in the total complex of intelligent behavior."

Spitz has also been appropriately concerned with the fact that the retest reliability of the scores of his retardates is not impressive and that the lack of any intercorrelation of individual scores among some of his tasks is troublesome for his position. Across modalities, and even in the same modality, correlations have been moderate or nonexistent. Spitz has also been sensitive to the issue of how accurately the subject's response, often a verbal report, reflects the perceptual response being investigated. (See Garner *et al.* (1956) and Goldiamond (1958) for a general discussion of this complex problem and Spivack (1963) for a discussion of the same problem in respect to research with the retarded.)

Adding to these difficulties is the fact that several investigators have now discovered that responses to cognitive and perceptual tasks are influenced by a variety of motivational factors (Cohen, 1956; Coons, 1956; Mayer and Coons, 1960; Zigler and DeLabry, 1962; Zigler and Unell, 1962). The relevance of these findings to Spitz's work will be made clear in the next section. In addition, certain aspects of Spitz's findings are inconsistent with those of other investigators. Spivack (1963) has voiced this concern in a review of research on perceptual processes in the retarded.

Of more importance to the central question of whether familial retardates are inherently different from normals of the same MA, we must conclude that Spitz's data throw little light on this issue. Like the Russians, Spitz believes that the distinction between familial and organic retardates is misleading. In his view, all retardates suffer from brain damage and belong to a common class (Garrison, in press). Therefore, his work has been characterized by a relative lack of concern with the problem of etiology, and we have little way of assessing whether the differences he reports are a product of gross organic pathology or may actually reflect the cortical phenomena he postulates.

That one gets differences between normals and retardates matched on chronological age (CA) is not very surprising since we are dealing with groups who are at different developmental levels (as defined by MA). One would be tempted to say that Spitz's work has little relevance to the question at hand except for the fact that he has been quite explicit in his view that the differences he obtains are not developmental phenomena, but reflect a physical defect that should manifest itself even in comparisons with MA-matched normals.

The Lewin-Kounin Formulation

The final defect position that we shall discuss is that of Lewin (1936) and Kounin (1941*a*, 1941*b*). This position is different from the other defect views in that the postulated defect is cognitive rather than physical. The Lewin-Kounin formulation has had considerable impact not only on our thinking about the retarded, but also on the treatment and training practices that have been employed over the years. (For a more complete historical review and critique of the Lewin-Kounin formulation, see Zigler, 1962.)

In Lewin's general theory of personality (1936), the individual is treated as a dynamic system and differences among individuals as resulting from differences in: (1) structure of the total system, (2) "material" and "state" of the system, or, (3) its meaningful content. The first two factors play the most important role in Lewin's theory of retardation. In respect to cognitive structure, Lewin viewed the retarded child as being less "differentiated," that is, having fewer "cells," than a normal child of the same age and therefore superficially resembling a normal younger child. In relation to the "material" and "state" of the system, Lewin stated that even though a retarded child corresponded in degree of "differentiation" to a normal *younger* child, these children still were not entirely similar. He considered

> the major dynamic difference between a feebleminded and normal child of the same degree of differentiation to consist in a greater stiffness, a smaller capacity for dynamic rearrangement in the psychical systems of the former.

(Degree of differentiation was later operationally defined as MA.)

The clearest experimental support for the position that the familial retarded are more rigid than normal individuals having the same degree of differentiation is contained in the work of Kounin (1941*a*, 1941*b*, 1948). Kounin, building upon Lewin's work, advanced the view that rigidity increases regularly with age. It is imperative to note that by "rigidity" Kounin, like Lewin, referred to "that property of a functional boundary which prevents communication between neighboring regions" and not to rigid behaviors as we usually think of them.

Kounin (1941*a*) offered the findings of five experiments in support of his theory. In these experiments he employed three groups: older familial retarded individuals, younger familial retarded individuals, and normals. He defined the degree of differentiation as the MA of an individual and equated the three groups on it. He also attempted to control behavioral rigidity by making each subject feel confident and secure in the experimental tasks. As predicted from the Lewin-Kounin formulation, the normals showed the greatest amount of transfer effects from task to task, the younger retarded a lesser amount of transfer, and the older retarded the least amount of transfer.

On one task, the lesser "rigidity" of the normals, as defined by Lewin and Kounin, results in a higher incidence of perseverative responses, which are often characterized as rigid in the conventional sense. Furthermore, this lack of influence of one "region" upon another in the performance of the retarded would only be predicted where the retarded individual is "psychologically" placed into a new "region" by an instructional procedure. In instances where the individual must move on his own from one region to another without instructions, the Lewin-

Kounin formulation would predict that movement would be more difficult for the retarded than for the normal individual. This prediction was also confirmed by Kounin in a concept-switching experiment in which the child was asked to sort a deck of cards which could be sorted on the basis either of color or of form. After doing it one way, he was then asked to put the cards together some other way. Here the normals evidenced the least difficulty in shifting, the older retarded the most difficulty, and the younger retarded group again fell between the other two groups. Thus, when a movement to a new "region" is self-initiated, it is the retarded who evidence the higher incidence of perseverative responses.

The Lewin-Kounin theory of rigidity is a conceptually demanding one in that it sometimes predicts a higher and sometimes a lower incidence of "rigid" behaviors in retarded as compared to normal individuals. However, the fact that it generates specific predictions as to when one or the other state of affairs will obtain is a tribute to the theory. Kounin thus offered impressive experimental support for the view that, with MA held constant, the older or more retarded an individual is, the more his behaviors will be characterized by dynamic rigidity, that is, greater rigidity in the boundaries between regions.

This model and its experimental support was so impressive that, until fairly recently, very few further tests of it were attempted. However, recent explicit tests of the model (Balla and Zigler, 1964; Plenderleith, 1956; Stevenson and Zigler, 1957; Zigler and Unell, 1962) and tangential studies as well (Capobianco, 1962; Osborn, 1960) have failed to provide support for it. Furthermore, a partial replication study (Zigler and Butterfield, in press) resulted in findings quite unlike Kounin's. Much evidence now indicates that the differences found by Kounin were not a product of the inherent rigidity of retardates but, rather, reflected a number of motivational differences between normal children and institutionalized retardates of the same MA. These motivational factors will be discussed in the final section.

MOTIVATION AND EMOTION IN RETARDED BEHAVIOR

A variety of nonintellective factors are important determinants of the level at which the retarded function. We shall never comprehend the behavior of the retarded if we assume that every behavior he manifests is the immutable product of his low intelligence. Furthermore, we must disavow the overly simplistic idea that all retardates manifest a highly similar pattern of behavior which is determined by their common defect. Indeed, a striking feature encountered when groups of retardates are observed is the variety of behavior patterns displayed. Clearly, we are not dealing with a homogeneous group of simple organisms. Once we concern ourselves with the total behavior of the retarded child, we find him an extremely complex psychological system. To the extent that his behavior deviates from the norms associated with his mental age, he is even more difficult to understand than the normal individual.

It is unfortunate that so little work bearing on personality has been done with the retarded. Some progress has been made, however, and much recent work supports the view that the same constructs used to account for the behavior of normal individuals can explain the behavior of the familial retarded. It appears that many of the differences between retardates and normals of the same MA are a result of motivational and emotional differences which reflect differences in environmental histories and not in innate capacities.

Several workers have noted that personality factors are as important as intellective factors in the retardate's adjustment (Penrose, 1963; Sarason, 1953; Tizard, 1953; see also, Windle, 1962, for an especially comprehensive review of the importance of nonintellective factors in the prognosis of mental retardation.) Many of the early workers in this country, such as Fernald and Potter, felt that the difference between social adequacy and inadequacy in borderline retardates was a matter of personality and character rather than of intelligence. A number of studies have confirmed this view. Perhaps the best of these is the comprehensive study by Weaver (1946) of the adjustment of 8000 retardates, mostly with IQ's below 75, inducted into the United States Army. Of the total group, 56 percent of the males and 62 percent of the females made a satisfactory adjustment to military life. The median IQ's of the successful and unsuccessful groups were 72 and 68, respectively. Weaver (1946) concluded that, "personality factors far overshadowed the factor of intelligence in the adjustment of the retarded to military service."

The tendency to overemphasize the importance of the intellect in adjustment has been made clear by Windle (1962), who found in a survey that most institutions assume that intelligence is the critical factor in adjustment following release. Windle points out that the vast majority of studies (over twenty) on outcome "after release from institutions have reported no relation between intellectual level and later adjustment." In examining this literature, we find that the factors which led to poor social adjustment include anxiety, jealousy, excessive-dependency, poor self-evaluation, hostility, hyperactivity, and failure to follow orders well within the range of intellectual competence.

It is hardly surprising that retardates evidence such difficulties in light of their atypical social histories. These vary, of course, from child to child. Two sets of parents who are themselves familially retarded may provide quite different socialization histories for their children. At one extreme we may find a familially retarded child who grows up in an abysmal home environment and who is ultimately institutionalized, not because of lack of intelligence, but because his own home is such a poor environment. That many borderline retardates are institutionalized for just such reasons has been confirmed by Kaplun (1935) in a study of 642 high-grade retardates; Zigler's recent finding (1961) of a positive relationship between the institutionalized familial retardate's IQ and the amount of preinstitutional deprivation he experienced provides further support for this claim. This does not mean, of course, that social deprivation produces greater intelligence, but rather that our institutions contain borderline retardates who would not be institutionalized except for their extremely poor home environments.

At the other extreme, the familially retarded parents of an institutionalized child may have provided a relatively normal home even though it might differ in some important respects from the typical homes of families with average or superior intelligence. The child from the troubled home not only experiences an unfortunate socialization history while he is still living with his parents, but also differs from the child in the second situation in that institutionalization itself affects his personality structure. Given the penchant of many investigators for comparing institutionalized retardates with children of average intellect who live at home, the factor of institutionalization becomes an extremely important one. One cannot help but wonder how many differences discovered in such comparisons really reflect some cognitive aspect of mental retardation rather than the effects of institutionalization, the factors that led to the child's institutionalization, or some complex interaction between these factors.

To add even more complexity, the socialization histories of both institutionalized and noninstitutionalized familial retardates differ markedly from the history of brain-damaged retardates. The brain-damaged do not show the same gross differences in environmental background as familials do. This complexity, though puzzling, does not make it impossible for us to isolate the development of factors which are important in influencing the retardate's level of functioning. Once we think of the retardate as occupying a position on a continuum of normality, our knowledge of normal development can give direction to our efforts.

We must not ignore the importance of the lowered intelligence per se, however, since personality traits and behavior patterns do not develop in a vacuum. But, in some instances the personality characteristics of the retarded reflect environmental factors that have little or nothing to do with intellectual endowment. For example, many of the effects of institutionalization may be the same regardless of the person's intelligence level, while others may reflect an interaction between lowered intellectual ability and the conditions of institutionalization. In the latter case, a retarded person will have experiences and develop certain behavior patterns that differ from those of a person with greater intellectual endowment. For example, the retardate typically experiences a greater amount of failure. Again, it must be emphasized that the behavior pattern developed by the retardate as a result of a history of failure will not differ essentially from that of an intellectually normal person who also experiences an inordinate amount of failure. By the same token, if the retardate can somehow be guaranteed a history more typical of success, we would expect his behavior to be more normal, regardless of his intellectual level. Within this framework, we will discuss some personality factors which have been known to influence the performance of the retarded.

Caution is needed in evaluating the role of motivational and emotional factors in the performance of the retarded. Performance on a task depends on two types of factors—intellective or cognitive, and nonintellective or motivational. The contribution of each factor will vary with the nature of the task. Motivational factors will more readily influence a perseveration task, such as continuing to put marbles into a box, than they will a discrimination-learning task or a concept-formation task, although performance on tasks of the latter type is also somewhat influenced by motivational factors (Butterfield and Zigler, 1965*a*; Zigler and DeLabry, 1962). Improving task motivation may help the mentally retarded to use their intellectual capacity to best advantage even though it cannot change that capacity.

Anxiety

Considerable evidence has now been collected showing the importance of anxiety on performance for a wide variety of tasks (Sarason *et al.*, 1960; Spence, 1958; Taylor, 1963). The disruptive effects of anxiety on performance appear to stem both from the task-irrelevant defensive responses employed by the person to alleviate his anxiety (Mandler and Sarason, 1952; Sarason *et al.*, 1960) and the drive features of anxiety itself. As we saw in Chapter 3, the drive approach to anxiety (Spence, 1958; Taylor, 1963) views high anxiety as helpful on nondemanding tasks but as detrimental on complex tasks where a variety of responses should be available to the person. The higher anxiety level of retardates, as compared to normals, has now been noted by several investigators (see Berkson, 1963; Cantor, 1963; Garfield, 1963; Spradlin, 1963; Stevenson, 1963), suggesting that heightened anxiety could well have produced certain of the differences between retardates and normals reported in the literature. Work with retardates that has been concerned with anxiety is of considerable value "in that it applies concepts and techniques to the study of retarded individuals, which for the most part had not been applied or seen as relevant for this group" (Garfield, 1963, p. 594).

That anxiety level affects the performance of retardates as much as that of normals and that retardates might have higher levels of anxiety than normals tells us little about the ontogenesis of anxiety in retardates. To understand the development of their atypical anxiety levels, we must examine the relatively atypical experiences of the retarded, as well as a variety of other motivational states which influence their performance.

Social Deprivation

It is clear that our understanding of the performance of institutionalized familial retardates will be enhanced if we consider the inordinate amount of preinstitutional social deprivation they have suffered (Clarke and Clarke, 1954; Kaplun, 1935; Zigler, 1961). A series of recent studies (Green and Zigler, 1962; Shepps and Zigler, 1962; Zigler, 1961, 1963*a*; Zigler *et al.*, 1958; Zigler and Williams, 1963) has indicated that one result of such early deprivation is heightened motivation to interact with a supportive adult. These studies suggest that, given this heightened motivation, retardates show considerable compliance with instructions when the effect of compliance is to increase or maintain social interaction with the adult. Compliance is reduced when it tends to terminate the interaction.

It now appears that the perseveration so frequently noted in the behavior of the retarded is primarily a function of this motivational factor rather than of the inherent cognitive rigidity suggested by Lewin (1936) and Kounin (1941*a*, 1941*b*). Evidence for this comes from findings that (1) the degree of perseveration is directly related to the degree of preinstitutional deprivation (Zigler, 1961), and (2) institutionalized children of normal intellect are just as perseverative as institutionalized retardates, while noninstitutionalized retardates are no more perseverative than noninstitutionalized children of normal intellect (Green and Zigler, 1962; Zigler, 1963*a*). The finding that institutionalization (or the social history factors leading to institutionalization) is the crucial factor in determining the child's response to social reinforcement on a simple task has also been reported by Stevenson and Fahel (1961). Heightened motivation to interact with an adult, stemming from a history of social deprivation, accounts for the frequent observation of certain marked behaviors in the retarded, such as seeking attention and affection (Cruickshank, 1947; Doll, 1962; Hirsh, 1959; Wellman, 1938*b*).

It is impossible to place too much emphasis on the role of excessive dependency in the institutional familial retarded and on the socialization histories that give rise to such dependency. The shift from dependency to independence is perhaps the most necessary condition of the retardate's becoming a self-sustaining member of society. It appears that the institutionalized retardate must satisfy certain affectional needs before he can cope with problems in the manner of individuals whose affectional needs have been relatively fulfilled. Unsatisfied affectional needs often interfere with his problem-solving activities. Because the retardate is highly motivated to satisfy such needs through maximizing interpersonal contact, he is relatively unconcerned with the specific solution to other problems. Of course, the two goals are not always incompatible, but in many instances they are. Some evidence that this aspect of retarded behavior can be overcome has been presented by McKinney and Keele (1963), who found improvement in a variety of behaviors in the mentally retarded after an experience of increased mothering.

Zigler and Williams (1963) have provided some evidence on the interaction between preinstitutional social deprivation and institutionalization in influencing the child's motivation for social interaction and support. It was found that although institutionalization generally increased this motivation, it was increased much more in children coming from relatively nondeprived homes than in those coming from more socially deprived backgrounds.

An unexpected finding of the Zigler and Williams study was that the IQ's of retardates generally declined between the administration of two IQ tests, one given at the time of admission and the other five years later. This change in IQ is reminiscent of a finding by Clarke and Clarke (1954) that changes in the IQ's of retardates following institutionalization were related to their preinstitutional histories. Children coming from extremely poor homes showed an *increase* in IQ which was not observed in children coming from relatively good homes. Zigler and Williams did not find that IQ change was significantly related to preinstitutional deprivation, but in their study also, the only children who evidenced an increase in IQ were the deprived ones. The failure of Zigler and Williams to replicate the exact findings of Clarke and Clarke may be due to differences in the studies, especially to the fact that the IQ changes reported by Clarke and Clarke took place during only two years of institutionalization, while those reported by Zigler and Williams occurred over a five-year institutionalization. This fact is important in view of Jones and Carr-Saunders' finding (1927) that the IQ of normal institutionalized children *increases* early in institutionalization but *decreases* with longer institutionalization.

The work of Clarke and Clarke, Jones and Carr-Saunders, and others (for example, Guertin, 1949) dealing with changes in IQ after institutionalization points up the importance of the intellectual stimulation provided by the institution in contrast to that provided by the original home. They suggest that the actual intellectual potential of the person is altered. The Zigler and Williams study, however, suggests that the change in IQ reflects a change in the child's motivation for social interaction. That is, as social deprivation resulting from long institutionalization increases, the desire to interact with the adult experimenter increases. Thus, for the deprived child the desire to be correct must compete in the testing situation with the desire to increase social interaction. This would explain Clarke and Clarke's finding that highly deprived subjects evidence an increase in IQ with relatively short institutionalization, while the less deprived subjects demonstrate no greater increase than a control group. One would further expect that with continued institutionalization all children would exhibit a decrease in IQ, the phenomenon found both by Jones and Carr-Saunders and by Zigler and Williams. Direct support for this view comes from the finding in the latter study that the amount of decrease in IQ was greatest among children whose motivation for social interaction was greatest.

It should be noted that the Jones and Carr-Saunders study (1927) involved institutionalized children of approximately average IQ, indicating that these dynamics are the same for both normal and retarded children. The position advanced here is also quite consistent with the findings obtained by Barrett and Koch (1930) and by Krugman (1939) on normal children; these investigators found that the greatest increase in IQ was obtained by children who showed the greatest improvement in personality traits or by children who evidenced a marked change in their relationship with the examiner. Conversely, what must be emphasized about lowered IQ's is not the test score per se, but rather that the factors which reduce the test score will, in all probability, reduce the adequacy of much social problem solving.

Although there is considerable evidence that social deprivation increases motivation to interact with a supportive adult, it appears to have other effects as well on retarded children, increasing their fearfulness, their wariness or avoidance of strangers, or their suspicion and mistrust (Hirsh, 1959; Wellman, 1938*b*; Woodward, 1960). The experimental work of Zigler and his associates on the behavior of the institutionalized retarded has indicated that social deprivation simultaneously produces a heightened motivation to interact with supportive adults (positive reaction tendency) and a reluctance and wariness to do so (negative reaction tendency). Both of these tendencies are influenced by the quality of past relationships with adults and are amenable to experimental manipulations, as has been demonstrated in recent studies of both normal and retarded children (Berkowitz and Zigler, 1965; McCoy and Zigler, 1965; Shallenberger and Zigler, 1961; Zigler, 1958). However, little work has been done to date on the range of behaviors that might be influenced by the negative reaction tendency.

Failure

Another determinant of the performance of the retarded is their high expectancy of failure (Cromwell, 1963), which is an outgrowth of a lifetime of frequent confrontations with tasks for which they are intellectually ill equipped. That failure experiences and the failure expectancies to which they give rise affect a wide variety of behaviors in the intellectually normal has now been amply documented (Atkinson, 1958*a*, 1958*b*; Katz, 1964; Rotter, 1954; Sarason *et al.*, 1960). Of special interest to workers in mental retardation is Lantz's finding (1945) that a relatively simple failure experience prevented children from profiting by practice of a kind which ordinarily leads to improvement on intelligence test scores.

The results of experimental work on success and failure experiences with retardates is still somewhat inconsistent. The work of Cromwell and his students (Cromwell, 1963) lends support to the general proposition that retardates have a higher expectation of failure than normals do. This results in a style of problem solving for the retardate which causes him to be much more motivated to avoid failure than to achieve success (compare Chapter 3). However, the inconsistent research findings suggest that this fairly simple proposition needs further refinement. One investigator found that retardates performed better following success and poorer following failure than a control group did (Gardner, 1957). Another (Heber, 1957) found that the performance of normals and retardates was equally improved after both a failure and a success, but that after a success the performance of retardates was more improved than that of normals.

Conversely, Kass and Stevenson (1961) found that success improved the performance of normals more than that of retardates. Another study found that failure also had a general improving effect for both normals and retardates, but that it improved the performance of normals more than that of retardates (Gardner, 1958). In a recent study by Butterfield and Zigler (1965), one factor which may have produced these inconsistencies was isolated. They found that both normal and retarded children reacted to both success and failure experiences according to their responsiveness to adults, that is, according to their desire to gain an adult's support and approval. Among highly responsive subjects, failure impaired the performance of retarded and improved the performance of normal subjects. Among poorly responsive subjects, failure impaired the performance of normals but improved that of retardates.

The debilitating effects of prolonged failure on the performance of the retarded have been documented by Zeaman and House (1960), who noted that it prevented retardates from solving a simple problem they had previously been able to do. Assuming a failure "mental set" in retardates, Stevenson and Zigler (1958) confirmed the prediction that these children would "settle for" a lower degree of success than normal children of the same mental age would. The fear of failure in the mentally retarded also appears to be an important factor in differences found between normals' and retardates' achievement motivation (Jordan and DeCharms, 1959).

Recent studies (Green and Zigler, 1962; Turnure and Zigler, 1964; Zigler *et al.*, 1958) have indicated that the high incidence of failure experienced by retardates generates a cognitive style of problem solving characterized by "outer directedness" (compare to the "outer-directed character" of Chapter 8). That is, the retarded child comes to distrust his own solutions to problems and therefore seeks guides to action in the immediate environment. This outer directedness may explain the great suggestibility so frequently attributed to the retarded child. Evidence has now been presented indicating that, compared to normals of the same MA, retarded children are more sensitive to verbal cues from adults, more imitative of the behaviors of both adults and peers, and more apt to engage in visual scanning. Furthermore, certain findings (Green and Zigler, 1962) suggest that the noninstitutionalized retardate is more outer directed in his problem solving than the institutionalized retardate is. This makes sense since the noninstitutionalized retardate does not reside in an environment adjusted to his intellectual shortcomings and therefore experiences more failures than the institutionalized retardate does.

Turnure and Zigler (1964) have suggested that the distractability so frequently encountered in the retarded reflects, in part, this outer-directed style of problem solving. This interpretation is of particular interest since distractability has often been viewed as a neurophysiologically determined characteristic of the retarded, rather than the reflection of a style of problem solving emanating from the particular experiential histories. Work on the outer-directedness of the retarded also appears related to the "locus of control" work done by Cromwell and his associates (reviewed in Cromwell, 1963). These investigators found that retardates, as compared to normals, manifest an external locus of control; that is, they attribute certain events, caused by their own behavior, to outside forces over which they have little control. (This internal versus external control dimension has been employed by Cromwell to bring some further order to the inconsistent findings in the success-failure literature.)

The Reinforcer Hierarchy

Another nonintellective factor important in understanding the behavior of the retarded is the retardate's motivation by various types of incentives. Performance by both normals and retardates on a variety of tasks is influenced by the nature of the incentive (Cantor, 1963). The social deprivation work discussed earlier in this section indicates that retardates have an extremely high motivation for attention, praise, and encouragement. Several investigators (Beller, 1955; Cromwell, 1963; Gewirtz, 1954; Heathers, 1955; Zigler, 1963*b*) have suggested that, in normal development, the effectiveness of attention and praise as reinforcers diminishes with maturity and is replaced by the reinforcement inherent in the information that one is correct. This latter type of reinforcer appears to serve primarily as a cue for self-reinforcement.

Zigler and his associates (Zigler, 1962; Zigler and DeLabry, 1962; Zigler and Unell, 1962) have argued that a variety of experiential factors in the history of the retarded cause them to be less motivated than normals of the same MA toward correctness for its own sake. Stated somewhat differently, they have argued that the position of various reinforcers differs in the reinforcement hierarchies of normal and retarded children of the same MA. To date, the experimental work of this group has centered around the reinforcement which inheres in being correct. This reinforcer is the most frequently dispensed and immediate incentive in most real-life tasks. Furthermore, it is a frequently used incentive in many experimental and assessment tasks on which retardates and normals are compared, and it is often the most important one. When such an incentive is employed in experimental studies, one wonders how many of the differences found result from differences in capacity between retardates and normals rather than from differences in the values the incentive has for the two types of subjects.

Clearest support for the view that the retardate is much less motivated to be correct than the middle-class child typically compared with him is contained in a study by Zigler and DeLabry (1962), who tested middle-class, lower-class, and retarded children equated for MA on a concept-switching task (Kounin, 1941*a*) under two conditions of reinforcement. In the first condition, as in that employed by Kounin, the only reinforcement dispensed was the information that the child was correct. In the second condition the child, was rewarded with a toy if he switched from one concept to another. In the "correct" condition, they found, as Kounin did, that retardates were poorer in concept switching than middle-class children were. This was not a simple matter of cognitive rigidity because lower-class children equated with the middle-class children on MA were also inferior to them. In the "toy" condition, this inferiority disappeared, and retarded and lower-class children performed as well as middle-class children. This study makes clear how erroneous the assumption is that the lower-class and the retarded child are motivated by the same incentives as the typical middle-class child.

General Effects of Institutionalization

No discussion of motivational factors in the performance of the retarded would be complete without some mention of the effects of institutionalization. The institutionalization variable has probably contaminated more research in mental retardation than any other single variable. Since we generally know little about the effects of institutionalization on human behavior, the extent of this contamination cannot be determined. Several in vestigators have suggested that the effects of institutionalization on the behavior of retardates are considerable (Guskin, 1963; Lipman, 1963; McCandless, 1964; Nye, 1958; Sarason and Gladwin, 1958; Spradlin, 1963; Windle, 1962). In view of the general consensus concerning their importance, it is amazing that more work has not been done to investigate these effects.

Some fairly clear findings with retardates have demonstrated that institutionalization causes a decrement in the quality of language behavior (Lyle, 1959; Schlanger, 1954), reduces the level of abstraction on vocabulary tests (Badt, 1958), interferes with the ability to conceptualize an emotional continuum (Iscoe and McCann, 1965), and increases the child's orientation toward punishment (Abel, 1941). These studies, though suggestive, have shed little light on the specific aspects of institutionalization which create these effects or on the exact nature of the process through which behaviors are affected. Whether the deficiencies in the behavior of the institutionalized retardate are motivational in nature or reflect an actual change in intellectual capacity is still an open question.

Evidence that institutions for the retarded differ in their effects on behavior has recently been reported by Butterfield and Zigler (1965*b*). They found that children residing in a cold, restrictive institution were more eager for adult support and approval than children in an institution having a warm, accepting social climate. These investigators are presently conducting a longitudinal study of six state schools for the retarded in an effort to isolate the institutional factors and psychological processes underlying such effects.

Much of this work on motivational and emotional factors in the performance of the retarded is very recent. The research on them discussed in this section is more suggestive than definitive. It is clear, however, that these factors are extremely important in determining the retardate's general level of functioning. Furthermore, they seem much more open to environmental manipulation than the cognitive processes discussed earlier. An increase in knowledge of motivational and emotional factors and their ontogenesis and manipulation holds considerable promise for alleviating much of the social ineffectiveness displayed by persons who must function at a relatively low intellectual level.

SUMMARY

This chapter has attempted to review the current status of thinking about the mentally retarded. The past decade has witnessed renewed interest in the problem of mental retardation, which has resulted in vigorous research and the construction of a number of theories that attempt to explain low level intellectual functioning. However, much of the research and many of the theoretical efforts are hampered by a variety of conceptual ambiguities. Workers in the area are not solely responsible for this state of affairs. Mental retardation is not a discrete, easily demarcated area of knowledge, but rather it is intimately related to the general field of developmental psychology. Advances in this larger area cannot help but bring further order to the smaller one. This is particularly true with respect to the refinement of views concerning the nature of intelligence.

There is a critical need for a comprehensive theory of intelligence, including an adequate definition of it. The psychometric approach, with its emphasis on the *contents* of behavior rather than on the cognitive *processes* which mediate behavior, is of limited value, and an inadequate definition of intelligence must inevitably result in an inadequate definition of mental retardation. Given the discontent with intelligence test scores as measures of retardation, many workers have championed the social competence criterion. Others have pointed out the inadequacy of such a criterion, and the area continues to suffer from the lack of a universally acceptable definition of mental retardation. This problem can be seen clearly in the inconsistent findings reported about the prevalence of mental retardation at different times and places.

Other ambiguities in the area do appear to be the result of the practices of certain workers rather than of a general knowledge lag in psychology. Thinking of the retarded as a homogeneous group, defined by some arbitrary IQ score, is a case in point. It is more valuable to clearly distinguish between the group of retardates who are known to suffer from some organic defect and the larger group referred to as the familial or cultural-familial. The familial retardate currently presents the greatest mystery to workers in the area, and it is no surprise to discover that where there is mystery, there are conflicting views. One approach to the familial retardate has emphasized the cultural and social deprivation experienced, stressing environmental causality. This approach remains a popular one, and it should be viewed within the framework of both the older and the more recent literature on the nature-nurture controversy, which, although it appears to have abated within the general field of psychology, remains a lively issue in the area of mental retardation. However, our review would appear to indicate that any simplistic view of the role of environment is inadequate to the task of explaining the etiology of familial retardation.

A number of authorities have emphasized the need for employing recent polygenic models of inheritance in understanding the familial retarded. While appreciating the importance of environment in affecting the distribution determined by genetic inheritance, these workers have argued that the familial retarded are not essentially different from individuals of greater intellect but rather represent the lower portion of the intellectual curve that reflects normal intellectual variability. Within such a framework, the familial retardate would be viewed as a perfectly normal expression of the population gene pool whose intellectual development is slower and more limited than the individual of average intellect, whose intellectual development, in turn, is slower and more limited than the individual of superior intellect. This viewpoint generates the proposition that retardates and normals of the same general cognitive level (MA) are similar in respect to cognitive functioning. Such a proposition runs headlong into the findings that retardates and normals, even though equated on MA, often differ in performance, and these findings have bolstered what is currently the most popular theoretical approach to retarded functioning, namely, the view that all retardates suffer from some specific defect which inheres in mental retardation and thus makes the retardate immutably "different" from normals.

The most recent approach to the study of retardation has been the systematic evalution of the role of experiential and motivational factors. This approach, which emphasizes the personality structure of the retardate, takes as its central thesis the view that performance on experimental and real-life tasks is never the single inexorable product of the retardate's cognitive structure, but rather reflects a wide variety of relatively nonintellective factors which greatly influence the general quality of performance. Anxiety, social deprivation, a high incidence of failure experiences, atypical reinforcer hierarchies, and institutionalization all influence the behavior of the retardate.

There is little question that we are presently witnessing a productive, exciting, and perhaps inevitably chaotic, period in the history of man's concern with the very human problem of mental retardation. Even the disagreements that presently exist must be considered rather healthy phenomena. These disagreements will unquestionably generate new knowledge which, in the hands of practitioners, may become the vehicle through which the performance of children, regardless of intellectual level, may be improved.

GLOSSARY

ABSOLUTE—a value that does not vary with time or circumstances; a moral absolute is a rule that the individual believes holds for all times, places, and conditions (see Chapter 8).

AMAUROTIC IDIOCY—a severe mental defect which usually leads to early death (see Chapter 2).

BORDERLINE RETARDATE—a person who is usually considered legally competent but slightly subnormal in intelligence.

BOUNDARY—in Lewinian theory, a region separating one cognitive or affective system from another; "a region between two systems within which information exchange or energy exchange is less than it is within either of the systems; a relation between psychological forces."[1]

CHROMOSOMAL DEFECT (CHROMOSOMAL ABERRATION)—nonlethal changes in the structure and number of chromosomes (see Chapter 2).

COGNITIVE STRUCTURE—according to Lewin, the psychological organization of the social and physical worlds; it includes the organization of facts, beliefs, expectations, and concepts and the patterns of their interactions.

CONCEPT FORMATION—the ability to organize individual instances under a general idea, including the ability to distinguish these instances from others; requires both abstraction and generalization.

CONCEPT-SWITCHING TASK—a task wherein a person is asked to group objects according to one concept and then to find another concept according to which the objects can be grouped.

DIFFERENTIATION—according to Lewin, the number of "cells"; operationally defined as mental age.

DOMINANT GENE—the member of a pair of alleles that predominates and is responsible for the phenotype of a heterozygous individual; thus, if we have two alleles, A and O, if an individual's genetic composition is AO (hyterozygous), and if the individual exhibits the phenotype A, A is called the dominant gene (see Chapter 2).

EEG (ELECTROENCEPHALOGRAPH)—a graphic recording of the wavelike changes of the electrical potential of the brain.

ENCEPHALITIS—an infectious disease of the brain, known also as sleeping sickness.

ETIOLOGY—the study of the origins or causes, especially of a disease.

FACTOR ANALYSIS—a statistical method for interpreting the correlations between scores from a number of tests.

FAMILIAL RETARDATE—a diagnosis made when examination fails to reveal any physiological causes for retardation and when retardation exists among parents, siblings, or other relatives of the person studied; familial retardates are usually only mildly retarded, with IQ's mainly above 50.

GAUSSIAN DISTRIBUTION—see NORMAL DISTRIBUTION.

GENERAL ABILITY—ability manifested across a wide variety of tasks.

GENOTYPE—the qualities or traits that are transmitted biologically (see Chapter 2).

IDIOT—technically, a person whose IQ is below 25; idiots cannot be taught connected speech and are unable to defend themselves against common dangers.

IMBECILE—technically, a person whose IQ is between 25 and 49; an imbecile is usually able to defend himself but cannot earn a living.

[1] This definition is taken from H. B. English and Ava C. English, *A Comprehensive Dictionary of Psychological and Psychoanalytical Terms*, New York: David McKay Company, Inc., 1958.

INTELLECTUAL CAPACITY—an "innate" potential for the development of intellectual functions.

INTELLIGENCE—a hypothetical construct which ultimately refers to the cognitive processes of the individual, that is, to the caliber of his memory, perceptual discriminations, concept formation, abstract reasoning, and such.

INTELLIGENT BEHAVIOR—refers to content of behavior, specifically to the appropriateness, however defined, with which an organism carries out an act.

LOCUS OF CONTROL—a concept developed by Rotter to describe the manner in which an individual perceives his relationship to his environment; external locus of control refers to the sense that, on balance, the environment controls the individual's behavior and fortunes; internal locus of control describes the relative feeling that the individual himself controls his fortunes.

MENTAL AGE (MA)—the level of development in intelligence, expressed as equivalent to the chronological age at which the average child attains that level.

MENTAL ORTHOPEDICS—techniques used by Binet to promote intellectual improvement in mentally retarded persons.

MENTAL SET—a readiness for, or sensitization toward, a particular event or stimulus.

MENTALLY RETARDED—conservatively falling in the lower 3 percent of the distribution of IQ score; the definition established by Heber (1959) includes all persons whose IQ falls below the population mean; the *social competence* definition includes all those who are unable to meet minimal societal demands.

MODALITY—sense data that resemble each other more than they resemble data from other senses; for example, vision, hearing, warmness and so on.

MONGOLISM—a congenital mental deficiency (see Chapter 2).

NEGATIVE REACTION TENDENCY—wariness of, or reluctance for, social interaction.

NEURAL SATIATION—a state of relative insensitivity in the nerve fibers (an inability to be stimulated) that follows a period of stimulation by a series of closely related stimuli.

NORMAL DISTRIBUTION—a frequency distribution characterized by a bell-shaped curve (see Chapter 1).

OLIGOPHRENIA—a generic term, preferred by Russian scientists, for mental retardation.

PERSEVERATION—a response characterized by inappropriate repetitiveness and stereotypy; it is often revealed by difficulty in shifting from one task to another, or in shifting from one method to another in a problem-solving task; response rigidity.

PHENOTYPE—the sum total of the observable characteristics of an individual (see Chapter 2).

PHENYLKETONURIA—a type of mental retardation, considered hereditary, that becomes evident only under certain environmental conditions (see Chapter 2).

PHYSIOLOGICALLY DEFECTIVE RETARDATES—a classification given to retarded persons when examination reveals specifically abnormal physiological processes; the defective retardate usually has an extremely low IQ (below 40).

POLYGENIC MODEL—a genetic model in which many different genes are involved in the expression of one phenotype (see Chapter 2).

POSITIVE REACTION TENDENCY—a heightened motivation for social interaction.

PSYCHOMETRICIAN—a psychologist skilled in the administration and interpretation of mental tests.

RECESSIVE GENE—the member of a pair of alleles that is subordinate and is not responsible for the phenotype of a heterozygous individual; where the individual's genetic composition is, say, AO, and the phenotype A is exhibited, O is called the recessive gene; in order for the phenotypic characteristics of O to be exhibited, the genetic composition would have to be OO (see Chapter 2).

RIGIDITY—relative inability to alter one's actions or attitudes in accord with changing conditions; according to Lewin, the property of a functional cognitive boundary which prevents communication between neighboring regions.

SPECIFIC ABILITY—an ability which is manifested in only a narrow range of tasks.

REFERENCES

Abel, T. M. Moral judgments among subnormals. *Journal of Abnormal and Social Psychology*, 1941, 36, 378–392.

Allen, G. Patterns of discovery in the genetics of mental deficiency. *American Journal of Mental Deficiency*, 1958, **62**, 840–849.

Anastasi, A. *Differential psychology*, Ed. 3. New York: Crowell-Collier and Macmillan, Inc., 1958.

Atkinson, J. W. Motivational determinants of risktaking behavior in J. W. Atkinson (ed.), *Motives in fantasy, action, and society*. Princeton, N. J.: D. Van Nostrand Company, Inc., 1958*a*, pp. 322–340.

———. Towards experimental analysis of human motives in terms of motives, expectancies, and incentives. In J. W. Atkinson (ed.), *Motives in fantasy, action, and society*. Princeton, N. J.: D. Van Nostrand Company, Inc., 1958*b*, pp. 288–305.

Badt, M. I. Levels of abstraction in vocabulary definitions of mentally retarded school children. *American Journal of Mental Deficiency*, 1958, **63**, 241–246.

Balla, D., and E. Zigler. Discrimination and switching learning in normal, familial, retarded, and organic retarded children. *Journal of Abnormal and Social Psychology*, 1964, **69**, 664–669.

Barrett, H. E., and H. L. Koch. The effect of nursery-school training upon the mental test performance of a group of orphanage children. *Journal of Genetic Psychology*, 1930, **37**, 102–122.

Beckham, A. S. Minimum intelligence levels for several occupations. *Personnel Journal*, 1930, **9**, 309–313.

Beller, E. Dependency and independence in young children. *Journal of Genetic Psychology*, 1955, **87**, 25–35.

Berkowitz, H., and E. Zigler. Effects of preliminary positive and negative interactions and delay conditions on children's responsiveness to social reinforcement. *Journal of Personality and Social Psychology*, 1965, **4**, 500–505.

Berkson, G. Psychophysiological studies in mental deficiency. In N. R. Ellis (ed.), *Handbook of mental deficiency*. New York: McGraw-Hill, Inc., 1963, pp. 556–573.

Bradway, K. P. An experimental study of factors associated with Stanford-Binet IQ changes from the preschool to the junior high school. *Journal of Genetic Psychology*, 1945, **66**, 107–128.

Bruner, J. The course of cognitive growth. *American Psychologist*, 1958, **13**, 1–15.

Burks, B. S. The relative influence of nature and nurture upon mental development; a comparative study of foster parent-foster child resemblance and true parent-true child resemblance. *Yearbook of National Social Studies Education*, 1928, **27** (I), 219–316.

———. Review of Marie Skodak, *Children in foster homes: A study of mental development*. *Journal of Educational Psychology*, 1939, **30**, 548–555.

Burr, E. T. Minimum intellectual levels of accomplishment in industry. *Personnel Journal*, 1925, **3**, 207–212.

Burt, C. The inheritance of mental ability. *American Psychologist*, 1958, **13**, 1-15.

——— and M. Howard. The multifactor theory of inheritance and its application to intelligence. *British Journal of Statistical Psychology*, 1956, **9**, 95–131.

——— and M. Howard. Heredity and intelligence: A reply to criticisms. *British Journal of Statistical Psychology*, 1957, **10**, 33–63.

Butterfield, E. C., and E. Zigler. The effects of success and failure on the discrimination learning of normal and retarded children. *Journal of Abnormal Psychology*, 1965*a*, **70**, 25–31.

——— and ———. The influence of differing institutional social climates on the effectiveness of social reinforcement in the mentally retarded. *American Journal of Mental Deficiency*, 1965*b*, **70**, 48–56.

Cantor, G. N. Hull-Spence behavior theory and mental deficiency. In N. R. Ellis (ed.), *Handbook of mental deficiency*. New York: McGraw-Hill, Inc., 1963, pp. 92–133.

Capobianco, R. J. Reasoning methods and reasoning ability in mentally retarded and normal children. In E. P. Trapp and P. Himelstein (eds.), *Readings on the exceptional child*. New York: Appleton-Century-Crofts, 1962, pp. 211–227.

Chein, I. On the nature of intelligence. *Journal of Genetic Psychology*, 1945, **32**, 111–126.

Clarke, A. D. B., and A. M. Clarke. Cognitive changes in the feebleminded. *British Journal of Psychology*, 1954, **45**, 197–199.

——— and ———. Some recent advances in the study of early deprivation. *Child Psychology and Psychiatry*, 1960, **1**, 26–36.

Clarke, A. M. Criteria and classification of mental deficiency. In A. M. Clarke and

A. D. B. Clarke (eds.), *Mental deficiency: The changing outlook*. New York: The Free Press of Glencoe, 1958, pp. 43–64.

Coffey, H. S., and B. L. Wellman. The role of cultural status in intelligence changes of preschool children. *Journal of Experimental Education*, 1936–1937, **5**, 191–201.

Cohen, B. Motivation and performance in schizophrenia. *Journal of Abnormal and Social Psychology*, 1956, **52**, 186–190.

Coons, W. Abstract ability in schizophrenia and the organic psychoses. *Canadian Journal of Psychology*, 1956, **10**, 43–50.

Cromwell, R. L. A social learning approach to mental retardation. In N. R. Ellis (ed.), *Handbook of mental deficiency*. New York: McGraw-Hill, Inc., 1963, pp. 41–91.

Cruickshank, W. M. Qualitative analysis of intelligence test responses. *Journal of Clinical Psychology*, 1947, **3**, 381–386.

Dahlberg, G. On the frequency of mental deficiency. *Uppsala Lakareforenings Förhandlingar*, 1937, **42**, 439.

Doll, E. E. A historical survey of research and management of mental retardation in the United States. In E. P. Trapp and P. Himelstein (eds.), *Readings on the exceptional child*. New York: Appleton-Century-Crofts, 1962, pp. 21–68.

Ellis, N. R. The stimulus trace and behavioral inadequacy. In N. R. Ellis (ed.), *Handbook of mental deficiency*. New York: McGraw-Hill, Inc., 1963, pp. 134–158.

Erlenmeyer-Kimling, L., and L. F. Jarvik. Genetics and intelligence: A review. *Science*, 1963, **142**, No. 3598, 1477–1478.

Ferguson, G. A. On learning and human ability. *Canadian Journal of Psychology*, 1954, **8**, 95–112.

———. On transfer and the abilities of man. *Canadian Journal of Psychology*, 1956, **10**, 121–131.

Flavell, J. H. *The developmental psychology of Jean Piaget*. Princeton, N.J.: D. Van Nostrand Company, Inc., 1963.

Fremming, K. H. *The expectation of mental infirmity in a sample of a Danish Population*. London: Cassell & Co., Ltd., 1951.

Fuller, J. L. *Nature and nurture: A modern synthesis*. New York: Doubleday & Company, Inc., 1954.

——— and W. R. Thompson. *Behavior genetics*. New York: John Wiley & Sons, Inc., 1960.

Gardner, W. I. Effects of interpolated success and failure on motor task performance in mental defectives. Paper read at meeting of Southeastern Psychological Association, Nashville, Tenn., 1957.

———. *Reactions of intellectually normal and retarded boys after experimentally induced failure: A social learning theory interpretation*. Ann Arbor, Mich.: Universal Microfilms, 1958.

Garfield, S. L. Abnormal behavior and mental deficiency. In N. R. Ellis (ed), *Handbook of mental deficiency*. New York: McGraw-Hill, Inc., 1963, pp. 574–601.

Garner, W. R., H. W., Hake, and C. W. Eriksen. Operationalism and the concept of perception. *Psychological Review*, 1956, **63**, 149–159.

Garrison, M. (ed.). Cognitive models and development in mental retardation. *American Journal of Deficiency*, in press.

Gewirtz, J. Three determinants of attention seeking in young children. *Monographs on Social Research in Child Development*, 1954, **19**, No. 59.

Goldiamond, I. Indicators of perception. I. Subliminal perception, subception, unconscious perception: An analysis in terms of psychophysical indicator methodology. *Psychological Bulletin*, 1958, **55**, 373–411.

Goldstein, K. Concerning rigidity. *Character and Personality*, 1942–1943, **11**, 209–226.

Gottesman, I. L. Genetic aspects of intelligent behavior. In N. R. Ellis (ed.), *Handbook of mental deficiency*. New York: McGraw-Hill, Inc., 1963, pp. 253–296.

Green, C., and E. Zigler. Social deprivation and the performance of feebleminded and normal children on a satiation type task. *Child Development*, 1962, **33**, 499–508.

Guertin, W. H. Mental growth in pseudofeeblemindedness. *Journal of Clinical Psychology*, 1949, **5**, 414–418.

Guskin, S. Social psychologies of mental deficiency. In N. R. Ellis (ed.), *Handbook of mental deficiency*. New York: McGraw-Hill, Inc., 1963, pp. 325–352.

Heathers, G. Emotional dependence and independence in nursery school play. *Journal of Genetic Psychology*, 1955, **87**, 37–57.

Hebb, D. O. *Organization of behavior*.

New York: John Wiley & Sons, Inc., 1949.

Heber, R. F. *Expectancy and expectancy changes in normal and mentally retarded boys.* Ann Arbor, Mich.: Universal Microfilms, 1957.

———. A manual on terminology and classification in mental retardation. *American Journal of Mental Deficiency, Monograph Supplements,* 1959, **64,** No. 2.

———. Mental retardation: Concept and classification. In E. P. Trapp and P. Himelstein (eds.), *Readings on the exceptional child.* New York: Appleton-Century-Crofts, 1962, pp. 69–81.

Hirsch, J. Behavior genetics and individuality understood. *Science,* 1963, **142,** 1436–1442.

Hirsh, E. A. The adaptive significance of commonly described behavior of the mentally retarded. *American Journal of Mental Deficiency,* 1959, **63,** 639–646.

Hogben, L. *Nature and nurture.* London: George Allen & Unwin Ltd., 1933.

Hunt, J. McV. *Intelligence and experience.* New York: The Ronald Press Company, 1961.

Hurst, C. C. A genetic formula for the inheritance of intelligence in man. *Proceedings of the Royal Society, London,* 1932, **112** (Series B), 80–97.

Iscoe, I., and B. McCann. The perception of an emotional continuum by older and younger mental retardates. *Journal of Personality and Social Psychology,* 1965, **1,** 383–385.

Itard, J. M. G. *The wild boy of Aveyron* (translated by G. and M. Humphrey). New York: Appleton-Century-Crofts, 1932.

Jervis, G. A. The mental deficiencies. In S. Arieti (ed.), *American handbook of Psychiatry,* Vol. 2. New York: Basic Books, Inc., 1959, pp. 1289–1313.

Jones, D., and A. Carr-Saunders. The relation between intelligence and social status among orphan children. *British Journal of Psychology,* 1927, **17,** 343–364.

Jones, H. E. The environment and mental development. In L. Carmichael (ed.), *Manual of child psychology,* (Ed. 2.) New York: John Wiley & Sons, Inc., 1954, pp. 631–696.

Jordan, T. E., and R. DeCharms. The achievement motive in normal and mentally retarded children. *American Journal of Mental Deficiency,* 1959, **64,** 457–466.

Kaplun, D. The high-grade moron: A study of institutional admissions over a ten year period. *Proceedings of the American Association for Mental Deficiency,* 1935, **40,** 68–89.

Kass, N., and H. W. Stevenson. The effect of pre-training reinforcement conditions on learning by normal and retarded children. *American Journal of Mental Deficiency,* 1961, **66,** 76–80.

Katz, I. Review of evidence relating to effects of desegregation on the intellectual performance of Negroes. *American Psychologist,* 1964, **19,** 381–399.

Kephart, N. C. *The slow learner in the classroom.* Columbus, Ohio: Charles E. Merrill Books, Inc., 1960.

Kirk, S. *Early education of the mentally retarded.* Urbana, Ill.: University of Illinois Press, 1961.

Kohlberg, L. Sex differences in morality. In E. E. Maccoby (ed.), *Sex role development.* New York: Social Science Research Council, in press.

Köhler, W., and H. Wallach. Figural aftereffects. *Proceedings of the American Philosophical Society,* 1944, **88,** 264–357.

Kounin, J. Experimental studies of rigidity: I. The measurement of rigidity in normal and feebleminded persons. *Character and Personality,* 1941*a,* **9,** 251–272.

———. Experimental studies of rigidity: II. The explanatory power of the concept of rigidity as applied to feeblemindedness. *Character and Personality,* 1941*b,* **9,** 273–282.

———. The meaning of rigidity: A reply to Heinz Werner. *Psychological Review,* 1948, **55,** 157–166.

Kraepelin, E. *Lehrbuch der psychiatrie.* Leipzig, Ger.: Barth, 1912.

Krugman, M. Some impressions of the revised Stanford-Binet scale. *Journal of Educational Psychology,* 1939, **30,** 594–603.

Lantz, B. Some dynamic aspects of success and failure. *Psychological Monographs,* 1945, **59,** No. 271.

Lashley, K. S., K. L. Chow, and J. Semmes. An examination of the electrical field theory of cerebral integration. *Psychological Review,* 1951, **58,** 123–136.

Laurendeau, M., and A. Pinard. *Causal thinking in the child.* New York: International Universities Press, 1962.

Leahy, A. M. Nature-nurture and intelligence. *Genetic Psychology Monographs*, 1935, **17**, 236–308.

Lewin, K. *A dynamic theory of personality*. New York: McGraw-Hill, Inc., 1936.

Lewis, E. O. *Report of the Mental Deficiency Committee*, Part IV. London: His Majesty's Stationery Office, 1929.

———. Types of mental deficiency and their social significance. *Journal of Mental Science*, 1933, **79**, 298–304.

Lipman, R. S. Learning: Verbal, perceptual-motor, and classical conditioning. In N. R. Ellis (ed.), *Handbook of mental deficiency*. New York: McGraw-Hill, Inc., 1963, pp. 391–423.

Liverant, S. Intelligence: A concept in need of re-examination. *Journal of Consulting Psychology*, 1960, **24**, 101–110.

Luria, A. R. Psychological studies of mental deficiency in the Soviet Union. In N. R. Ellis (ed.), *Handbook of mental deficiency*. New York: McGraw-Hill, Inc., 1963, pp. 353–387.

Lyle, J. The effect of an institution environment upon the verbal development of imbecile children. I. Verbal intelligence. *Journal of Mental Deficiency Research*, 1959, **3**, 122–128.

Maher, B. A. Intelligence and brain damage. In N. R. Ellis (ed.), *Handbook of mental deficiency*. New York: McGraw-Hill, Inc., 1963, pp. 224–252.

Mandler, G., and S. B. Sarason. A study of anxiety and learning. *Journal of Abnormal and Social Psychology*, 1952, **47**, 166–173.

Masland, R. L. Methodological approaches to research in etiology. *American Journal of Mental Deficiency*, 1959, **64**, 305–310.

Mayer, E., and W. Coons. Motivation and the spiral aftereffect with schizophrenic and brain damaged patients. *Canadian Journal of Psychology*, 1960, **14**, 269–274.

McCandless, B. R. Relation of environmental factors to intellectual functioning. In R. Heber and H. Stevens (eds.), *Review of research in mental retardation*. Chicago: University of Chicago Press, 1964, pp. 175–213.

McClearn, G. E. The inheritance of behavior. In L. Postman (ed.), *Psychology in the Making*. New York: Alfred A. Knopf, 1962, pp. 144–252.

———. Genetics and behavior development. In M. L. Hoffman and L. W. Hoffman (eds.), *Review of child development research*, Vol. 1. New York: Russell Sage Foundation, 1964, pp. 433–480.

McCoy, N., and E. Zigler. Social reinforcer effectiveness as a function of the relationship between child and adult. *Journal of Abnormal and Social Psychology*, 1965, **1**, 604–612.

McKinney, J. P., and T. Keele. Effects of increased mothering on the behavior of severely retarded boys. *American Journal of Mental Deficiency*, 1963, **67**, 556–562.

Mental retardation in the Soviet Union. *Canada's Mental Health Supplement*, 1964, No. 42.

Milgram, N. A., and H. G. Furth. The influence of language on concept attainment in educable retarded children. *American Journal of Mental Deficiency*, 1963, **67**, 733–739.

Newman, H. H., F. N. Freeman, and K. J. Holzinger. *Twins: A study of heredity and environment*. Chicago: University of Chicago Press, 1937.

Nye, F. I. *Family relationships and delinquent behavior*. New York: John Wiley & Sons, Inc., 1958.

O'Connor, N., and B. Hermelin. Discrimination and reversal learning in imbeciles. *Journal of Abnormal and Social Psychology*, 1959, **59**, 409–413.

Osborn, W. Associative clustering in organic and familial retardates. *American Journal of Mental Deficiency*, 1960, **65**, 351–357.

Penrose, L. S. *The biology of mental defect*. London: Sidgwick & Jackson, Ltd., 1963.

Pevsner, M. S. *Oligophrenia: Mental deficiency in children*. New York: Consultants Bureau Enterprises, Inc., 1961.

Phillips, L., and E. Zigler. Social competence, the action-thought parameter and vicariousness in normal and pathological behaviors. *Journal of Abnormal and Social Psychology*, 1961, **63**, 127–146.

——— and ———. Role orientation, the action-thought parameter and outcome in psychiatric disorder. *Journal of Abnormal and Social Psychology*, 1964, **68**, 381–389.

Piaget, J. *The moral judgment of the child*. New York: The Free Press, 1948.

Pickford, R. W. The genetics of intelligence. *Journal of Psychology*, 1949, **28**, 129–145.

Plenderleith, M. Discrimination learning and discrimination reversal learning in normal and feeblemindead children. *Journal of Genetic Psychology*, 1956, **88**, 107–112.

President's Panel on Mental Retardation. *A proposed program for national action to combat mental retardation.* Washington, D.C. U. S. Government Printing Office, 1962.

Riber, M. Verbal mediation in normal and retarded children. *American Journal of Mental Deficiency*, 1964, **68**, 634–641.

Roberts, J. A. F. The genetics of mental deficiency. *Eugenics Review*, 1952, **44**, 71–83.

Rotter, J. B. *Social learning and clinical psychology*. Englewood Cliffs, N.J.: Prentice-Hall, Inc., 1954.

Sarason, S. B. *Psychological problems in mental deficiency*. New York: Harper & Row, Publishers, 1953.

———, K. S. Davidson, F. F. Lighthall, R. R. Waite, and B. K. Ruebush. *Anxiety in elementary school children*. New York: John Wiley & Sons, Inc., 1960.

——— and T. Gladwin. Psychological and cultural problems in mental subnormality: A review of research. *Genetic Psychology Monographs*, 1958, **57**, 3–290.

Schlanger, B. B. Environmental influences on the verbal output of mentally retarded children. *Journal of Speech and Hearing Disorders*, 1954, **19**, 339–345.

Shallenberger, P., and E. Zigler. Rigidity, negative reaction tendencies, and cosatiation effects in normal and feebleminded children. *Journal of Abnormal and Social Psychology*, 1961, **63**, 20–26.

Shepps, R., and E. Zigler. Social deprivation and rigidity in the performance of organic and familial retardates. *American Journal of Mental Deficiency*, 1962, **67**, 262–268.

Siegel, P. S., and J. G. Foshee. Molar variability in the mentally defective. *Journal of Abnormal and Social Psychology*, 1960, **61**, 141–143.

Sjögren, T. Genetic-statistical and psychiatric investigations of a West Swedish population. *Acta Psychiatrica et Neurologica Scandinavica*, Supplement, 1948, **52**, 1.

Skeels, H. M., R. Updegraff, B. L. Wellman, and H. M. Williams. A study of environmental stimulation. *University of Iowa Studies in Child Welfare*, 1938, **15**, No. 4.

Smedslund, J. The acquisition of conservation of substance and weight in children. *Journal of Scandinavian Psychology*, 1961, **2**, 71–87.

Smith, S. Language and non-verbal test performance of racial groups in Honolulu before and after a fourteen-year interval. *Journal of Genetic Psychology*, 1942, **26**, 51–98.

Spence, K. W. A theory of emotionally based drive (D) and its relation to performance in simple learning situations. *American Psychologist*, 1958, **13**, 131–141.

Spiker, C. C., and B. R. McCandless. The concept of intelligence and the philosophy of science. *Psychological Review*, 1954, **61**, 255–266.

Spitz, H. H. Field theory in mental deficiency. In N. R. Ellis (ed.), *Handbook of mental deficiency*. New York: McGraw-Hill, Inc., 1963, pp. 11–40.

Spivack, G. Perceptual processes. In N. R. Ellis (ed.), *Handbook of mental deficiency*. New York: McGraw-Hill, Inc., 1963, pp. 480–511.

Spradlin, J. E. Language and communication of mental defectives. In N. R. Ellis (ed.), *Handbook of mental deficiency*. New York: McGraw-Hill, Inc., 1963, pp. 512–555.

Stevenson, H. W. Discrimination learning. In N. R. Ellis (ed.), *Handbook of mental deficiency*. New York: McGraw-Hill, Inc., 1963, pp. 424–438.

——— and L. Fahel. The effect of social reinforcement on the performance of institutionalized and noninstitutionalized normal and feebleminded children. *Journal of Personality*, 1961, **29**, 136–147.

——— and E. Zigler. Discrimination learning and rigidity in normal and feebleminded individuals. *Journal of Personality*, 1957, **25**, 699–711.

——— and ———. Probability learning in children. *Journal of Experimental Psychology*, 1958, **56**, 185–192.

Strömgren, E. *Beiträge zur psychiatrischen erblehre*. Copenhagen: Munksgaard, 1938.

Taylor, J. A. Drive theory and manifest anxiety. In M. T. Mednick and S. A. Mednick (eds.), *Research in personality*. New York: Holt, Rinehart & Winston, 1963, pp. 205–222.

Thorndike, E. L. Measurements of twins. *Columbia University Contributions to Philosophy and Psychology*, 1905, **13**, 1–64.

Thorpe, L. P. *Child psychology and development*. New York: The Ronald Press Company, 1946.

Tizard, J. The prevalence of mental subnormality. *Bulletin of the World Health Organization*, 1953, **9**, 423–440.

Tredgold, A. F. *A textbook of mental deficiency*, Ed. 8. Baltimore: The Williams & Wilkins Company, 1952.

Tuddenham, R. D. The nature and measurement of intelligence. In L. Postman (ed.), *Psychology in the making*. New York: Knopf, 1962, pp. 469–525.

Turnure, J., and E. Zigler. Outerdirectedness in the problem solving of normal and retarded children. *Journal of Abnormal and Social Psychology*, 1964, **69**, 427–436.

Tyler, L. E. *The psychology of human differences*, Ed. 2. New York: Appleton-Century-Crofts, 1956.

Weaver, T. R. The incidence of maladjustment among mental defectives in a military environment. *American Journal of Mental Deficiency*, 1946, **51**, 238–246.

Wellman, B. L. The effect of preschool attendance upon the IQ. *Journal of Experimental Education*, 1932–1933, **1**, 48–69.

———. Growth in intelligence under differing school environments. *Journal of Experimental Education*, 1934–1935, **3**, 59–83.

———. Mental growth from preschool to college. *Journal of Experimental Education*, 1937–1938, **6**, 127–138.

———. The intelligence of preschool children as measured by the Merrill-Palmer scale of performance tests. *University of Iowa Studies in Child Welfare*, 1938*a*, **15**, No. 3.

———. Guiding mental development. *Childhood Education*, 1938*b*, **15**, 108–112.

Werner, H. Process and achievement—a basic problem of education and developmental psychology. *Harvard Education Review*, 1937, **7**, No. 3, 353–368.

Wheeler, L. R. A comparative study of the intelligence of East Tennessee mountain children. *Journal of Educational Psychology*, 1942, **33**, 321–334.

Whitney, E. A. Mental deficiency—1955. *American Journal of Mental Deficiency*, 1956, **60**, 676–683.

Windle, C. Prognosis of mental subnormals. *American Journal of Mental Deficiency, Monograph Supplements*, 1962, **66**, No. 5.

Wohlwill, J. E., and R. C. Lowe. Experimental analysis of the development of the conservation of number. *Child Development*, 1962, **33**, 153–167.

Woodward, M. Early experiences and later social responses of severely subnormal children. *British Journal of Medical Psychology*, 1960, **33**, 123–132.

———. The application of Piaget's theory to research in mental deficiency. In N. R. Ellis (ed.), *Handbook of mental deficiency*. New York: McGraw-Hill, Inc., 1963, pp. 297–324.

Woodworth, R. S. *Heredity and environment*. New York: Social Science Research Council, 1941.

Zeaman, D., and B. J. House. Approach and avoidance in the discrimination learning of retardates. In D. Zeaman *et al.* (eds.), *Learning and transfer in mental defectives*. Progress Report No. 2, National Institute of Mental Health, 1960, pp. 32–70.

Zigler, E. The effect of pre-institutional social deprivation on the performance of feebleminded children. Unpublished doctoral dissertation, University of Texas, Austin, 1958.

———. Social deprivation and rigidity in the performance of feebleminded children. *Journal of Abnormal and Social Psychology*, 1961, **62**, 413–421.

———. Rigidity in the feebleminded. In E. P. Trapp and P. Himelstein (eds.), *Readings on the exceptional child*. New York: Appleton-Century-Crofts, 1962, pp. 141–162.

———. Rigidity and social reinforcement effects in the performance of institutionalized and noninstitutionalized normal and retarded children. *Journal of Personality*, 1963*a*, **31**, 258–269.

———. Social reinforcement, environment and the child. *American Journal of Orthopsychiatry*, 1963*b*, **33**, 614–623.

——— and E. Butterfield. Rigidity in the retarded: A further test of the Lewin-Kounin formulation. *Journal of Abnormal Psychology*, in press.

——— and J. DeLabry. Concept-switching in middle-class, lower-class, and retarded children. *Journal of Abnormal and Social Psychology*, 1962, **65**, 267–273.

———, L. Hodgen, and H. Stevenson. The effect of support on the performance of normal and feebleminded children. *Journal of Personality*, 1958, **26**, 106–122.

——— and E. Unell. Concept-switching in normal and feebleminded children as a function of reinforcement. *American Journal of Mental Deficiency*, 1962, **66**, 651–657.

——— and J. Williams. Institutionalization and the effectiveness of social reinforcement: A three year follow-up study. *Journal of Abnormal and Social Psychology*, 1963, **66**, 197–205.

SUGGESTED READINGS

1. Anastasi, Anne. *Differential psychology*, Ed. 3. New York: Crowell-Collier and Macmillan, 1958. A text that, concerned with the differences between people, devotes several excellent chapters to considerations of both mental retardation and of genius.
2. Ellis, N. R. (ed.). *Handbook of mental deficiency*. New York: McGraw-Hill, Inc., 1963. A collection of theories and research papers on mental retardation.
3. Flavell, J. H. *The developmental psychology of Jean Piaget*. Princeton, N.J.: D. Van Nostrand Company, Inc., 1963. A comprehensive summary and evaluation of Piaget's endeavors by a man who is both sympathetic to his views and concerned about the research documentation that supports them. Piaget is an enormously prolific and complicated writer whose works now extend over nearly five decades.
4. Hirsch, J. Behavior genetics and individuality understood. *Science*, 1963, **142**, 1436–42. An important contribution on the biological bases of individual differences. The paper is relevant to the polygenic model of retardation that is presented here.
5. Lewin, K. *A dynamic theory of personality*. New York: McGraw-Hill, Inc., 1936. A classic in personality theory that describes Lewin's theories of boundaries, permeability, and rigidity.
6. Zigler, E., and J. Williams. Institutionalization and the effectiveness of social reinforcement: A three year follow-up study. *Journal of Abnormal and Social Psychology*, 1963, **66**, 197–205. An examination of the effects of institutionalization on the responsiveness of mentally retarded children to social reinforcement. Children who had come from "good" homes (that is socially nurturant ones) evidenced less need for social reinforcement initially, but considerably more after three years. On the other hand, those who came from relatively impoverished social backgrounds responded strongly to social reinforcement from the time of admission to the institution.

15

Therapy and Remediation

DAVID ROSENHAN

PERRY LONDON

There is no shortage at all of methods and techniques for helping people with psychological problems; but there is a terrible shortage of methods that work with any certainty, and an even greater shortage of knowledge about what makes any technique work successfully when it does. Either way, any simple overview of the educational and healing methods applied to the wide variety of known personal problems is likely to be misleading. If it is comprehensible, then the very size of the catalogue of treatments creates the mistaken impression that the field is better studied and understood than it really is. If the list of treatments is brief, on the other hand, and more attention is paid to the processes of remediation which are evidently used in treatment, the impression is given that these processes are less speculative and more real than is, in fact, known to be the case.

The problem is not so much one of exposition as it is of the very nature of remedial work in this field. The organizer of textbook material on therapy is almost faced more with the question of how to do least disservice to the reader than of how to make the most through presentation of the subject matter.

Since there does not seem to be an altogether satisfactory solution to the problem, we have decided, for the purposes of this chapter, to concentrate on the ways in which treatment procedures can be organized and understood rather than to elaborate what all of them are. To this end, the chapter is divided into three parts. The first concerns the nature of treatment, the problems to which it is addressed, and the categories into which treatments can most conveniently be divided. The second section gives a brief description of the different techniques and systems which may be regarded as, respectively, *medical* and *educational*. The third part, which contains the bulk of the subject matter, focuses on the particular set of treatments called *psychotherapy*; it presents an intellectual scheme for understanding them and offers some description of the actual techniques and practices of different schools and practitioners.

THE NATURE OF MENTAL TREATMENT

It should be clear from the material of earlier chapters that there is no clear-cut agreement about the precise nature of psychological disorders. "Mental illness" is not an acceptable term for many conditions because illness or disease is plainly not involved; "learning problem" does not apply to other conditions because they seem to involve so much more or less than learning. Some physical ailments are evidently learned in the sense that one or another habit pattern has disposed the individual to them, as with headaches or ulcers, and some disorders of behavior stem directly from physical illness, such as some mental retardations or paresis or epilepsy. As we saw in Chapter 13, there is no clear way to distinguish between psychological and physical disorders if one requires an absolute and firm distinction. And the conflict over whether so-called mental illness is really illness or not can, if taken too seriously, produce more confusion than understanding.

For the most part, there is no need to be very precise about the distinction between the categories of disorder (psychological versus physical), any more than there is a need to decide whether the soul and the body are really separate or separable. Most physical ailments, regardless of how they originated, are treated most readily by one or another medical means. Most behavior disorders, on the other hand, yield more readily or permanently to psychological or behavioral kinds of treatment, although medicine is sometimes a helpful adjunct. What is important to understand is the nature of the different problems and ailments that come within the common purview of the mental health disciplines and professions and the strengths and weaknesses of the different methods used to help resolve them.

Historically, virtually all disorders of the brain or central nervous system fell within the province of psychiatry, but most of these are properly relegated to neurology, medicine, and surgery today. Conditions like paresis, encephalitis, meningitis, brain tumors, and toxic, metabolic, and nutritional deficiencies are clearly within the scope of medical rather than psychological treatments. These will not be discussed further here.

The conditions which are most clearly in the province of the mental health disciplines are those which are most clearly functional in origin and for which strictly medical treatment may or may not be of any value. There are many different ways of classifying these problems. The most familiar one, of course, is the conventional trichotomy of (1) neuroses, (2) psychoses, and (3) character disorders, but as we have seen, the utility of these classifications is questionable; they do not always imply a clear distinction of kind or of severity of the problems involved. What is more, neither psychosomatic nor some mental retardation problems can be classified as "functional," strictly speaking, but they certainly are mental health problems.

It should be quite apparent from the previous six chapters that, traditionally, different problem categories were composed on the basis primarily of *symptom similarity* and secondarily of *probable etiology* (origins), *not* on the basis of amenability to one or another kind of treatment. Indeed, it was long taken for granted that many problems could not be treated by *any* means; on the other hand, many mental health experts naively try to use one kind of pet treatment for a whole variety of problems. The truth is that just about every kind of treatment tends to be used by one or another practitioner for just about every kind of disorder, and it is important to understand that this happens because the disorder implies nothing about the treatment. In other words, the classification of a disorder does not dictate its cure, regardless of whether the classification is based on symptoms or on cause. Psychosomatic *symptoms* like asthma or hypertension may respond very nicely to psychotherapy and may not respond as well to medicines, although the opposite is probably more often true. Mental retardation is most often approached by educational techniques, although sometimes by medicine, and psychosis, neurosis, and character disorders are commonly attacked by all three modes of treatment. Genetic *causes* of things like some kinds of retardation or possibly schizophrenia do not imply either that the conditions are untreatable or that educational techniques are useless in their treatment. Nor does the fact that many disorders have *dynamic*, that is psychological, causes suggest that they cannot be treated by physical means.

The most sensible way to classify disorders, if one wishes to relate type of problem to type of treatment, is in terms of the functional problem involved, that is in terms of what needs to happen to somebody for him to be considered free of a given disorder or, conversely, what it is about his *behavior* that makes us consider him disordered to begin with. This is precisely what is attempted for many disorders in Chapter 9 under "Social-Learning Taxonomy of Deviant Behavior." Unfortunately, a comprehensive classification by functional analysis is not possible because too many kinds of different problems can be defined as psychological. If it were possible, moreover, its usefulness would be limited by the fact that some effective treatments are not aimed directly at the disorder but at some underlying attribute of it. A functional analysis of depression, for example, would not necessarily indicate that electric shock was a good treatment for it, nor could anybody guess, from functional analysis of phenylketonuric mental deficiency, that drugs and diet can be used to control it (see Chapter 2). Functional analysis is still the best single means of classification for treatment purposes, however; the point is that *no completely* satisfactory scheme exists.

Categories of Treatment

The study of treatments is saved from being a hopeless mess because they do not have to be classified by disorders in order to be intelligible. Just as there are conventions for categorizing disabilities, there are conventional ways of classifying the things that are done to relieve them. These conventions typically revolve around the kinds of personnel who treat psychological disorders, the kinds of techniques they use, and the situations in which they use them. Pooling these together yields three inexact categories: (1) medical treatments, (2) educational treatments, and (3) psychotherapy. These categories are anything but mutually exclusive; psychotherapy, in particular, overlaps the other two. But medical treatments do include a number of things which are ordinarily handled only by physicians and a few things which are illegal for anyone else to administer. Educational treatments include a number of techniques which involve specialized training ordinarily possessed only by educational specialists. Professional trade and technical treatment get mixed up by our classification, but they are all mixed up among the professions anyway, and you can be spared some confusion by recognizing in advance the profusion of names and confusion of titles and functions that characterize the field. By *medical* treatments, we mean only the use of *chemical* or *physical* manipulations of the body, but some physicians consider psychotherapy a form of medicine. By *educational* treatments, we mean the use of *instructions* and *demonstrations* to alleviate fairly specific and concrete disabilities, but some kinds of educational treatments, called "guidance" and "counseling," can be considered forms of psychotherapy. And psychotherapy can inevitably be regarded as a special case of educational treatment, although it is more often viewed as a separate discipline which is not exactly the practice of medicine, not just the same as teaching, more than merely giving advice, and less than religious revivalism—but still a means of changing people's lives.

Assessing treatment effects. Regardless of how they are classified, all kinds of treatment must confront the same problems of evaluation. Are they effective? But that simple question is considerably more complex than it appears, for what do we mean by "effective"? One can judge a treatment by a variety of means:

How many of the patient's symptoms abate?
How long does he stay in the hospital, or in treatment?
Once discharged from treatment or the hospital, how long does he stay out, and if he returns, how much further treatment does he require?
Quite apart from symptom remission, does the patient feel well?
How long does it take for the treatment to begin to work?
How expensive is the treatment?
Even if one treatment takes a longer time to work than another, can it be utilized outside the hospital whereas the other can only be used with hospitalization?
Might the patient have "gotten well" as rapidly without the treatment? And even if not, might it have been better to extend the illness somewhat by withholding treatment in order to reduce the expense and potential dangers of treatment?

Clearly these are not easy questions, and most often the study that addresses itself to one overlooks the others. Moreover, there is no simple correlation between one criterion and another: one cannot assume that because a treatment reduces symptoms, it also has reduced the probability, say, that the patient will require rehospitalization. Making general comparisons of the relative effectiveness of two kinds of treatment is no easier. Treatment A can be more effective than B according to one criterion, less effective according to another, and equally effective with regard to a third.

The difficulties, moreover, are not simply limited to finding a criterion or a set of criteria against which a particular treatment can be evaluated. In addition, it is difficult to separate the treatment from *the person* who administers it and *the context* in which it is administered. During the early days of chlorpromazine, for example, when it was being used experimentally to treat schizophrenia, the drug was introduced to a group of some two hundred chronic schizophrenics all of whom had been hospitalized for at least five years and many of whom were seriously regressed. Before the initiation of drug therapy, the building they lived in had been understaffed. But once the drug was introduced, staff from the entire hospital was brought to examine the effects and to assess the action of the drug against a large number of criteria. Data on the patients were collected daily, and in general there was an atmosphere of considerable optimism. After all, chronic schizophrenia had been resistant to all forms of treatment, and this particular drug had excellent references.

It did not take long before the effects of the drug were visible. Patients became more manageable and rational, bizarre symptoms were disappearing, and some patients were moving towards discharge. In less than six months, the staff was sufficiently optimistic that it began to use the drug with other patients in the hospital with the same fine results. The discharge rate climbed, and with it, the sense that some important psychiatric problems had been all but solved.

Not very long thereafter, when the excitement abated and the drug was beginning to be taken as a matter of course, the staff noticed that the discharge rate was beginning to fall. For some reason, patients were not improving so well as they had during the prior year. Having ascertained that the chemical formula of the drug had not been altered, the search for the sources of reduced effectiveness led inevitably to the conclusion that the effects of the drug were inextricably bound to the attitudes of the staff. During the experimental period, the staff interacted vigorously with the patients, some of whom had not spoken to a physician or psychologist for a long time. The slightest minutiae of patient progress became matters of considerable interest. But once the utility of the drug was "established," the staff returned to its former chores and habits, and the rate of patient recovery declined. At it happens, even with less concentrated staff attention, the rate of recovery stabilized at a higher level than it had been before the use of the drug, but not at nearly as high a level as had occurred during the early days of experimentation.

In sum, human beings are such complicated creatures that their disorders and repairs take complicated forms. The proper evaluation of any treatment, therefore, requires not merely that it work but that it work better than an alternative might. Specifically, an effective treatment must produce a higher rate of recovery than could be obtained *spontaneously*, that is, without any treatment at all. And it must also work better than a *placebo*, that is, a phony technique which bears a superficial resemblance to treatment but which takes effect, if at all, only because it has some of the properties of treatment without the same substantive characteristics. The best single method which has been evolved for testing these effects is that of the *double-blind*.

The double-blind method. One of the main reasons why many therapies retain an image of much greater effectiveness than they actually have is that there is a tremendous medical literature attesting to their efficacy. The scientific utility of much of that literature, however, is at best quite weak, and the image it propels is maintained by bulk rather than by substance. Its main shortcomings consist in (1) the failure to employ control groups and (2) the failure to employ a double-blind design.

In the typical evaluation, a researcher treats a group of patients with a particular technique and assesses its effects without using another group of similar patients who receive placebo or no treatment. If a researcher finds that some 50 percent of his patients improve under this particular treatment, how do we know that they would not have improved without treatment or with placebo treatment?

Even where control groups are employed, the fact that the researcher knows which patient is in the experimental group and which on placebo is likely to affect the outcome of the study. Clearly, where the doctor knows that the patient is receiving the drug, he will be inclined, in his subsequent evaluations, to favor the drug over the placebo. And of course, should the patient know that he is getting placebos, he is not likely to improve. The double-blind method consists of withholding from doctor and patient alike knowledge of which pill is drug and which placebo, so that the subsequent evaluations are made only with reference to the patient's progress and with no contaminating foreknowledge. In the abundant literature on treatment methods, such studies are rare indeed.

The double-blind method, however, is by no means foolproof. Drug treatments have side effects, for example, while placebos commonly do not, and over a period of time it is quite likely that a thoughtful doctor will detect that some of his patients are receiving the "real thing." In some hospitals, nursing staffs charged with the administration of drugs in a double-blind experiment make something of a game out of discerning which is the drug and which the placebo. Thus, even the double-blind procedure has hazards.

It is clear, in short, that one cannot consider the effects of treatments apart from the context in which they are administered and the agents who administer them. While it has sometimes seemed that drugs are a medical rather than a psychological treatment, they clearly involve both, and in this sense, are truly psychosomatic. The social psychology of the administration of a treatment is as relevant to the health of the patient as is the chemistry of a pill.

To make things even more difficult, it is not always easy to say what kinds of treatment effects are desirable or undesirable even when it is possible to specify exactly what the effects are. This is often a moral question to which scientific answers are irrelevant, but it comes up all the time in connection with mental health problems (London, 1964; in press). If an alcoholic who is treated medically with Antabuse (a drug that causes violent vomiting if alcohol is taken while it is in the body) gives up drinking but takes up marijuana instead, how does one evaluate the treatment? Good, bad, or nil? If a sexually frigid woman undergoes psychotherapy and, freed of her fears of sex, becomes promiscuous, shall we consider her improved or impaired? The answer depends on the moral perspective of the patient, the therapist, and society, but since these may all be at cross-purposes, it is necessarily an ambiguous answer.

FOCUSED TREATMENTS: MEDICAL AND EDUCATIONAL

Medical Procedures

A large number of medical treatments are used for several different disorders. Their effectiveness is less than their profusion. Considering the ways they are used and the kinds of effects they are intended to have, medical treatments fall into two general groups: (1) *assault* treatments, which mainly include shock therapies and surgery; and (2) *tranquilizing* treatments, which nowadays are limited almost entirely to two kinds of drugs—"energizers," which lift the spirits, and "tranquilizers," which soothe them.

Assault treatments. Colloquially known as "shock" treatments, assault therapies are generally used only with patients whose disabilities are serious enough to require hospitalization, although electric shock treatments ("electroconvulsive therapy" or ECT), the most widely used assault method, are occasionally used in office practice as well. As currently practiced, ECT consists of applying a small electric current (60 cycles a.c.) to the front part of the patient's head. This produces unconsciousness and a convulsion, with some slight risk of wrenching muscles or breaking bones. At its best, the process is very distasteful to those who undergo it because, although it seems to be painless, patients awaken afterwards with frightening feelings of disorientation in time and space. At its worst, it can have dangerous side effects in damaged muscles, bones, or brain tissue.

The use of electricity in the treatment of physical and psychological disorders has a fairly long history, dating almost from the discovery of electricity; it has been applied to the cure of almost everything, and with little success. Its modern use dates from the discovery by Cerletti and Bini, in 1938, that convulsions could be produced electrically in dogs without causing apparent damage to brain tissue.

Later, similar findings were established for humans, along with clinical observations that they appeared to be relieved of symptoms of psychological disorders.

Until 1950, ECT was the primary and often the sole treatment for schizophrenia, but it is now clear that schizophrenics are not responsive to the treatment. The major area in which effectiveness has been reported is in the treatment of depression, and particularly of severe or agitated depression. Here, there seems to be some advantage of ECT over no treatment, drug treatment, or placebo, although the evidence is difficult to evaluate for several reasons. In the first place, where ECT is concerned, it is not possible to perform a "double-blind" study, where neither the patient receiving the treatment nor the person evaluating it is aware of what has been administered. Moreover, where ECT seems to be more effective than other procedures, it is difficult to know what it is that makes it more effective. There is some evidence that ECT widely affects the entire autonomic nervous system and lowers the blood-brain barrier, enabling chemical substances to pass more readily from the circulatory system into the brain, but it is not clear how such events might be responsible for the alleviation of depression. Conceivably, the very pain of receiving ECT might be sufficient to abate depression, as indicated in Chapter 11.

With the advent of antidepressant drugs in the 1950's, the use of ECT was greatly curtailed, perhaps by as much as 50 percent (Impastato, 1962). The treatment seemed altogether too traumatic, the effects on memory too substantial, and the difficulty of administration too great. However, antidepressant drugs were not as successful as had been expected, and within a short period of time, physicians were again using ECT for the treatment of depression. Smith and Biddy (1964) claim that ECT, compared to drugs, is the more effective, reliable, and rapid method for alleviating severe depression. Lingl (1964), on the other hand, reports that drug-treated patients begin to improve earlier than those treated with ECT, although both of his groups remained hospitalized for essentially the same period of time.

While both ECT and antidepressant drugs have been shown to be significantly more effective than placebo or no treatment at all, we need to bear in mind that a high percentage of patients improve without treatment. Because of the high incidence of spontaneous improvement, it has been thought advisable to withhold shock therapy from patients who complain only of mild depression in order to avoid the risks of side effects associated with it. In cases of severe depression, however, especially where the possibility of suicide exists, immediate treatment with ECT or drugs has commonly been recommended.

The use of chemical shocking agents preceded the use of electricity as a means of inducing convulsions to treat mental illness. There is even some evidence that efforts to treat mental illness with chemically induced convulsions date back to the eighteenth century.

Von Meduna is credited with being the first to systematically investigate the effectiveness of chemically induced convulsions in treating mental illness. The results of his work were made public in 1935, three years before electroconvulsive therapy was introduced. In his early work, von Meduna used 25 percent camphor in oil, injected intramuscularly, to induce convulsions. Because of difficulties associated with this method, he later used injections of Metrazol, a soluble, synthetic camphor preparation. Despite the superiority of Metrazol injections over the earlier method, several difficulties still remained. The most serious drawback was that the patient remained conscious until the convulsions took place, and many experienced what they described as a feeling of impending death and sudden annihilation during the interval between the Metrazol injection and the convulsions. In some cases, a convulsion failed to occur at all after injections of Metrazol, and the patients often experienced anxiety, restlessness, nausea, and general discomfort which lasted for several hours. By and large, Metrazol therapy, like insulin, has been abandoned in favor of strong tranquilizing drugs.

Insulin coma treatment was actually the earliest of the modern methods of shock treatment for mental illness. Before 1933, it was used for the symptomatic treatment of various types of psychiatric patients, such as morphine addicts, but it was then administered in small doses, and pains were taken to avoid inducing a hypoglycemic coma. Sakel, however, observed that schizophrenic patients often showed significant improvement after accidentally experiencing coma during insulin treatment. This observation led him to treat schizophrenics by deliberately inducing comas with larger doses of insulin. Following its introduction in 1933, insulin coma treatment became very popular, and at the International Congress of Psychiatry in 1950, it was accepted as the best available treatment of early schizophrenia. Insulin coma has also been used to treat other mental illnesses, such as involutional melancholia, but its effectiveness remains greatest in schizophrenia.

With the advent of tranquilizers in the early 1950's, the use of insulin coma was greatly curtailed. Most controlled studies have found no difference in effectiveness between insulin coma treatment and tranquilizers, but administering tranquilizer pills is a far simpler procedure than administering insulin, which requires close and continuous observation of the patient for a period of a month or more, and tranquilizers are much cheaper to boot. They have not, however, completely replaced insulin coma treatment, which is still used in mental hospitals when such methods as tranquilizers prove ineffective.

Most people do not think of *surgery* as a method of psychiatric treatment, but "prefrontal lobotomy," where the patient's frontal brain lobes are partially separated from the thalamus, was fairly widely practiced during the late thirties and forties. Its effect was to calm an aroused patient (and often to arouse a calmed one) and to make him more manageable in the hospital. Unintended side effects were often dramatic, and death resulted in from 1 to 4 percent of the surgeries performed. While variations of the prefrontal lobotomy have been introduced and promoted, especially by Freeman and Watts (1942; Freeman, 1949), the general opinion of psychiatrists is that their risks far outweigh their potential benefits, particularly since the damages inflicted by brain surgeries are not reversible.

Although it is not widely discussed as such, some mention might be made of *plastic surgery* as a treatment for psychological conditions. Often, people will request cosmetic surgery and doctors will undertake it in order to alleviate anxieties or difficulties in life which result from a marred appearance. The utility of this treatment is another story. In some instances, it is really of immense value to the individual. In others, especially where the desire for surgery reflects an unrealistic fantasy that changing appearance will somehow provide or restore a new and happier personality, the results are nil or worse. On rare occasions, the fact that the person's difficulties are not relieved one iota may cause even more severe disturbances than were evident originally, since the fantasy no longer shields the individual from the source of his or her difficulties.

Tranquilizing treatments. Although some kinds of physical restraints—like *hydrotherapy*, a compulsory long-lasting warm bath—were once thought of as having a soothing therapeutic effect, such techniques are no longer used much in enlightened institutions. Tranquilizer pills, which were rapidly accepted by the medical profession after their introduction in 1953, have made them unnecessary. Uhr and Miller (1960) estimate that tranquilizers are the third most common kind of drug dispensed by general practitioners and that they appear in more than 10 percent of all prescriptions —in more than 65 million prescriptions a year.

Drugs are certainly by now the most common form of medical treatment for *all* psychological disabilities, and they are becoming more common all the time as hard-working drug companies proliferate research which produces more and more of them and promotions which sell more and more of them. They have wrought a real revolution in the management of mental disorders, especially in hospitals; but in and of themselves, they generally do not produce cures of any kind.

There are several different technical categories of psychiatric drugs. The main ones are *ataractics* or "strong" tranquilizers, most common of which is chlorpromazine; "minor" or "weak" *tranquilizers*, best represented by meprobamate (which you may know as Equanil or Miltown, its commercial names); *antidepressants*, which tend to induce euphoria; and *sedatives*, such as phenobarbital. In terms of what they do, they can all be divided into "tranquilizers" and "energizers." All of them work on the central nervous system, and their overall effect is just what the class name suggests. They are obviously of particular value for people whose symptoms include lethargy, on the one hand, or agitation, on the other. Sometimes they help to alleviate feelings of depression and very often of anxiety. In a hospital situation, this makes it much more possible for hospital personnel to manage their routines and, to that extent, to be more sympathetic and helpful to their patients. Both in and out of hospitals, the equilibrating effect of the drugs, particularly the strong ones, may make it easier for a patient to be receptive to psychological treatments.

Less is known about the drugs than would seem to be the case from either the ease with which doctors sometimes prescribe them or the exorbitant prices the public is made to pay for them. In some cases, they have no demonstrable effects at all; in still others, the effects are just the opposite of those expected. A hyperactive child, for example, who is absolutely uncontrollable by means of tranquilizers or sedatives may be considerably calmed by the administration of benzedrine, one of the most powerful energizing drugs. No good reason for this phenomenon is known, and the selection of particular drugs for particular conditions is often done on a purely and rudely experimental basis.

Research on psychiatric drugs is often of poor quality also. Drug companies are not always eager to sponsor research they cannot control, and sponsored research sometimes appears to provide very little definitive information about the value of a drug.

Most prescriptions for psychological drugs are for the weaker tranquilizers, but there is really no substantial evidence for their effectiveness (Kramer *et al.*, 1964). They are *less* effective than barbiturates for reducing anxiety (although they are also less dangerous), and most controlled studies suggest that meprobamate, the most commonly prescribed of the weaker tranquilizers, is no more effective than simple placebo. Also, adaption to meprobamate occurs in a relatively short time, usually within two or three weeks, so that even the few benefits it may confer are short-lived.

Evidence for the utility of strong tranquilizers is better than that for the weaker ones, but it is still quite mixed. Since tranquilizers have been widely used, the rate of discharge from psychiatric hospitals has risen and the resident patient population has declined in spite of a rise in admissions. Moreover, while in the hospital, patients are more manageable, evidencing fewer bizarre symptoms and constituting less of a problem to the staff, than they formerly had been. These data are not altogether compelling evidence in favor of drugs, however, since during this very same period, other changes have been introduced to psychiatric hospitals, such as increased staff and new psychotherapy techniques. Moreover, patients have come to expect better treatment from a more sympathetic public after they are discharged, and this may have increased their motivation for discharge. Even so, Wortis (1965) and Cole (1964) conclude that schizophrenic patients have been relieved of a variety of symptoms by tranquilizers, particularly chlorpromazine. The evidence with regard to rehospitalization is not as clear, but informed opinion appears to conclude that if tranquilizers do not reduce rehospitalization, they at least delay it, allowing a patient to stay outside the hospital for a longer period of time (Englehardt, 1963; Gittleman *et al.*, 1964).

The revolution in hospital care that has resulted from the strong tranquilizers is less a product of the curative effect the drugs have on patients than of the humanizing effect they promote among hospital staffs. Even though it is the patient who takes the drug, its soothing effects on him permit the hospital staff to be more relaxed and congenial, to make less use of restrictive or punitive custodial methods, and to be generally more premissive and humane in their treatments. Despite their limited value as direct treatments, therefore, the drugs have provided a major service in the institutional care of psychiatric cases.

The weak tranquilizers have not demonstrated such value, however, and their widespread use must be seriously challenged, *especially* their use outside the hospital by people who may not only fail to benefit from them, but who may be damaged financially by their exorbitant cost (the margin of profit on many drugs is so high that American drug companies have been subjected to congressional investigation) and psychologically by inappropriately relying on them to do what they cannot—solve problems.

There seem to be three main reasons why the profligate use of these drugs continues to increase: (1) *doctors* think they work and lack both facilities and sophistication to critically examine their belief; (2) *pharmaceutical* manufacturers are making money hand over fist from them and therefore promote their use beyond reasonably conservative limits and without sufficiently critical evidence of value or safety; and most important of all, (3) the *public* demands pills. People are more aware of their anxieties and tensions today than ever before, but they are probably no more willing than they ever were to examine their lives critically or to radically change them as a result of self-examination. Pills sound like an easy solution, and both physicians and patients are easily misled into thinking their results are valuable without inquiring whether another kind of treatment might have done as well or whether no treatment at all might have produced identical results. Since everybody knows that experience is the best teacher, few people, especially people in need, stop to notice that uncritical acceptance of one's experience may teach lies instead of truth.

The very novelty of the psychiatric drugs is somewhat misleading. For many people who suffer the garden variety of personal difficulties, anxieties, and headaches, no drugs are of any particular value, and aspirin may very well do as much as a very expensive tranquilizer. While the use of these drugs under medical supervision is ordinarily not likely to be harmful, it is not likely to be very beneficial either. The important thing to remember about them is that while they may temporarily reduce some of the distressing symptoms of a psychological conflict or problem, they are not likely to have any effect at all on the problem! The proper view towards taking them should therefore be one of caution.

Educational Treatments

Educational treatments are distinguished easily enough from medical ones, on the whole, by virtue of the fact that they do not involve medicine or surgery. As will be seen, they are not so easily distinguished from psychotherapy. The usual thing that identifies a treatment procedure as educational is that it is used in connection with a specific educational problem, more often than not in the physical setting or under the formal auspices of an educational institution, and generally involves some specific technical instruction. The most common kinds of educational treatments are (1) remedial teaching of subject matter skills, especially reading, and (2) speech therapy.

Remedial reading. Any kind of remedial teaching can be considered an educational treatment, but remedial reading is by far the best studied and most widely and formally practiced. The techniques of remedial reading are, with few exceptions, unconcerned with the theory of language acquisition or symbol comprehension; they are directed simply to remedying known deficiencies, largely by means of techniques that are also considered useful in other academic areas. Reading deficiencies fall into four broad categories: (1) word recognition, (2) vocabulary, (3) reading comprehension, and (4) reading speed; and specialized techniques have been devised for coping with each kind of problem. Training in remedial reading is highly differentiated according to the specific problem involved, and most therapists are competent at a variety of training skills.

Most reading deficiencies are probably the result of bad training and, to that extent, might seem unrelated to the psychological disabilities under consideration here. Indeed, there is little evidence to support the once popular idea that most reading disabilities are rooted in personal anxieties which manifest themselves in this symptom. On the other hand, it is undoubtedly true that reading handicaps in children often *create* emotional problems with potentially serious consequences for their lives. As a result of his disability, the retarded reader receives considerable negative reinforcement in school and may have already acquired a profound sense of failure by the time he comes for reading remediation. For this reason, most reading clinics concern themselves with allaying the reader's anxieties by presenting him with graded materials designed to ensure gradual success. The diagnostic reading process is critical for this purpose in that appropriate remedial techniques can be subsequently applied without prolonging the failure experiences in which the reader has been involved.

Speech therapies. It is possible to classify speech therapies under psychotherapy rather than educational treatments, considering both the kinds of problems usually involved and the techniques used in their resolution, but they are contained with educational treatments here because there is an important professional subspecialty which deals entirely in speech problems, and also because the techniques for dealing with these problems are commonly taught in special programs for training *speech therapists* rather than in general psychotherapeutic training programs.

Much of our interpersonal competence depends on our ability to speak, so much, in fact, that we take our complex speaking abilities for granted. We may, at times, feel that we say too much or too little, or wish that we had said it differently, but the capacity for speech itself is taken as a matter of course by most adults. This is not so for those suffering speech impediments. These people are so painfully aware of their stuttering and stammering that they often weigh the desire to say something against the anxiety and embarrassment of speaking at all.

It has been estimated that nearly 1 percent of the people in the United States stutter. Of these, more than 75 percent are men. Stuttering appears to begin before the age of six, often shortly after the child has learned to speak.

The dynamics of stuttering are unclear. Some theorists have argued for a hereditary disposition, and others have emphasized brain damage and other neurological disorders as the source of this disturbance. But the most popular view has been that stuttering is a manifestation of emotional conflict. Psychoanalysts, for example, see stuttering as a manifestation of psychological immaturity involving oral needs. Nonpsychoanalysts have tended to describe stuttering in terms of an approach-avoidance conflict (see Chapters 3 and 10): for some reason, the stutterer fears speaking and would like to avoid it, but the social necessities of everyday living compel him to speak. The two tendencies, to speak and to avoid speaking, are equally strong, and the conflict is manifested in the marked speech hesitancy that characterizes stuttering.

Until recently, the primary treatment for stuttering consisted of some kind of verbal psychotherapy directed to the presumed sources of anxiety and conflict, particularly as they manifested themselves in interpersonal behavior. But many stutterers were refractory to verbal psychotherapeutic methods, and such success as was achieved was often transitory; the stutterer frequently relapsed into stuttering when later faced with emotional crises.

Recently, several psychologists have attempted to apply principles drawn from theories of learning to the treatment of speech disorders. Flanagan *et al.* (1958), for example, sought to modify stuttering by altering the reinforcements related to it (compare the techniques of "stimulus control" in Chapter 9). Their subjects were three stutterers attending a speech clinic. Each subject was seen twice, and on both occasions a base rate of stuttering was ascertained. In one session, a loud noise was played every time the subject stuttered, while in the other session, the noise was played continuously *except* when the subject stuttered. When stuttering was followed by the loud noise, its rate decreased for all three subjects. When it was followed by a cessation of the loud noise, the three subjects showed an increase in stuttering.

In later research, Goldiamond attempted to replicate the study described above, but this time he substituted delayed auditory feedback for the loud noise. (Delayed auditory feedback involves recording a subject's voice as he speaks and playing it back to him through earphones a fraction of a second later than he would normally hear himself—very annoying!) He discovered that continuous delayed auditory feedback could induce a stutterer to use slow prolonged speech without stuttering and that, when the subject was encouraged to speed up this new speech pattern, he eventually was able to attain almost normal, fluent speech. Goldiamond subsequently used this method and variations of it to treat several other stutterers. Once they were able to speak fluently in the experimental situation, they were given exercises to help them outside the laboratory. The technique seems promising, although it needs further verification with large groups of stutterers.

Adjunctive therapies. Some educational treatment procedures are virtually never used alone because they have no *direct* bearing on the problem at hand. The best known of these are *occupational* or *industrial therapy* and *vocational rehabilitation.*

Industrial therapy consists mainly of instructing people in the techniques and skills of work. It is used primarily in mental hospitals, but has been extended to persons discharged from hospitals. Its initial purpose was probably only to provide some interesting diversions for patients with nothing to do, although in "moral treatment" (see Bockoven, 1963), it was very much a part of treatment. Since work was deemed "good for the soul" and busyness supposedly worked against anxiety, industrial therapy (it was then called "occupational therapy") consisted largely of engaging patients in the busywork of the hospital. It was subsequently observed that patients ready to be discharged from the hospital often lacked the necessary skills to obtain jobs on the outside. This situation was discouraging to the patient; it reduced his capacities for adaption and frequently brought him right back to the hospital. Thus hospitals acquired a second function in addition to treating the psychological disorder: to prepare the patient to adjust to the outside community after he is discharged. The vocational rehabilitation program was developed for this purpose.

Three kinds of programs have evolved under the heading of industrial therapy:

Hospital work programs involve assigning patients to hospital jobs such as clerical work, gardening, housekeeping, and carpentry. Factors like the patient's intelligence and social class, his emotional stability, the difficulty of the task, and the kind of supervisor he will be working with are considered in making assignments. Gradually he is assigned to more difficult and challenging jobs and to jobs that may be like those he will find outside the hospital.

Member-employee programs are another innovation in industrial therapies. A patient lives inside the hospital while working outside of it, and the aim is to gradually introduce him into ordinary society while still providing him with whatever supports he requires before making the full adjustment. The patient leaves the hospital to go to work in the morning and returns to the hospital in the evening. Quite commonly a cooperative arrangement between the hospital and the patient's employer allows the job itself to be temporarily modified and made less demanding. Occasionally these modifications permit the patient to work under the supervision of hospital personnel. Further improvement enables his total discharge and return to the community, where he can continue his employment (Ewalt, 1959).

The sheltered workshop resembles a small factory in both its working conditions and regimen. The workshop produces salable products and the patient is paid for his work. Unlike the ordinary factory, however, in the workshop supervisors are mainly hospital personnel and working hours are shorter, although the patient commonly remains at the workshop for the full day. As in the hospital program, the patient is assigned to increasingly more responsible jobs as his work skills improve.

The final step in most vocational rehabilitation programs is that of assisting the patient to find permanent full-time employment in the community at a job that is consistent with his needs and abilities. It can be very difficult, however, to find employers who can be induced to hire former hospital patients and to tolerate such of their oddities as still remain. Of 200 businessmen interviewed in a large metropolitan area, less than 15 percent had ever hired any known former psychiatric (hospital) patients, and only 2 percent had hired a sizable proportion of former patients (Olshansky, 1959). As might be expected, it is the stereotypic image of the former psychiatric patient—a violent, uncontrollable, and unpredictable person whom you have to "watch like a hawk" or "treat with kid gloves"—that contributes most to employers' reluctance to hire.

PSYCHOTHERAPY

The aim of this section is to describe what psychotherapy is, how it got its present forms, what directions it is taking, and what some of its implications are for modern man. This is not easy.

Thousands of books and articles about psychotherapy are read by millions of people, many of whom have personally experienced it, but the nature of the enterprise still eludes straightforward explication. To be precise, the same thing can be said about medicine or other crafts. Concepts like "health" and "illness," for example, become quite elusive if one requires great exactness in defining them. But this is not a very serious problem in the practice of medicine, for rather good reasons, and it is a very critical one in the practice of psychotherapy, for equally good reasons. These reasons have to do with what may be labeled the *criterion problem.*

There is considerable agreement among all parties to the medical enterprise about the criteria of medical involvement, even when explicit definition of those criteria is lacking. In other words, there is some consensus among doctors, patients, and society about what it is like to be sick, or to be well, or to be subjected to medical treatment of one or another kind, even though these are not clear in every case or situation.

If anything, the opposite may be said in psychotherapy. There is not very much agreement about what it is like to need psychotherapy, or not to need it, or to properly administer it or satisfactorily respond to it. And this uncertainty is almost as great among the people who teach and practice it as among those to whom it is addressed, despite some instances of clarity and agreement.

> First and least important, there are several different professions with strong vested interests in the public practice of psychotherapy: Psychiatry, Psychology, and Social Work all officially use it. Most people do not know the difference between these professions and indeed, with respect to the practice of psychotherapy, most differences that are not financial are probably ficticious; psychiatrists earn more than psychologists, who earn more than social workers.
>
> Second and more confusing, perhaps, is the fact that psychotherapy is practiced by many more different kinds of professionals who, unlike those above, differ in most functions as well as in their titles. Some of these find it impolitic to identify their therapeutic work with this label. Ministers who do psychotherapy call it "pastoral counseling," educators do therapy called "guidance," and a host of persons with credentials in any or all or none of these professions label their particular therapeutic practices "marital counseling" or "psychoanalysis" or some such term which refers to no formal profession and overlaps in meaning with several other terms all properly equivalent to psychotherapy. (London, 1964, pp. 29–30.)

From the perspective of the specialist involved, the explanation of his therapeutic practice is likely to reflect the jargon of his professional training, regardless of the term he uses to name his work. The *medical* psychotherapist views his work as the treatment of mental illness.

The *educational* psychotherapist sees himself as teaching the correction of bad habit patterns or the techniques of developing good ones. The *pastoral* psychotherapist sees his work as a means for helping people "seek relatedness" or perhaps "justification."

In terms of its origins, it would be appropriate to say that the medical view is the most correct one, but the term "mental illness," as we have seen, has itself been used ambiguously to refer both to peculiarities of thought or feeling which result from some physical disturbance of the body and to peculiarities of bodily function which apparently result from some irregularities of thought and feeling. Neither of these concepts is adequate to describe the great bulk of conditions for which people seek psychotherapy in modern times. Especially in the case of educated and sophisticated people, it is probably fair to say that they seek help mostly for irregularities of thought and feeling which result from irregularities of thought and feeling. Simply stated, they have "psychological problems" or "emotional difficulties" or "disordered personalities," or they are just "maladjusted" or unhappy.

In practice, regardless of the professionalism which dictates one or another "point of view," therapy reduces to a means of attacking personal problems and trying to solve them largely by talking and related processes, whether they are called psychotherapy, psychoanalysis, counseling, or guidance.

And regardless of the particular ideology of the practitioner, most advocates of most systems treat most people for most problems for which most therapists of most other systems would treat them. Such differences in clientele as exist among therapists are generally matters of preference, sources of referral, and the like, and not the studied consequences of any special orientation or system.

But far from being altogether bad, the very indifference in fact to differences in theory on the part of most therapists makes it possible for clients to find help without first either having to learn much about psychotherapy or be shunted around from one specialist to another. And the willingness of most therapists to take on most patients for most conditions reflects what is probably the chief article of faith of the profession, namely that the skillful application of psychotherapy by a trained practitioner is of definite value to most patients.

This would seem to suggest that it is clear what training in psychotherapy ought to be like, but that is far from a clear-cut matter—again, because of the criterion problem. Just as there is no clear-cut notion of who ought to practice it on whom for what purpose, there is no clear way of evaluating training in it either. Essentially, training in psychotherapy is a matter of apprenticeship in which one learns to perform in accord with the demands of his teacher.

> This is most unlike training in engineering in which the person of the teacher has no great bearing on the performance of what is learned. Bridges stand or fall in their own right. Neither is it entirely like learning to play the piano, paint pictures, or carve furniture, for performance in these arts can be repeatedly submitted for judgment to very large audiences. Nor is it even quite like learning medicine, in which a goodly number of erstwhile patients may, through incompetent performance, become patent victims. In psychotherapy, there is no clear body of truth which stands apart from its discoverer and no great audience to listen all at once to its performance; evidently, too, nobody dies from it. Finally, if one is not entirely sure the patient is sick before treatment, how can he be judged to be well after it? (London, 1964, p. 23.)

The upshot of this situation is that the field of psychotherapy is so scattered and intellectually disordered, at first glance, that it appears almost impossible to survey intelligently. This is not necessarily so, however; the problem is really that one can view the field from several different perspectives, and confusion results only from trying to see it from all of them at once. To straighten matters out, it is necessary to do three things: (1) set psychotherapy in historical perspective, (2) spell out the dimensions of discourse which can be used to help understand it; and (3) describe the systems which characterize it. The remainder of this chapter is directed towards these purposes.

The History of Psychotherapy

There are two mainstream traditions from which modern forms of psychotherapy evolved: a medical one and an educational one. The medical tradition differs considerably from hospital to office practice.

Medieval mental hospitals were little more than prisons which served the immediate purpose of isolating deranged people from society at large. Were this isolation devoid of efforts at treatment, its effects on both the individuals and society might have been less harmful than they actually were. Without efforts at treatment, the normal conditions of filth and decay in hospitals assured that the patients would become ill and die in reasonably short order. As it was, attempts at treatment further assured that, should patients show any semblance of sanity at the time of admission, there would be none at all soon thereafter.

The prevailing theory of insanity in medieval and well into modern times was that its victims suffer from "possession" by demons. Efforts at treatment were largely directed towards exorcising these demons one way or another—and a commonly elected way was by beating, starving, or otherwise torturing the vessel in which they were hiding (Figure 15.1). The "vessel" would suffer, often intolerably in the process, but the technique remained popular for some time nevertheless.

By the eighteenth century, with the coming of the "age of reason," the demonology theory was thoroughly discredited, but the harsh treatments it had fostered remained popular for some time, although they were now, of course, rationalized differently. Benjamin Rush (1745–1813), the "father of American

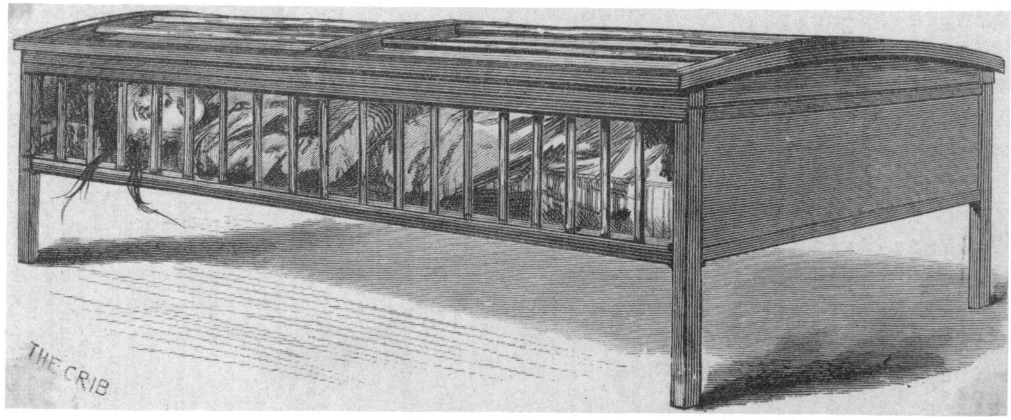

Figure 15.1a Insane patient in "The Crib" at a New York institution, 1882. Photo courtesy The Bettmann Archive.

psychiatry," was a forerunner of more humane treatment for the mentally ill. Relying on "scientific" theories of astrology, rather than demonology, he recommended bloodletting, food deprivation, threats of death, and purgatives for his patients. Although his reforms were not as extensive as those of Phillipe Pinel (1745–1826), they paved the way for the eventual acceptance of Pinel's theory of "moral treatment" in America.

The mental hospital practices of the middle ages were not altogether unique to that period. It is not widely realized that conditions in American mental hospitals were often just as bad, especially with respect to leaving patients helplessly isolated, not only from any kind of intelligent treatment, but also from the normal amenities of civilized existence. In some parts of the United States, primitive hospital conditions have existed until quite recently (Deutsch, 1948), while in most areas, hospital environments fail even today to approach the optimal.

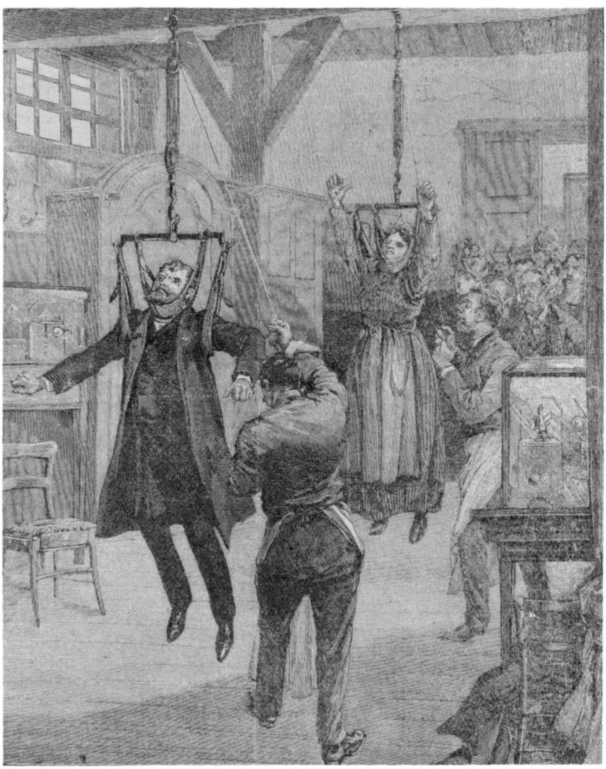

Figure 15.1*b* Suspensory treatment for nervous ataxia at the Salpêtrière, Paris. Photo courtesy The Bettmann Archive.

Pinel. The critical shift in hospital care of the mentally ill which anticipated the best psychotherapeutic techniques of modern times were originated by Pinel, the director of the Bicêtre and later of the Salpetrière hospital in Paris. Pinel's theory, in brief, was that the mentally ill could be resurrected from their depraved condition if they were allowed to observe and emulate the most wholesome, rational, and kindly behavior of others. He consequently enjoined the personnel of his hospital to engage in "moral treatment" of a kind which would exemplify to the patients how they themselves could profitably comport their lives. This meant, of course, that it was necessary to treat patients kindly and considerately, and at the same time to communicate expectations to them that they would themselves assume increasing responsibility for their lives. Pinel's scheme was a wonderful success, and it was rapidly borrowed for the treatment of the mentally ill in England, Italy, and Germany. In 1817, under Rush's guidance, an American hospital was founded for the specific purpose of providing moral treatments for the psychologically disturbed. Within the next four years, several other such hospitals were founded, and gradually these institutions began to affect the manner in which the mentally ill were treated in all hospitals.

Almost two hundred years ago, Pinel's hospital, and those which followed its example, began to achieve successful treatments of disturbed people that have not been excelled by even the best mental hospitals to this very day.

Unfortunately, Pinel's techniques not only failed to overtake the psychiatric industry engaged in hospital treatment, but were largely abandoned within sixty years. Bockoven (1963) suggests that one contributing factor to this abandonment was the failure of the innovators to provide for their own succession in numbers that were adequate to accommodate the growing needs of the country. Other factors seemed equally important, especially the reemergence of a "new" viewpoint in European psychiatry: that the disturbed person was suffering from a physical disease rather than a psychological disorder, and therefore needed to be treated with physical rather than psychological techniques. This ancient view (see Chapter 1) was propounded with renewed vigor after European scientists discovered that paresis had a physiological basis: syphyllis. The discovery constituted one of the most thrilling chapters in the history of psychiatric research, climaxing more than a century of work in laboratories throughout Europe. But with it grew the belief that all mental disturbance had a physical basis and should be treated physically, implying that the treatment techniques of moral psychiatry were misdirected. Physical techniques also reduced the amount of time personnel needed to spend with patients, and thus alleviated much of the social, economic, and manpower dilemma in the United States, a fortunate coincidence for those who found moral psychiatry burdensome. Moral treatment was abandoned to be rediscovered several decades later.

"Organic psychiatry," as the disease theory of mental illness is now called, fathered the medical treatment techniques referred to in the previous section. Although it never showed very strong evidence of being effective, in the sense of increasing the rates of discharge from hospitals, it remained the dominant trend in hospital treatment for close to one hundred years.

Office Practice. What was later to become the office practice of psychotherapy originated in the form of gadgetry and problem-solving therapy techniques of one or another kind in the wealthy salons and courts of Europe. The kinds of operations involved in "therapy" in those days were not always much like the kinds used today, but the kinds of problems they addressed were recognizably similar. Leaving aside the practice of frankly occult therapeutic arts like witchcraft and black magic, there were still any number of practices which would today seem more like selling snake oil (what we would now call "placebo treatment") than like psychotherapy. Without a doubt, the most glamorous of these was the "celestial magnetico-electro bed" of John Graham, O.W.L. (Oh Wonderful Love). Invented in the seventeenth century, the purpose of Graham's bed was to restore sexual potency to the flagging roués of Restoration England.

The oldest form of treatment which preceded what we would now call office psychotherapy was probably the "animal magnetic" treatments of Anton Mesmer. This was the term with which Mesmer identified the effect of various hand movements, such as waves and passes, which he would make in front of the faces and around the afflicted body parts of patients suffering from a variety of aches, pains, and paralytic conditions. Mesmer's movements would induce a trancelike condition in the patient, after which the ailment would frequently disappear. Himself an Austrian, Mesmer became famous in the court of Louis XVI of France for his enormous successes both in the wealthy salons of Versailles and in the free clinic which he operated, where he would treat whole crowds of people at once. He became so famous for his successes, in fact, that a royal commission was appointed in 1784 to investigate the scientific status of Mesmer and of animal magnetism. Benjamin Franklin, then in France as the ambassador of the Continental Congress to raise money and military support for the American Revolution, was a member of the commission. Its findings discredited Mesmer thoroughly, claiming that there was no such thing as animal magnetism and that his cures were achieved merely "by suggestion." This put him out of business, of course—but it actually had no bearing on the evident effectiveness and genuineness of the cures he had achieved. Mesmer is regarded as the father of modern hypnotism, which for some time was known as mesmerism, after him.

Modern psychotherapy stems most immediately from the office psychiatry of the late nineteenth century, which gave rise to psychoanalysis, and from the psychoeducational clinic, an institution which originated in the United States at the same time. The first of these clinics was created by Lightner Witmer at the University of Pennsylvania in 1896. It has gradually become the prototype of such facilities for the development of remedial techniques for school problems, and for guidance and counseling organizations within school systems. Almost every major university in the United States today maintains a counseling center to assist its own students with both personal and educational problems which interfere with the successful achievement of a higher education.

From the beginning of this century until World War II, supporters of psychoanalysis fought a largely uphill battle to establish it as a legitimate form of therapy. They were eventually so successful that by now, for all practical purposes, psychoanalysis is commonly regarded as the prototype of psychotherapy, and most new forms of treatment are compared with it as a measure of their adequacy. Other modes of treatment have been available for at least as long as analysis, which itself was not originally designed as a therapy for most kinds of outpatient troubles. But for a number of good reasons, interest in analysis has dominated that in all other forms of therapy until very recently, and it may now be considered the orthodoxy of psychotherapy. Conflicts over the efficacy of psychotherapy, which have become increasingly widespread since about 1950, have largely been conflicts about the effectiveness of psychoanalysis. As it turns out, the problem of effectiveness of any kind of psychotherapy is more complicated than it appears at first, as will be apparent below.

The term *psychoanalysis* originally referred to a form of psychotherapy developed and expounded by Sigmund Freud and his students. Only a few years after psychoanalysis became formalized as a treatment method, however, it became subject to a variety of heresies, both theoretical and practical. A number of important offshoots of psychoanalysis developed as therapeutic techniques in the period from about 1910 until shortly after World War II. Some of these variant therapies are themselves identified with psychoanalysis in greater or lesser measure by name, such as *analytical psychotherapy*, the technique of C. G. Jung. Some of them, on the other hand, have no evident origins in psychoanalysis but are still descendants of it, as the *will therapy* of Otto Rank, or the *client-centered therapy* of Carl Rogers.

The influence of therapies derived from psychoanalysis has been so great in America and Western Europe that many people are still unfamiliar with the forms of psychotherapy that have arisen from the work of Ivan Pavlov in Russia and E. L. Thorndike (and later others) in the United States, both working at the same time that Freud was formulating psychoanalytic theory in Vienna. Pavlov and Thorndike were themselves laboratory scientists rather than clinical practitioners, which is one reason why their work was not translated into clinical situations for some time. Currently, however, and based on the novelties and refinements which two generations of scientists have added to their early findings, the psychotherapy systems derived from their studies are arousing increasing interest in universities, clinics, schools, and hospitals everywhere.

At the present time, there are two types of psychotherapy in fairly widespread use: the more common type takes the psychoanalytic work of Sigmund Freud as its prototype (sometimes without admitting it), and the other can be traced to the "conditioning" studies of Pavlov and "learning" research of Thorndike.

The actual forms in which these systems are applied varies considerably. Many people are seen individually for therapy, some are seen only in group therapy situations, and still others in a combination of the two. Similarly, therapy is accompanied by a wide variety of adjuncts. Sometimes dramatic acting called "psychodrama" provides the context of treatment. Sometimes hypnosis is used to facilitate therapy. Occasionally drugs are employed, as in the case of D-lysergic acid diethylamide (LSD). In such instances, however, the drug does not itself serve as the therapy, which makes it different from the medical treatments described earlier. Nor are any of the adjunctive methods of treatment particularly more applicable to one therapy system than the other; both use all of them.

Though the different types of psychotherapy have some importance in their own right, and may very well make critical differences in the outcome for the patient, no discussion of them is very useful without first understanding the different dimensions of discourse which are available for examining this discipline. Thinking about the different schemes of psychotherapy in terms of dimensions permits them to be understood in relation to each other and in terms of a limited set of factors that contribute to them, rather than requiring that they be understood individually and in all respects at once. The dimensional scheme used here is by and large the one used in *The Modes and Morals of Psychotherapy* (London, 1964), but it is not identical with it.

There appear to be two critical dimensions for the understanding of psychotherapy systems. One of them can be looked upon as a *scientific* dimension because it can be discussed and evaluated entirely in terms of its factual characteristics. The second is an *evaluative* or *moralistic* dimension because it refers to the desirability of a therapy rather than to its validity. The scientific value of psychotherapy is judged by how well it accomplishes what it sets out to do; to the extent that it does, it may be said to be true. Its moral value, on the other hand, is judged by the extent to which the theoretical goals or factual accomplishments of a therapy are desirable, even if they are clearly attainable. It is easier to agree on scientific than on moralistic judgments, of course, because there is generally more agreement about the criteria for what is *true or false* than for what is *good or bad.*

It is generally the case that responsible members of any trade or profession which offers public services are concerned to see to it that their skills are used for desirable purposes, but the moral concerns of psychotherapists are greater than those in many other professions because the enterprise is by nature largely a moralistic one. The disorders to which psychotherapy is applied are largely moral disorders in the sense that they are defined by some assumptions about the way people ought to live rather than by any physical disabilities, and it is often impossible to aid their solution without assuming or communicating some moral stance. There has been relatively little discussion of the morals of psychotherapy in the therapeutic literature, and some confusion about the difference between the two dimensions of concern has hampered both the scientific development of the field and the determination of its proper function as a social instrument.

The Scientific Dimensions

From the scientific point of view, systems of psychotherapy must be examined with respect to (1) the principles of behavior or theories of personality which underlie them, (2) the technical focus of activity which characterizes them, including both the procedures and operations of the psychotherapist and the immediate goals he expects to achieve by their means, and (3) the "locus of disorder" to which the principles and techniques apply.

Of these, the examination of techniques is perhaps most important, or at least serves as a convenient springboard from which to view both underlying principles and loci of application.

The immediate objectives of virtually all therapeutic systems, viewed in terms of their operations (as opposed to their ultimate goals), tend to be either (1) to foster *insight* into an aspect of the patient's life, or (2) to produce some definite change in his *actions*. The many individual operations which characterize a single therapy system, moreover, tend to be so consistent with each other that they permit a taxonomy on whose basis any system can be classified as leaning towards either the insight or the action pole of a technical dimension. Accordingly, a system may be fairly labeled either an insight or an action therapy. There are some important differences between them.

In terms of the underlying theories and principles of behavior by which they are rationalized, *insight* therapies tend to be based upon derivatives of the psychoanalytic tradition indicated above and *action* therapies to be related to the "learning theories" of Pavlov, Thorndike, and others.

Insight Therapy

If there is a single basic idea which guides all insight therapies, it is the notion that motives dictate behavior, that is, that psychologically disordered behavior is the direct or oblique consequence of peculiarities in the motivational system that arouses people to action of any kind. In order to treat such disorders successfully, it is argued, the therapist must seek out the particular motives which underly the observed difficulties and, by bringing them to light, loosen the otherwise inevitable bond between them and the disordered behavior they produce. Stated differently, this means that the therapist engages in procedures which eventually will give the patient *insight* into the relationship between his motivations and his behavior, the assumption being that this insight will give him greater control over his behavior than was hitherto the case.

Still another way of putting it is that the techniques of insight therapy are designed to lead the patient to greater understanding of himself, particularly those aspects of himself which have not been fully conscious or which he has been unable to confront previously in a direct and forthright manner. Understanding the basis of one's own behavior, of course, makes that behavior more meaningful. This makes it easy to see how insight therapy comes to be regarded by most of its adherents as a technique which not only frees the patient of disabling symptoms but which also offers him the opportunity to seek the meaning of his acts and, in so doing, to make his whole life more meaningful. It is precisely this characteristic of insight therapy which gives it its greatest appeal in modern times, especially in the form of *existential psychotherapy* for, as we shall see, its actual potency as a means of reducing troubling symptoms is questionable.

The details of technique vary considerably among insight therapists, but there are two vital features of procedure which tend to be common to them all: (1) patient responsibility and (2) therapist anonymity. The patient is generally required to assume responsibility for virtually all the subject matter that is discussed in the therapy sessions. In the ordinary course of events, the onus rests with him to initiate discourse and to conduct it, and the therapist serves more to guide the stream of the patient's consciousness than to interfere with it. The therapist generally refrains from any significant disclosure of his own characteristics. Both of these procedures are obviously designed to encourage and reinforce the patient's exploration of himself rather than to compel him to follow a train of thought which is actually the therapist's or, by "knowing too much" about the therapist's personal characteristics, patterning his own life after this potential model. Both patient responsibility and therapist anonymity are seen in the different kinds of insight therapy, but they do not serve quite the same purposes in every system. This becomes clearer by looking at some of the techniques used more specifically in *psychoanalysis* and in *client-centered* therapy, the two most popular kinds of insight treatment. In psychoanalysis, (3) free association and (4) transference are important, and in client-centered therapy, (5) reflection, a variant of what analysts call interpretation, is an important special technique.

Free association is the main psychoanalytic method for uncovering unconscious motives (see Chapter 10). The analyst tells the patient to utter everything that comes into his mind, then sits back, usually out of sight, and waits for him to do so. It is quite difficult to do, as you can see for yourself if you just lie down, close your eyes, and try to keep track of every trace of thought that flashes through your mind. Revealing those thoughts to another person is even harder to do. One function of the couch is to relax the patient, so that it is easier for him to freely associate. The analyst may occasionally make remarks intended to stimulate the patient's associations, but until the patient has developed some skill at freely associating, the analyst probably will not make any interpretive remarks. And the responsibility for developing this skill rests on the patient. The same thing that makes it hard to learn to freely associate also makes it valuable; one converses differently here than in ordinary discourse. In the latter, the speaker is obliged to retain a train of thought and to move logically from item to item so as not to wander from the point at hand. In psychoanalysis, it is precisely the chain of thoughts that would ordinarily be suppressed as irrelevant or embarrassing or inappropriate that is especially useful and germane. It is useful for two reasons. First, thoughts occur in associative chains, those that we are more aware of coming first, and those that are more repressed (and hence closer to central discomforting motivations) coming later. Free association permits one to go gradually from the more to the less available, uncovering ideas, affects, and experiences that are more laden with anxiety and less available to consciousness.

But free association is useful also because it violates ordinary "conversation manners." By encouraging in the patient the "urge to utter" (Ford and Urban, 1963), regardless of the listener's response, the patient is led to value and to explore his ideas and feelings.

Transference is the phenomenon of *projecting* onto the analyst the attributes of other people who are important in one's life and then experiencing towards him the emotions the other people arouse. A patient may come to believe, for example, that the psychoanalyst is just like his father, and then to have the same emotions towards the analyst that he feels towards his father. To some extent, transference occurs in any intimate relationship between people, but psychoanalysis makes deliberate and ingenious use of the phenomenon. By encouraging transference, the analyst helps the patient to expose many feelings towards others that have been frightening him and impairing his relationships with them, and that he may not have been aware of. Once exposed, they can be analyzed and the transference resolved.

It is his personal anonymity which enables the therapist to recognize a transference reaction when it occurs. Since the patient does not know much about the analyst's real life or what he is really like, the traits he attributes to the analyst must be taken from his experience with other people, and the emotions he has towards him must be emotions he has had towards others. It is therefore important for psychoanalysts to avoid social relations with their patients in order to help the transference develop.

Other insight therapists avoid social relationships more because they do not want to exercise undue influence on their patient's course of self-discovery. It is, after all, probably easier to borrow a respected therapist's style of living and thinking than it is to find one's own; but insight therapists generally hold that it is much less worthwhile. One reason Freud thought of having his patients lie down while he sat out of sight was to minimize the influence of his own expressive gestures and reactions on the course of the patient's thoughts (he also found it wearing to have to look at and be looked at for hours and hours every day). In short, therapist anonymity serves to focus the patient's attention on himself and his own psychological processes.

Reflection, the main technique of client-centered therapy, is a single kind of interpretive response which serves some of the combined purposes aimed for in psychoanalysis by free association, transference, and interpretation. Reflection is the therapist's restatement of what the patient has said in such a way that he exposes the feelings underlying the content of the patient's statement and communicates his understanding and acceptance of them. Among other things, this has the effect of reinforcing the patient in the pursuit of his own ideas and associations and in taking responsibility for the therapeutic discourse. Interpretation, which is more widely practiced among therapists of analytic persuasion, has the same effect: by timing interpretations so that they do not go beyond what a patient is prepared to understand and accept, the therapist communicates that he is "following" his patient and thereby encourages him to continue his self-initiated exploration.

Despite its continued great popularity, there are three important criticisms to which insight therapies have been chronically susceptible:

1. However much it may be true that problems of motive underly the symptoms of distress that bring people into psychotherapy, it is the symptoms, not the motives, that bring them. Since this is the case, the insight therapist inevitably engages in activities designed to persuade or otherwise orient the patient towards a concern with his motivations.

But unless there is no doubt whatsoever about the exact relationship of motives to behavior, the therapist is put in the position of "selling" a product which the patient did not intend to "buy." In that event, he runs the risk of deceiving the patient and perhaps himself.

2. There is some evidence that the therapeutic uncovering of motives does not really have as much power to remove symptoms as we would hope. Since insight therapies are almost seventy years old, the lack of firm indications that they are really effective is cause for great concern. A primary justification for focusing attention on motives is that it helps to relieve symptoms. If it does not do so, an important purpose of therapy has been defeated.

Studies of the effectiveness of insight therapy have proved equivocal, by and large; some have turned up fairly good results (Knight, 1941; Weinstock, 1960) and others have reported very few acceptable indications that therapy works (Eysenck, 1960; Astin, 1961). Evaluative studies of psychotherapy, however, are even harder to do than drug studies. Some of the major difficulties are: (1) *the base rate problem,* that is the tendency of some people to improve spontaneously with or without treatment (see Chapter 11); (2) individual differences among patients, that is, the fact that therapy inevitably works better for some people than for others, so that it is hard to know whether a given sample of patients provides a fair test of the treatment method; and (3) individual differences among therapists, which paralleling the differences among patients, suggests that some therapists will be better than others in using particular techniques or, for that matter, in doing any kind of therapy at all.

3. Insight therapists sometimes argue, not without merit, that therapy helps to resolve people's *existential dilemmas* even when it fails to relieve their symptoms. This is not mere rationalization, for many patients who originally enter insight therapy with the desire only to be free of their symptomatic difficulties discover that "the quest for meaning" or "search for authenticity" (Bugental, 1963) is really of more central importance in their lives. But this argument does create an embarrassing paradox—for the patient is now in the position of saying that, though the symptom has not been treated, he is no longer troubled by it. Such a situation can be described as one where therapy, instead of changing the symptom to fit the patient's needs, has changed the patient to suit the requirements of the symptom.

Action Therapy

The various action therapies may be conveniently understood as falling at the opposite pole of technical procedures from the *insight* therapies. Instead of concerning themselves primarily with the motivational states that may have given rise to a person's symptoms, they tend to focus on the symptoms themselves, limiting their goals to treatment of the symptom without much concern about its origins or "meaning." Instead of seating the responsibility for the content of treatment with the patient, they place it entirely in the hands of the therapist. Instead of concentrating on the patient's existential concerns, they pay attention only to his functioning and to how his symptoms interfere with it. Finally, and perhaps most important, instead of handling therapy as a process for aiding the acquisition of insight or self-understanding, they view it as *planful* attack on symptoms of disorder without regard to whether any self-understanding is likely to come about.

Action therapists, who are also called "behavioristic" both because they focus on observable behavior and because they claim a historical indebtedness to the psychology of behaviorism of John B. Watson, are less concerned theoretically with motivation than with the "conditioning of habit patterns. One of their foremost modern exponents, Hans Eysenck

> defined neurotic behavior as maladaptive habits formed through a process of conditioning and capable of being extinguished through several techniques of demonstrated effectiveness in the laboratory. There is no complex, no illness, and treatment is directed entirely to the symptoms, as distinguished from psychotherapy with its stress on hypothetical underlying complexes and disease processes. (Grossberg, 1964, p. 74.)

Action therapists and theorists make a point of insisting that their work is based on "modern learning theory" (Grossberg, 1964), but there is no *one* modern learning theory on which such therapies can be based. Action therapists do take their inspiration from learning theory, and do depend upon more recent studies of learning than those of Thorndike and Pavlov or even Hull and Skinner, but they are not really as thoroughly dependent on experimental studies of learning as they would like to believe, and their theories certainly do not always agree with each other.

> While Eysenck, Wolpe, and Skinner are in accord with respect to the emphasis on direct behavior modification as the focus of remedial efforts, Eysenck and Wolpe employ a Hullian behavior theory with constructs such as inhibition and drive which are rejected by Skinner. (Grossberg, 1964, p. 75.)

In addition to the practical agreement concerning focus of treatment, however, actionists also agree among themselves in

> the rejection of traditional psychodynamic personality theories, . . . consists of the application of the principles of modern learning theory to the treatment of behavior disorders. (Grossberg, 1964, p. 75.)

They are, by and large, less concerned with the specific theoretical origins of a technique than with inventing new methods for treatment of the psychologically distressed. Their approaches fall into the area of action, rather than insight, therapy, and they commonly agree that their approaches are "a welcome contrast to the convolutions of other psychotherapeutic theories" (Rachman and Eysenck, 1966), though their inspirations come from a variety of sources.

There are three main types of action therapy in common use: (1) counterconditioning techniques, (2) extinction techniques, and (3) behavior-shaping (or operant) techniques. Counterconditioning and extinction are both used primarily for the treatment of extreme fears (phobias), anxiety, sexual problems, and their like, while behavior-shaping methods are designed primarily for the teaching of skills and fostering the development of desirable habit patterns.

Counterconditioning techniques. To countercondition means to replace an existing feeling or behavior with one that is antithetical to it. Anxiety, as we shall see, can be replaced by anger or by a feeling of calm. Desire for a forbidden object can be replaced by fear or by nausea.

Counterconditioning techniques include essentially three different methods, all of which are associated with the work of Joseph Wolpe (1958). Many of them are older than they appear to be from the literature of the action therapists, having in some cases been first suggested by Guthrie (1935, 1938) and Bagby (1928). The techniques discussed here are (1) conditioned avoidance, (2) discriminative responses, and (3) assertive responses.

Conditioned avoidance responses are used either to make an unpleasant state more tolerable or to reduce the pleasure associated with an undesirable habit. The first is rarely used in practice: in order to alleviate the anxiety caused by a particular behavior, the patient is continuously subjected to a harmless but quite painful electric shock. Before shocking him, however, the therapist tells the patient that if he finds the shock excessive, he can terminate it by saying the word "calm." Continued over many trials, the word "calm" becomes associated with (conditioned to) pain reduction. It is anticipated that this form of conditioning will be generalized to other painful states, such as anxiety, so that whenever the patient is confronted with intense anxiety he can reduce it by saying "calm." Note that the source of the anxiety is of little concern here.

The same method can be used to reduce the pleasure associated with some undesirable behavior patterns. To free somebody of homosexual arousal, for example, the electric shock might be associated with pictures of a nude model of the same sex. Each time the patient is aroused by the picture, he is shocked until eventually the pairing of the negative reinforcer (pain) with an arousing stimulus (the nude picture) reduces the pleasure of it.

Discriminative approach and avoidance responses are used almost exclusively for sexual problems, and then only when the patient is either impotent or unable to have complete sexual relations. Wolpe's treatment (1958) consists of training the patient to attempt sexual relations *only* when "he has an unmistakable, positive, desire to do so, for otherwise he may very well consolidate, or even extend his sexual inhibitions" (p. 130). The training requires that he be able to discriminate between situations that are anxiety arousing and those that are not, and that he avoid the former and pursue the latter. A patient would then seek out people with whom he can be aroused in

> a desirable way . . . and when in the company of one of them, to "let himself go" as freely as the circumstances allow. . . . If he is able to act according to plan, he experiences a gradual increase in sexual responsiveness to the kind of situation of which he has made use . . . [and] the range of situations in which lovemaking may occur is thus progressively extended as the anxiety potentials of stimuli diminish. (P. 131.)

Assertive responses are aggressive acts a patient learns to use in situations where he experiences interpersonal anxiety which results in his being intimidated and taken advantage of. Wolpe (1958) assumes that the presence of anxiety inhibits all kinds of appropriate interpersonal expression. Assertion inhibits the anxiety, allowing the patient greater interpersonal latitude in his dealings with others.

Extinction techniques. Unlike counterconditioning methods, in which anxiety is weakened indirectly by learning responses which are antagonistic to it, extinction techniques try to attack anxiety directly by any of three methods: (1) reinforcement withdrawal, (2) desensitization, and (3) implosive therapy.

Reinforcement withdrawal makes use of a long-known learning principle: "When a learned response is repeated without reinforcement, the strength of the tendency to perform that response undergoes a progressive decrease" (Dollard and Miller, 1950). When, for example, patients reveal thoughts or experiences for which they expect others to condemn them, they tend to become anxious. If the expected condemnation does not occur, their anxiety over self-revelation diminishes or disappears (is extinguished). The notion of extinction has been applied in this way to insight therapies (Dollard and Miller, 1950), but it is taken up more vigorously and flexibly in the action therapies.

The treatment of tantrum behavior in children is an excellent example of one use of reinforcement withdrawal. Some children, for example, have tantrums at bedtime. They scream and rage after their parents have left the room, which brings their parents back and permits them to stay up longer. The reinforcing properties of tantrums are clear: each time the child rages, he gets attention and has his way. After ascertaining that there was nothing physically wrong with a tantrumming child, Williams (1959) advised the parents to put him to sleep in a leisurely fashion, leave the room, and then not return when the child raged. Figure 15.2 shows what occurred. On the first night, the boy screamed for forty-five minutes before going to sleep. On the second, he went to sleep immediately. By the tenth night, he no longer whimpered or cried but even smiled as his parents left.

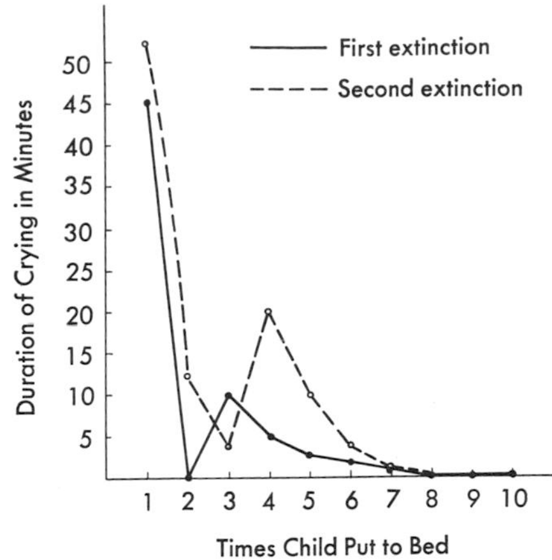

Figure 15.2 Duration of crying during extinction procedures aimed at eliminating tantrums. From Williams (1959).

The reintroduction of reinforcement following extinction brings the original behavior back in full measure. This happened in Williams' case some time later when the child's aunt put him to bed, returned to the room when he raged, and stayed with him until he fell off to sleep. The extinction curve for this second period is shown on the dotted lines in Figure 15.2. The form of the curve is similar to that of the first extinction, but the second extinction procedure took less time.

In action therapies, extinction is often combined with what is called *negative practice,* which means overdoing a bad habit until it becomes unpleasant and "worn out." Yates (1958) required a patient to voluntarily produce a tic many times within a fairly brief period of time (massed trials). Gradually, the patient became fatigued, which is a negative affective state. After doing this procedure many times, the tic became associated with the negative state and was gradually decreased.

Desensitization is a way of using imagination to extinguish anxiety, particularly in phobias. It was developed by Joseph Wolpe (1958). The patient and therapist jointly compose a list of things that arouse anxiety, ranking them from least to most anxiety provoking. The patient is trained, sometimes with hypnosis, to relax deeply and the therapist then presents the least anxiety-provoking situation and asks him to imagine it vividly. If he can do so without getting upset, he is then told to imagine the next item, and so on. When an item begins to provoke tension, the patient signals the therapist, who returns him to an earlier item in the list. Anxiety cues are increased from session to session until the most intense stimulus in the hierarchy fails to disturb the patient's relaxed state. The extinction of anxiety presumably is generalized from the vividly imagined fears in the consulting room to the real-life fears outside of it.

Implosive therapy is aimed entirely at combatting anxiety; it is something like reinforcement withdrawal in principle, but it looks very different. Instead of letting the undesirable behavior wear itself out naturally, this method tries to create an explosion inwards (implosion) of anxiety, frightening the patient as much as possible in situations where his fears cannot be reinforced by an actually experienced harm. This is done in a fashion similar to desensitization; that is, the therapist and patient first decide what things are more and less anxiety arousing, and the therapist then asks the patient to imagine them. What is unlike desensitization, however, is that he presents the most frightening events very quickly and intensively, seeking to arouse rather than to soothe the patient. The repeated experience of intense anxiety without harm causes gradual extinction of the anxiety, and treatment is complete when the therapist's provocative stories no longer arouse the patient. The technique of implosion was devised by Thomas Stampfl, but it is not yet widely known in psychotherapy literature (London, 1964, pp. 95–109).

There is no reason why neuroses of the kind Stampfl describes could not be treated by Wolpe's desensitization method. There is not much difference between the two men's theories of the neurotic process and how to approach it therapeutically. They agree that anxiety is at the core of neurotic behavior, that motive analysis and insight are irrelevant to its remediation, and that what is called for is a direct attack on the anxiety itself. But the techniques they employ to extinguish anxiety are diametrically opposed. Wolpe begins with the least, and works upward to the most, anxiety-provoking stimulus. Stampfl starts with the most terrifying stimulus he can find and constantly exposes the patient to it. Which is the better and more effective technique is a matter for empirical research, but it is clear that learning theory per se is of no immediate help here.

Behavior shaping. Behavior-shaping techniques are associated with the work of B. F. Skinner, who, though not a psychotherapist, has been instrumental in devising methods for altering behaviors that have been applied with some promise to psychotherapy. Counterconditioning and extinction methods are used chiefly against disorders believed to have traumatic origins, while behavior-shaping methods can be used more effectively for conditions which are chronic in nature and require broader changes in behavior. Skinnerian views are nontheoretical in the sense that they are not very much concerned with nonobservable experiences like anxiety. If a person behaves neurotically, therapists commonly assume he is experiencing anxiety. Skinner and his students will have none of this. Rather, they consider that certain behaviors need to be changed, regardless of their origin, and they set about changing them by relying mainly on the principles of *reinforcement* and *learning by successive approximations,* that is, learning in gradual steps where each new step towards the desired behavior is positively rewarded. These principles together constitute *behavior shaping.* Both principles and some therapeutic techniques derived from them have been discussed in detail in Chapters 5 and 9.

To shape behavior, the therapist needs to know what his patient finds rewarding and what aversive, and that is all he needs to know. By providing rewards, he can increase the incidence of desirable behavior, and by withholding rewards, he can decrease the incidence of undesirable behavior. He might also, of course, administer punishment to control undesirable behavior. But the effects of punishment, unless it can be applied with great skill, are often unpredictable. The Skinnerian psychotherapist therefore commonly works by rewarding positive behaviors.

This can be done with many neuroses and psychoses. Bachrach *et al.* (1965) have been able to induce a person suffering from anorexia nervosa (a form of depression in which the person refuses to eat) to eat and gain weight by controlling the availability of things she found rewarding. At first, a survey was made of the pleasurable aspects of her hospital environment:

> The patient was in an attractive hospital room with pictures on the wall, flowers available and usually present, a lovely view of the verdant grounds visible through the window. She had free access to visitors; a radio, books, records and a record player, television, and magazines were present, although she had considerable difficulty in reading because of her generalized debility. People would visit her and read to her as well as provide television control and record play. In discussion with her it was found that she enjoyed these activities and seemed to enjoy visitors as well. Because these activities apparently provided enjoyment for her and could thus be considered positively reinforcing to her behavior, she was removed from her pleasant hospital room and transferred to the psychiatric ward, to a private room from which all attractive accountrements had been removed. The room was barren, furnished only with a bed, nightstand and chair. . . .
>
> At first, any portion of the meal that was consumed would be a basis for a postprandial reinforcement (a radio, TV set, or phonograph would be brought in by the nurse at a signal from the experimenter); if she did not touch any of the food before her, nothing would be done by way of reinforcement and she would be left until the next meal. More and more of the meal had to be consumed in order to be reinforced until she eventually was required to eat everything on the plate. The meals were slowly increased in caloric value, . . . with the menu her own choice from several alternative menus, as was true of all the other patients on the ward. (Pp. 156–157.)

This patient had been admitted to the hospital weighing 47 pounds. She was discharged after two months of treatment, having gained 17 pounds, most of it during the course of treatment. Follow-up indicated that her progress continued to be excellent one and a half years later, when she weighed 85 pounds and was engaged in a full round of social and professional activities.

Success Rates of Action and Insight Therapies

The claims of action therapies have to be justified in terms of the economics of treatment; that is, they have to be equally or more successful than insight therapies in the same or shorter periods of time and to be equally or more easily applied by clinical practitioners with equal or less training. Otherwise, if there is no net gain in their use, then the polemic which action therapists level against insight therapists is without foundation.

Although some studies of the effectiveness of insight therapy have been done, action therapy has been more frequently studied. Because the relative success of each approach seems to be largely related to the type of problem to which it is applied, it is useful to examine some of their specific applications.

Fear reactions. Of all the action treatments, *desensitization* seems to be the most powerful in the treatment of phobias. Perhaps the earliest case study in desensitization is that reported by Mary Cover Jones (1924*a* and *b*). Jones treated a young child who was afraid of rabbits and whose fear had not only been generalized to other furry animals but also to such things as cotton and soft toys. The treatment consisted of inducing relaxation in the child by feeding him, and then gradually bringing the feared rabbit

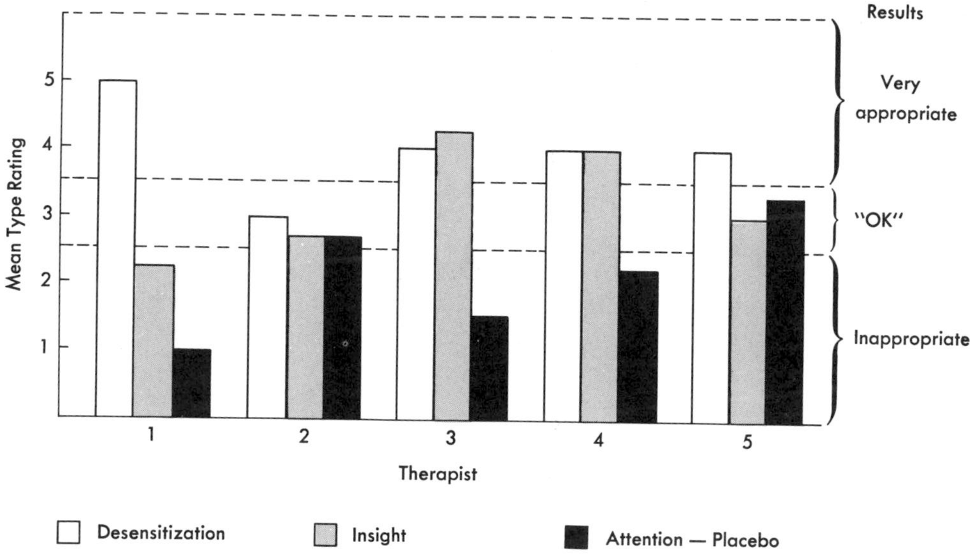

Figure 15.3 Mean therapist ratings of appropriateness of type of treatment for subjects within each treatment group. From Paul (1966).

closer and closer. Jones reported considerable success after a relatively brief treatment, as have other therapists who have worked with this particular phobia (Lang and Lazovik, 1963; Lazarus, 1959; Lazarus and Abromovitz, 1962; Lazarus and Rachman, 1957).

A study of the treatment of fear of public speaking by Gordon Paul (1966) contains one of the most careful comparisons yet reported between the effects of insight and action therapy. Paul's subjects were divided into four groups. The first received insight psychotherapy, the second desensitization, and the third placebo treatment consisting of reassurance that the procedures they were undergoing (swallowing a placebo and listening to taped noise over earphones) would help them with their public-speaking phobia. Finally, a fourth group served as a "no-treatment" control: apart from the initial contact, they were not seen until the posttherapy evaluation. All subjects were seen by the same five psychotherapists, who were experienced insight therapists carefully trained to administer the desensitization and placebo procedures. Students in these three groups were all seen for five fifty-minute sessions over a six-week period. Compared to the untreated controls, all treated groups, including the placebo group, showed some improvement. Fully 100 percent of the patients in desensitization (action) improved in therapy, while less than 50 percent of the insight and placebo subjects were found in the highest improvement categories. Clearly, at least as far as *this symptom* is concerned, action therapy was the more appropriate and successful treatment (Figure 15.3). In terms of *feelings of improvement*, on the other hand, members of all three treatment groups reported that they were much improved, and in relation to areas other than the specific symptom of anxiety about public speaking, the therapists rated subjects in the insight group as most improved and subjects in the desensitization group as least in need of further treatment (Paul, 1966, p. 53).

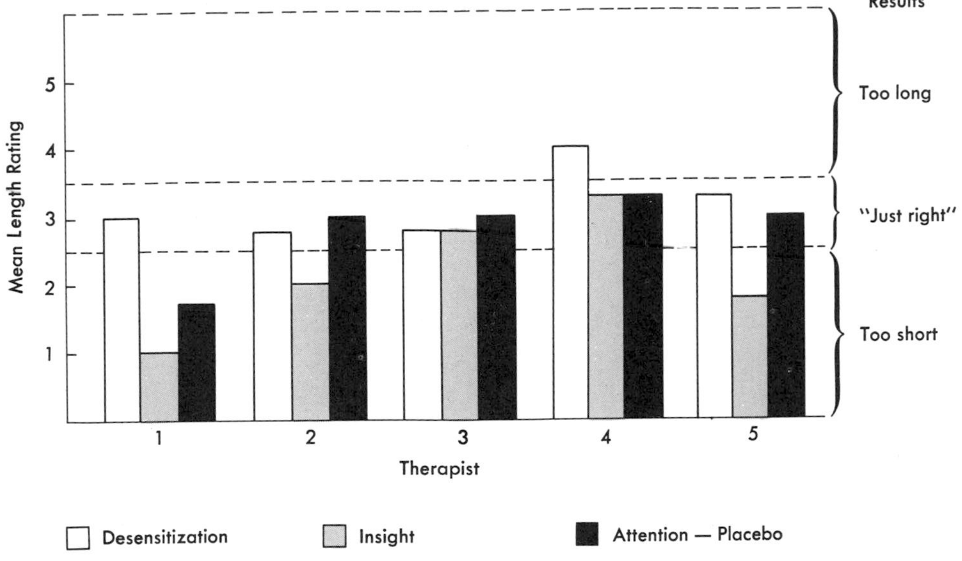

Figure 15.4 Mean therapist ratings of appropriateness of length of treatment for subjects within each treatment group. From Paul (1966).

These results, which are shown in Figure 15.4, further demonstrate how the effectiveness of a treatment method depends on what specific problem is examined.

Anxiety reactions. Wolpe (1958) reported on the treatment of 210 patients, more than half of whom presented symptoms of pervasive anxiety. After treatment with desensitization, 90 percent were either cured or much improved, although Breger and McGaugh (1966) point out that improvements are recorded only for those who had remained in treatment for fifteen sessions or more. Since some patients terminated treatment before the fifteenth session, the true improvement figures are less than 90 percent.

Sexual disorders. The effects of action therapies on sexual problems, especially homosexuality and other deviations, are quite equivocal. Freund (1960) reported that conventional insight psychotherapy was no less effective than action therapies that employed nauseant drugs among sixty-seven male homosexuals. Similar results are found in other case reports (Clark, 1963; Cooper, 1963; Morgenstern *et al.*, 1965), and electric shock works no better than drugs (Thorpe *et al.*, 1964). Feldman (1966), who has summarized the literature with a view to finding why these therapies have failed, suggests that the classical conditioning paradigm is not the one of choice, because classically conditioned responses of this sort yield rapidly to extinction. He suggests that operant, rather than classical, conditioning might be the treatment of choice for sexual deviance.

Enuresis. Enuresis is the inability to contain one's urine during sleep. It is a particular problem among children, especially boys, but it sometimes troubles adults as well. Mowrer and Mowrer (1938) investigated whether it was symptomatic of underlying pathology, as insight therapists ordinarily believe, or merely the result of faulty habit training. They invented an electrical device to condition bladder pressure to a stimulus for waking up. The first drop of urine would activate a bell, which would wake the patient up and send him to the bathroom. Eventually, pressure in the bladder alone would be sufficient to awaken him. A thorough follow-up of the children revealed no symptom substitution, which might have occurred if there were some underlying pathology of motivation.

Jones (1960) reviewed several studies in which this treatment, or variants of it, had been applied to nearly 1500 people. He indicates that some 76 percent were "cured" while 14 percent were failures. There were no reports of symptom substitution, and there was some evidence of positive personality change in successful cases. Because enuresis is a nasty symptom that is likely to bring on problems of its own, relief from it probably helps alleviate the problems associated with it.

Alcoholism. The primary action therapy for alcoholics consists of some kind of aversive procedure. Franks (1958), reviewing the large-scale sample studies, finds that average total abstinence rates several years after treatment are approximately 50 percent, which does not exceed the cures reported for various other treatments, including psychotherapy, religious conversion, and Alcoholics Anonymous methods. Grossberg (1964) points out, however, that aversion therapies may be faster and less expensive than other forms of treatment.

Psychoses. No form of psychotherapy has been particularly successful in treating psychoses, and action therapies, though effective in producing some kinds of behavior change among psychotic children and adults, have not yet produced cures.

In working with psychotics, action therapists have tended to rely almost solely on behavior-shaping (operant) techniques like those described in Chapter 9. The reason for the choice of operant techniques over other forms of action therapy is that the other forms require the patient's cooperation, and psychotic patients are often unable to cooperate. With operant techniques, however, one simply identifies behaviors that are to be modified, along with reinforcements the patient responds to, and proceeds without necessarily engaging the patient's cooperation or interest.

The importance of the behaviors that have thus far been amenable to behavior shaping is questionable. For example, Isaacs, *et al.* (1960) induced a mute schizophrenic to speak by giving him chewing gum as a reinforcer, but they could not get very extensive speech from him. Ayllon (1965) describes how two schizophrenic women were trained to give up being spoonfed and dallying over food by reinforcement with candy as they gradually performed more desirable behaviors. And Ayllon and Michael (1959) succeeded in greatly reducing long-standing psychotic talk and producing more normal talk in a schizophrenic woman by teaching ward nurses to disregard the one and reinforce the other.

Other investigators have reported similar kinds of successes with psychotic adults and children, but the most favorable conclusion that seems justified from this work is that these techniques are mainly useful for making patients more manageable on the ward and less of a general nuisance. A practical problem in their use, moreover, is that operant techniques essentially require that the entire hospital staff be highly conversant with and able to implement the method, and that they be able to adapt it to the needs of each patient. Given the state of the art and the state of institutions for the psychologically disturbed, action therapy has thus made only a small beginning toward the treatment of psychoses. But no other form of therapy has made major strides either.

Existential problems. The trouble with symptomatic treatments, such as the action therapies, is that no matter how successful they are for the problems they attack, they do not resolve the existential problems which may continue to arise even after phobias, inhibitions, and the like are successfully treated. Insight therapies are no substitute for symptom removal techniques, but the very fact that they aim at helping people to make their entire life meaningful gives them a potential value which action therapies do not necessarily even claim.

Problems of meaning or existential problems are psychological problems in which a person is concerned to understand his values, his personal identity, his aspirations, and his commitments. He may be deeply troubled by these concerns without having any of the symptoms usually associated with disorder. Action therapies that are concerned with symptoms and their removal are not easily adaptable to these kinds of problems.

A few students of therapy have been particularly concerned with the problem of simultaneously changing action patterns *and* resolving existential crises. Some of the best known among them are Carl Jung, Alfred Adler, Erich Fromm, and O. H. Mowrer. Mowrer's *integrity* therapy, which has been discussed in Chapter 11, is a good example of the attempt to relate disordered behavior patterns, like those found in depression, to the violations of values which may stimulate them. *Insight* into these values and their transgression elicits curative *action*. Jung's therapy differs both in language and technique from Mowrer's, but it too seeks to produce behavior change as a result of a kind of religious commitment. Adler and Fromm relate positive behavior to social commitments. The principle of all these systems, despite their differences, is that action is only curative in relation to *a meaningful life*, however that is defined.

Picturing the Scientific Dimension

Perhaps the easiest way to summarize the scientific or technical dimension of psychotherapy is to picture it as a continuum whose two extremes are *insight* and *action* therapies. Towards the insight end of the continuum are techniques in which the therapist devotes most of his efforts to enhancing the self-awareness and understanding of the patient without trying to actually manipulate the pattern of his acts. Therapists towards the action end aim at influencing action patterns without much concern for the cognitive or intellectual processes of the patient, and especially not with his existential concerns. In the middle are treatments that try to comprehend both kinds of therapy in a single system (Figure 15.5).

Existential, Rogerian, and classical psychoanalytic therapies fall at the insight end of the scientific dimension. They are concerned almost entirely with the individual's experience and cognitions, the ways he feels and thinks about himself, significant others, and his universe. If behavioral change comes about at all, it comes by way of changes in the individual's experience, perceptions, and cognitions.

At the other end of the technical dimension are the operant therapies and such therapies as those propounded by Wolpe and Stampfl. Although they differ in significant ways, all share the common concern with action—altering the patient's behavior. Their concerns with individual experience and cognition, except as these reflect symptoms, are minimal, and their therapies reflect it.

Somewhere towards the middle of this dimension are the therapies of O. H.

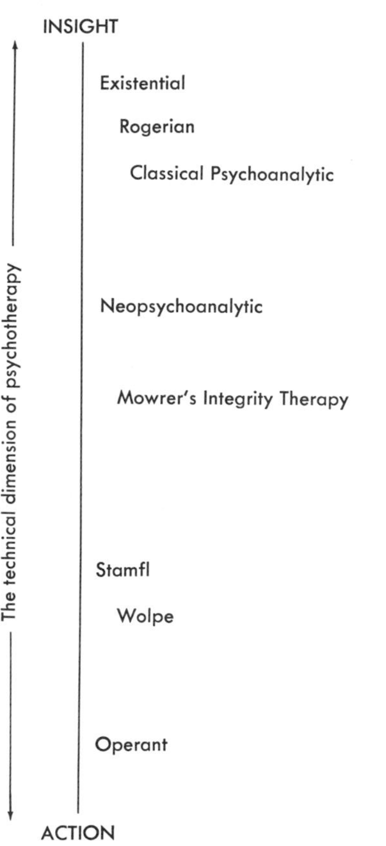

Figure 15.5 The technical dimension of psychotherapy.

Mowrer and of the neopsychoanalysts. Their concerns are for both insight and behavior change; they hold that behavior change cannot occur without insight, but that insight alone is clearly not enough.

The Locus of Disorder

In evaluating systems of psychotherapy, it is important to remember that the applicability of a particular technique depends on what is wrong with the patient in the first place. Whether existential therapy or counterconditioning or integrity therapy is any good does not necessarily depend as much on the intrinsic properties of the technique as on its relevance to the condition for which it is being used. In general, it seems clear that action therapies are more or less uniquely equipped to address disorders which can be defined by their symptoms, such as phobias. Insight systems may be more suited to disorders of meaning and feeling. Neither mode by itself seems adequate to cope with disorders which combine distressed behavior with disordered meanings or values, such as alcoholism, sexual deviations, or the host of less dramatic but equally painful problems of existence, which may, in fact, be most characteristic of most troubled people in modern times. For these, it seems that therapies are needed which integrate the properties of insight and action.

Another dimension of importance for understanding psychotherapy is thus the "locus of disorder" dimension; that is, the position that a particular individual's difficulties occupy on a continuum of problems whose two extremes are symptomatic disturbance and existential crises (Figure 15.6). In cases occurring toward the symptomatic disturbance end, there is something clearly disordered in the person's functioning, and an effective therapy aims toward alleviating this symptom. Its objective is, so to speak, to repair his behavior. In cases occurring toward the existential crisis end, the problem revolves around the total meaning of the person's life, and a therapeutic system which tries to deal with it must be concerned with his broadest values. Its objective is more like the objective of a clergyman than like that of either a doctor or a mechanic. Between these two ends of the continuum fall most of the "character disorders" (Chapter 11), those problems where the "symptoms" observed may represent disorder only because of a social convention which disdains the behavior in question, such as homosexuality, or where the symptom reflects a lack of personal values which might permit an individual to control

Locus of Disorder Dimension

SYMPTOM BEHAVIOR _ _ _ _ _ _ _ SOCIAL BEHAVIOR _ _ _ _ _ _ _ _ MOTIVE MEANING

Figure 15.6 The "locus of disorder" dimension of psychotherapy.

it or to be free of it, such as alcoholism. Disorders in the middle group ordinarily involve infringements of social norms whether they involve discomfort to the individual or not.

The *technical* and *locus of disorder* dimensions should not be treated as completely independent of each other in evaluating a therapy's effectiveness because some therapies are more suited to disorders at some loci than at others. The fact that some techniques tend to be applied to problems anywhere at all along the disorder dimension reflects both the complexity of human difficulties and the fact that therapists have not always examined the limitations of their schemes very thoroughly.

The Valuative Dimension

Clarification of the scientific characteristics of psychotherapy makes clearer than ever that there is a moral side to this discipline as well. Therapy techniques, by and large, are means of controlling and altering behavior, and the possession of techniques of control is useless or dangerous and harmful without wisdom and decency to dictate what behaviors to control and towards what end. Ultimately, therapists must base their decisions about how to treat people on some assumptions or beliefs about how people ought to live. Such beliefs may be formulated into any of a number of different systems, which are variously labeled "religious," "political," and "philosophical." Regardless of the label, however, they may all be regarded as *moral codes*.

Moral codes differ vastly among psychotherapists, but some critical moral problems are intrinsic to the therapeutic enterprise and need to be confronted by everybody involved in it. The most important of these problems is that of *individual, social,* and *normative* standards of morality.

Psychotherapists with *individualistic* moral orientations tend to believe that the main objective of therapy is to guide people toward living in ways that are individually satisfying to them. If these ways of living put the individual in conflict with other people or with social conventions, the individually oriented psychotherapist would argue that the patient's own needs have legitimate priority, and he would direct his therapeutic be havior toward supporting that view, probably justifying it in the name of personal liberty.

The *social* moral orientation is one that sees the purpose of therapy as the teaching of social adjustment, that is of reconciling the needs of the individual to those of social convention. If the satisfaction of society's demands requires that the individual change some of his values, the socially oriented therapist would work to induce such change, probably arguing that it is his chief job to help secure the happiness of his patient.

The *normative* moral orientation is a modified social orientation. It proposes that the individual should conform to the demands of society, but that there are good and bad societies, and he is obligated to oppose the demands of a wicked society.

Each of these positions has its own problems. The individualistic psychotherapist does not usually justify personal aggression in his patients, but his moral stance makes it hard for him to justify his arguments against such behavior. The socially oriented psychotherapist tends to promote conformism at the price of individual liberty and of the traditional values which individuals often enter therapy with and which often set them in conflict with society. The normative orientation presents difficulties because it may set the therapist's values against both the individual impulses of the patient and the social conventions at the same time. Besides, it is not easy to decide in all cases what constitute good and bad social norms or who is entitled to make such decisions.

Regardless of his personal orientation, every psychotherapist is faced repeatedly with all of these moral problems in the course of his daily work. There are no completely satisfactory resolutions, and most therapists are therefore very cautious about taking a firm moral position in relation to most of the problems their patients discuss. This does not mean that they lack moral perspective, but only that they recognize, if they are sensitive and conscientious, that they have responsibilities both to the individual they serve and to the society that sanctions their service.

SUMMARY

There is no completely satisfactory means of classifying all the different mental disorders, but the great variety of methods that have been devised to treat them can be divided into three inexact categories: (1) medical treatments, (2) educational treatments, and (3) psychotherapy.

Medical treatments fall into two general groups: (1) assault methods, which are mainly shock therapies and surgery; and (2) tranquilizing methods, which mainly use "energizing" drugs to lift the spirits and "tranquilizing" drugs to calm them. Electric shock therapy has been used primarily for the treatment of schizophrenia and depression. It seems to be useless for the former but quite effective for the latter. Chemical shock therapies are chiefly injection of Metrazol or the induction of insulin coma. These have been used mostly for schizophrenia; but their effects are questionable, they are rather dangerous, and the tranquilizing drugs have made them generally unnecessary. Surgical treatments are not common today, but prefrontal lobotomy was widely used less than a generation ago to calm unmanageable psychotics. Plastic surgery is not generally a psychiatric treatment, but it is sometimes used to relieve anxieties or personal difficulties that stem from a marred appearance.

Tranquilizing drugs are among the most common medical treatments in use today. Ataractics, or strong tranquilizers, are commonly used for severe anxiety and functional psychosis, especially in hospitalized patients. So-called weak tranquilizers are used more for outpatients. Antidepressant drugs like Dexedrine and sedatives such as phenobarbital are not often thought of as psychiatric drugs, but they certainly belong among the tranquilizers. Despite their widespread use, relatively little is known about the value of the weak tranquilizers. Ataractic drugs have been valuable in hospital treatment because of their soothing influence on severely disturbed patients; they make these people easier to manage and thus permit hospital personnel to behave more therapeutically than was once true. But by and large, no drugs can solve personal problems.

The most important educational treatments are (1) remedial reading techniques, (2) speech therapy, and (3) occupational therapy. Reading disabilities are mostly the result of bad learning experiences, but they sometimes have an emotional basis, and they often create emotional problems even when they do not result from them. Speech therapy is often considered a special form of psychotherapy, but it is usually taught in programs especially designed for the purpose and practiced by people trained exclusively for such work. Stuttering is the most common speech disorder. Occupational therapy is considered an adjunctive educational therapy because it is not used to attack psychological problems directly, but as a peripheral means of facilitating other treatments.

Psychotherapy is the term for most nonmedical forms of psychological treatment. It evolved from two distinct traditions, a medical tradition of mental hospital care and a mixed medical and educational tradition of outpatient treatment and guidance, which evolved into office practice. Psychoanalysis, the invention of Sigmund Freud at the turn of the century, is today considered the prototype of psychotherapy, but it only became very popular after World War II. Behavioristic psychotherapy has become well known since about 1960, but its roots extend back as far as psychoanalysis in the experimental studies of Ivan Pavlov and E. L. Thorndike.

The many different kinds of psychotherapy can be best understood in terms of two-dimensional schemes, a scientific or technical dimension and a moralistic or evaluative dimension. The two extremes of the scientific dimension are *insight* and *action* therapies. Insight therapies are aimed at increasing self-understanding by such techniques as "free association" and "transference," chiefly used in psychoanalysis, and by "reflection of feelings," chiefly used in client-centered therapy. Action therapies are aimed at changing behavior patterns by such methods as "counterconditioning," chiefly associated with Joseph Wolpe, "extinction techniques," like the implosive therapy of Thomas Stampfl, and "behavior shaping," as in the operant methods of B. F. Skinner. Some therapy methods, like the integrity therapy of O. H. Mowrer, attempt to combine insight and action techniques. The value of a particular method depends somewhat on the kind of problem to which it is applied. Insight therapies may be most effective for existential problems of values and goals, action therapies may be best for treating specific symptoms, such as anxiety, phobias, and habit disorders, and integrative therapies may be best for treating so-called disorders of character.

All psychotherapies involve moral problems because they concern the ways people ought to conduct their lives. Therapists vary in their personal and professional moral orientations, but they are commonly very conservative about communicating their orientations to their patients. The most common moral dilemmas which appear in psychotherapy involve the potential conflict between individual desires and the demands of society.

GLOSSARY

ACTION THERAPIES—therapies that concentrate on changing behavior (see Chapter 15).

ADJUNCTIVE THERAPIES—educational procedures, such as occupational therapy, used in conjunction with therapies that are directed at symptoms or their causes.

ANALYTICAL PSYCHOTHERAPY—the psychotherapeutic technique devised by C. G. Jung; an insight therapy that derives, but is quite different, from Freudian psychoanalysis.

ANXIETY—an unpleasant feeling state usually characterized by increased motility of the gastrointestinal tract, increased heart rate, palmar sweating, shivering, flushing, and muscular contractions (see Chapters 4 and 10).

APPROACH-AVOIDANCE CONFLICT—conflict produced by the fact that a particular goal is, at the same time, both attractive and aversive.

ASSAULT TREATMENTS—medical procedures used in the treatment of psychological disorders; shock therapies and surgery are the most common of the assault treatments.

ASSERTIVE RESPONSES—commonly, aggressive acts a patient learns to use in situations where he feels intimidated and taken advantage of; assertive responses inhibit anxiety and thus allow the patient greater latitude in his dealings with others.

BASE RATE PROBLEM—the tendency of some people to improve spontaneously with or without treatment.

BEHAVIORISM—the view that psychology as a science is concerned only with behavior; it does not use introspection or deal with mental processes or contents.

BEHAVIOR SHAPING—teaching, in gradual steps, the new and desired behavior by reinforcing each response that approximates the desired behavior.

CHARACTER DISORDERS—psychopathological conditions whose symptomatic behaviors include antisociality, aggression, dishonesty, and deception.

CHLORPROMAZINE—a strong tranquilizer.

CLASSICAL CONDITIONING—the process of establishing "connections" between a neutral stimulus (like a bell) and a meaningful one (like delicious food which makes one salivate) such that the neutral stimulus now evokes the meaningful response (salivation).

CLIENT-CENTERED PSYCHOTHERAPY—a nondirective therapy, devised by Carl Rogers, which places great stress on enabling the client to understand himself by "reflecting" the client's feelings and observations and by accepting him on his own terms.

CONDITIONED AVOIDANCE RESPONSES—a technique used by action therapists primarily for reducing the pleasure associated with an undesirable habit.

CONDITIONING—the learning of a particular response as a consequence of specific stimuli which either elicit or reward it.

CONTROL GROUP—persons who are not exposed to the experimental variable but are exposed to as many as possible (and ideally, all) of the other conditions in the experiment in order to ensure that the effects of the experiment are not the result of irrelevant or unnoticed considerations.

CORRELATION—the relationship of two variables such that a change in one is accompanied by a corresponding change in the other.

COUNTERCONDITIONING—replacing a feeling or behavior with one that is antithetical to it; anxiety can be replaced by anger or by a feeling of calm.

DEPRESSION—an emotional state of great sadness often accompanied by guilt and anxiety, gloomy ruminations, lassitude, inability to respond to pleasant stimuli, and suicidal impulses.

DESENSITIZATION—the process devised by Joseph Wolpe (1958) of reducing sensitivity to anxiety-provoking stimuli; having ordered these stimuli from least to most anxiety provoking, the patient vividly imagines the least noxious stimulus until it no longer troubles him; he then goes to the next item, and so on until the most distressing stimulus fails to disturb him.

DISCRIMINATIVE APPROACH AND AVOIDANCE RESPONSES—a training procedure used by action therapists that trains the patient to discriminate carefully between situations that are anxiety arousing and those that are not.

DOUBLE-BLIND METHOD—a technique for ensuring that the experimenter's knowledge of the purpose of the experiment will not influence his assessment of the outcome; knowledge of which subject is receiving treatment and which is the control is concealed from the experimenter and the subject alike (hence, double-blind).

EDUCATIONAL TREATMENTS—treatment procedures used in connection with a specific educational problem; a specific technical instruction, such as reading or speech therapy, is usually involved.

ELECTRIC SHOCK (ELECTROCONVULSIVE) THERAPY (ECT)—an assault treatment consisting of the application of electric current to the front part of the patient's head.

EPILEPSY—a general name for a group of neurological disorders marked primarily by convulsions.

EXISTENTIAL PROBLEMS — psychological problems centering about the meaning of life, including understanding values, personal identity, aspirations, and commitment.

EXISTENTIAL PSYCHOTHERAPY—psychotherapy that is primarily addressed to problems of meaning.

EXTINCTION—progressive reduction in the response, achieved by withholding the rewards or reinforcements which usually follow the response.

Extinction techniques—techniques used by action therapists to attack anxiety directly by one of three methods: (1) reinforcement withdrawal, (2) desensitization, and (3) implosive therapy.

Feedback—information obtained by an organism as a consequence of his own action.

Free association—a psychoanalytic (insight therapy) method for uncovering unconscious motives; the patient utters everything that comes to mind, allowing thoughts that are ordinarily suppressed as irrelevant, embarrassing, or inappropriate to be verbalized and examined.

Functional disorder—a disorder in which there is no evidence of organic malfunctioning or structural pathology.

Generalization—the transfer of learnings acquired in one context to another one that bears some resemblance to it (see Chapters 3, 9, and 10).

Hypnotism (hypnosis)—a little understood state characterized by relaxation, concentration, and heightened susceptibility to the hypnotist's suggestions.

Implosive therapy—a technique devised by Stampfl for reducing sensitivity to anxiety-provoking stimuli; the patient is asked to vividly imagine the *most* anxiety arousing stimulus, but since the anxiety aroused goes unreinforced, it is gradually extinguished.

Inhibition—suppression of a response, often unconsciously, even though the stimuli that would ordinarily elicit it are present.

Insight therapies—therapies based upon, or derived from, the psychoanalytic tradition of Freud; insight therapies have in common the notion that motives determine behavior, and that proper understanding of motives will itself lead to altered behavior.

Involutional melancholia—depressive psychotic reaction, occurring mainly during menopause.

LSD—lysergic acid diethylamide.

Mentally retarded—conservatively, falling in the lower 3 percent of the distribution of IQ scores; the definition established in the *Manual on Terminology and Classification in Mental Retardation*[1] includes all persons whose IQ falls below the population mean; the *social competence* definition classifies all those who are unable to meet minimal societal demands (see Chapter 14).

Negative practice—a therapy, often combined with one of the extinction techniques, involving the overdoing of a bad habit till it becomes unpleasant or "worn out."

Neopsychoanalysis—a version of psychoanalysis which rejects its instinctual and biological emphasis and holds that insight alone is insufficient to provoke changes in behavior.

Neurosis—a negative abnormality ill-defined in character but milder than psychosis.

Operant conditioning—the process of learning to operate on the environment in order to gain reward.

Organic psychiatry—a disease theory of mental illness, upon which medical techniques for the treatment of negative abnormality are based.

Paresis—a progressive organic psychosis and paralysis resulting from a syphilitic infection of the brain.

Phenylketonuric mental deficiency—a type of mental retardation, usually considered hereditary, that becomes evident only under certain environmental conditions (see Chapters 2 and 14).

Phobia—any irrational fear.

Placebo—a "nondrug" or "nontreatment"; an inactive substance which looks like a real medicine; where the placebo is effective it is because it has some of the same *suggestive* properties of the treatment, but not its substantive characteristics.

Psychiatrist—a medical doctor who specializes in the diagnosis and treatment of nervous and mental disorders.

Psychoanalysts—psychotherapists who adhere to the body of doctrine set forth by Freud, and its modifications by his close disciples.

Psychodrama—the enactment before a participating audience of roles and dramatic incidents in order to reveal to the client the meaning and effects of his behavior.

Psychologist—one who has studied psychology, commonly at the graduate level.

Psychosis—an ill-defined term generally meaning any severe, negative psychological abnormality.

[1] By R. F. Heber. See the *American Journal of Mental Deficiency, Monograph Supplements,* 1959, 64, No. 2.

PSYCHOSOMATIC DISORDERS—physical symptoms resulting from psychological stress or conflict (see Chapter 13).

PSYCHOTHERAPY—the use of any psychological technique in the treatment of mental disorder or maladjustment.

REFLECTION—used in insight therapies, it is the therapist's restatement of what the patient has said in such a way that he exposes the feelings underlying the content of the patient's statements and communicates his understanding and acceptance of them.

REINFORCEMENT—that which strengthens a response.

REINFORCEMENT WITHDRAWAL—as used in this chapter, a therapeutic technique based on the principle that if a response is repeated without reinforcement, the probability that it will occur again is diminished.

SCHIZOPHRENIA—one of the psychoses, characterized by generalized withdrawal from reality, blunted and distorted affect, regression, and disorganized thought processes.

SOCIAL WORKER—a person who engages in professional services, concerned with the investigation, treatment, and material aid of the economically underprivileged and socially maladjusted.

STIMULUS—an internal or external event.

SYMPTOM REMISSION—temporary abatement or cessation of the symptoms of a disorder.

TRANQUILIZING TREATMENTS—medical procedures which involve the administration of "energizing" drugs, which lift the spirits, and "tranquilizers," which soothe them.

TRANSFERENCE—the attribution to someone in the present of traits and feelings that characterized a significant person in the past; considered an important ingredient in psychoanalytic psychotherapies.

TRAUMATIC EVENT—anything that inflicts serious psychological damage upon the organism.

WILL THERAPY—Otto Rank's variant of psychoanalysis.

REFERENCES

Astin, A. W. The functional autonomy of psychotherapy. *American Psychologist*, 1961, **16**, 75–78.

Ayllon, T. Some behavioral problems associated with eating in chronic schizophrenic patients. In L. P. Ullmann and L. Krasner (eds.), *Case studies in behavior modification*. New York: Holt, Rinehart & Winston, 1965.

——— and J. Michael. The psychiatric nurse as a behavioral engineer. *Journal of the Experimental Analysis of Behavior*, 1959, **2**, 323–334.

Bachrach, A. J., W. J. Erwin, and J. P. Mohr. The control of eating behavior in an anorexic by operant conditioning techniques. In L. P. Ullmann and L. Krasner (eds.), *Case studies in behavior modification*. New York: Holt, Rinehart & Winston, 1965.

Bagby, E. *The psychology of personality: An analysis of common emotional disorders*. New York: Holt, Rinehart & Winston, 1928.

Bockoven, J. S. *Moral treatment in American psychiatry*. New York: Springer Publishing Company, Inc., 1963.

Breger, L., and J. L. McGaugh. Learning theory and behavior therapy: A reply to Rachman and Eysenck. *Psychological Bulletin*, 1966, **65**, 170–173.

Bugental, J. F. T. Humanistic psychology: A break-through. *American Psychologist*, 1963, **18**, 563–567.

Cerletti, U., and L. Bini. Electric shock treatment. *Bulletin Accademia Medica Roma*, 1938, **64**, 36.

Clark, D. F. Fetishism treated by negative conditioning. *British Journal of Psychiatry*, 1963, **109**, 404–408.

Cole, J. O. Phenothiazine treatment in acute schizophrenia. *Archives of General Psychology*, 1964, **10**, 246–261.

Cooper, A. J. A case of fetishism and impotence treated by behavior therapy. *British Journal of Psychiatry*, 1963, **109**, 649–652.

Deutsch, A. *The mentally ill in America*, Ed. 2. New York: Columbia University Press, 1948.

Dollard, J., and N. E. Miller. *Personality and psychotherapy: An analysis in terms of learning, thinking, and culture*. New York: McGraw-Hill, Inc., 1950.

Engelhardt, D., N. Freedman, L. Hernkoff, D. Mann, and R. Margolis. Long term induced symptom modification in schizophrenic out-patients. *Journal of Nervous and Mental Disease*, 1963, **137**, 231–241.

Ewalt, J. R. National aspects. In M. Greenblatt and B. Simon (eds.), *Rehabilitation of the mentally ill*. Washington, D. C.: American Association for the Advancement of Science, 1959, pp. 3–12.

Eysenck, H. J. The effects of psychotherapy. In H. J. Eysenck (ed.), *Handbook of abnormal psychology*. New York: Basic Books, Inc., 1960, pp. 697–725.

Feldman, M. P. Aversion therapy for sexual deviations: A critical review. *Psychological Bulletin*, 1966, **65**, 65–79.

Flanagan, B., I. Goldiamond, and N. Azrin. Operant stuttering: The control of stuttering behavior through response contingent consequences. *Journal of Experimental Analysis of Behavior*, 1958, **1**, 73–77.

Ford, D. H., and H. B. Urban. *Systems of psychotherapy*. New York: John Wiley & Sons, Inc., 1963.

Franks, C. M. Alcohol, alcoholism and conditioning: A review of the literature and some theoretical considerations. *Journal of Mental Science*, 1958, **104**, 14–33.

Freeman, W. Psychosurgery: Retrospects and prospects based on twelve years' experience. *American Journal of Psychiatry*, 1949, **105**, 581–584.

——— and J. W. Watts. *Psychosurgery*. Springfield, Ill.: Charles C Thomas, Publisher, 1942.

Freund, K. Some problems in the treatment of homosexuality. In H. J. Eysenck (ed.), *Behavior therapy and the neuroses*. New York: Pergamon Press, Inc., 1960, pp. 312–326.

Gittleman, R. K., D. F. Klein, and M. Pollack. Longterm effects of psychotropic drugs on adjustment. *Psychopharmocologia*, 1964, **5**, 317–338.

Grossberg, J. M. Behavior therapy: A review. *Psychological Bulletin*, 1964, **62**, 77–88.

Guthrie, E. R. *The psychology of learning*. New York: Harper & Row Publishers, 1935.

———. *The psychology of human conflict*. New York: Harper & Row Publishers, 1938.

Inpastato, D. J. Effect of drug therapy on the frequency of EST. *American Journal of Psychotherapy*, 1962, **16**, 387–396.

Isaacs, W., J. Thomas, and I. Goldiamond. Application of operant conditioning to reinstate verbal behavior in psychotics. *Journal of Speech and Hearing Disorders*, 1960, **25**, 8–17.

Jones, H. G. The behavioural treatment of enuresis nocturna. In H. J. Eysenck (ed.), *Behavior therapy and the neuroses*. New York: Pergamon Press, Inc., 1960, pp. 377–403.

———. Specific conditioning treatment of enuresis nocturna. *Cerebral Palsy Bulletin*, 1961, **3**, 227–236.

Jones, Mary C. Conditioning and reconditioning: An experimental study in child behavior. *Proceedings and Addresses of the National Education Association*, 1924*a*, **62**, 585–590.

———. The elimination of children's fears. *Journal of Experimental Psychology*, 1924*b*, **7**, 382–390.

Knight, R. P. Evaluation of the results of psychoanalytic therapy. *American Journal of Psychiatry*, 1941, **98**, 434–446.

Kramer, M., P. Ornstein, and R. Whitman. Drug therapy. In E. A. Spiegel (ed.), *Progress in neurology and psychiatry*, Vol. 20. New York: Grune & Stratton, Inc., 1964, pp. 723–753.

Lang, P. J., and A. D. Lazovik. Experimental desensitization of a phobia. *Journal of Abnormal and Social Psychology*, 1961, **66**, 519–525.

Lazarus, A. A. The elimination of children's phobias by deconditioning. *South African Medical Proceedings*, 1959, **5**, 261–265.

———. Group therapy of phobic disorders by systematic desensitization. *Journal of Abnormal and Social Psychology*, 1961, **63**, 504–510.

——— and A. Abramovitz. The use of "emotive imagery" in the treatment of children's phobias. *Journal of Mental Science*, 1962, **108**, 191–195.

Lingl, F. A. Combined drug therapy compared with electric shock in psychotic depressions. *American Journal of Psychiatry*, 1964, **120**, 808–810.

London, P. *The modes and morals of psychotherapy*. New York: Holt, Rinehart & Winston, 1964.

———. Morals and mental health. In R. Plog, R. Edgerton, and R. Beckwith (eds.), *Determinants of mental illness*. New York: Holt, Rinehart & Winston, in press.

Morgenstern, F. S., J. F. Pearce, and L. W. Rees. Predicting the outcome of behavior therapy by psychological tests. *Behavior Research and Therapy*, 1965, **2**, 191–200.

Mowrer, O. H., and W. M. Mowrer. Enuresis: A method for its study and treatment. *American Journal of Orthopsychiatry*, 1938, **8**, 436–459.

Olshansky, S. Employer receptivity. In

M. Greenblatt and B. Simon (eds.), *Rehabilitation of the mentally ill.* Washington, D.C.: American Association for the Advancement of Science, 1959, pp. 213–221.

Paul, G. L. *Insight versus desensitization in psychotherapy: An experiment in anxiety reduction.* Stanford, Calif.: Stanford University Press, 1966.

Rachman, S., and H. J. Eysenck. Reply to a "critique and reformulation" of behavior therapy. *Psychological Bulletin,* 1966, **65,** 165–169.

Smith, K., and R. L. Biddy. Shock therapy. In E. A. Spiegel (ed.), *Progress in neurology and psychiatry,* Vol. 19. New York: Grune & Stratton, Inc., 1964.

Thorpe, J. G., E. Schmidt, P. T. Brown, and D. Castell. Aversion-relief therapy: A new method for general application. *Behavior Research and Therapy,* 1964, **2,** 71–82.

Uhr, L., and J. Miller. Prologue. In L. Uhr and J. Miller (eds.), *Drugs and behavior.* New York: John Wiley & Sons, Inc., 1960.

Williams, C. D. The elimination of tantrum behavior by extinction procedures. *Journal of Abnormal and Social Psychology,* 1959, **59,** 269.

Wolpe, J. *Psychotherapy by reciprocal inhibition.* Stanford, Calif.: Stanford University Press, 1958.

Wortis, J. Psychopharmacology and physiological treatment. *American Journal of Psychiatry,* 1965, **121,** 648–652.

Yates, A. J. The application of learning theory to the treatment of tics. *Journal of Abnormal and Social Psychology,* 1958, **56,** 175–182.

SUGGESTED READINGS

1. Dollard, J., and N. E. Miller. *Personality and psychotherapy.* New York: McGraw-Hill, Inc., 1950. A brilliant examination of psychoanalytic therapy and diagnosis from the point of view of modified learning theory.
2. Freud, S. *General introduction to psychoanalysis.* New York: Permabooks, 1956, Chapters 27–28. A solid introduction to Freud's own views on psychotherapy.
3. Krasner, L., and L. P. Ullman (eds.). *Research in behavior modification.* New York: Holt, Rinehart and Winston, 1965. A theoretical presentation of various techniques of action therapy. For the application of action therapy to negative psychological abnormalities see L. P. Ullman, and L. Krasner, *Case studies in behavior modification,* New York: Holt, Rinehart, & Winston, 1965.
4. McCary, J. L., and D. L. Scheer (eds.). *Six approaches to psychotherapy.* New York: Holt, Rinehart & Winston, 1955. An overview of insight therapies and their modifications.
5. Wolpe, J. *Psychotherapy by reciprocal inhibition.* Stanford, Calif.: Stanford University Press, 1958. An important treatise on action therapies, particularly those involving counterconditioning and desensitization.

16

Mental Health: The Promise of Behavior Science

PERRY LONDON
DAVID ROSENHAN

It is much easier to discuss psychopathology intelligently than it is to talk about *mental health* because *health* is an ambiguous term in a way that *illness* is not. Illness can be identified by the presence of symptoms of disorder; but health can be understood either as the *absence* of symptoms or the *presence* of some condition, and both definitions make sense. If a person has been ill, for example, and then recovers, we say that he has recovered his health, meaning that the symptoms of his disorder have disappeared and that no others have cropped up in their place. On the other hand, one obviously does not have to become ill first in order to be healthy. The absence of symptoms of illness can be considered a definition of health even when there have been no symptoms to begin with. Still, if health is defined in such a narrow way, then some absurd propositions become possible, like, "He was healthy (free of symptoms) in the kidneys, but died of cancer." In the same way, it is absurd to say that a person has regained his mental health (from schizophrenia) but continues to be hospitalized (for manic-depressive psychosis). Clearly we use the term *health* to mean general rather than specific freedom from symptoms.

General freedom from symptoms is a negative definition of health and a tricky one at that, for it is often difficult to separate it from the positive implication that a person who lacks pathological symptoms must be functioning effectively. This is especially true with psychological disorders, where the symptoms themselves are often purely functional. In other words, mental health can be equated with the mere absence of mental illness.

Many professional students of mental health have come to believe that the mere absence of illness does not connote health in any meaningful way (see Jahoda, 1959; Offer and Sabshin, 1966). It is undoubtedly true, for example, that the 97-pound weakling of advertising fame is not ill in the usual sense of the word, but to equate his effectiveness in any positive sense with that of his adversary in the "before" picture is quite absurd.

It may not be possible to produce a more useful definition of mental health at the present time. But it will be helpful to bear in mind throughout any discussion of the concepts of illness and health that these terms do not have absolute meanings but are only convenient labels which we use to identify relatively different conditions. While the definition of health as the absence of illness lacks comprehensiveness, it still can serve the convenient purpose of describing a relatively distinct state.

ENVIRONMENT AND MENTAL HEALTH

All the determinants of behavior are conventionally described in two broad categories: the *genetic* and the *environmental*. The former were reviewed mainly in Chapter 2. Much of the rest of this book has focused on the effects of *local* environment, especially interpersonal interactions and their effects. Most of the study of environmental determinants, as of genetic ones, has been concerned with their *pathogenic* role in *producing* mental illness rather than with their *prophylactic* role in *preventing* it. This has been particularly emphasized in Chapter 12. Also, little attention has been paid thus far to the implications of the *broader* environment, particularly the social and economic setting in which the individual finds himself, for mental health and illness.

The definition of mental health as the absence of symptoms is most difficult to interpret in situations where the general environment is conducive to the development of symptoms or restricts the development of normally socialized individuals. The concept of mental health usually implies a reasonably stress-free environment; where such environs are absent, it is not very meaningful to speak of mental health in any terms other than those of *resistance to stress.*

In the presence of a favorable social environment, mental health is reflected less in a person's ability to *withstand* the pressure of events than in his ability to actively control his relationship to them. To some extent, these may be the same thing, in that both refer to a person's ability to maintain equilibrium between himself and the external world. But more likely they involve somewhat different personal skills or characteristics. The man who survives by bending with the storms passively accepts whatever comes, while the person who seeks to master situations may act most effectively in opposite directions. Both types fall within the conventional definitions of normality discussed in Chapter 5.

Whether a positive concept of mental health involves mastery of the environment or merely the ability to tolerate it (to resist stress) may depend as much on the environment as on the concept, at least when the stresses the environment poses are severe ones. Suppose a person is subjected to economic exploitation, persecution, or another form of duress over which he has no control. This is precisely the case in racial and religious discrimination. It makes no sense to require, in the name of mental health, that the Negro change his color or learn to live without a job. In the long run, mastery of the situation, that is, behavior that will change the environment to correspond to the needs of the individual, is desirable. But at any given time, it is necessary for the person to manage somehow to survive the duress he is under and adapt to it as best he can.

Resistance to stress and mastery are not antagonistic concepts, of course. Even in an underprivileged and harsh environment, one may find both characteristics in the same person (see Harrington, 1962; Hobbs, 1964; Reissman *et al.*, 1964). But for the most part, extreme stress reduces people's efforts to master their environments or severely distresses people by frustrating their efforts. Numerous writers, for example, have observed that the discrepancy between level of aspiration and opportunities for fulfilling aspirations is a major source of psychological distress among minority groups, especially Negroes (Horney, 1939; Kardiner and Ovesey, 1951; Hollingshead *et al.*, 1954; Parker and Kleiner, 1966). And such attempts at mastery as do occur often take the form of antisocial behavior. Clark (1965) suggests that the lack of social status and of opportunity is a major determinant of both psychological disorder and antisocial activity among Harlem Negroes. These deficiencies in the social structure are often so great that most Negroes are unable to overcome them: the social structure simply does not permit it. Adaptation, when it occurs, must for them consist primarily of resistance to stress.

The excessively punitive environments in which the racially and religiously persecuted live constitute extreme stresses on mental health, but the lower socioeconomic classes in general, be they white or Negro, have greater difficulty achieving mental health than the more fortunate members of the middle and upper social strata (Srole *et al.*, 1962). As we saw in Chapter 12, the stresses of war and the ravages of economic depression have similar debilitating effects. Some have argued, in fact, that the very structure of certain societies predisposes their members to various forms of insanity by promiscuously endorsing irrational behavior and attitudes, such as fanatical nationalism, economic competition, or interpersonal aggression (Fromm, 1941; Koestler, 1945, 1955).

If the environment is simply too consistently harsh to support individuals in a way which is reasonably free of anxiety or discomfort, then the notion of mental health becomes meaningless altogether. The actual use of the term seems always to imply the possibility that most people can realize a relatively unburdened and comfortable existence in a society which is free of drastic poverty and brutal social discrimination. The other side of that coin is that, where such an existence is possible, as it is for many Americans, the problem of *anxiety* in response to stress may be replaced by the problem of *ennui*, that is, the distress of boredom, or of *anomie*, the lack of identity—problems of finding meaning in life or, as they are often called, *existential crises*.

Some people argue that there is a kind of ideal or optimal tension level, in relation to both one's environment and one's own feelings. Societies that fulfill economic objectives, providing their members with relative freedom from the environment, but that are unable to provide goals which satisfy people's needs for a purposive existence are, from this point of view, "sick" (see Chapter 5).

PREVENTIVE MENTAL HEALTH

The achievement of mental health in a society requires the *prevention* of disorders, not merely the discovery of ways to treat them once they have occurred. The situation for mental health is much the same as for physical health, in that prevention requires a different professional technology and body of personnel from the kind required for treatment. Protection of the public health is vested largely in the hands of sanitary engineers, quarantine officers, and the research personnel who study such problems as air pollution, the purity of food and drugs, and the consumption and distribution of food and water. The prevention of mental disorders cannot be vested in precisely the same people because these conditions differ from disorders to which the skills of sanitary engineers and epidemiologists are applicable, and the requirements for protection from them are likewise different.

On the whole, the problems which commonly fall under the purview of mental hygienists develop in connection with the processes of learning rather than with those of physical growth. For that reason, they also tend to originate during childhood rather than adulthood, so that the best modes of preventing them necessarily require extensive mental hygienic work with children more than with any other segment of the population.

On the face of it, this would make it seem that parents and teachers should be the primary social agents for fostering positive mental health and that professional persons like psychiatrists, psychologists, and social workers should assume only a secondary role in this connection. Indeed, no other solution seems very possible if the mental hygiene needs of the nation are to be confronted with any real hope of resolution, for the available numbers of psychiatrists, psychologists, and social workers are pitifully small in relation to the nation's needs, and there is no prospect whatsoever of substantially increasing these numbers in the forseeable future.

A survey of mental health manpower needs (Albee, 1959) offered some indication of how critical these shortages are. Increasing demands for psychological services both inside and outside hospitals have so strained current resources that some hospitals and clinics, particularly among those operated by states and counties, have almost no professionally trained personnel. This is not only because recalcitrant legislatures have failed to make necessary budgetary provisions for mental health, but also because few trained people can be found even when there is money to pay them. Albee found that 25 percent of budgeted positions for psychiatrists and psychologists among state and county hospitals always remain unfilled, and his figures for psychiatric social workers and for nurses were similar.

The vacancies in budgeted positions tell only a small part of the story, however, because the number of budgeted positions is itself far less than the *minimal* number required for adequate care, let alone the optimal number (Joint Information Service, 1960*a* and *b*). And this shortage is for treatment personnel, not prevention specialists. There are simply not enough psychiatrists, psychologists, social workers, and nurses to go around, nor are there likely to be unless some radical efforts at massive training programs are undertaken.

If it is correct that the focus of public attention with respect to preventive mental health must be on children, then regardless of who assumes the responsibility for administering to them, it is important to find out just what it is that children must be taught to best prepare them to cope effectively with the vicissitudes of life. This brings us back to the question of what we mean by positive mental health, a problem we can evade somewhat when we are concerned with the treatment of already existing disorders, but one which must be confronted in any intelligent discussion of prevention.

As usual, a comprehensive answer is not possible, but it is possible to provide a useful and practical list of things which can be taught to children and which will help secure their mental health. Many of them have already been indicated in previous chapters:

1. Chapter 4 emphasized the critical effect of parental training on personality

development, especially the effects of toilet training, punishment and reward, and parental sex role models at different critical periods of growth. The chapter also lays heavy emphasis on the importance of developing *standards* for evaluating one's thoughts and actions in order to have a positive ideal for onself.

2. Chapter 5 emphasizes the flexible behavior patterns which the normal man must develop in order to maintain a balanced relationship with society, one in which he is usually invisible but still able to pursue his individual goals. It also specified the critical roles of *competence* and *integrity* in establishing a personal sense of fulfillment or well-being, especially in the face of social opposition.

3. Chapter 6 emphasized that identifying genius is a "chancey" thing but that learning habits of skilled work is not. Such learning can and should be planned for by society.

4. Chapter 8 emphasized the importance of the many components of *identification* for building positive character traits in children.

5. Chapter 10, although it generally emphasized the banal results of excessive reliance on ego defenses, pointed out very clearly that they also have positive values under many circumstances.

Considering the great differences in subject matter and perspective which appear in these chapters, let alone the differences in interests and biases of their authors, some very striking common implications for child training can be derived from them.

The idea of *standards* in Chapter 4 is similar to the concepts of *integrity* or *responsibility* in Chapter 5, which are in turn like the *moral judgment* and *moral feeling* of Chapter 8. The critical training experiences of Chapter 4, the "planning for genius" recommendations of Chapter 6, and the positive side of learning ego defenses of Chapter 10 can all be neatly summarized in the terminology of Chapter 5 as the learning of *competencies*. Taken all together, these ideas appear to fall into two broad kinds of education which serve the interests of positive mental health: (1) acquiring a *moral disposition*, that is an evaluative, personal, subjective and affective set of attitudes for judging oneself and others and for establishing relationships, and (2) acquiring a body of *technical skills* for manipulating the environment and one's relationship to it. Freud summarized these objectives as the capacity for "love and work." Modern psychologists might lump them together less simply as "the process of socialization." What is important is the common view among students of behavior that both kinds of training are vital to positive mental development.

The processes by which skills are developed can all be described as the learning of *control*, from which a child gains the ability to regulate his autonomy in the environment and his dependency on it. The development of moral dispositions seems to occur through the mechanisms of *identification*, from which a person formulates the goals and values that permit a rewarding feeling of well-being from the exercise of his skills.

Control

The learning of control refers both to self-control and to control over the environment. There is probably no need to make any distinction between them as far as young children are concerned. Although adolescents and adults are sharply aware of the difference between controlling themselves (especially their feelings and sometimes their thoughts) and mastering their surroundings (which usually means performing well at some task), small children are not. Their natural egocentrism (Piaget, 1932) inclines them to view the world as an extension of their own experience. It is precisely this view that makes necessary the learning of control, that is, the separation of themselves from the environment and the techniques for mastering their relationships with it.

The mechanics of control are learned in the same sequence as any other kind of learning; they include (1) interactions with the environment, (2) processing information from those interactions, and (3) experiencing reinforcements. The only respects in which learning control differs from other kinds of learning are that (1) the interaction with the environment must be one in which the child's own role is *active* or *manipulative* rather than merely attentive, and (2) the reinforcements he experiences must generally be positive and rewarding rather than painful and fearful. There must be some correspondence between the child's intended and achieved learning if he is to develop the sense of competence (White, 1959, 1960) or mastery which will permit him to exercise his controls most effectively.

The same sense of mastery that is familiar to most of us in the learning of motor skills can also be developed over internal processes. An extreme form of such control is familiar in the behavior of yogis, fakirs, and other religious adepts. And in more common experience, although we are often unaware of the learning which has gone into it, we all recognize the differences in degrees of control which people have developed over every aspect of behavior. For *cognition,* this is the ability to concentrate or, conversely, to free one's imaginative faculties and to have unusual, even bizarre hallucinatory experiences. For *emotions,* as for *senses,* we are all acquainted with the different abilities of people to exert control over their responses, expressing or inhibiting themselves as seems appropriate to different situations. Apparently, the mechanics of control over thoughts and over emotions are similar to or identical with the mechanics of control over motor skills, so that children who learn early in life to apply the same kinds of discipline toward cognitive and affective processes as toward motor development are more likely than others to be spared the feeling later on that they are victims of their own internal states.

Excessive control. There is a popular notion that some people are too much controlled emotionally, implying some defect in their personalities which requires therapeutic correction. This idea leads some people to be wary of teaching children to be "controlled" rather than "spontaneous" in expressing their emotions. Actually, there is some confusion in this controversy, and it is important to understand the relationship between control and spontaneity.

People who are concerned about "excessive control" generally use the term to mean the "*inhibition of behavior,*" and they use *spontaneity* to mean the "expression" of it. Neither of these uses is quite accurate, however, or by itself implies either a desirable or an undesirable way of acting. The "natural" expression of impulses is indeed spontaneous, but it is often undesirable, and a large part of socialization training must be directed towards teaching children to control such expressions. And while control does imply restraint or inhibition of some expressive inclinations, it also implies the positive ability to express others. Actually, control should not be equated with inhibition so much as with *volition,* because it properly refers to *skilled voluntary* behavior, sometimes involving inhibition and restriction of activity but sometimes involving exhibition and expression. As used here, the essence of control is not the inhibition of impulses (though that is often a necessary part of it), but the inhibition or expression of oneself in ways that are best suited to particular goals. In this sense, there is no such thing as "excessive control."

There certainly *is* such a thing as excessive inhibition, that is of behavior so severely restrained that a person lacks the ability to express himself appropriately, perhaps repressing his thoughts, withholding his feelings, and even constricting his movements. Such a person might appear to others to be intellectually disorganized, as in "flighty" or "scatterbrained" behavior, emotionally aloof, sexually frigid, shy or diffident, physically awkward, ungainly, or tense. Such symptoms do represent disturbed behavior; they do not reflect an excess of control, however, but a deficiency of it, in which the victim is unable to control his responses to appropriate stimulation by performing the acts or expressing the sentiments the situation demands. Such problems of inhibition are probably learned in the course of learning socially desired restraints, but they are more likely a result of bad teaching tactics, especially excessive use of humiliating and anxiety-arousing punishments, than of the effort to teach controls as such.

Identification

The critical role of personal identifications both in the general development of personality and the particular development of positive character has been discussed at sufficient length in Chapters 4 and 8, respectively, so that there is no need to belabor it here. What is important here is to emphasize that identification is vital to preventive mental health.

As indicated earlier, identification is the basis for the moral or evaluative disposition from which a person formulates his life goals and judges his success in reaching them. This means not only that he develops *standards* for rating his skills, but also that he develops *feelings* of satisfaction or despair with which he rewards or punishes himself for his judgment. More important still, in the long run, the very *choice of skills* a child attempts depends very much on the identifications he has formed—and at such an early age that his choices are necessarily irrational and often irrevocable. Identifying themselves with significant other people and the roles they seem to play in life gives children a model of activity from which they orient their own lives and base plans for action. Such models tend to guide much of their behavior during childhood and through adolescence and the vicissitudes of young adulthood, including the selection of occupation and marital partner. They are particularly valuable, moreover, as points of behavioral and ideological reference under enduring stressful conditions. Firm personal identifications provide the guidelines for channeling behavior as the child gains control over it.

It is not easy to tell what a child's interests will be, in most respects, merely from knowing that he has firm positive identifications with his parents because although these identifications, especially with the parent of the same sex, may be the most important ones a child forms, they are far from being the only ones. Children identify with many people they come into contact with in real life, like teachers and peers, and with many more who are *culture heroes* (or villains) and with whom their contact is only vicarious, through movies, TV, and comic books (see Chapter 8). All these models serve the same general purpose in the identification process: they enable the child to idealize and emulate specific characteristics of behavior, integrating them into his own personality to form what is called his "ego identity" (Erickson, 1959). The development of stable ego identity does *not* depend on a positive identification with any single person, which is why children from broken homes where the parent of the same sex is missing or from orphanages where they never know any parents can grow up to be mentally healthy adults—they take their identification models where they find them, often with much success.

Firm positive identifications in childhood are perhaps the best protection against later psychological disorder, but it is hard to be precise or statistical about this because nobody can keep count of how many people might-have-but-did-not develop pathologies. On the other hand, there are a number of increasingly evident behavior disorders in modern times that seem to be related to *identity crises,* that is, conflicts in adolescence and adulthood that seem to result from the absence of an adequate sense of personal identity. This is one category of *existential crisis,* and some of its consequences may be seen in rising juvenile crime rates, suicide rates, and problems of *anomie* and ennui that preoccupy people whose life circumstances should otherwise leave them fulfilled. As indicated in Chapter 10, some of the common neurotic troubles of our time also may be attributed to problems of identification, and since identification is ultimately only a refined sort of imitation, the *aggressive* and *aversive self-reinforcement* problems in Chapter 9 resulting from vicarious learning by observation of models may also be considered disorders of identification. Finally, some skill deficiencies, such as those described in Chapter 15 or implied in Chapter 5, may also be related to identification problems. The absence of firm and consistent identifications can easily undermine a person's confidence in his ability to learn and thus inhibit the development of *competence.*

Although identification is discussed here as a mental health prophylactic, it has been discussed at greater length as the principle means of building positive character traits (Chapter 8). The agents of identification, in fact, are identical with the agents of character building, that is, the family, peers, teachers, and culture heroes. This implies, in effect, that *preventive mental health, as we have envisioned it, is the very same thing as positive character education.* The reason for this is plain if you think back on the attributes of positive character: they are the things that make a person simultaneously able to resist stress and to seek mastery over his environment—the same qualities we have described as the apotheosis of mental health.

If you return now to examine the notion of *personality traits* implied in Chapter 1 and explicated in Chapter 4 and the parallel notion of *behavioral predispositions* or *subject variables* in Chapter 9, you may recognize that a concern with identification processes and character education is an attempt to attack the subject-variable aspect of mental health.

Competencies are also traits, but the development of competencies, from the mental health viewpoint, is an attempt to deal with what Chapter 9 calls *stimulus situations.* As indicated above, an individual does not have much control over the broad external environment; war, pestilence, and poverty, let alone accidents of birth and religion, automatically pit the individual against stressful stimulus situations which must consume a large part of his life energies. Learning competencies gives him the tools to resist some of these stresses and, with luck, persistence, and the help of others, perhaps to master his situation and change the stimulus conditions of his own or his childrens' lives. Viewed this way, some of the most important preventive mental health programs are those which aim to give people competence, that is, means of control over the environment, rather than aiming at their psychological conditions per se. Birth control programs, "head start" nurseries, job training, neighborhood action committees, and their like, which often go under the label of social welfare work, rather than of education or psychology, are among the most important mental health operations in America.

EMERGING PROBLEMS OF MENTAL HEALTH

Although few people would disagree that the most fruitful area for preventive mental health work lies in work with children, other significant segments of the population are becoming targets of mental health endeavors either because they have increased in size, which makes their long-standing mental health needs more noticeable, or because they have become objects of increasing public attention on fronts other than public health. Old people and discordant families illustrate the former, and poor people, especially urban minorities and residents of economically deprived regions, are good examples of the latter. Many programs are underway to help such people, but many more are needed, along with great increases in the numbers and perhaps kinds of helping professions and personnel.

The Elderly, Discordant Families, and the Poor

Age. The psychological problems of the elderly are probably the same now as they have been for many years in the United States, but the proportion of elderly people has increased so greatly in recent years that they have attracted more attention than ever before. Because of medical advances and the general rise in the standard of living, more people live beyond retirement age, and for more years, than ever did before. The *economic* problems of old people have been matters of public concern ever since the pattern of family life changed from one in which a large number of relatively immobile progeny took care of their progenitors after retirement to one where the elderly were left to fend for themselves. The Social Security laws first passed during the depression and progressively extended down to Medicare today have attempted to aid in this problem. But the psychological changes and difficulties that naturally accompany the aging process and that are magnified by changes in the status of aging people have become more evident to more people, even though they are often the same ones that existed when the population of people over sixty-five was five million instead of twenty million.

The most important psychological problem of the elderly is undoubtedly that of adjusting to retirement (Birren, 1959; Birren *et al.*, 1963). Work has been a source of special status and individual purpose as well as of income, and it is difficult for many to give up their jobs without giving up their self-esteem as well. Concern with impending death is another problem for many elderly people. Even those in vigorous health, observing the infirmities and deaths of their contemporaries, sometimes become so preoccupied with these matters that they magnify their own minor ailments and may even develop new ones (Yarrow *et al.*, 1963).

Family discord. The problems of families are similar to those of the aged in the sense that the psychological events which precipitate discord and divorce between married people and conflict between parents and children are not necessarily different now than they were a generation ago. But the number of marriages, divorces, and conflict-ridden families has increased enormously, if for no other reason than that the population has expanded greatly since World War II.

The fact that there is some tendency for the elderly to congregate in geographically favored areas, and that almost all of them continue to vote after retirement, guarantees that their needs come speedily to the attention of political aspirants and responsible government officials. This same truism applies to the nation's poor, recently perhaps even more than to the aged, because so many poor people are Negro. Both the absolute and proportionate size of impoverished and socially oppressed groups in the United States is almost certainly less now than ever before in American history, but this makes their plight more noticeable rather than less so, particularly in an age of compassion and concern for promoting the rights and opportunities of individuals.

Poverty. The idea that psychological disorders of varying degrees of severity are related to social disorganization, economic deprivation, and irrational oppression is a relatively old and established one. Formal studies like those reviewed in Chapter 12 have verified that social problems ranging from crime to mental illness can be understood and predicted largely on the basis of the socioeconomic conditions of people's lives. It hardly requires the formalities of social science, however, to recognize the inherent relationships between general human misery and the particular miseries which are sometimes glamorized or depersonalized with the label "mental illness." From Dostoyevsky's Raskolnikov to the brutally plaintive adolescents of Bernstein's *West Side Story* who chant, "We're depraved on account of we're deprived!", it is plain enough that a crying need for preventive mental health work exists among the socially and economically deprived. Competence-oriented programs to that effect are rapidly developing all over the United States as part of the "Great Society" political program.

What is not so apparent is the fact that, with few exceptions, mental health facilities for dealing directly with these massive problems either do not exist yet or cannot be used properly by the people who need them most. So little is known about the problems of aging that a virtually new profession, probably eventually to take the name "gerontology," is developing to study and cope with them. Marital counseling and family and child guidance personnel and techniques already exist, but their numbers are pitifully small relative to the need, and the resources at their disposal are few. Some hopeful attempts to develop new facilities for this purpose are being made by domestic relations courts, which in some places are making marital counseling a routine prerequisite to legal divorce and separation proceedings, and by clinic and guidance facilities which are trying to develop new modes of operation that can provide more realistic services than those they now have. The traditional pattern of clinic procedure, for example, requires people seeking help to make advance appointments and to maintain a rather rigorous schedule of continuous meetings with professional people over long periods of time. Many people simply cannot make use of the clinics under such conditions. Pioneering "emergency" and "drop-in" clinics are exploratory attempts to provide a more usable service. Many people are also experimenting with the development of more rapid treatment techniques than those used in most psychotherapeutic and counseling practices today. "Conjoint family therapy," in which parents and children are seen simultaneously by a counselor, "limited-term therapy," in which a termination date is stipulated at the *beginning* of treatment, and "crisis therapy," usually on a drop-in basis, are efforts in this direction.

It is not very clear at the present time just what kinds of direct mental health efforts will be most useful in connection with anti-poverty programs because very little in the field of mental health has been directed towards that aim until very recently. But there is no question but that the efforts of mental health experts will be engaged increasingly in work with the underprivileged and with other special groups.

Developing New Professionals

It is much easier to see where the needs for mental health work lie than it is to figure out who is going to meet them. At the present time, there are only three kinds of professional people—psychiatrists, psychologists, and social workers—whose training is devoted primarily to work in this field. Special training programs in pastoral counseling and in guidance have been designed to further the abilities of clergymen and of high school and college counselors to cope with the many mental health problems they inevitably confront in the course of their work. But all such programs, though of unquestioned value, must still fail to contribute very much to the enormous pool of unattended mental health needs in this country. The problem is more one of *manpower shortage* than of insufficient training in the mental health professions or the many occupations peripherally related to them.

We have earlier discussed the critical shortage of trained manpower to deal with the mental health and illness problems of the population. There are only 13,000 psychiatrists in the United States at this time, and twice that number are needed. Of these, fewer than 200—an appallingly low figure—are *child psychiatrists*. Similar shortages exist among clinical psychologists and psychiatric social workers. The annual crop of psychiatric nurses is approximately 1000, while the annual need is for 4000.

It takes a very long time to train a mental health professional. From the time he graduates from high school, the budding *psychiatrist* commonly requires four years of undergraduate work, four years of medical study, a one- or two-year internship, and three additional years of specialized training in psychiatry—twelve or thirteen years of training in all. He will require even more schooling if he aspires to be a psychoanalyst.

Clinical psychology likewise requires extensive training. Beyond the four years of undergraduate work, there lie some four to six years of graduate and practical training in psychology, before the Ph.D. is achieved. And additional postdoctoral work in diagnosis, therapy, and research are becoming quite common. It takes two or three years beyond the bachelor's degree to train a *psychiatric social worker*. Here too, additional schooling beyond the graduate degree is often useful.

Beyond the time required for training and the consequent difficulty of attracting people into these professions, the expense of training both for the sponsoring institutions and the student is so enormous that medical and graduate facilities have had to expand quite slowly, despite the pressing social need (Albee, 1959) and extensive government support. It is quite unlikely that they will be able to expand enough in the foreseeable future to meet society's minimal needs, let alone those of optimal prevention and treatment.

One answer to the problem of manpower shortage may be the creation of new professional groups whose training would equip them for mental health work without demanding the many years of arduous preparation that now go into the training of psychiatrists, psychologists, and social workers. Within these professions, there has been increasing fractionation of training in recent years designed to make it more consonant with the work the individuals will actually do. *School psychology*, for example, has developed as a branch of clinical and educational psychology devoted exclusively to personal, familial, and learning disorders which may be identified and aborted more quickly in the school setting than in any other. Some thought has recently been given to creating a new discipline of *medical psychology* that would combine the specialized training of psychologists and psychiatrists into a new profession especially equipped to deal with disorders that appear in or require a medical setting. Finally, since the shortage of clinical psychologists is severe, and since training in the discipline is very largely scientific and academic rather than practical and applied, attention has recently been addressed to the creation of a new training program for clinical psychologists which would be concerned primarily with the practical applications of the profession and for which a specialized doctorate (rather than the Doctor of Philosophy degree that is presently offered) would be invented. The University of Illinois is actually pioneering such a program.

While all of the possibilities indicated here have some virtues, the sheer size of the problem makes it plain that none of them will make any very large contribution to its solution. The amount of time and effort required by advanced graduate and professional work is so great that only a very small number of people can reasonably be expected to pursue it. If the personnel problem is capable of solution, the solution must necessarily involve training large numbers of people to do good quality mental health work without having to undergo the expense, rigor, or long duration of time which must be invested in a program leading to an advanced degree.

Mental health counselors. The most important possibilities in this connection thus far are promising not only for the creation of a large corps of mental health workers, but for the solution of problems of surplus manpower as well. This is the training of mature, responsible, housewives and retired people as mental health counselors (Rioch *et al.*, 1963).

Women who have completed their major child-rearing tasks often find themselves, usually in their early forties, in the peculiar position of having nothing to do with their time. Often there is no special need for them to contribute to the family coffers. Without the prospect of something useful and demanding to do, it is understandable that women are likely to find themselves bored and unhappy, especially if they have led busy and productive lives until then.

There are at least several hundred thousand such women in the United States today with the very attributes that could best serve the needs of a massive mental health program. They are intelligent and educated, and they have considerable life experience that makes up in wisdom what they lack in formal training and that may be even more valuable in many counseling situations. They also have time to devote to further training and are not necessarily restricted in the work they can do by the need for high income. A program for training such people as counselors could eliminate much of what now constitutes the curriculum of the mental health professions and still be of high academic caliber, since the participants in the program would be reasonably well educated to begin with. In fairly short order, with adequate professional supervision these women could enter the ranks of professional mental health work in precisely those places where they are most needed and where, largely for economic reasons, fully trained professions do not tread. It seems reasonable that this large corps could become the bulwark of mental health service work in the United States. A pilot program for training such women has been completed successfully by Margaret

Rioch and her colleagues at the University of Maryland.

Exactly the same kind of program could make use of people who are retired and past the age of sixty or sixty-five. Quite often the retired person has years of vigor ahead of him and years of wisdom and experience behind him, and, in addition, no important defects of intelligence or personality. Many of them need an activity that will prolong their usefulness and status in society. The supply of vigorous retired people is growing daily, and several hundred thousand are probably able and willing to undertake this work, which would simultaneously contribute to the general welfare and foster their own well-being.

Resistances to professional innovation. Whether such programs for mental health counselors will ever come into being on a large scale is quite another matter, for in addition to the problems that normally accompany the creation of new technical and professional disciplines, the mental health field is peculiarly beset by resistance to new developments from the people who are most directly responsible for them—the professional workers themselves!

At first blush, this may not seem to make sense, because one would expect the professional workers in the field to understand the scope of the nation's mental health problems best and to be even more diligent than anyone else in seeking solutions to them. Unfortunately, this is not always the case. Some professional workers are not very sensitive to the proportions of the problem. Others, who are both knowledgeable and concerned, are sometimes more afraid of solutions that will work than of ones that won't, especially if the ones that work threaten the professional status and incentives that they have worked throughout their careers to establish. The truth is that even though the mental health professions today are considered among the nation's most important ones, their recognition is very recent, and they have not yet learned to accept it with equanimity. *Psychiatry* has been among the lowest status branches of the medical profession for a long time; *social work* has long been the lowest paid and lowest esteemed division of the mental health profession; and *clinical psychology*, which only came into existence as an independent profession after World War II, has had an unclear professional identity and role, with origins and traditions of activity that stem from some unspecified mixture of the medical clinic, the educational and academic setting, and the scientific laboratory.

Without demeaning either the importance or the vitality of these professions, it is still plain that they are all "immature" professions in the sense that they are still struggling for status, public recognition, and satisfactory earnings. Struggles for these prerogatives occur among professionals in the same way as among entrepreneurs of other kinds and make them reluctant to risk hard won professional gains on untried innovations.

Despite these conservative forces, the problems of innovation have not gone unnoticed by the mental health profession and, indeed, are discussed at length in their report to Congress entitled *Action for Mental Health* (Ewalt *et al.*, 1961). Under the circumstances, it is surprising that these professions have done as well as they have, for most proposals for the enlargement of manpower pools so far have come from their members, and probably will in the future, too.

Nonprofessional Treatments

Despite the attention which is increasingly paid to the problems of special segments of the population and the need for mental health manpower, the main focus of attention in this field remains for the present, as in the past, on the *professional* treatment of existing disorders in "respectable" facilities. A huge industry exists for this purpose, operating through the institutional facilities of federal, state, and local governments, the dedication of laymen who sponsor and support professional treatment facilities, and individual psychiatrists, psychologists, social workers, and others who set up offices for the private practice of counseling or psychotherapy. Because these agencies are almost all controlled or endorsed either by government or professional organizations, they have considerable social status. Some of the most important mental health facilities, however, are purely voluntary organizations created and operated by laymen, and they often have an "offbeat" reputation. Their widespread public acceptance and demonstrable effectiveness in some cases, has lent them at least the quasi-official blessing of the American mental health establishment. The two most important organizations of this kind are probably *Alcoholics Anonymous* and *Synanon.*

Alcoholics Anonymous. The discussions of alcoholism in Chapters 9, 11, and 12 concerned the origins, severity, and prevalence of this condition but had nothing important to say about its treatment. The reason is that virtually nothing important is known about its treatment except that none of the innumerable methods that have been tried have turned out very well. Perhaps the most successful effort at curing alcoholism has been that of Alcoholics Anonymous, a therapeutic club founded by a group of cured alcoholics to help others and to reinforce their own abstinence. Membership in A.A. is open to anybody who defines himself as alcoholic. One of the main activities of the organization is conducting regular group therapy meetings in which people discuss their addiction along with other problems, reinforce each other's efforts to be free of alcohol, and provide each other with general social support. Another critical aspect of A.A.'s operation is a "buddy system" in which a long-abstinent member is constantly available to newer or less fortunate members who are going through the travail of withdrawal from alcohol. The buddy may be called on in the middle of the night to attend a member who is gripped by the desire to drink and to help him withstand the temptation. The combined effects of active models who have overcome the addiction, assistance in constructing a new life while abandoning an old one, and active sympathy and support seem to be critical factors in the success of A.A.

Two important principles of A.A.'s operation may simultaneously enhance its effectiveness for some people and dissuade others from joining it. These are (1) the doctrine that once an alcoholic, always an alcoholic, regardless of how long one refrains from drinking, and (2) the doctrine that help with alcoholism ultimately depends on God, not on the personal resources of the victim alone. The *permanency* doctrine implies that total abstinence is necessary rather than mere controlled alcoholic intake and also that affiliation with A.A. should be a lifetime activity. The *religious* doctrine implies that disbelievers cannot benefit very much from the therapeutics of A.A. and, by its Protestant fundamentalist tone, discourages people of other faiths from participation, although the organization is not restricted to people of one creed.

Synanon. Giving up addicting drugs is a painful matter. The withdrawal symptoms that follow "cold turkey" (sudden and complete abstinence from drugs) are severe enough to send most addicts to a hospital for treatment. Even the less painful techniques of withdrawal, which

clusively as an intimate interpersonal encounter find the idea repulsive. In recent years, some psychotherapists have moved from describing their work in terms of mechanical models (Krasner, 1962) to actually constructing therapeutic machinery. This is not new to *action* therapies, which have long used things like electric shock and candy dispensers as reinforcing instruments. Experimentation is now underway, however, on the use of computers for *insight* therapy. Dr. Kenneth M. Colby (1965) of Stanford University has devised an experimental "therapeutic person-computer conversation," basing his work on the earlier efforts of Joseph Weizenbaum of the Massachusetts Institute of Technology. Although the technique is still very primitive, its intent is clear. Colby writes:

> Our aim . . . is ultimately to provide a type of psychotherapy for thousands of mental hospital or psychiatric center patients for whom there are no human therapists available. . . . Our intent is not to replace the psychotherapist, but to place one in environments where none are available or to utilize therapists more efficiently by extending their abilities to monitor and regulate the therapy of dozens of patients. . . . The man-power shortage will not be relieved by any foreseeable increase in the number of therapists trained by medicine, psychology, or social work. . . . The power of computers in extending the skills of a therapist is that . . . dozens and perhaps hundreds of patients an hour can be treated.

Physical control of the brain. Computer psychotherapy does not yet have any practical applications, but control of behavior through surgical implantation of radio transmitter-receivers in the brain is already a reality. Electrical stimulation of the brain has been done experimentally since the late nineteenth century, but developments in modern surgery and in the miniaturization of electronic equipment have made it possible to implant very small permanent transceivers in some brain centers and to control behavior by electrically stimulating these centers. Radio controls of this kind have already been successfully used to increase the speech and improve the mood of an eleven-year-old boy with uncontrollable epileptic seizures, and to induce various thought patterns, hallucinations, and pleasant shifts of mood in a number of patients (Delgado, 1965). Even more elaborate controls of complex social behavior have been exerted on monkeys, and there is no doubt but that the improvement of techniques and equipment will enable these controls to be applied to human beings. The leading student of this important field is Dr. José Delgado of Yale University.

No one can say for sure what the limits of surgical controls will be, but there is no doubt, upon examining Delgado's work to date that it will eventually be possible to use both chemical and electrical stimulation to control very refined human behavior. This would be wonderful for helping people with epilepsy, mental retardation, and perhaps the functional psychoses as well, but it could also be used unscrupulously for tyrannical political or individual purposes. In any case, these controls are rapidly being developed, and conscientious students of mental health problems must consider how their use can be restricted to the benefit of humanity.

MENTAL HEALTH PROBLEMS VERSUS OTHER MISERIES

The fact that people generally experience misery and unhappiness from mental health problems does not mean that every source of unhappiness or misery should be treated as a matter of mental health. It is important to understand the distinction in order to avoid the absurd idea that psychological treatment is needed every time a person experiences conflict, frustration, or grief. Even though we cannot find an entirely adequate positive definition of mental health, some intelligent basis for making practical decisions about the quality of one's own difficulties must be available to people if they are to take intelligent steps towards their solutions.

The most commonly accepted basis for evaluating mental health status is implied by the statistically oriented approach to normality which dominates most of this book (see Chapter 1) and it is explicated briefly in Chapter 11. This involves the comparison of individual experience with that of "people in general" and of the subgroup of people the person is most like in some important ways, such as other Americans, Negroes, Catholics, children, middle-income people, and so forth. If there is a *hypothetical consensus* between him and others about the nature of reality, which means that he and others understand many of their individual experiences in the same way, then his unhappy states of guilt, anxiety, or conflict will not be considered psychological disorders provided that (1) similar states are commonly experienced by other people in response to similar stimuli, and (2) the unhappy state is resolved spontaneously in due time without permanent disability. This *consensual* definition of mental disorder, despite its abstract sound, is precisely the one that most of us use most commonly in our daily lives.

If a person experiences protracted and intense grief over the death of a loved one, for example, we generally expect that he will be absent from work for several days, that he will be morose, unhappy, and depressed for some time after that, and that he may be generally listless and without interest in his usual activities. Nobody would be particularly surprised, further, if doing this period, he were occasionally to burst into tears or otherwise manifest grief in some extreme form. This behavior contains the main components of clinical depression (see Chapter 11), but it is not considered disordered or pathological in this case because it reflects a social consensus that such public behavior is acceptable or even desirable in connection with mourning. Were he, on the contrary, to show some signs of pleasure at the loss of a near kin, he would be the object of opprobrium—and much more likely to be considered deranged than if he mourned extravagantly.

The same convention that sanctions mourning, however, also sets limitations on it, especially limitations of time. If the same mourning goes on for more than a few weeks, for example, people will almost certainly begin to express concern about why the person is not "coming out of it," judging the proper limits of his mourning by their expectations of others in the same situation. Their implied consensus is only hypothetical, of course, for nobody even pretends to know the precise point at which normal mourning turns into clinical depression. But the limits are as real as they are imprecise. At some point, continuation of this once acceptable behavior will cause people to judge the individual disordered because continued mourning demonstrably interferes with his functioning.

It is important to keep clearly in mind that no behavior is considered pathology if it is common enough that people can assume, in its early stages, on a purely statistical basis (that is, judging entirely from their previous experience), that it will resolve itself spontaneously with time. It is only this assumption which prevents parents from running immediately to psychiatrists when their children reach teen age and begin indulging in what look like lunatic practices. The same expectation of eventual spontaneous recovery keeps young lovers from being jailed or hospitalized and makes society a good deal more tolerant of many kinds of deviations than might otherwise be true.

The consensual definition of disorder places the great majority of adjustment problems outside the official framework of "mental health" concern, for by this definition, most conflict, frustration, and unhappiness probably should be considered part of the ordinary provocations of life rather than the province of special experts in living. It is only when such unhappy events are unusual or persistent for one individual more than for others with equal provocations that they fall into the province of mental health problems.

As a practical matter, this approach suggests that you should be wary of interpreting every psychological problem as a "mental health" problem in the sense that it is unique, that it necessarily requires expert attention, or that it has all kinds of hidden meanings beyond the obvious ones. As a matter of intellectual concern, it suggests that you be careful not to cheat yourself of understanding the richness and complexity of human behavior at its heights and at its depths by thoughtlessly reducing every conspicuous act to such vague and often irrelevant pigeonholes as "health" and "illness." These terms have their uses, but as we have seen, they are not adequate to describe much of human behavior, even of eccentricity and misery, much less of joyous madness. The hermit who withdraws from society to spend his life alone seeking God in a cave, the passionate suicide, the professional thief, the fanatical evangelist preaching the world's imminent end, the saint who resurrects it by feeding birds but does not preach at all, the kamikazes of every war, the frenzied artists who write immortal novels in three days or compose messianic oratorios in endless hallucination or chip at marble blocks in frenzied eagerness to find the lovely images hidden there—all the abnormals, quietly preoccupied or else consumed by the divine fire or the flames of hell, are the proper objects of our inquiry. The mentally ill and healthy are contained among them but do not contain them.

GLOSSARY

ACTION THERAPY—therapies that focus mainly on symptoms and behaviors and are less concerned with the origins and meanings of such symptoms; these therapies tend to be derived from various learning theories.

ADAPTATION—diminution in strength of response upon repeated presentation of a stimulus.

ALCOHOLICS ANONYMOUS—a therapeutic club founded by a group of cured alcoholics to help others toward a cure and to reinforce their own abstinence.

ANOMIE—the feeling that one lacks an identity.

AUTOMATED PSYCHODIAGNOSIS—diagnosis of mental disorders by machinery which can elicit and record diagnostic information.

AUTOMATED PSYCHOTHERAPY — man-computer interactions for the purpose of treating psychological distress.

CONJOINT FAMILY THERAPY—therapy in which parents and children are seen simultaneously by a counselor.

CONTROL—as used in this chapter, the ability to regulate one's self and one's environment—akin to volition.

CRISIS THERAPY—therapy on a "drop-in" basis for people experiencing psychological emergencies.

EGO IDENTITY (ERIKSON)—the characteristics of models which the child chooses to idealize, emulate, and integrate into his own personality and with his earlier learnings.

ENNUI—boredom.

EPIDEMIOLOGIST—one who studies the incidence, distribution, and control of disease in a population.

EXCESSIVE CONTROL—as used in this chapter, excessive inhibition of behavior or thought.

EXISTENTIAL CRISIS—a crisis centering about the problem of finding meaning in life.

FUNCTIONAL SYMPTOMS—symptoms that have no organic basis.

GERONTOLOGY—the study of the problems of the aged.

IDENTIFICATION—the process by which a person comes to believe that he possesses some of the attributes of a revered model; it involves vicarious sharing in the affective states of the model (see Chapters 4 and 10).

IDENTITY CRISIS—conflicts in adolescence and adulthood that seem to result from the absence of an adequate sense of personal identity.

INSIGHT THERAPY—psychotherapy that is based upon or derived from the psychoanalytic tradition of Freud; insight therapies have in common the notion that motives determine behavior and that proper understanding of motives will itself lead to altered behavior.

LEVEL OF ASPIRATION—ambition; the standard by which a person judges his own performance as a success or failure.

LIMITED-TERM THERAPY—therapy in which the termination date is stipulated at the beginning of treatment.

MORAL DISPOSITION—an evaluative set of attitudes for judging oneself and others.

NATURAL EGOCENTRISM (PIAGET)—the inclination (in young children) to view the world as an extension of their own experience (see Chapter 4).

OPTIMAL TENSION LEVEL—the amount of tension, in relation to both environment and one's internal state, that some people argue is most conducive to mental health (see Chapter 5).

PATHOGENIC—causing disease.

PROPHYLACTIC—preventive.

PSYCHIATRIC SOCIAL WORKER—a social worker trained to work with patients and their families on psychological problems.

SOCIAL STATUS—the position accorded to a person in his own group.

SOCIAL STRUCTURE—the pattern of relationships by which a social group or culture is organized and sustained.

STIMULUS SITUATIONS—situations to which individuals are responsive.

SUBJECT VARIABLES—characteristics of individuals.

SYNANON—a residential treatment center for drug addicts.

REFERENCES

Ackerman, E. Computers and medical research. In "Symposium on applications of digital computers," *Mayo Clinic Proceedings*, 1964, **39**, 815–817.

Albee, G. W. *Mental health manpower trends*. New York: Basic Books, Inc., 1959.

Birren, J. E. (ed.). *Handbook of aging and the individual*. Chicago: University of Chicago Press, 1959.

———, R. N. Butler, S. W. Greenhouse, L. Sokoloff, and Marian R. Yarrow. Human aging: A biological and behavioral study. Public Health Service Publication No. 986, U. S. Department of Health, Education and Welfare, 1963.

Clark, K. B. *Dark ghetto*. New York: Harper & Row Publishers, 1965.

Colby, K. Therapeutic person-computer conversation. Unpublished manuscript, 1965.

Delgado, J. M. R. *Evolution of physical control of the brain*. James Arthur Lecture on the evolution of the human brain, 1965. New York: American Museum of Natural History, 1965.

Erikson, E. H. *Identity and the life cycle*. New York: International Universities Press, Inc., 1959.

Ewalt, J. R., *et al*. *Action for mental health*. New York: Basic Books, Inc., 1961.

Fromm, E. *Escape from freedom*. New York: Holt, Rinehart & Winston, 1941.

Harrington, M. *The other America*. New York: Crowell-Collier and Macmillan, Inc., 1962.

Hobbs, N. Mental health's third revolution. *American Journal of Orthopsychiatry*, 1964, **34**, 822–833.

Hollingshead, A. B., R. Ellis, and E. Kirby. Social mobility and mental illness. *American Sociological Review*, 1954, **19**, 577–584.

Horney, Karen. *The neurotic personality of our time*. New York: W. W. Norton & Company, Inc., 1939.

Hunt, G. H., and M. E. Odoroff. Followup study of narcotic drug addicts after hospitalization. *Public Health Reports*, 1962, 77, 41–54.

Jahoda, Marie. *Current concepts of positive mental health*. New York: Basic Books, Inc., 1959.

Joint Information Service. Fifteen indices: An aid in reviewing state and local mental health and hospital programs. American Psychiatric Association and National Association for Mental Health, 1960*a*.

———. Fact Sheet No. 12. American Psychiatric Association and National Association for Mental Health, 1960*b*.

Kardiner, A., and L. Ovesey. *The mark of oppression: A psychological study of the American Negro*. New York: W. W. Norton & Company, Inc., 1951.

Koestler, A. The Yogi and the commissar. In *The Yogi and the commissar and other essays*. New York: Crowell-Collier and Macmillan, Inc., 1945.

———. Guide to political neurosis. In *The trail of the dinosaur and other essays*. Port Washington, N.Y.: Kennika Press, 1955.

Krasner, L. The therapist as a social reinforcement machine. In H. H. Strupp and L. Luborsky (eds.), *Research in psychotherapy*, Vol. II. Washington, D.C.: American Psychological Association, 1962, pp. 61–94.

Mutual aid in prison. *Time*, 1963, **81**, 45.

Offer, D., and M. Sabshin. *Normality: Theoretical and clinical concepts of mental health*. New York: Basic Books, Inc., 1966.

Parker, S., and R. J. Kleiner. *Mental illness in the urban Negro community*. New York: The Free Press of Glencoe, 1966.

Pearson, J. S., W. M. Swenson, H. P. Rome, P. Malaya, and T. L. Brannick. Automated personality inventory. In "Symposium on applications of digital computers," *Mayo Clinic Proceedings*, 1964, **39**, 823–829.

Piaget, J. *The moral judgment of the child*. London: Routledge and Kegan Paul, Ltd., 1932.

Reissman, F., J. Cohen, and A. Pearl (eds.). *Mental health of the poor: New treatment approaches for low income people*. New York: The Free Press of Glencoe, 1964.

Rioch, Margaret J., Charmian Elkes, Arden A. Flint, Blanche S. Usdansky, Ruth G. Newman, and E. Silber. National Institute of Mental Health pilot study in training mental health counselors. *American Journal of Orthopsychiatry*, 1963, **33**, 678–689.

Srole, L., T. S. Langner, S. T. Michael, M. K. Opler, and T. A. C. Rennie. *Mental health in the metropolis: The midtown Manhattan study*, Vol. 1. New York: McGraw-Hill, Inc., 1962.

White, R. W. Motivation reconsidered: The concept of competence. *Psychological Review*, 1959, **66**, 297–333.

———. Competence and the psychosexual stages of development. In M. R. Jones (ed.), *Nebraska Symposium on Motivation*. Lincoln, Neb.: University of Nebraska Press, 1960, pp. 97–141.

Yarrow, M. R., P. Blank, O. W. Quinn, E. G. Youmans, and J. Stein. Social psychological characteristics of old age. In J. E. Birreb *et al.* (eds.), *Human aging*. Bethesda, Md.: U.S. Department of Health, Education, and Welfare, 1963.

SUGGESTED READINGS

1. Delgado, J. M. R. *Evolution of physical control of the brain*. James Arthur lecture on the evolution of the human brain. New York: American Museum of Natural History, 1965. An examination of the possibilities of electronically controlling the mind and behavior.
2. Fromm, E. *Escape from freedom*. New York: Holt, Rinehart & Winston, 1941. A historical examination of the varieties and sources of personal freedom for the light they cast on the nature of modern man and his societies.
3. Jahoda, Marie. *Current concepts of positive mental health*. New York: Basic Books, Inc., 1959. An examination of conceptions of psychological well-being.
4. Offer, D., and M. Sabshin. *Normality: Theoretical and clinical concepts of mental health*. New York: Basic Books, Inc., 1966. An integrated review of concepts of mental health.

Name Index

Subject Index